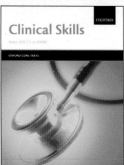

Clinical Skills

Edited by Cox and Roper

"Feels as though you are at the bedside being taught by a doctor."

Medical Student, Manchester

978-0-19-262874-9

Human Physiology*

Third Edition

Pocock and Richards

This established textbook provides medical students and others in health-related disciplines with the essential information and learning tools necessary to understand human physiology.

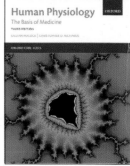

978-0-19-856878-0

Psychiatry

Third Edition

Gelder, Mayou and Geddes

"For students of any mental health profession, this is an excellent text ... Get it!"

Amazon.co.uk reviewer

978-0-19-852863-0

Surgery

Edited by Stonebridge, Smith, Duncan and Thompson

Surgery takes a patient-centred approach, using clinical scenarios to anchor surgical knowledge in an applied clinical context.

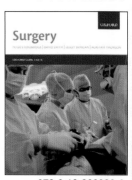

978-0-19-262990-6

Neurology

Second Edition

Donaghy

"I would strongly recommend this text to medical students looking for a good introduction to the subject of neurology."

Amazon.co.uk reviewer

978-0-19-852636-0

Oncology*

Second Edition

Watson, Barrett, Spence and Twelves

Oncology presents a clear and compact survey of the subject, equipping students for their oncology attachment, and informing the study of cancer in related disciplines.

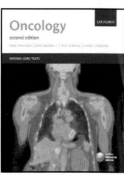

978-0-19-856757-8

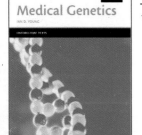

Medical Genetics*

Young

"A remarkable achievement and one which should be warmly commended to all students."

Journal of Medical Genetics

978-0-19-856494-2

Epidemiology and Prevention*

Yarnell

"This book promises to be a good companion to epidemiology courses."

Medical Student, Imperial College

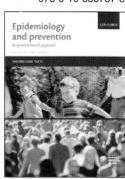

978-0-19-853014-5

Also available: Clinical Dermatology, Fifth Edition, by MacKie (978-0-19-852580-6)
Health and Illness in the Community, by Taylor, Smith and Teijlingen (978-0-19-263168-3)
Palliative Care, by Faull and Woof (978-0-19-263280-9)

Clinical Pathology

James Carton

Specialist Registrar in Cellular Pathology
John Radcliffe Hospital,
Oxford, UK

Richard Daly

Consultant Pathologist
Weston General Hospital,
Weston-super-Mare, UK

Pramila Ramani

Consultant Histopathologist (Paediatric)
Bristol Royal Infirmary,
Bristol, UK

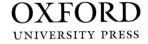

OXFORD
UNIVERSITY PRESS

OXFORD

UNIVERSITY PRESS

Great Clarendon Street, Oxford OX2 6DP

Oxford University Press is a department of the University of Oxford.
It furthers the University's objective of excellence in research, scholarship,
and education by publishing worldwide in

Oxford New York

Auckland Cape Town Dar es Salaam Hong Kong Karachi
Kuala Lumpur Madrid Melbourne Mexico City Nairobi
New Delhi Shanghai Taipei Toronto

With offices in

Argentina Austria Brazil Chile Czech Republic France Greece
Guatemala Hungary Italy Japan Poland Portugal Singapore
South Korea Switzerland Thailand Turkey Ukraine Vietnam

Oxford is a registered trade mark of Oxford University Press
in the UK and in certain other countries

Published in the United States
by Oxford University Press Inc., New York

British Library Cataloguing in Publication Data

Data available

Library of Congress Cataloging in Publication Data

Data available

Typeset by Cepha Imaging Pvt. Ltd., Bangalore, India
Printed in Spain
on acid-free paper by
Graficàs Estella

ISBN 0-19-856946-7 (Pbk.)   978-0-19-856946-6 (Pbk.)

1 3 5 7 9 10 8 6 4 2

Preface

Clinical Pathology was written with the following aims:

♦ To write a sensibly sized textbook focusing on the pathology relevant to the 99 per cent of medical students who will go on to become clinicians and not specialist pathologists.

♦ To cover all common and important diseases, even those where pathologists themselves play little role in their management.

♦ To integrate all the pathology disciplines together in one book (cellular pathology, haematology, clinical biochemistry, microbiology, and immunology).

♦ To address commonly faced problems, particularly terminology, head on rather than ignore them.

♦ To write in a friendly and engaging way in an attempt to make the subject enjoyable.

We hope we have gone some way to achieving these ambitious aims. We welcome all comments, good or bad, from our readers. We certainly hope that we will have the opportunity to address them in a future edition.

James Carton and Richard Daly

To our families and close friends. We are back in your lives again!

Acknowledgements

We acknowledge the following individuals for providing images: Dr Ian Roberts, Consultant Pathologist, Department of Cellular Pathology, John Radcliffe Hospital, Oxford (Figs. 6.18, 11.14, 12.8, 12.14, 12.16, 14.7); Dr Juan Piris, Consultant Pathologist, Department of Cellular Pathology, John Radcliffe Hospital, Oxford (Figs. 8.1(a), 8.2, 8.5, 8.6, 8.8(b), 9.9, 9.14); Dr David Ferguson, EM Unit, Nuffield Department of Pathology, John Radcliffe Hospital, Oxford (Fig. 1.4); Professor Barbara Bain, Professor in Diagnostic Haematology, Department of Medicine, Imperial College Faculty of Medicine, St Mary's Hospital, London (Fig. 15.9); St. John's Institute of Dermatology, London (Figs. 12.1, 12.2, 16.9, 16.15); Dr Maggie Kirkup, Consultant Dermatologist, Weston General Hospital, Weston-super-Mare (Figs. 16.7, 16.10, 16.11); Dr Olaf Ansorge, Consultant Neuropathologist, & Dr Lisa Browning, Specialist Registrar, Department of Neuropathology, Radcliffe Infirmary, Oxford (Figs. 18.10, 18.12, 18.13); Mr G. A. Shun-Shin, Nuffield Hospital, Wolverhampton (Fig. 20.3); Dr Neel Patel (Fig. 9.1), and the staff of the pathology department at Weston General Hospital.

A huge thank you to Helene Beard, Illustration Services, Department of Cellular Pathology, John Radcliffe Hospital for converting legions of 35 mm slides into digital images and cleaning up our own photos.

Thanks to everyone who read the chapters or answered any niggling questions we had: Dr Andrew Bell, Dr Frank Booth, Mr Nicholas Gallegos, Dr Grahame Gould, Dr D. Grier, Dr Y. Ho, Dr A. Jain, Mr F. John, Dr A. Joshi, Mr A. Parry, Mr John Probert, Mr M. Saunders, Mr R. Spicer, Professor L. Spitz, Dr J. Tooley, and all the anonymous reviewers (you know who you are, but we don't!).

Finally, thanks to everyone at Oxford University Press who believed in us and helped bring this project to fruition, particularly Catherine Barnes who first got the project off the ground, and Ruth Craven, Colin McDougall, and Caroline Connelly who kept it in the air!

Figure acknowledgements

Fig. 3.6 Reproduced with permission from Warrell DA, Cox TM, Firth JD (2003). *Oxford Textbook of Medicine*, 4th edn, Vol. 3. Oxford University Press, Oxford.

Fig. 6.2 Adapted from Haslett C et al (2002). *Davidson's Principles and Practice of Medicine*, 19th edn. Churchill Livingstone, copyright (2002) with permission from Elsevier.

Fig. 6.14 Reproduced with permission from Scally P (1999). *Medical Imaging*. Oxford University Press, Oxford.

Fig. 6.21 Reproduced with permission from Warrell DA, Cox TM, Firth JD (2003). *Oxford Textbook of Medicine*, 4th edn, Vol. 2. Oxford University Press, Oxford.

Fig. 7.4 Reproduced with permission from Scally P (1999). *Medical Imaging*. Oxford University Press, Oxford.

Fig. 8.4 Adapted from Calam J, Baron JH (2001). Pathophysiology of duodenal and gastric ulcer and gastric cancer. *British Medical Journal*; 323: 980–982, with permission from the BMJ Publishing Group.

Fig. 8.17 Adapted from Fearon ER, Vogelstein B (1990). A genetic model for colorectal carcinogenesis. *Cell*; 61, 759–767, copyright (1990), with permission from Elsevier and reproduced with permission from Warrell DA, Cox TM, Firth JD (2003). *Oxford Textbook of Medicine*, 4th edn, Vol. 2. Oxford University Press, Oxford.

Fig. 9.8 Reproduced with permission from Warrell DA, Cox TM, Firth JD (2003). *Oxford Textbook of Medicine*, 4th edn, Vol. 2. Oxford University Press, Oxford.

Fig. 11.12 Reproduced with permission from Scally P (1999). *Medical Imaging*. Oxford University Press, Oxford.

Fig. 12.3 Reproduced with permission from Warrell DA, Cox TM, Firth JD (2003). *Oxford Textbook of Medicine*, 4th edn, Vol. 1. Oxford University Press, Oxford.

Fig. 14.12 Reproduced with permission from Davidson AM *et al.* (2005). *Oxford Textbook of Clinical Nephrology*, 3rd edn, Vol. 3. Oxford University Press, Oxford.

Fig. 15.4 Reproduced with permission from Warrell DA, Cox TM, Firth JD (2003). *Oxford Textbook of Medicine*, 4th edn, Vol. 2. Oxford University Press, Oxford.

Fig. 15.6 Reproduced with permission from Warrell DA, Cox TM, Firth JD (2003). *Oxford Textbook of Medicine*, 4th edn, Vol. 3. Oxford University Press, Oxford.

Fig. 15.8 Reproduced with permission from Warrell DA, Cox TM, Firth JD (2003). *Oxford Textbook of Medicine*, 4th edn, Vol. 2. Oxford University Press, Oxford.

Fig. 15.11 Reproduced with permission from Gatter K, Delsol G (2002). *Atlas: The Diagnosis of Lymphoproliferative Diseases*. Oxford University Press, Oxford.

Fig. 16.3 Reproduced with permission from MacKie R (2003). *Clinical Dermatology*, 5th edn. Oxford University Press, Oxford.

Fig. 16.4 Reproduced with permission from MacKie R (2003). *Clinical Dermatology*, 5th edn. Oxford University Press, Oxford.

Fig. 16.5 Reproduced with permission from MacKie R (2003). *Clinical Dermatology*, 5th edn. Oxford University Press, Oxford.

Fig. 16.6 Reproduced with permission from MacKie R (2003). *Clinical Dermatology*, 5th edn. Oxford University Press, Oxford.

Fig. 16.8 Reproduced with permission from MacKie R (2003). *Clinical Dermatology*, 5th edn. Oxford University Press, Oxford.

Fig. 16.13 Reproduced with permission from MacKie R (2003). *Clinical Dermatology*, 5th edn. Oxford University Press, Oxford.

Fig. 16.16 Reproduced with permission from MacKie R (2003). *Clinical Dermatology*, 5th edn. Oxford University Press, Oxford.

Fig. 16.17 Reproduced with permission from Ledingham JGG, Warrell DA (2000). *Concise Oxford Textbook of Medicine*. Oxford University Press, Oxford.

Fig. 16.18 Reproduced with permission from MacKie R (2003). *Clinical Dermatology*, 5th edn. Oxford University Press, Oxford.

Fig. 16.19 Reproduced with permission from MacKie R (2003). *Clinical Dermatology*, 5th edn. Oxford University Press, Oxford.

Fig. 16.20 Reproduced with permission from MacKie R (2003). *Clinical Dermatology*, 5th edn. Oxford University Press, Oxford.

Fig. 16.21 Reproduced with permission from MacKie R (2003). *Clinical Dermatology*, 5th edn. Oxford University Press, Oxford.

Fig. 17.5 Reproduced with permission from Scally P (1999). *Medical Imaging*. Oxford University Press, Oxford.

Fig. 17.7 Reproduced with permission from Warrell DA, Cox TM, Firth JD (2003). *Oxford Textbook of Medicine*, 4th edn, Vol. 3. Oxford University Press, Oxford.

Fig. 17.8 Reproduced with permission from Warrell DA, Cox TM, Firth JD (2003). *Oxford Textbook of Medicine*, 4th edn, Vol. 3. Oxford University Press, Oxford.

Fig. 17.9 Reproduced with permission from Ledingham JGG, Warrell DA (2000). *Concise Oxford Textbook of Medicine*. Oxford University Press, Oxford.

Fig. 18.7 Reproduced with permission from Scally P (1999). *Medical Imaging*. Oxford University Press, Oxford.

Fig. 18.8 Reproduced with permission from Scally P (1999). *Medical Imaging*. Oxford University Press, Oxford.

Fig. 19.3 Reproduced with permission from Soames JV, Southam JC (2005). *Oral Pathology*, 4th edn. Oxford University Press, Oxford.

Fig. **19.4** Reproduced with permission from Soames JV, Southam JC (2005). *Oral Pathology*, 4th edn. Oxford University Press, Oxford.

Fig. **19.5** Reproduced with permission from Soames JV, Southam JC (2005). *Oral Pathology*, 4th edn. Oxford University Press, Oxford.

Fig. **19.6** Reproduced with permission from Soames JV, Southam JC (2005). *Oral Pathology*, 4th edn. Oxford University Press, Oxford.

Fig. **20.5** Reproduced with permission from Warrell DA, Cox TM, Firth JD (2003). *Oxford Textbook of Medicine*, 4th edn, Vol. 3. Oxford University Press, Oxford.

Fig. **23.1** Reproduced with permission from Scally P (1999). *Medical Imaging*. Oxford University Press, Oxford.

Contents

List of figures

from normal epithelium to adenoma to carcinoma as genetic mutations accumulate.

Fig. 8.18 This polyp was present in a colectomy specimen performed for colonic carcinoma, at a site distant from the carcinoma. Microscopy showed it to be a tubular adenoma with mild dysplasia.

Fig. 8.19 On the left is a picture of a severely dysplastic adenomatous polyp. In one area (dark blue), severely dysplastic glands have breached the basement membrane and infiltrated the lamina propria of the large bowel mucosa within the polyp. However, because the muscularis mucosae has not been breached, this lesion is still called a severely dysplastic adenomatous polyp. Only once the muscularis mucosae has been infiltrated is the term adenocarcinoma used (right).

Fig. 8.20 Adenocarcinoma of the caecum. This is a right hemicolectomy specimen in which a small piece of terminal ileum, the caecum, the appendix, and ascending colon have been removed. A large tumour is seen in the caecum which was confirmed on microscopy to be an adenocarcinoma. This tumour was picked up at colonoscopy performed because the patient was found to have an unexplained iron deficiency anaemia.

Fig. 8.21 Transverse section of the midrectum in the male. At this level, the rectum lies below the peritoneal cavity completely surrounded by mesorectal fat. Rectal tumours have a potential for spread throughout the mesorectum, so it is vital that surgical resection of the rectum for rectal cancer includes the whole mesorectum with an intact mesorectal fascia.

Fig. 8.22 Diverticular disease. Diverticula are outpouchings of mucosa that herniate through the circular muscle layer of the large bowel. Their tips are separated from the pericolic fat by only a thin layer of longitudinal muscle.

Fig. 8.23 Anatomy of the anal canal. Note the location of the submucosal anal cushions that give rise to haemorrhoids. Infection tracking down the anal glands can give rise to abscesses and perianal fistulas.

Chapter 9

Fig. 9.1 Microanatomy of the liver. The liver is composed of one cell thick liver cell plates surrounded by venous sinusoids. Blood flows from the portal veins and hepatic arteries towards the central veins. Bile formed from hepatocytes flows in the opposite direction in canaliculi to drain into bile ducts in the portal triads.

Fig. 9.2 Bilirubin metabolism. Haemoglobin derived from senescent erythrocytes is converted in the splenic macrophages to unconjugated bilirubin which travels in the blood to the liver where it is conjugated in hepatocytes and excreted in bile into the intestine.

Fig. 9.3 Routes to hepatic failure. Hepatic failure may occur following massive damage to a normal liver (acute hepatic failure) or following a minor insult to a chronically damaged liver (decompensated hepatic failure).

Fig. 9.4 Cardinal features of hepatic failure.

Fig. 9.5 Diagram comparing outcomes of infection with hepatitis A, B, and C viruses.

Fig. 9.6 Serology in hepatitis B virus infection. (a) Most patients with acute hepatitis B infection successfully clear the virus, with disappearance of HBsAg, resolution of abnormal liver enzyme levels, and appearance of serum anti-HBsAg antibodies. (b) Patients with a weak immune response to HBV develop chronic HBV infection. HBsAg levels remain high, and persistent liver cell damage results in persistently raised liver enzymes. Note that people vaccinated against HBV have anti-HBsAg antibodies but not HBsAg.

Fig. 9.7 Features of chronic liver disease. Patients with chronic liver disease may show a variety of clinical signs. Note that patients may exhibit some or all of these features, and that many patients with chronic liver disease may show none at all.

Fig. 9.8 Typical endoscopic retrograde cholangiographic findings in primary sclerosing cholangitis showing stricturing and dilation of the intra- and extrahepatic biliary tree.

Fig. 9.9 Cirrhotic liver. This liver was removed at post-mortem from a patient known to abuse alcohol. The whole of the liver is studded with nodules. Microscopically, the liver showed nodules of regenerating hepatocytes separated by dense bands of fibrosis, confirming established cirrhosis.

Fig. 9.10 Pathogenesis of liver fibrosis. In the normal liver, only delicate collagen fibres are present and the hepatic stellate cells are quiescent cells in the space of Disse. In the setting of chronic liver disease, Kupffer cells lining the vascular sinusoids release cytokines which activate the hepatic stellate cells. Activated hepatic stellate cells proliferate and secrete large quantities of dense collagen, leading to irreversible liver fibrosis.

Fig. 9.11 Clinical features of cirrhosis. Patients with cirrhosis may show any of the features of chronic liver disease, together with features of portal hypertension, i.e. splenomegaly, caput medusae, and ascites. Note that some patients with cirrhosis may show none of these features at all.

Fig. 9.12 Clinical features of decompensated cirrhosis. Patients with decompensated hepatic failure show the features of advanced cirrhosis together with the features of hepatic failure such as deep jaundice, hepatic encephalopathy, and a severe coagulopathy.

Fig. 9.13 Diseases caused by gallstones.

Fig. 9.14 Chronic cholecystitis. This is a microscopic image from a gallbladder specimen removed from a patient several weeks after an attack of acute cholecystitis. The gallbladder wall shows the features of chronic cholecystitis, with hypertrophy of the muscular layer of the wall, chronic inflammation, and formation of Rokitansky–Aschoff sinuses (pouches of epithelium which have herniated through the muscular layer of the gallbladder wall—arrows).

Fig. 9.15 Carcinoma of the head of the pancreas. The head of this pancreas is replaced by a large white tumour. Microscopically this was shown to be an adenocarcinoma.

Chapter 10

Fig. 10.1 Nephron structure.

Fig. 10.2 Graphical representation of acute renal failure. In acute renal failure, a massive insult to previous healthy kidneys causes them suddenly to fail. If acute renal failure is due to hypoperfusion alone and circulating volume is restored before intrinsic kidney damage occurs, then renal function may rapidly return to normal. If, however, intrinsic renal damage occurs (e.g. acute tubular necrosis), then renal failure will be prolonged and the patient will need support until regeneration occurs.

Fig. 10.3 Graphical representation of chronic renal failure. Chronic renal failure is the result of a gradual insidious decline in renal function. No symptoms occur until chronic renal failure is relatively advanced, so the diagnosis will only be picked up if renal function is measured for another reason. Lost nephrons in chronic renal failure can never be recovered.

Fig. 10.4 Symptoms and signs of advanced chronic renal failure.

Fig. 10.5 Normal glomerulus.

Fig. 10.6 The glomerular filtration barrier. There are three elements to the glomerular filter: the fenestrated endothelium of the capillary loops, the thin glomerular basement membrane, and the foot processes of the podocytes which line the urinary space.

Fig. 10.7 (a) Proliferative responses show increased cellularity of the glomerulus and tend to cause dominant haematuria. (b) Structural responses may include thickening of the glomerular basement membrane or glomerular sclerosis. These are associated with podocyte foot process fusion which causes proteinuria. (c) A necrotizing response is associated with glomerular capillary thrombosis and rupture, stimulating the formation of crescents which compress and obliterate the capillary tuft. Widespread crescent formation is associated with the development of acute renal failure.

Fig. 10.8 Reflux nephropathy. Unilateral reflux nephropathy typically presents with hypertension. Provided the other kidney is normal and compensates, renal function remains normal. Bilateral reflux nephropathy initially causes hypertension but eventually leads to chronic renal failure. This is one of the most common causes of chronic renal failure in children and young adults.

Fig. 10.9 Polycystic kidneys. Typical appearance of polycystic kidney disease with bilateral replacement of the kidneys with numerous fluid-filled cysts.

Chapter 11

Fig. 11.1 Urinary tract and male genital tract.

Fig. 11.2 Common causes of obstruction in the urinary tract.

Fig. 11.3 Diagram of a prostate gland showing the arrangement of acini and ducts with intervening fibromuscular stroma.

Fig. 11.4 A huge benign nodular hyperplastic prostate gland bulging up into the base of the bladder. The bladder wall is trabeculated due to hypertrophy of the smooth muscle layer developing in response to the bladder outflow obstruction.

Fig. 11.5 Prostate chippings from a transurethral resection of the prostate in a patient with benign nodular hyperplasia.

Fig. 11.6 This patient presented with macroscopic haematuria and was found to have a solid renal mass on CT imaging. A nephrectomy was performed and sent to pathology. The kidney has been sliced open by the pathologist to reveal a large tumour in the upper pole of the kidney. Subsequent microscopic examination of samples of the tumour revealed this to be a clear cell renal cell carcinoma.

Fig. 11.7 Typical appearance of a clear cell renal carcinoma. Note the strikingly clear cytoplasm of the malignant cells. These tumours are typically highly vascular, and this can also be appreciated here; look at all the red blood cells in the background.

Fig. 11.8 Urine cytology from a patient with a high grade transitional cell carcinoma of the bladder. Clusters of malignant transitional epithelial cells are seen with large irregular nuclei filling the cells (arrow).

Fig. 11.9 Types of bladder transitional cell carcinoma. Superficial transitional cell carcinomas are usually frond-like lesions made up of bland looking cells with no invasion or minimal invasion. Muscle invasive transitional cell carcinomas are usually solid lesions which infiltrate into the muscle coat of the bladder wall. Carcinoma in situ is a flat lesion in which the full thickness of the urothelium is replaced by malignant appearing cells but with no invasion.

Fig. 11.10 Bladder cancer staging.

Fig. 11.11 Evolution of prostate cancer. Prostatic adenocarcinoma develops from a precursor stage known as prostatic intraepithelial neoplasia (PIN) which microscopically shows neoplastic cells confined to the duct system.

Fig. 11.12 A bone scan from a patient with a very high prostate specific antigen level shows multiple metastatic bony deposits in the vertebral bodies and ribs.

Fig. 11.13 Development of the testis showing the origin of the cells giving rise to testicular tumours.

Fig. 11.14 This is a testis from a young man who presented with an enlarging testicular lump. Following an ultrasound scan which was suspicious for a neoplasm, he underwent orchidectomy. The testis has been sliced in the pathology department revealing this white solid mass in the testis. This appearance is typical of a seminoma and microscopic examination confirmed this.

Chapter 12

Fig. 12.1 Psoriasis of the vulva, flexural variant. Note the well demarcated, intensely erythematous eruption involving the vulva and groins. Scaling is typically absent in flexural disease.

Fig. 12.2 Lichen sclerosus of the vulva. Note symmetrical white lesions with marked atrophy and spots of haemorrhage.

Fig. 12.3 Cervicitis. The cervix is inflamed and there is mucopurulent material exuding from the external os.

Fig. 12.4 Transformation zone of the cervix. (A) Before puberty, the ectocervix covered by squamous epithelium meets the endocervical epithelium at the external os. (B) At puberty, the lower endocervix becomes exposed to the vagina and is visible as a rough red area (ectropion). (C) The endocervical epithelium undergoes squamous metaplasia in response to the acidic environment of the vagina, creating the transformation zone where squamous epithelium overlies endocervical glands. It is this process which is diverted into a potentially neoplastic pathway by persistent infection with high risk types of human papillomavirus. The transformation zone is visible and must be completely sampled when taking a cervical smear. (D) After the menopause, the cervix involutes such that the transformation zone is drawn up into the endocervical canal.

Fig. 12.5 Infection of immature squamous metaplastic epithelium of the transformation zone by high risk types of human papillomavirus (HPV) diverts the metaplastic process into a neoplastic process. Persistent infection in some women leads to the development of increasing degrees of cervical intraepithelial neoplasia (CIN). In a small minority of untreated women, an invasive squamous cell carcinoma develops.

Fig. 12.6 Common sites of endometriosis in the pelvis.

of angiotensin II. Angiotensin II stimulates the release of aldosterone from the adrenal cortex, which causes reabsorption of sodium and water by the kidneys to restore circulating volume.

Fig. 14.5 Clinical features of Cushing's syndrome.

Fig. 14.6 Control of thyroid hormone release. TRH from the hypothalamus stimulates release of TSH from the anterior pituitary which drives T3 and T4 production in the thyroid gland. The thyroid hormones then provide negative feedback on release of TRH and TSH to maintain normal levels of thyroid hormones.

Fig. 14.7 Multinodular goitre. This massive multinodular goitre was removed from an elderly lady because it was compressing her trachea.

Fig. 14.8 Clinical features of thyrotoxicosis.

Fig. 14.9 Clinical features of hypothyroidism.

Fig. 14.10 Follicular neoplasm. This patient presented with a solitary thyroid nodule. A fine needle aspiration cytology preparation diagnosed a 'follicular neoplasm' so the tumour was removed. Macroscopically, a well circumscribed tumour is seen surrounded by a thin capsule. This is likely to be a follicular adenoma, however microscopic examination of the edge of the tumour at the capsule must be carefully carried out to detect evidence of capsule invasion or vascular invasion diagnostic of a follicular carcinoma.

Fig. 14.11 Papillary carcinoma. This histological image from a papillary carcinoma of the thyroid shows the diagnostic nuclear features of nuclear clearing, nuclear grooving, and intranuclear inclusions (arrow).

Fig. 14.12 Hyperparathyroid bone disease. Radiographic features of hyperparathyroid bone disease in a patient with chronic renal failure. There is erosion of the edges of the bones, most marked in the middle phalanges.

Fig. 14.13 Mechanism of hyperglycaemia in diabetes mellitus. Lack of insulin causes breakdown of protein in muscle and of triglyceride in fat, providing substrates for gluconeogenesis in the liver. This, together with glucose formed from glycogen in the liver, causes hyperglycaemia.

Fig. 14.14 Long-term complications of diabetes mellitus.

Chapter 15

Fig. 15.1 Haematopoiesis.

Fig. 15.2 Haemoglobin molecule composed of four polypeptide globin chains, each of which contains a haem molecule. The iron atom at the centre of the haem group binds to oxygen.

Fig. 15.3 Blood film in iron deficiency anaemia showing pale and distorted red blood cells.

Fig. 15.4 Blood film in megaloblastic anaemia showing a hypersegmented neutrophil and oval macrocytes.

Fig. 15.5 Typical sequence of events leading to a diagnosis of pernicious anaemia.

Fig. 15.6 Haemoglobin electrophoresis in sickle cell disorders. The following are shown from left to right: (1 and 2) sickle cell trait; (3) normal; (4) sickle cell anaemia; (5) normal.

Fig. 15.7 Haemostasis. Following vascular injury, platelets bind to exposed collagen, forming the primary haemostatic plug. Simultaneously, the coagulation system is activated, leading to the deposition of fibrin on the platelets, forming the secondary haemostatic plug.

Fig. 15.8 Peripheral blood film from a patient with chronic lymphocytic leukaemia showing small neoplastic lymphocytes, some of which have formed smear cells.

Fig. 15.9 Peripheral blood film from a patient with chronic myeloid leukaemia showing large numbers of neutrophils and neutrophil precursors.

Fig. 15.10 Normal B lymphocyte development, showing postulated neoplastic counterparts.

Fig. 15.11 Microscopic image of Hodgkin–Reed–Sternberg cells seen in Hodgkin lymphoma.

Fig. 15.12 Pathogenesis of bone disease in multiple myeloma. Lytic bony lesions in myeloma result from the interaction of myeloma cells with bone marrow stromal cells and the release of cytokines that stimulate osteoclast formation and activation.

Fig. 15.13 Clinical features of myeloma.

Fig. 15.14 A histological image of a bone marrow trephine biopsy taken from a patient with multiple myeloma. The white spaces represent fat cells in the bone marrow space which has been nearly completely replaced by large numbers of neoplastic plasma cells.

Chapter 16

Fig. 16.1 Structure of the skin.

Fig. 16.2 Diagram of melanocytic nevi. Junctional nevi result from proliferating nests of melanocytes confined to the dermoepidermal junction. Some of the melanocytes then migrate into the dermis, forming a compound nevus. Once all of the melanocytes have migrated into the dermis, the lesion becomes an intra-dermal nevus.

Fig. 16.3 Compound nevus on the neck of a young woman. The lesion is uniformly pigmented, slightly raised, and measures about 4 mm in diameter.

Fig. 16.4 Intradermal nevus. Note the lack of pigmentation.

Fig. 16.5 Dermatofibroma on the leg of a young woman.

Fig. 16.6 Pyogenic granuloma. Typical vascular appearance of a pyogenic granuloma arising on a digit.

Fig. 16.7 Multiple actinic keratoses on the scalp of an elderly woman. These yellow scaly lesions on an erythematous base show the typical appearance of an actinic keratosis.

Fig. 16.8 Intraepidermal carcinoma. This scaly lesion on the lower leg of an elderly woman was excised. Microscopic examination showed full thickness dysplasia of the epidermis.

Fig. 16.9 Dysplastic nevus showing irregular borders and a diameter greater than 6 mm. Symmetry remains preserved and the pigmentation is even.

Fig. 16.10 Nodular basal cell carcinoma showing the characteristic telangiectatic vessels over the surface.

Fig. 16.11 Ulcerated basal cell carcinoma with characteristic rolled edges.

Fig. 16.12 Microscopic image of a basal cell carcinoma. The tumour, composed of nests of small blue neoplastic cells embedded in a loose stroma, is seen growing down from the epidermis at the top of the image.

Fig. 16.13 Ulcerated squamous cell carcinoma of the skin.

Fig. 16.14 Diagrammatic representation of different stages of melanoma. Melanoma in situ comprises malignant melanocytes confined to the epidermis. In radial growth phase invasive melanoma, malignant melanocytes invade the dermis but the growth of the tumour is still confined to the epidermis. In vertical growth phase invasive melanoma, the growth of the tumour switches from the epidermis to the dermis.

Fig. 16.15 Superficial spreading melanoma. Note the large nodule representing the vertical growth phase arising from a surrounding flat component of the preceding radial growth phase.

Fig. 16.16 Psoriatic plaque. Classical appearance of untreated psoriatic plaque topped with silvery scales.

Fig. 16.17 The rash of lichen planus favouring the wrists. The lesions are flat topped, violet, and shiny.

Fig. 16.18 Ring-like lesion of granuloma annulare on the dorsum of the hand.

Fig. 16.19 Erythema multiforme on the leg showing typical target lesions.

Fig. 16.20 Large, tense, raised blisters of pemphigoid.

Fig. 16.21 Scaling lesion of tinea corporis on the trunk.

Chapter 17

Fig. 17.1 Anatomy of a long bone.

Fig. 17.2 Microarchitecture of normal and osteo-porotic bone showing marked loss of trabecular bone.

Fig. 17.3 Examples of pathways to osteoporosis. (a) Peak bone mass is achieved in early adulthood followed by slow age-related bone loss. In women, there is an accelerated period of bone loss during the menopause. (b) This male patient develops osteoporosis due to therapeutic administration of glucocorticoids. (c) This female patient develops osteoporosis because she failed to reach peak bone mass for genetic reasons and had an early menopause.

Fig. 17.4 Common fragility fractures in osteoporosis.

Fig. 17.5 This right femur shows a thickened cortex and bone sclerosis caused by Paget's disease. Incidentally, the hip joint also shows the features of osteoarthritis with loss of the joint space.

pressure, rapidly deteriorated, and died. There is an ill defined tumour with areas of haemorrhage. Microscopy revealed this to be a glioblastoma which was much more extensive than was apparent macroscopically.

Fig. 18.16 Meningioma. This very well circumscribed tumour (arrow) has the typical macroscopic appearance of a meningioma, a suspicion which was confirmed microscopically.

Chapter 19

Fig. 19.1 Anatomy of the head and neck.

Fig. 19.2 (a) Dental caries. Dental plaque erodes through tooth enamel. If the pulp cavity is entered, acute pulpitis leads to throbbing pain related to the tooth and risks the development of a deep periapical abscess. (b) Chronic periodontal disease. Dental plaque eroding down the sides of a tooth destroys the periodontal ligaments that hold the tooth in the socket. Over many years, the tooth becomes gradually loosened and is eventually lost.

Fig. 19.3 Oral candidiasis. This infection was due to oral deposition of steroid in an asthmatic patient with a poor inhaler technique.

Fig. 19.4 Early squamous cell carcinoma of the oral cavity presenting as a persistent ulcerated lesion on the undersurface of the tongue.

Fig. 19.5 This firm lesion on the lower gum was excised and shown to be a fibroepithelial polyp on microscopic examination.

Fig. 19.6 This vascular lesion on the lower gum was excised and shown to be a lobular capillary haemangioma (pyogenic granuloma) on microscopic examination.

Fig. 19.7 Pleomorphic adenoma. Typical microscopic appearance of a pleomorphic adenoma with an intermingling of epithelial elements (arrow) set within a mesenchymal component.

Fig. 19.8 Warthin's tumour. Classical microscopic appearance of a Warthin's tumour with a double layer of eosinophilic epithelial cells (bright pink cells) overlying a dense lymphoid stroma (dark blue area).

Fig. 19.9 Common origins of lumps in the neck.

Chapter 20

Fig. 20.1 Anatomy of the eye.

Fig. 20.2 Open angle and closed angle glaucoma. In open angle glaucoma, aqueous humour can reach the trabecular meshwork but is unable to drain through it. In closed angle glaucoma, the iris becomes pushed up against the cornea, preventing aqueous humour from reaching the trabecular meshwork.

Fig. 20.3 Cataract.

Fig. 20.4 Structure of the retina. The retina is composed of a neurosensory layer comprising rods, cones, and neurones, which sits on the retinal pigment epithelium.

Fig. 20.5 Proptosis in a patient with Graves' ophthalmopathy.

Chapter 21

Fig. 21.1 Postulated pathogenesis of systemic lupus erythematosus. Defective phagocytosis of apoptotic bodies leads to priming of the immune system to intracellular antigens and activation of autoreactive B and T lymphocytes. Circulating immune complexes formed between autoantibodies and self-antigens then become deposited in various tissues around the body (skin, joints, kidneys), stimulating inflammation and tissue damage.

Fig. 21.2 Clinical features of generalized amyloidosis.

Chapter 22

Fig. 22.1 Effects of placental insufficiency on the fetus and correlation with diagnostic features.

Fig. 22.2 Chest radiograph in respiratory distress syndrome showing diffuse fine shadowing throughout both lungs.

Fig. 22.3 Congenital heart disease. Summary of pathophysiological and clinical features of the common congenital heart diseases.

Fig. 22.4 Ventricular septal defect. In the presence of a ventricular septal defect, blood flows from the higher pressure left ventricle into the right ventricle, resulting in a left-to-right shunt.

Fig. 22.5 Tetralogy of Fallot. Tetralogy of Fallot comprises pulmonary stenosis, a ventricular septal defect, an over-riding aorta, and right ventricular hypertrophy.

PART I

Getting to grips with pathology

CHAPTER 1

Introducing pathology

Chapter contents

Introduction

Pathology is the study of disease and therefore forms a central part of medicine. A sound knowledge of the pathology of a disease allows the clinician to understand its symptoms and signs, potential complications, the basis of its treatment, and its likely course.

Nomenclature of disease

Pathology has a language of its own and it is necessary to familiarize yourself with some of the common terms used when discussing diseases.

The **aetiology** of a disease is its underlying *cause*. A number of aetiological agents are known to cause disease (Table 1.1). Nowadays we recognize that most diseases are caused by the interaction of several different aetiologies all acting together. For instance, an infection may cause disease in patient A but not in patient B due to differences in their genetic makeup. There remain many diseases whose aetiology is completely unknown, and these may be described using terms such as **idiopathic**, **cryptogenic**, or **essential**.

The **pathogenesis** of a disease is the *mechanism* by which the aetiological agent leads to the manifestations of the disease. Even if the aetiology of a disease is not known, much can still be learnt about its pathogenesis, and this knowledge may be used to design treatments. A good example here would be rheumatoid arthritis, where we know plenty about the sequence of events that leads to joint destruction but not what triggers it off in the first place.

TABLE 1.1	Aetiologies of disease
Genetic	
Infective	
Environmental, e.g. diet, smoking, sunlight	
Physical, e.g. trauma	

The **incidence** of a disease is the number of *new* cases of the condition occurring in a population over a set period of time. Incidence, therefore, refers to the rate at which new cases are being diagnosed. The **prevalence** of a disease is the total number of cases of a condition in a population at any one time.

The **prognosis** of a disease is a prediction of its likely course. Whilst a patient with a common cold is likely to recover completely with no residual problems, the patient with metastatic small cell carcinoma of the lung is likely to be dead within only a few months.

The **morbidity** of a disease refers to the extent of the reduction in the patient's health as a consequence of the disease. A good example of a disease associated with much morbidity is diabetes mellitus, a common cause of ischaemic heart disease, chronic renal failure requiring dialysis, and blindness.

The **mortality** of a disease reflects the likelihood that a patient will die from that disease. For instance, the mortality of lung cancer is very high, whereas the mortality of chronic lymphocytic leukaemia is low as most patients die with the disease rather than from it.

Acute and **chronic** refer to the time course of a disease. Acute diseases have a rapid onset and often a rapid resolution. Chronic conditions tend to have a gradual onset with a prolonged course over many months or years. Chronic conditions are more likely to cause irreversible damage.

A **syndrome** is a set of symptoms and signs which, when occurring together, suggest a particular underlying cause. A syndrome therefore indicates the possibility of a particular disease, but is not a disease in itself. For example, the combination of breathlessness on lying flat, fatigue, a raised jugular venous pressure, and oedema is typical of chronic heart failure which may be caused by a number of diseases including coronary artery atherosclerosis, hypertension, and valvular heart disease.

Classification of disease

Many different classifications of disease have been devised, though none is perfect as we do not know everything about every disease to create an all-encompassing scheme. As such, commonly used classification systems tend to use a mixture of aetiological and pathogenetic labels.

- **Genetic** diseases are inherited conditions in which a defective gene leads to disease, e.g. cystic fibrosis, haemophilia, or sickle cell disease.
- **Infective** diseases are the result of invasion of the body by microorganisms, e.g. pneumonia and malaria.
- **Inflammatory** diseases are due to excess inflammatory activity in an organ, e.g. acute appendicitis, atopic dermatitis, or rheumatoid arthritis.
- **Neoplastic** diseases are due to uncontrolled growth of cells, e.g. lipoma, breast carcinoma, or acute lymphoblastic leukaemia.
- **Vascular** diseases are due to disorders of blood vessels. They often present with symptoms related to inadequate blood supply to a tissue, e.g. ischaemic heart disease or cerebrovascular disease.
- **Metabolic** diseases are due to abnormalities in metabolic pathways, e.g. diabetes mellitus.
- **Degenerative** diseases occur due to loss of specialized cells, e.g. Alzheimer's disease due to loss of neurones from the cerebral cortex, and osteoarthritis due to degeneration of articular cartilage in joints.
- **Iatrogenic** disease is due to the effects of treatment, e.g. iatrogenic osteoporosis caused by glucocorticoid treatment.

Diseases may also be divided into **congenital** or **acquired**. Congenital diseases are present at birth, although they may not be recognizable at the time. Acquired diseases only occur after birth. Note that whilst many congenital diseases are inherited, not all are. For instance, intrauterine infection with organisms such as *Toxoplasma* or rubella can lead to severe congenital abnormalities.

Cellular adaptations

Diseases occur because of injury to cells of the body

Our current understanding of disease processes is firmly placed at the cellular level. In order to understand why disease comes about, one needs to have a basic understanding of how cells can be damaged and how they respond to such damage.

Cells need to be able to adapt to cope with the demands placed on them

The conditions to which cells are exposed are constantly changing. Cells therefore need to be adaptable units in order to survive in the face of such changes. Marked physiological or pathological demands on a cell may bring about a number of adaptive responses (Fig. 1.1):

♦ Atrophy

♦ Hypertrophy

♦ Hyperplasia

♦ Metaplasia

A key feature of these adaptations is that the altered pattern of growth is reversible following removal of the underlying stimulus. This distinguishes them from neoplastic processes where cell growth is unregulated and does not regress.

Atrophy

Atrophy is a reduction in size of a tissue or organ

A tissue or organ that has reduced in size is said to have undergone **atrophy**. Atrophy may come about through a reduction in cell *number* by cell deletion (**apoptosis**) or a reduction in cell *size* by shrinkage. Which modality is used depends on the type of tissue undergoing atrophy.

Atrophy may occur as a normal physiological process when the functional demand on a tissue is reduced. For instance, the thymus undergoes atrophy during adolescence, and the ovaries and testes shrink in old age.

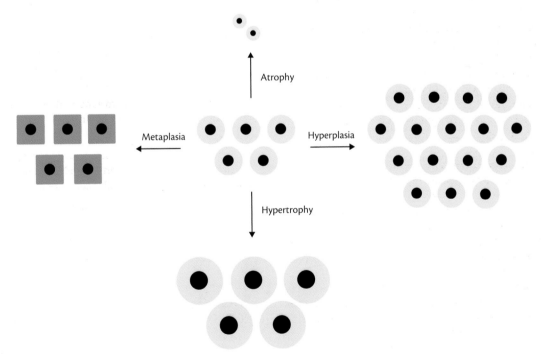

Fig. 1.1 Cellular adaptations.

Pathological causes of atrophy include muscle atrophy following denervation, and cerebral atrophy due to atherosclerosis of the blood vessels supplying the brain.

Hypertrophy

Hypertrophy is an increase in size of individual cells

In **hypertrophy**, cells increase in size due to an increase in the number of cell proteins and organelles, leading to an overall increase in the size of the organ. Hypertrophy is seen in organs containing terminally differentiated cells that cannot multiply, e.g. cardiac and skeletal muscle. Physiological causes of hypertrophy include the myometrium of the uterus in pregnancy and the muscles of a bodybuilder. Pathological causes of hypertrophy include left ventricular hypertrophy due to hypertension or aortic stenosis.

Hyperplasia

Hyperplasia is an increase in the number of cells

In **hyperplasia**, the number of cells increases due to increased cell division, leading to an increase in size of the tissue or organ. Many tissues undergo physiological hyperplasia in response to stimuli, e.g. the endometrium and the terminal duct lobular units of the breast both undergo hyperplasia in response to oestrogen. A pathological cause of hyperplasia would be nodular hyperplasia of the prostate in response to increased local androgen levels in the prostate.

Some diseases are characterized by hyperplasia, but the stimulus for the hyperplasia is unknown. For example, in psoriasis, there is marked hyperplasia of the epidermis, and one form of primary hyperparathyroidism is due to sporadic hyperplasia of all four parathyroid glands for no apparent reason.

Metaplasia

Metaplasia is a change in which one cell type is replaced by another

Metaplasia refers to a switch from one cell type to another. The precise mechanism underlying metaplasia is still not known for certain, but it is thought to be the result of progenitor cells differentiating into a new type of cell rather than a direct metamorphosis of cells from one type to another (Fig. 1.2). Metaplasia only occurs in cells that can divide, reinforcing the theory that metaplasia is a form of abnormal regeneration.

Metaplasia is almost exclusively seen in epithelial cells, which undergo metaplasia in response to chronic irritation. A very common type of metaplasia is the replacement of glandular type epithelium by the more robust multilayered squamous epithelium (**squamous metaplasia**). Common sites of squamous metaplasia include the bronchi in cigarette smokers and the endocervix in response to exposure to the acidic environment of the vagina.

The reverse situation can also occur whereby a squamous epithelium becomes replaced by glandular epithelial cells (**glandular metaplasia**). This is seen in some patients with gastro-oesophageal reflux disease, where part of the native squamous epithelium of the lower oesophagus switches to a columnar type of epithelium in response to persistent injury from gastric acid.

Metaplasia is a particularly important adaptation to understand as it is a marker that there is chronic damage at work to an area of epithelium which, over a long period of time, *may* lead to the development of malignancy. Several important epithelial malignancies are well known to develop in areas of metaplasia

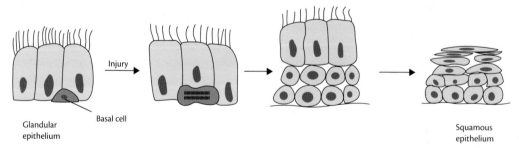

Fig. 1.2 Postulated mechanism of epithelial metaplasia. Injury to this glandular epithelium has stimulated the basal cells to divide. The progeny from the basal cells have then differentiated into squamous type epithelium, replacing the original glandular type.

including squamous cell carcinomas of the bronchus and cervix, and adenocarcinomas of the oesophagus.

> ## Key points: Cellular adaptations
>
> ◆ Cells are able to adapt to demands placed upon them.
>
> ◆ Atrophy refers to a reduction in size and number of cells.
>
> ◆ Hypertrophy refers to an increase in the size of cells.
>
> ◆ Hyperplasia refers to an increase in the number of cells.
>
> ◆ Metaplasia occurs when one cell type is replaced by another cell type. Metaplasia is usually seen in epithelial cells, and is an important early stage in the development of some malignancies.

Cellular death

Cellular death occurs when a cell is damaged beyond its abilities to adapt

Cell death is potentially a very dangerous event. All cells are loaded with lysosomal proteolytic enzymes ready to self-digest the cell as soon as the cells begin to die (**autolysis**). Uncontrolled autolysis leads to liberation of highly irritant cell contents into the surrounding environment and a self-perpetuating cycle of cell death and inflammation. Furthermore, priming of the immune system to intracellular proteins could potentially lead to autoimmune attack against the body's own cells.

Preventing or minimizing these consequences is the most important final job a dying cell has to complete. The principle difference between the two modes of cell death, **necrosis** and **apoptosis**, is the degree of control that the cell has over its own death.

LINK BOX

Biochemical markers of necrosis

Proteins liberated from dead cells can be measured in the blood and can be useful blood tests for diagnosing necrosis of particular cell types. For instance, a rise in cardiac troponin levels in the blood is highly specific for the diagnosis of myocardial infarction (p. 88).

Necrosis

Necrosis is a poorly controlled form of cell death

Necrosis is the result of severe forms of cellular injury in which the cells have little time or energy to control their death. Membrane integrity is inevitably compromised, with leakage of cellular contents and an inflammatory response in the surrounding area. Cells undergoing necrosis, however, attempt to minimize this by uncoiling the tertiary structure of their proteins, a process known as **denaturation**.

Denaturation reduces the formation of proinflammatory peptides by inactivating autolytic enzymes (remember enzymes are themselves proteins) and by rendering their target protein an unsuitable substrate. In addition, denaturation makes intracellular proteins non-antigenic so they will not be recognized as self by the immune system.

The fate of a tissue undergoing necrosis depends on the overall balance between the amount of denaturation and the amount of autolysis. If denaturation prevails, the area of necrosis is converted into a pale firm mass called **coagulative necrosis**. If autolysis wins, the area turns into a semisolid mass called **liquefactive necrosis**.

Coagulative necrosis is the most common form of necrosis

In most tissues, protein denaturation prevails in necrotic cells and coagulative necrosis is the result. Macroscopically, the dead area appears pale and feels firm. Microscopically, the cells lose the structural detail of their cytoplasm and often the nucleus is lost, but the general architecture of the tissue is preserved and the cellular outlines are retained.

Liquefactive necrosis is usually seen in the brain

Liquefactive necrosis is typically seen in the brain. Because neurones have a much higher lysosomal content, autolysis dominates, leading to liquefaction. Macroscopically, necrotic brain tissue is therefore soft and semisolid. Liquefactive necrosis may also be seen in other organs following severe bacterial infections due to massive outpouring of enzymes from neutrophils destroying the tissue.

Caseous necrosis is a mixture of coagulative and liquefactive necrosis

Caseous necrosis is a special type of necrosis due to a mixture of coagulative and liquefactive necrosis. It was named because it looks like cream cheese to the naked eye. Although this may be seen in many conditions, it is most commonly associated with tuberculosis.

Key points: Necrosis

- Necrosis is a poorly controlled form of cell death which involves large numbers of cells in a tissue.

- Necrotic cells start to denature their own proteins to minimize the amount of inflammation and to prevent an immune response to intracellular antigens.

- The type of necrosis a tissue undergoes depends on the balance between denaturation and autolysis.

- Coagulative necrosis is the most common form of necrosis. Macroscopically the dead tissue is firm and pale. Microscopically the dead tissue retains its architecture and cell outlines.

- Liquefactive necrosis occurs if autolysis prevails over denaturation and is most often seen in the brain because neurones have a very high lysosomal content.

- Caseous necrosis is a mixture of coagulative and liquefactive necrosis which resembles soft cheese macroscopically. Caseous necrosis is most commonly seen in tuberculosis but can be seen in a number of other conditions.

Apoptosis

Apoptosis is a highly controlled form of cell death

Apoptosis is a form of cell death that is quite distinct from necrosis (Table 1.2). In apoptosis, cells bring about their own death in an orderly manner by activating enzymes that degrade the cell's own DNA and proteins. No cellular contents are released from an apoptotic cell, a key distinguishing feature from necrosis.

Whereas necrosis is always a pathological process, apoptosis has many important normal functions. Death by apoptosis is an important way to eliminate cells that are no longer needed, e.g. cell loss during embryogenesis, elimination of potentially self-reactive lymphocytes, and removal of cells with DNA damage.

TABLE 1.2 Comparison of apoptosis and necrosis

Apoptosis	Necrosis
Well controlled	Poorly controlled
Membrane integrity preserved	Membrane breached
No inflammation	Inflammatory response
Single cells	Groups of cells

Apoptosis is induced by a cascade of molecular events culminating in the activation of caspases

Apoptosis may be induced by two main pathways (Fig. 1.3). The *extrinsic* pathway is initiated by engagement and activation of surface 'death' receptors such as Fas and the tumour necrosis factor-α (TNF-α) receptor. The *intrinsic* pathway is a reflection of cellular injury and is mediated by proapoptotic molecules released from inside mitochondria that have become abnormally permeable due to cell damage.

Whichever way apoptosis is stimulated, the end result is the same. Protease enzymes called **caspases** become activated, and these dismantle all the working parts of the cell leading to breakdown of the cytoplasm and nucleus.

Apoptotic cells fragment into apoptotic bodies which are targeted for rapid removal

Apoptotic cells shrink down and then fragment into small pieces called **apoptotic bodies**, each of which retains an intact cell membrane (Fig. 1.4). Apoptotic bodies express markers on their surface which target them for cannabilization by adjacent cells ('eat me signals'). Prompt removal of apoptotic bodies is important to prevent their contents from diffusing out and stimulating an inflammatory response.

Disordered apoptosis is believed to be central to many important diseases

Defects in apoptosis have been implicated in a variety of important disease processes. An inability to eliminate cells with DNA damage via apoptosis is believed to be central to the accumulation of mutations in the genesis of malignant neoplasms.

Defects in the 'hoovering up' of apoptotic bodies may be relevant in the development of autoimmunity against normal cellular and nuclear proteins that may be vital to the pathogenesis of multisystem immune disorders such as systemic lupus erythematosus.

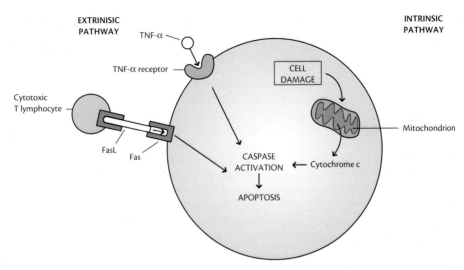

Fig. 1.3 Mechanisms leading to apoptosis. Apoptosis may be triggered extrinsically by ligation of death receptors' such as TNF-α receptor and Fas, or intrinsically if cell damage causes release of cytochrome c from mitochondria.

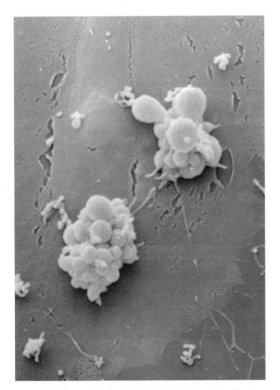

Fig. 1.4 Apoptosis. This scanning electron micrograph shows two cultured endothelial cells undergoing apoptosis. The apoptotic cells have formed numerous blebs which will eventually dissociate into apoptotic fragments for phagocytosis by nearby cells.

Key points: Apoptosis

◆ Apoptosis is a controlled form of cell death in which a cell brings about its own death in an orderly manner without stimulating inflammation.

◆ Apoptosis may be stimulated by extrinsic or intrinsic pathways.

◆ Both pathways culminate in the activation of enzymes called caspases which dismantle the cell into numerous membrane-bound fragments called apoptotic bodies. Apoptotic bodies are then rapidly taken up by adjacent cells.

◆ Defective apoptosis is a central part of carcinogenesis and may also be relevant in the pathogenesis of multisystem autoimmune diseases.

Inflammation

Introduction

Inflammation is the body's response to cellular injury. It serves to dilute and remove injurious agents and trigger healing of the damaged tissue. Although inflammation is intended to be a protective response, it may also be harmful when inappropriately activated.

Inflammation is elicited by any form of cellular damage including infection, physical injury, chemical injury, and ischaemia. Be careful not to equate inflammation with infection. Whilst infection is often accompanied by inflammation, there are many diseases characterized by inflammation which are not caused by infection, such as autoimmune diseases, and even some infectious diseases where inflammation is absent, e.g. variant Creutzfeldt–Jacob disease.

There are two main types of inflammation which differ in their time course and the inflammatory cells involved. Acute inflammation is usually a transient phenomenon involving neutrophils, whereas chronic inflammation is a more persistent reaction involving cells such as macrophages and lymphocytes.

JARGON BUSTER

Nomenclature of inflammation

Tissues which show inflammation are given the suffix '-itis' to indicate the presence of inflammation and are designated as acute or chronic, e.g. acute appendicitis, chronic pancreatitis.

TABLE 2.1 Diseases characterized by acute inflammation
Acute appendicitis
Acute pneumonia
Acute pancreatitis
Acute cholecystitis

Acute inflammation

Acute inflammation is the initial response to tissue damage. It is a non-specific reaction which serves to clear away any dead tissue, fight off any infection, and set the scene for attempted healing. Clinically, inflamed tissues are swollen, red, warm, and painful. A number of common diseases are characterized by acute inflammation (Table 2.1).

A range of chemical mediators stimulate acute inflammation

The process of acute inflammation is orchestrated by a number of chemical mediators called **cytokines** released from cells in areas of injury (Table 2.2).

- **Histamine** and **serotonin** are two particularly important mediators of acute inflammation which are stored in mast cells and platelets ready for immediate release.

- **Prostaglandins** and **leukotrienes** are groups of long chain fatty acids synthesized from a phospholipid called arachidonic acid in response to tissue damage. Prostaglandins are synthesized using an enzyme called cyclooxygenase, whereas leukotrienes are synthesized by the action of an enzyme called lipooxygenase.

- **Platelet-activating factor**, as well as causing platelet stimulation as its name suggests, is also a potent stimulator of acute inflammation.

TABLE 2.2 Mediators of acute inflammation
Histamine
Serotonin
Prostaglandins
Leukotrienes
Platelet-activating factor

Knowledge about the chemical mediators of acute inflammation is important as drugs which block their actions have anti-inflammatory activity. Examples include the widely used non-steroidal anti-inflammatory drugs which inhibit cyclooxygenase.

Activation of endothelial cells is a crucial event in acute inflammation

One of the most critical actions of the mediators of acute inflammation is to activate capillary endothelial cells in the area of damage. Activated endothelial cells swell and retract from their neighbours, so the vessel becomes leaky to fluid and small proteins. Fibrinogen is one of the important proteins to leak out. Activation of the coagulation cascade in the area of cell damage leads to the production of thrombin which converts fibrinogen into insoluble fibrin.

Activated endothelial cells also express particular types of adhesion molecules on their surface which allow circulating neutrophils to stick to them, and pass into the area of damage. Once in the area of damage, it is thought that the large polymers of fibrin act as a scaffold which neutrophils can use to move around the area of inflammation. Neutrophils engulf and kill microorganisms, and release enzymes to break down the damaged tissue.

Acute inflammation is characterized by formation of the acute inflammatory exudate

The end result of endothelial cell activation is that the area of injury becomes occupied by fluid, fibrin, and neutrophils. These three components make up the **acute inflammatory exudate** which is the hallmark of acute inflammation (Fig. 2.1).

The relative amounts of fluid, neutrophils, and fibrin within an exudate can vary, giving rise to different types of exudate known as **serous exudates**, **purulent exudates**, and **fibrinous exudates**, respectively.

Severe acute inflammation may lead to abscess formation

An **abscess** is a localized collection of pus in a necrotic cavity which is usually the result of bacterial infection. Large abscesses are often difficult to treat with antibiotics because the bacteria within the abscess are inaccessible to the drugs. Surgical incision and drainage of the abscess is often needed to collapse the cavity and promote healing.

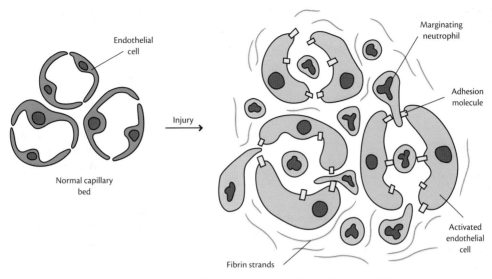

Fig. 2.1 Formation of the acute inflammatory exudate. Release of chemical mediators following cell injury stimulates endothelial cell retraction and expression of neutrophil adhesion molecules, leading to formation of an acute inflammatory exudate containing fluid, fibrin, and neutrophils.

JARGON BUSTER

Pus

Pus is a thick yellow fluid which consists of living, dying, and dead neutrophils together with cell debris.

Acute inflammation may resolve, heal with scarring, or progress to chronic inflammation

There are three main outcomes of acute inflammation, depending on the nature and intensity of the injury and the type of tissue that has been damaged (Fig. 2.2):

◆ Complete resolution. If acute inflammation disappears within a few days and the tissue returns to normal, then resolution is said to have occurred.

◆ Repair with scarring. If there is substantial tissue destruction, or destruction in tissues incapable of regeneration (e.g. heart muscle), then fibrous tissue is laid down in a process called **organization**.

◆ Progression to chronic inflammation.

JARGON BUSTER

Systemic inflammatory response syndrome

Under normal circumstances, activation of endothelial cells and the inflammatory response occurs in a controlled manner localized only to the area of damage. In certain severe clinical conditions, widespread systemic activation of endothelial cells leads to generalized vasodilation, circulatory collapse, and multiple organ failure. This is called the **systemic inflammatory response syndrome** and carries a high mortality. It is most often caused by circulating bacterial products in bacterial septicaemia.

Chronic inflammation

Chronic inflammation is said to occur when inflammation persists for weeks, months, or longer. There is ongoing active inflammation with tissue destruction and attempts at repair all proceeding simultaneously. Chronic inflammation may arise from unresolved acute inflammation or occur from the outset.

Key points: Acute inflammation

♦ Acute inflammation is a rapid, non-specific response to cellular injury.

♦ A variety of chemical mediators released from injured cells leads to a vascular response which leads to the release of fluid and fibrin into the site of injury. Upregulation of adhesion molecules on endothelial cells causes neutrophils to marginate into the area of damage.

♦ The combination of fluid, fibrin, and neutrophils defines the acute inflammatory exudate.

♦ The aim of acute inflammation is to dilute and wall off the injurious stimulus and set in motion the healing response.

♦ The ideal outcome of acute inflammation is resolution in which the tissue returns to normal.

♦ If there is severe destruction, or inflammation in a tissue incapable of regeneration, then healing occurs by fibrosis with formation of scar tissue.

♦ Acute inflammation which fails to terminate progresses to chronic inflammation.

Chronic inflammation is characterized by the presence of chronic inflammatory cells, namely macrophages, lymphocytes, and plasma cells. Chronic inflammation is important as it is much more likely to cause tissue destruction and heal with irreversible scarring rather than resolve.

Chronic inflammation may occur in response to an injurious agent that cannot be cleared, e.g. a microorganism resistant to the immune response or foreign material that cannot be degraded such as a surgical suture. Alternatively, chronic inflammation may occur due to an inappropriate inflammatory response either to environmental agents that should not normally evoke a response (e.g. hayfever) or to the body's own tissues (autoimmunity). A number of common diseases are characterized by chronic inflammation (Table 2.3).

The macrophage is the key inflammatory cell in chronic inflammation

Macrophages are a type of phagocyte derived from blood monocytes that migrate into tissues and differentiate into tissue macrophages (**histiocytes**). Macrophages become activated in chronic inflammation and secrete a number of products which are intended to help eliminate injurious agents (e.g. reactive oxygen intermediates) and initiate the process of repair (e.g. proteases, transforming growth factor-β). Prolonged release of these products, however, results in the tissue injury and fibrosis characteristic of chronic inflammation.

Interaction between macrophages and T lymphocytes is important in sustaining chronic inflammation

The interaction between macrophages and T lymphocytes, particularly CD4+ T helper lymphocytes, is crucial to persistence of chronic inflammation. CD4+ T lymphocytes release cytokines such as interferon-γ which is a powerful activator of macrophages. Activated macrophages then present antigens to CD4+

TABLE 2.3 Diseases characterized by chronic inflammation

Helicobacter pylori-associated gastritis
Inflammatory bowel disease
Rheumatoid arthritis
Chronic hepatitis

Key points: Chronic inflammation

♦ Chronic inflammation is a persistent form of inflammation in which there is simultaneous tissue destruction and attempted repair.

♦ Chronic inflammation is typically seen in response to organisms that have evolved to resist removal by the acute inflammatory response, foreign material that cannot be removed, or an inappropriate response to environmental agents or the body's own tissues.

♦ The key inflammatory cell in chronic inflammation is the macrophage which becomes activated and releases products that cause tissue destruction and stimulate fibrosis.

♦ Ongoing activation of macrophages is the result of a mutually activating relationship between CD4+ T lymphocytes and macrophages.

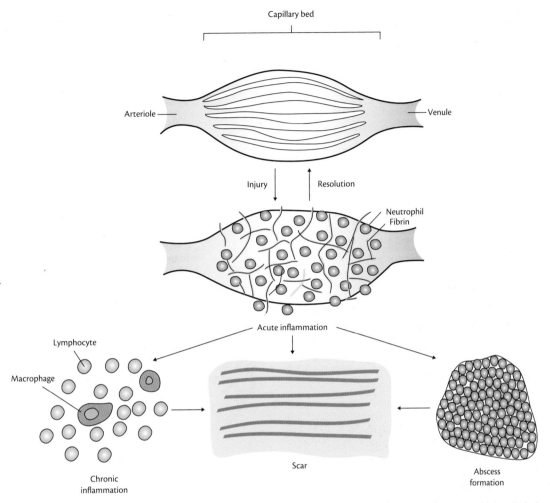

Fig. 2.2 Outcomes of acute inflammation. Acute inflammation may resolve with restoration of the original anatomy. Alternatively, it may progress into chronic inflammation or evolve into an abscess, both of which heal by repair with formation of a collagen-rich scar.

T helper lymphocytes and secrete cytokines such as interleukin-12 which activate T lymphocytes. This self-sustaining interaction allows persistence of the inflammatory activity (Fig. 2.3).

Granulomatous inflammation

Granulomatous inflammation is a special type of chronic inflammation. It is characterized by the presence of large numbers of activated macrophages called **epithelioid histiocytes**. This term was coined because the large nuclei and abundant cytoplasm of activated macrophages make them look a bit like

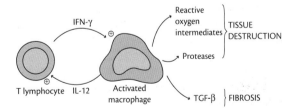

Fig. 2.3 Mechanism of tissue damage and fibrosis in chronic inflammation. A self-sustaining cycle of activation between T lymphocytes and macrophages causes release of large quantities of macrophage products which cause tissue destruction and fibrosis. IFN-γ, interferon-γ; IL-12, interleukin-12; TGF-β, transforming growth factor-β.

epithelial cells down the microscope. Sometimes, a group of epithelioid histiocytes within an area of granulomatous inflammation cluster together into a well defined collection of cells called a **granuloma** (Fig. 2.4).

Granulomatous inflammation tends to occur in response to persistent stimuli such as:

- Foreign bodies. These often incite a granulomatous response. Common examples include suture material following surgery and inhaled carbon in pulmonary lymph nodes of smokers.

- Persistent infections. Mycobacterial infections cause a granulomatous response because the organisms are resistant to normal phagocytic killing.

- Mysterious diseases. Granulomas are a feature of many diseases whose cause is still unknown. Sarcoidosis is a good example, a disease in which several tissues become filled with numerous well formed granulomas.

Be careful not to confuse either granulomatous inflammation or a granuloma with **granulation tissue** which is the special component of the healing response.

Healing

Healing must occur in all damaged tissues, and is a general term for the process of replacing dead and damaged tissue with healthy tissue. Healing may occur through either regeneration or repair.

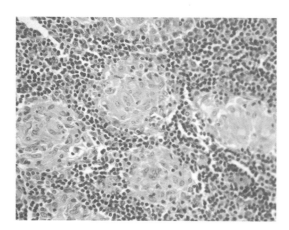

Fig. 2.4 Granulomas. This is a microscopic image of a group of granulomas, each composed of a well defined cluster of epithelioid macrophages with abundant pink cytoplasm.

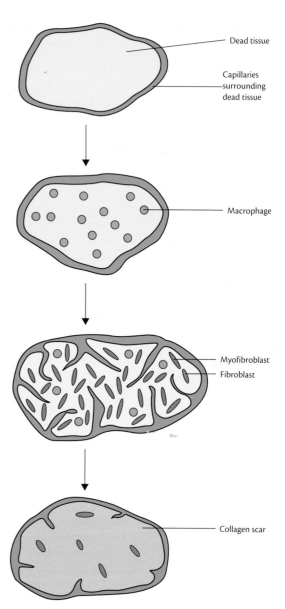

Fig. 2.5 Granulation tissue and repair by fibrosis. Repair begins with removal of cellular debris by macrophages, followed by formation of vascular granulation tissue containing sprouting capillaries, myofibroblasts, and fibroblasts. Over time, a poorly cellular collagen-rich scar remains.

Regeneration (resolution) is the replacement of damaged cells with exactly the same type of cell. Regeneration is therefore the ideal outcome of tissue injury. Regeneration can occur provided the injury is mild, the connective tissue framework is not disrupted, and the tissue is capable of regeneration. An example of healing by regeneration is acute pneumonia, in which the inflammatory exudate is cleared and the alveolar epithelial cells proliferate to restore the normal anatomy.

Regeneration is not possible if the connective tissue framework has been significantly damaged or if there is damage to cells incapable of dividing to replace the lost cells. Under these circumstances, healing takes place by **repair** (Fig. 2.5). Repair begins with the formation of **granulation tissue** which is composed of small blood vessels, fibroblasts, myofibroblasts, and inflammatory cells.

Myofibroblasts have contractile properties and act to contract the wound, whilst the fibroblasts release collagen. Over a period of a few weeks, the granulation tissue is eventually converted into a poorly cellular **scar** rich in collagen. Although structural integrity is maintained, there is a loss of function of the tissue that is scarred.

LINK BOX

Scarring

Important diseases due to scarring following chronic inflammation include cirrhosis of the liver due to chronic liver disease (p. 185) and lung fibrosis due to a diffuse parenchymal lung disease (p. 126).

Key points: Healing

- Healing is the process by which dead and damaged tissue is replaced by healthy tissue.

- Regeneration is replacement of damaged cells with exactly the same cell type and represents the ideal outcome of tissue injury.

- If regeneration is not possible, then repair occurs. Repair begins with the laying down of granulation tissue which is converted into a fibrous scar.

Infections

Introduction

Infections occur when a microorganism invades the body and causes disease. Despite immunization and the development of antimicrobial agents, infectious diseases still cause more illness worldwide than either cardiovascular disease or cancer.

An organism capable of causing disease is a **pathogen**. The **pathogenicity** of an organism refers to the severity of disease it causes compared with other organisms. For example, human immunodeficiency virus (HIV) is more pathogenic than a rhinovirus. **Virulence**, however, compares the severity of disease caused by different strains of the same microorganism. The attributes possessed by a particular strain of an organism that dictate its virulence are called **virulence factors**. As an example, the bacterium *Escherichia coli* O157 is more virulent than other strains of *E. coli* because it produces a toxin that can lead to haemolytic uraemic syndrome.

Some pathogens always cause infection if they gain access to a host; these are known as **obligate** pathogens. Others may only be able to cause disease in individuals with impaired immunity; these are known as **opportunistic** pathogens.

Acquisition of infection

One of the most important sources of microorganisms causing human disease are the indigenous bacteria that normally colonize the skin, mouth, and colon. Under normal circumstances, these bacteria exist harmlessly in the body, and indeed may have beneficial functions. However, in certain settings, these organisms can cause disease, e.g. colonic flora can cause urinary tract infection, skin flora can cause surgical wound infection, and oral flora can cause endocarditis and pneumonia.

Pathogens may also be acquired from external sources, the major sources of transmission being inhalation, ingestion, sexual contact, inoculation into the blood, and transplacental (Table 3.1).

Microorganisms

Microorganisms can be divided into five groups:

◆ **Bacteria**

◆ **Viruses**

◆ **Fungi**

◆ **Protozoa**

◆ **Helminths**

All living organisms have a scientific name, composed of the **genus** followed by the **species**. This name is printed in italics with the initial of the genus name in upper case, for instance *Streptococcus pneumoniae*. When bacterial names are used as adjectives or are used collectively, the names are not italicized and do not begin with an upper case letter, e.g. streptococci, streptococcal.

Some organisms may have other commonly used abbreviations or familiar names. As an example, the bacterium *Streptococcus pneumoniae* is also often referred to as *Strep. pneumoniae*, *S. pneumoniae*, and pneumococcus.

Bacteria

Bacteria are single-celled organisms containing DNA but no nucleus

Bacteria are single-celled organisms that have a cell membrane and contain double-stranded DNA. However, there is no nucleus and the cytoplasm contains no organelles except for ribosomes. All bacteria also possess a cell wall external to their cell membrane which provides a structural and physiological barrier between the bacteria and the external environment.

Most bacteria grow in air (**aerobes**) but can grow without it (**facultative anaerobes**). Some bacteria will only grow in the absence of oxygen (**strict anaerobes**).

TABLE 3.1	Major routes of transmission of infection			
	Bacteria	**Viruses**	**Fungi**	**Protozoa**
Respiratory	M. tuberculosis	Rhinovirus	H. capsulatum	
		Influenza virus		
Faecal–oral	H. pylori	Hepatitis A virus		G. lamblia
				T. gondii
Saliva		Herpes simplex virus		
		Epstein–Barr virus		
Sexual	C. trachomatis	Human papillomavirus		T. vaginalis
	N. gonorrhoeae	HIV		
		Hepatitis B virus		
Skin	S. aureus	Varicella zoster virus	Dermatophytes	
Blood		HIV		Plasmodium
		Hepatitis B virus		
		Hepatitis C virus		
Transplacental		Cytomegalovirus		T. gondii

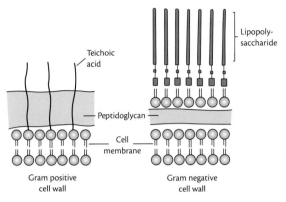

Fig. 3.1 Bacterial cell walls. Diagrammatic representation of the structure of Gram positive and Gram negative bacterial cell walls.

TABLE 3.2	Common bacterial pathogens
Gram positive cocci	*Staphylococcus aureus, Streptococcus pneumoniae*
Gram negative cocci	*Neisseria meningitidis, Neisseria gonorrhoeae*
Gram positive bacilli	*Clostridium difficile*
Gram negative bacilli	*Escherichia coli, Haemophilus influenzae*
Gram negative spiral	*Helicobacter pylori, Campylobacter jejuni*

Bacteria are classified according to the Gram stain and their shape

The Gram stain is the most widely used staining procedure in bacteriology. This technique divides bacteria into Gram positive or Gram negative according to the structure of their cell wall (Fig. 3.1).

The **Gram positive** bacterial cell wall is a thick structure composed of **peptidoglycan** and a second polymer which is often a **teichoic acid**. Gram positive bacteria stain dark violet with the Gram stain.

The **Gram negative** bacterial cell wall also has a layer of peptidoglycan, but this is much thinner and is overlaid by an outer lipid membrane. The outer lipid membrane is distinctive as the sole lipid component of the outer leaflet is **lipopolysaccharide**. Gram negative bacteria stain pink with the Gram stain.

There are three fundamental shapes of bacteria: spherical (coccus), straight rod (bacillus), and curved or spiral rods. One of the most common ways of categorizing bacteria is into groups according to their Gram staining and their shape (Table 3.2).

Pathogenic bacteria have a number of virulence factors which allow infection

In order to establish infection, pathogenic bacteria must be able to bind to host cells and overcome the immune system. A number of virulence factors may help them to achieve this.

Pili or **fimbriae**, are hair-like structures that protrude from the outer surface of some bacteria and are used to adhere to other surfaces. Pili are predominantly found on Gram negative bacteria, a good example being the P pili on strains of *E. coli* that allow them to adhere to urothelial cells and cause urinary tract infection. Gram positive bacteria do not have classical fimbriae, but many possess a fine fibrillar arrangement of proteins on their surface which bind to host cells. A notable example is the M protein of β-haemolytic streptococci which allows adherence to epithelial cells of the pharyngeal mucosa.

Flagella are long, thin structures protruding from the surface of some bacteria that can produce movement. Motile bacteria are able to migrate to areas where they are most likely to be able to colonize successfully. For example, *Helicobacter pylori* moves to the antrum of the stomach where gastric acidity is at its lowest.

The **lipopolysaccharide** molecule of Gram negative bacterial cell walls helps protect against complement-mediated lysis by activating complement at a distance from the cell membrane, thus preventing insertion of the membrane attack complex.

A **capsule** is a layer of polysaccharide that surrounds some bacteria and serves as a barrier to phagocytosis. Examples of encapsulated bacteria include *S. pneumoniae* and *Neisseria meningitidis*, both of which may survive in the blood stream because their capsule protects them from phagocytosis and complement-mediated lysis.

Bacteria cause disease due to toxins and enzymes

Toxins secreted by bacteria may have a number of effects. Examples of important toxins include the *Clostridium difficile* toxin and the heat labile toxin of enterotoxigenic *E. coli*, both of which cause diarrhoea.

Bacteria may secrete a number of enzymes which cause tissue destruction. **Collagenase** and **hyaluronidase** enzymes digest connective tissue, helping invasion of host tissues by the bacteria. **Streptokinase** released from certain streptococci digests fibrin in the acute inflammatory exudate, collapsing the scaffolding needed by neutrophils to move around an area of inflammation.

LINK BOX

Streptokinase

The enzyme **streptokinase** has found great use in the treatment of acute myocardial infarction by dissolving the fibrin-rich thrombus blocking the coronary artery and restoring perfusion to the myocardium (p. 90).

Spread of bacteria into the blood stream is a potentially serious event

Most bacterial infections remain localized to the initial site of infection. If bacteria gain access to the blood, the patient is said to have **bacteraemia**. Patients with bacteraemia are at risk of developing a systemic inflammatory response due to the potent proinflammatory effects of lipopolysaccharide, peptidoglycan, and teichoic acid. Patients with bacteraemia and signs of a systemic inflammatory response such as tachycardia, hypotension, and confusion are said to have **septicaemia**, a serious condition with a high mortality.

Special types of bacteria

Mycobacteria have a thick waxy cell wall that stains bright red with the Ziehl–Neelsen stain

Mycobacteria are a type of bacteria with a thick waxy cell wall which renders them impervious to the Gram stain. Special staining procedures are needed to highlight these bacteria, such as the **Ziehl–Neelsen** stain. In this technique, a bright red carbol fuschin stain is driven into the mycobacteria with heating and then the background is decolorized with dilute acid in alcohol. Because mycobacteria resist decolorization they are sometimes called **acid-fast bacilli** or **acid alcohol-fast bacilli** (Fig. 3.2).

The most well known mycobacteria are *Mycobacterium tuberculosis*, the organism which causes tuberculosis, and

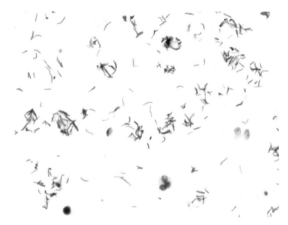

Fig. 3.2 Acid-fast bacilli. This tissue specimen from a case of tuberculosis has been stained with the Ziehl–Neelsen stain, revealing numerous bright red acid-fast mycobacteria.

Mycobacterium leprae which causes leprosy. There are also a number of less famous mycobacteria known as 'atypical', 'environmental', or 'opportunistic' mycobacteria. In healthy people, these organisms rarely cause disease, but over 50 per cent of acquired immune deficiency syndrome (AIDS) patients are infected with non-tuberculous mycobacteria, and the disease is usually disseminated.

Mycoplasma, Chlamydia, and *Rickettsia* are intracellular bacteria

Mycoplasma, Chlamydia, and *Rickettsia* are small bacteria which lack a cell wall and are obligate intracellular organisms. Because they do not stain with the Gram stain and will not grow on agar plates, they require tissue culture or molecular techniques to identify them.

Key points: Bacteria

◆ Bacteria are single celled organisms. Their double-stranded DNA is not contained within a nucleus and the only cytoplasmic organelles are ribosomes.

◆ The staining properties of the bacterial cell wall define the two major types of bacteria: Gram positive (violet) and Gram negative (pink).

Key points: Bacteria—cont'd

- Typical virulence factors found in pathogenic bacteria allowing them to colonize the body include pili, flagella, lipopolysaccharide, and capsules.

- Disease is caused by the release of bacterial enzymes and toxins.

- Most bacterial infections remain localized. Spread of bacteria into the blood with a systemic inflammatory response (septicaemia) is a serious condition with risk of septic shock, multiorgan failure, and death.

- Mycobacteria have a thick waxy cell wall which only stains with special techniques such as the Ziehl–Neelsen stain.

- *Mycoplasma*, *Chlamydia*, and *Rickettsia* species are small bacteria that lack a cell wall and are obligate intracellular organisms.

Viruses

Viruses are tiny organisms composed of nucleic acid and a protein capsid

Viruses are the smallest and simplest microorganisms, yet the most common cause of human infections (Table 3.3). Viruses consist of genetic material in the form of either DNA or RNA (but not both) enclosed in a protein shell called the **capsid** (Fig. 3.3).

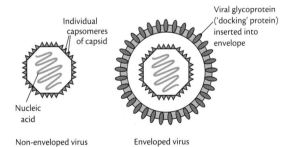

Fig. 3.3 Structure of a virus. Viruses are composed of a nucleic acid core surrounded by a protein capsid. Enveloped viruses also have an outer lipid envelope derived from the host cell which contains viral proteins.

In addition to the nucleic acid and capsid, some viruses have an outer lipid envelope which they acquire from the plasma membrane or nuclear membrane of the host cell they were spawned in. In general, enveloped viruses are less resistant to environmental factors such as drying and gastric acidity. This is probably because they are prone to losing the lipid envelope which contains the docking proteins the virus needs to infect host cells.

Viruses may be transmitted by a number of routes

The possible routes of viral infection are similar to those for other microorganisms (Table 3.1). The respiratory tract represents a major route for infection with viruses following inhalation of infected droplets. Salivary transmission is a particularly important route for some of the herpes viruses. Sexual transmission is the dominant mode of transmission of HIV. Transplacental spread of cytomegalovirus is now one of the most common causes of congenital anomalies.

Viruses are obligate intracellular organisms

Viruses are unable to synthesize their own proteins from their genetic material; they have no ribosomes or other organelles. For this reason, they can only replicate by infecting a host cell and hijacking its metabolic apparatus. Viruses enter host cells by first attaching to them using surface receptors which recognize proteins on the host cell, and then penetrating the cell. Many viruses have a specific preference for certain host cells ('tropism'). For instance, rhinoviruses infect the epithelium of the upper respiratory tract, and HIV infects CD4+ cells of the immune system.

Some viruses can remain completely quiescent within host cells

Some viruses are able to infect host cells and remain completely quiescent in the cell with no active viral replication. These are known as **latent** infections. The genetic material may remain free in the cytoplasm of the host cell or become incorporated into the genome of the host cell. Replication does not occur until some signal triggers release from latency. A good example of latent virus infection is herpes simplex virus which establishes latent infection in sensory nerve cell bodies of the dorsal root ganglion, reactivating intermittently to cause a crop of herpes simplex vesicles.

TABLE 3.3 Common viral pathogens
Hepatitis A, B, C
Human immunodeficiency virus
Herpes simplex virus
Varicella zoster virus
Epstein–Barr virus
Human papillomavirus

Viruses cause disease by destroying the cell they infect or by inducing an immune response

Replication of a virus within the host cell often leads to destruction of the cell ('direct cytopathic effect'). For example, influenza virus kills respiratory epithelial cells, and poliovirus kills neurones. Other viruses may not harm the cell they infect directly but still cause tissue damage because host CD8+ cytotoxic T lymphocytes recognize infected cells and destroy them. For example, most of the liver damage caused by hepatitis B virus infection is the result of the immune response to infected hepatocytes; the virus itself is not cytopathic.

Some viruses are carcinogenic

Certain viral infections have been shown to affect the function of important cell cycle proteins in the host cell, and are implicated in transformation of the host cell and the development of malignancy. Important examples include human papillomavirus in cervical carcinoma, hepatitis B virus in hepatocellular carcinoma, and Epstein–Barr virus in nasopharyngeal carcinoma.

- Some viruses can become latent, existing in the host cell in a completely quiescent state with no active replication. Reactivation may occur in response to certain triggers at a later date.

- Some viruses have been shown to interfere with cell growth and have a carcinogenic effect.

Fungi

Fungi are organisms which contain DNA within a nucleus and have a cell membrane and outer cell wall (Table 3.4). The fungal cell membrane differs from human cell membranes in that the predominant component is **ergosterol**. The outer cell wall is composed mostly of **chitin**. Fungi are widely distributed in the environment and can survive in extreme conditions where nutrients are limited.

There are two major types of fungi:

- **Yeasts** are small unicellular fungi that reproduce by budding. In some yeasts, such as *Candida*, the buds elongate to form long filaments called **pseudohyphae**.

- **Moulds** grow as branching filaments called **hyphae** (Fig. 3.4) that interlace to form a tangled mass known as a **mycelium**. Mycelia produce spores which are disseminated into the atmosphere, allowing colonization of new environments.

Key points: Viruses

- Viruses are infectious organisms which are totally dependent on living cells for replication.

- Viruses possess one type of nucleic acid, either DNA or RNA, surrounded by a protein capsid. They also have receptors which allow them to attach to and enter host cells.

- Viruses cause disease either by directly lysing the cell they infect or by inducing an immune response which kills the host cell.

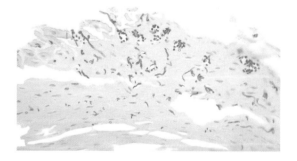

Fig. 3.4 Fungal hyphae. This is a high power view of a superficial fungal skin infection stained to make fungal cell walls appear purple. The hyphae of the dermatophyte fungi can be clearly seen.

TABLE 3.4	Common fungal pathogens
Dermatophytes	
Candida albicans	
Pneumocystis carinii	
Histoplasma	
Cryptococcus neoformans	

Some fungi can exist in both forms (dimorphic), being a yeast when invading tissues but a mould when living in the environment. A good example of a dimorphic fungus is *Histoplasma capsulatum*.

Fungal infections are divided into superficial mycoses and deep mycoses

Despite the many species of fungi present in the environment and on body surfaces, fungal infections (known as **mycoses**) are less common than viral or bacterial infections. Mycoses are classified into superficial mycoses and deep mycoses, depending on the site of infection.

Superficial mycoses are the more common fungal infections, typical sites being the skin (dermatophytoses) and genital tract. **Deep**, or **systemic**, **mycoses** in otherwise healthy people are caused by dimorphic fungi found in soil and are caused by inhalation of their spores. The lungs are therefore the main site of infection. The most common example of a deep mycosis in an otherwise healthy person is histoplasmosis caused by *Histoplasma capsulatum*, though this is virtually confined to North and South America.

Deep fungal infections in immunosuppressed people may be life threatening

Deep fungal infections are particularly important in immunocompromised people, in whom they can be life threatening. Examples of opportunistic fungi include *Cryptococcus neoformans*, *Pneumocystis carinii*, and *Aspergillus fumigatus*.

Until recently, *P. carinii* was thought to be a protozoan because it responds to antiprotozoal agents but not to antifungal agents. However, further study into the organism showed that its RNA genes are similar to fungal sequences and so it is now considered a fungus. It is not typical fungus, however, as it lacks ergosterol in its cell membrane and does not have a well developed cell wall.

Key points: Fungi

- Fungi are organisms with a thick cell wall. They are divided into yeasts and moulds.
- Yeasts are small unicellular fungi that reproduce by budding.
- Moulds grow as branching hyphae which reproduce by forming spores.
- Superficial mycoses are common, particularly of the skin and genital tract.
- Deep mycoses in healthy people are usually caused by inhalation of spores and therefore cause lung disease, e.g. histoplasmosis.
- Deep mycoses in immunocompromised people may be extremely severe. Important examples include *Pneumocystis carinii* pneumonia and *Cryptococcus neoformans* meningitis.

Protozoa

Protozoa are single-celled organisms which may live inside host cells or exist in the extracellular environment (Table 3.5). Intracellular protozoa enter host cells and derive nutrients from them, e.g. *Plasmodium* infects hepatocytes and red blood cells, and *Leishmania* and *Toxoplasma* both infect macrophages. Extracellular protozoa feed by direct nutrient uptake and/or by ingestion of shed epithelial cells, e.g. *Giardia lamblia* in the intestine (p. 153) and *Trichomonas* in the genital tract (p. 255).

TABLE 3.5	Common protozoal pathogens
Plasmodium falciparum	
Trichomonas vaginalis	
Toxoplasma gondii	
Giardia lamblia	

Malaria

Malaria is the most important protozoan disease

Malaria is caused by protozoa of the genus *Plasmodium*, which are transmitted to humans by the bite of the female *Anopheles* mosquito. The male mosquito does not transmit infection because it feeds only on plant juices.

Malaria is restricted to areas where *Anopheles* mosquitoes breed, such as tropical areas of Africa, Asia, and South America. Infected travellers may not present with symptoms until they have returned to their home country, and the increasing accessibility of air travel means that malaria is being seen more frequently in developed countries. Malaria is one of the most serious global health problems, with 10 million new cases and 2 million deaths each year.

Plasmodium species proliferate within hepatocytes and red blood cells

Four species of *Plasmodium* can cause malaria in humans: *P. falciparum*, *P. vivax*, *P. ovale*, and *P. malariae*. Infection with malaria begins when an infected mosquito feeds off a human and in doing so injects parasites directly into the blood. The parasites first infect hepatocytes and proliferate rapidly within them into a form which is then able to infect red blood cells. The parasite proliferates again in erythrocytes until the red cell explodes, releasing yet more parasites into the blood (Fig. 3.5).

Malaria should be suspected in any patient with fever and a history of possible exposure

The classical symptoms of malaria are cycles of fever with profuse sweating followed by shaking chills, related to the repeated rounds of erythrocyte invasion. Any patient with fever and an appropriate history of possible exposure to malaria must have the diagnosis excluded by repeated examination of blood films searching for the parasite in red blood cells (Fig. 3.6).

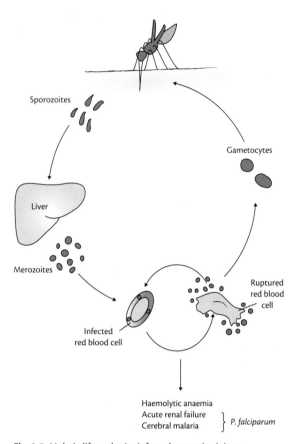

Fig. 3.5 Malaria life cycle. An infected mosquito injects sporozoites into the blood which home to the liver and multiply in hepatocytes, forming merozoites. Merozoites released into the blood infect red blood cells and multiply again, rupturing the red cells and infecting more red cells. Some merozoites mature into gametocytes which newly infect a mosquito, completing the life cycle.

Examination of a thick film is used to determine the presence of parasites. In positive cases, a thin blood film should then be used to determine the species and, in the case of *P. falciparum*, assess the severity of infection by counting the percentage of infected red blood cells.

Most fatal cases of malaria are caused by infection with *Plasmodium falciparum*

Making the distinction between an infection caused by *P. falciparum* and one caused by one of the other three *Plasmodium* species is particularly important.

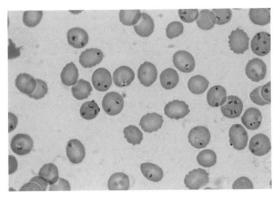

Fig. 3.6 *Plasmodium falciparum* seen in red cells on a blood film.

Plasmodium falciparum malaria is associated with severe haemolysis leading to renal failure due to toxic acute tubular necrosis caused by the large amounts of haemoglobin passing through the tubules. *Plasmodium falciparum*-infected red cells may also become blocked in cerebral capillaries causing **cerebral malaria** with progressive headache, convulsions, and coma.

Leishmaniasis

Leishmaniasis is caused by infection with *Leishmania* species transmitted by the bite of an infected sandfly. The disease is seen mostly in Africa, India, and Central and South America. Following inoculation into the skin, the parasite is phagocytosed by dermal macrophages. *Leishmania* is resistant to the killing mechanisms of the macrophages and can survive inside the macrophage, giving rise to a large ulcerated lesion in the skin at the site of the bite (**cutaneous leishmaniasis**). Most cases of cutaneous leishmaniasis eventually spontaneously heal when macrophages are strongly activated by interferon-γ and eventually kill the parasite.

In a minority of patients infected with certain species of *Leishmania*, the organism is not contained and it spreads, in macrophages, to other regions of the body including the liver, spleen, lymph nodes, and bone marrow (**visceral leishmaniasis**). Visceral leishmaniasis develops slowly, with weight loss, fever, lymphadenopathy, and massive hepatosplenomegaly. Untreated, the disease is fatal due to liver failure and bone marrow failure.

> ### Key points: Protozoa
>
> - Protozoa are single celled organisms which may infect humans as intracellular or extracellular parasites.
> - Intracellular protozoa include *Plasmodium*, *Leishmania*, and *Toxoplasma*.
> - Extracellular protozoa include *Cryptosporidium*, *Giardia*, and *Trichomonas*.
> - The most important protozoan disease is malaria, which should be suspected in any patient with fever and an appropriate history of possible exposure.
> - Malaria is diagnosed by repeated examination of blood films searching for the parasite in red blood cells.
> - *Plasmodium falciparum* causes the most severe form of malaria, associated with marked haemolysis and a risk of acute renal failure and cerebral malaria.
> - Leishmaniasis is caused by infection with *Leishmania* following a bite from an infected sandfly.
> - Cutaneous leishmaniasis is the commoner form of the infection. It causes a large ulcerated skin lesion at the site of the sandfly bite which slowly heals over a period of months.
> - Visceral leishmaniasis occurs if the organism spreads in macrophages to the liver, spleen, bone marrow, and lymph nodes. Untreated, it is a fatal disease due to liver and bone marrow failure.

Helminths

Helminths are complex multicellular parasitic worms which range in size from microscopic organisms to giant organisms measuring several metres in length. Many helminths have complex life cycles which often involve more than one host. Human helminth disease occurs worldwide, but is most prevalent in countries with poor socio-economic development. They seldom cause acute disease, but often cause severe chronic conditions. Helminths are divided into nematodes, cestodes, and trematodes.

Nematodes

Nematodes (roundworms) are worms with long cylindrical bodies which possess a mouth, digestive tract, anus and sexual organs. Most important nematode infections involve the gastrointestinal tract.

Enterobius vermicularis, or pinworm, is transmitted by hand to mouth transfer of eggs. The larva matures into an adult in the lumen of the gastrointestinal tract. The adult organisms are mainly located in the caecum. At night, the adult organisms migrate to the anus where the female deposits its eggs. Eggs on the anus and perianal skin cause perianal itching which may be extremely troublesome. The diagnosis is best made by using sticky tape on the anus to pick up the eggs and visualizing them under the microscope. A faecal sample is not helpful as the eggs are not usually found in faeces.

LINK BOX

Enterobius vermicularis and acute appendicitis

Pinworm organisms can also become lodged in the lumen of the appendix causing acute appendicitis (p. 159).

Necator americanus and *Ancylostoma duodenale* are both hookworms, which are so named because they are flexed dorsally giving them a hooked appearance. The organisms attach themselves to the jejunum by drawing mucosa into their mouths. A pump mechanism is then used to ingest blood and interstitial fluid from the host. *Ancylostoma duodenale* ingests about 0.15 ml of blood daily, and *N. americanus* 0.05 ml. Because worm loads may be high (over 500!) the cumulative effect of blood loss can be significant. Hookworm infection is the most common cause of iron deficiency anaemia worldwide.

Cestodes

Cestodes (tapeworms) are flat worms that can grow up to 10 m in length. Humans become infected after ingesting the eggs or larvae of the organism. Cestodes have no mouth or digestive tract but attach to the intestinal wall by suckers and absorb nutrients directly through their body surface.

Echinococcus granulosus is a minute tapeworm responsible for hydatid disease. Dogs are the primary host, and infection results from hand to mouth transmission of eggs from their faeces. Larvae hatch from the eggs in the small intestine, penetrate the gastrointestinal wall, and travel in the blood until they lodge in the capillaries of distant organs and form cysts (**hydatid cysts**). Hydatid cysts are most frequently seen in the liver where they cause epigastric pain and hepatomegaly. Hydatid cysts may also occur in the lungs, causing cough, haemoptysis, and breathlessness.

Taenia saginatum, or the beef tapeworm, is acquired by ingesting infected undercooked beef containing the larval form of the organism. No significant symptoms result from infection, though passing segments of the worm can cause understandable distress to the sufferer!

Taenia solium, or the pork tapeworm, is acquired following ingestion of the larvae in infected undercooked pork. The larvae mature into adult forms which attach to the small intestine. The clinical importance of the pork tapeworm is related to the fact that the larval forms can penetrate the intestinal tract and form cysts in tissues (**cysticercosis**) particularly skeletal muscle, subcutaneous tissue, the nervous system, and the eye.

INTERESTING TO KNOW

Cysticercosis

Recognized since the Hippocratic era, it has been suggested that suspicion of the origins of cysticercosis in pigs is what led some cultures to forbid the consumption of pork.

Trematodes

Trematodes (flukes) are flat, leaf-like organisms which live off cells, tissue fragments, fluid, and blood derived from the host. They have a mouth which leads into a blind-ending digestive tract with no anus. Waste material must therefore be regurgitated back out of the mouth!

The most important trematodes are the *Schistosoma* species which cause **schistosomiasis** (bilharzia). This disease occurs predominantly in sub-Saharan Africa. Infection results from contact with water containing larvae which burrow through the skin and develop into blood-dwelling worms. Schistosomiasis is most often an insidious and chronic disease with a range of manifestations involving the intestine and liver or urogenital tract, depending on the species type.

Schistosoma haematobium has a predilection for colonizing the veins of the genitourinary system. Disease results from deposition of eggs in the bladder wall. In the early active stage, there is typically painless haematuria caused by inflammation around the eggs. As the infection progresses, there is fibrosis around the eggs. Importantly, the epithelium lining the bladder may undergo metaplasia from the normal transitional epithelium to squamous epithelium. Malignant changes may then follow, culminating in a squamous cell carcinoma of the bladder (p. 237).

Schistosoma mansoni and *S. japonicum* have a predilection for colonizing the mesenteric veins of the intestine. Their eggs are swept into the liver via the portal vein where the inflammatory response leads to liver fibrosis and portal hypertension. Hepatosplenic disease is the most severe manifestation of *S. mansoni* and *S. japonicum* infection, as 80% of patients develop oesophageal varices which can cause death from massive haemorrhage.

Key points: Helminths

♦ Helminths are parasitic worms that may infect many organs of the body. Helminths are divided into nematodes, cestodes, and trematodes.

♦ Common nematode infections include *Enterobius vermicularis* which causes perianal itching in children, and hookworms which are the most common cause of iron deficiency anaemia worldwide.

♦ Cestodes may inhabit the intestinal tract with no significant symptoms, e.g. *Taenia saginatum*. Other cestodes cause disease because the larval forms penetrate the gut wall and enter tissues, e.g. *Echinococcus granulosus* (hydatid disease) and *Taenia solium* (cysticercosis).

♦ The most important trematode infection is schistosomiasis, caused by *Schistosoma* species. The organisms live in blood vessels and shed their eggs into tissues where they incite an inflammatory reaction that causes disease.

TABLE 3.6 Antibacterial agents

Inhibitors of cell wall synthesis
β-lactams, e.g. penicillins, cephalosporins
Glycopeptides, e.g. vancomycin, teicoplanin
Inhibitors of protein synthesis
Aminoglycosides, e.g. gentamycin
Tetracyclines, e.g. doxycycline
Macrolides, e.g. erythromycin, clarithromycin
Inhibitors of nucleic acid synthesis
Sulphonamides, e.g. sulphamethoxazole
Trimethoprim
Quinolones, e.g. ciprofloxacin
Rifamycins, e.g. rifampicin
Nitroimidazoles, e.g. metronidazole

Antimicrobial agents

Antimicrobial agents are one of the main armaments in the treatment and prevention of infectious disease. Most antimicrobials are designed to exploit differences between the microbial cells and host cells, so they only affect the microbe with minimal effects on the host (**selective toxicity**).

Antibacterial agents

Because bacteria are structurally distinct from human cells, there are a number of targets which can be exploited for the development of antibacterial agents with selective toxicity. There are now a vast number of different antibacterial agents in common use, and these are best classified according to their target site (Table 3.6).

Inhibitors of cell wall synthesis

Peptidoglycan is a vital component of bacterial cell walls and is not found in human cells, making it an ideal target for antibacterial agents. The two most important groups which target peptidoglycan are the β-lactams and the glycopeptides.

The **β-lactams** are a large family of compounds which include the **penicillins** and the **cephalosporins**. Structurally these agents all contain the β-lactam ring (Fig. 3.7). They act by inhibiting enzymes required for peptidoglycan synthesis. Accumulation of precursor

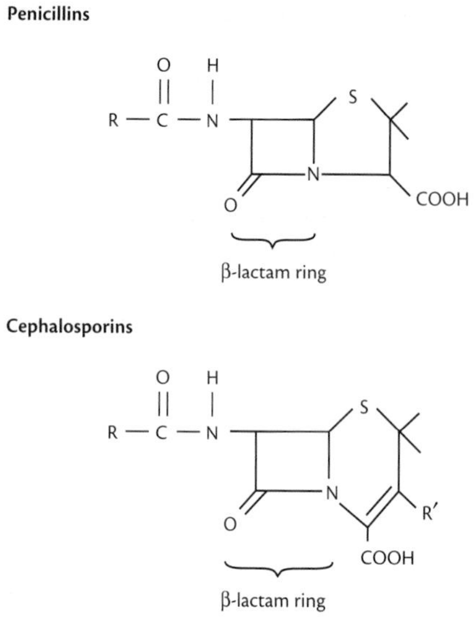

Penicillins

β-lactam ring

Cephalosporins

β-lactam ring

Fig. 3.7 β-Lactam ring.

units in the cell leads to cell lysis. β-lactams are mainly active against Gram positive bacteria.

Glycopeptide antibacterial agents interfere with cell wall synthesis by binding to the end of peptide chains that are part of the growing bacterial cell wall and preventing incorporation of new subunits into the growing cell wall. Vancomycin and teicoplanin are examples of glycopeptide antibacterial agents. Both must be given intravenously and are only active against Gram positive bacteria.

Inhibitors of protein synthesis

Although the mechanisms of protein synthesis are similar in bacteria and human cells, there are certain differences which have been exploited for antibacterial agents. Most of them act by binding to bacterial ribosomes and preventing elongation of protein chains.

Aminoglycosides are toxic antibacterial agents with activity against some Gram positive bacteria and many Gram negative bacteria. They are generally reserved for serious life-threatening infections such as Gram negative septicaemia. They are also used in combination with a penicillin for the treatment of infective endocarditis. Aminoglycosides can lead to renal failure and deafness, so patients receiving them require regular monitoring of blood levels of the drug to ensure the level is within the therapeutic range. Aminoglycosides are not

absorbed from the gut and must therefore be given either intravenously or intramuscularly.

Tetracyclines are broad-spectrum antibiotics but their value has decreased due to increasing bacterial resistance. They are now mostly used for infections caused by intracellular bacteria such as *Chlamydia*.

Macrolides are active against Gram positive bacteria and are a useful alternative to penicillin in patients who are penicillin allergic. Macrolides are concentrated intracellularly where they remain biologically active and so are useful against intracellular bacteria such as *Mycoplasma* and *Chlamydia*.

Inhibitors of nucleic acid synthesis

Antibacterial agents that inhibit nucleic acid synthesis generally act by interfering with the synthesis of DNA precursors or inhibiting bacterial enzymes involved in DNA replication.

Sulphonamides act by inhibiting synthesis of folic acid and thereby inhibit synthesis of purines and pyrimidines. Selective activity against bacteria depends on the fact that most bacteria must synthesize their own folic acid and cannot utilize exogenous sources. Human cells, however, rely on external sources of folic acid.

Trimethoprim is a pyrimidine-like structure which also acts by blocking the synthesis of folic acid, but acts later in the synthetic pathway by inhibiting the enzyme dihydrofolate reductase. Although this enzyme is also found in human cells, the antibiotic has a far greater affinity for the bacterial enzyme. Trimethoprim is mainly used for the treatment of urinary tract infections.

LINK BOX

Cotrimoxazole

Trimethoprim and sulphamethoxazole are believed to act synergistically against some bacteria when given simultaneously as **cotrimoxazole**. One of the main uses of cotrimoxazole is for prophylaxis and treatment of *P. carinii* pneumonia in patients with HIV (p. 50).

Quinolones act by inhibiting the enzyme DNA gyrase which is required to supercoil the bacterial chromosome. Inhibition of the enzyme means the bacterial genetic material cannot be packed into the cell.

The most commonly used quinolone is **ciprofloxacin** which has good activity against Gram negative bacteria. Quinolones are concentrated intracellularly, making them useful against intracellular bacteria such as *Mycoplasma* and *Chlamydia*.

Rifamycins act by binding to bacterial RNA polymerase, thus preventing synthesis of mRNA. The most important antibacterial in this group is **rifampicin** which has little affinity for human RNA polymerase. The main use of rifampicin is as part of the treatment regime for tuberculosis. It is also given prophylactically to close contacts of patients with meningococcal meningitis to eradicate nasopharyngeal carriage of the organism.

Metronidazole enters bacteria and is activated by a reduction process, yielding a product which binds to, and breaks, bacterial DNA. Metronidazole has high activity against anaerobic bacteria and protozoa, and is used widely for the treatment of trichomonal vaginosis, *Giardia lamblia* diarrhoea, and for prophylaxis of infection in colorectal and gynaecological surgery.

Antiviral agents

Compared with the vast number of antibacterial agents, there are very few antiviral drugs. This is because it is difficult to devise mechanisms that selectively attack viruses because they replicate within host cells. Most antiviral agents are nucleoside analogues which are incorporated into viral DNA and terminate DNA chain replication.

Aciclovir is a guanosine analogue which is phosphorylated into aciclovir triphosphate by the viral thymidine kinase enzyme. Aciclovir triphosphate is then incorporated into the viral DNA and terminates chain replication. Aciclovir is particularly active against herpes simplex virus because the herpes simplex thymidine kinase enzyme is particularly efficient at phosphorylating aciclovir.

Ganciclovir is related to aciclovir but is more active against cytomegalovirus. It is, however, much more toxic than aciclovir and should only be prescribed when the potential benefits outweigh the risks.

Interferon-α and **ribavirin** (a guanoside analogue) can be used in combination for patients with chronic hepatitis C who have high inflammatory activity on a liver biopsy.

Antiretroviral drugs have improved life expectancy in patients with HIV considerably. The drugs target the viral reverse transcriptase and protease enzymes required for viral replication. Treatment regimes for HIV usually comprise combination therapy with a mixture of **nucleoside reverse transcriptase inhibitors** such as didanosine or lamivudine, and **non-nucleoside reverse transcriptase inhibitors** such as efavirenz or nevirapine. **Protease inhibitors** such as indinavir or ritonavir may also be used. The precise combinations used vary considerably depending on the individual patient and on emerging data from clinical trials.

Antifungal agents

Only a small number of antifungal agents are available, as it is difficult to achieve selective toxicity. Most of them act on the synthesis or function of the fungal cell membrane.

The **azoles** are a group of agents which act by blocking the synthesis of ergosterol, thus interfering with the formation of the fungal membrane. Fluconazole is widely used for the treatment of oral or vaginal candidiasis.

The **polyene** group of agents bind avidly to sterols in the fungal cell membrane resulting in impairment of its barrier function. Amphotericin B has a wide spectrum of antifungal activity and is the treatment of choice for systemic fungal infections. Nystatin is too toxic for intravenous administration but is commonly used as a topical agent for oral candidiasis.

> ## Key points: Antimicrobial agents
>
> - The most important property of antimicrobial agents is selective toxicity, meaning that they target the microbe but not the host.
>
> - Antibacterial drugs are best classified according to their mode of action into those that inhibit cell wall synthesis, protein synthesis, and nucleic acid synthesis.
>
> - β-Lactam antibacterials such as penicillins and cephalosporins act by inhibiting bacterial cell wall synthesis.
>
> - Aminoglycosides, tetracyclines, and macrolides act by inhibiting protein synthesis.

Continued

Key points: Antimicrobial agents—cont'd

- Sulphonamides, trimethoprim, quinolones, and rifamycins act by inhibiting nucleic acid synthesis.

- Metronidazole has specific activity against anaerobic bacteria.

- Antiviral drugs are difficult to design due to toxicity to the host as well as the virus. Most antiviral drugs are nucleoside analogues.

- Aciclovir is a structural analogue of guanosine, and is very active against herpes simplex virus.

- Ganciclovir is similar to aciclovir but more active against cytomegalovirus.

- Antiretroviral treatment has considerably prolonged life expectancy in patients with HIV.

- The two main groups of antifungal agents, azoles and polyene, act by interfering with formation of the fungal cell wall.

Immunology

Introduction

Immunology is the study of the defences of the body against foreign materials and infections. The collection of tissues, cells, and molecules that mediate immunity is called the **immune system**, and the integrated reaction of this system is called the **immune response**.

Although the main role of the immune system is the prevention and eradication of infection, the immune response also has other important functions such as the killing of tumour cells and rejection of foreign tissue such as organ transplants. A more complete understanding of immunology and an ability to manipulate the immune system could therefore have wide-reaching implications in medicine.

Anatomy of the immune system

The immune system has two main 'arms': innate immunity and adaptive immunity. Innate immunity is ready to act as soon as a pathogen is encountered, but it is not specific and has no memory. The adaptive immune system, however, is highly specific and carries memory of its exposure enabling it to mount a quicker, more powerful response if the body is re-exposed to the same agent.

Although the division into innate and adaptive immunity is convenient conceptually, it is important to emphasize that the two components are inextricably interlinked.

Innate immunity

Innate immunity is an ancient form of host defence shared by almost all multicellular organisms. The innate immune system not only provides the first line of defence against microbes but also has a vital role in the establishment of the adaptive immune response. The innate immune system consists of a variety of mechanisms including epithelial barriers, phagocytes, and plasma proteins.

Epithelial surfaces

The principal portals of entry into the body by invading pathogens are the skin, respiratory tract, gastrointestinal tract, and genitourinary tract. All of these sites are lined by a continuous surface layer of epithelial cells which form a physical barrier against infection. In addition, each site has its own specific mechanisms of defence.

The low pH of the skin surface and the presence of fatty acids in sebum inhibits growth of microbes. The gastrointestinal tract has gastric acid, pancreatic enzymes, mucosal IgA antibodies, and the normal colonic flora. The respiratory tract secretes mucus which traps organisms; the beating action of cilia on the epithelial cells then transports the trapped organisms to the back of the throat where they are swallowed. The continuous flushing effect of urine in the urinary tract prevents microbes from adhering to the epithelium.

Phagocytes

If an epithelial surface is breached, then the microbe encounters tissue macrophages which recognize the invader and secrete cytokines that 'sound the alarm' to attract neutrophils to the site of attack. Macrophages and neutrophils are **phagocytes** that can ingest microbes by phagocytosis.

Phagocytosis is the process by which a phagocyte surrounds and encloses a microbe by extensions of its cell membrane, internalizing the organism within a vesicle in the cell called a **phagosome**. The phagosome is then fused to cytoplasmic lysosomes which contain toxic substances such as protease enzymes and reactive oxygen intermediates that kill the microbe.

Phagocytes recognize microbes via surface pattern recognition receptors

Recognition of foreign organisms by neutrophils and macrophages is achieved by a group of molecules known as **pattern recognition receptors**. These receptors bind to structures common to many microbial surfaces but which are absent from host cells, such as lipopolysaccharide and peptidoglycan which are components of bacterial cell walls. Examples of pattern recognition receptors include **mannose receptors** and **Toll-like receptors** (Fig. 4.1).

Binding of microbes to mannose receptors stimulates phagocytosis of the organism

Mannose receptors bind terminal mannose and fructose residues found at the ends of glycoproteins and glycolipids on microbial, but not human, cells. Binding of a microbe to a mannose receptor initiates the process of phagocytosis leading to engulfment of the organism. Activation of the phagocyte then stimulates efficient killing of the ingested organism.

Binding of Toll-like receptors activates phagocytes and enhances adaptive immunity

Activation of Toll-like receptors on phagocytes leads to the production of cytokines such as interleukin-1 (IL-1), IL-6, and tumour necrosis factor-α (TNF-α), all of which stimulate inflammation and enhance phagocytosis. The Toll pathway also leads to the expression of important co-stimulatory molecules essential for the induction of the adaptive immune response. This is an important example of how activation of adaptive immunity depends on molecules induced as a consequence of signalling via the innate immune system.

INTERESTING TO KNOW

Toll-like receptor agonists

Pharmacological compounds which stimulate Toll-like receptors and boost the immune system are being assessed as possible therapeutic agents for neoplasms. One such compound, **imiquimod**, has shown promising results in clinical trials as a topical treatment for pre-malignant and malignant cutaneous diseases such as actinic keratosis, superficial basal cell carcinoma, and lentigo maligna.

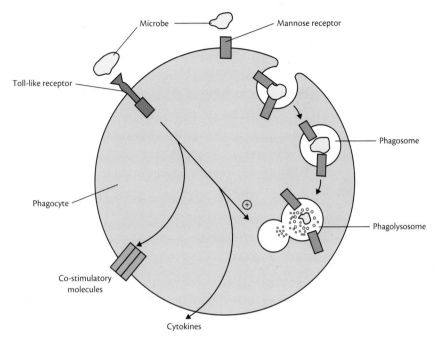

Fig. 4.1 Pattern recognition receptors on phagocytes. Microbes attaching to mannose receptors become a target for phagocytosis and intracellular killing. Toll-like receptors act to enhance phagocytic killing mechanisms and upregulate co-stimulatory molecules and cytokines for interaction with the adaptive immune system.

Acute phase proteins

The acute phase proteins also contribute to innate immunity

Following infection, cytokines produced by macrophages at the site of infection stimulate the liver rapidly to synthesize and release circulating plasma proteins known as **acute phase proteins** which contribute to innate immunity.

Mannose-binding lectin recognizes sugar structures containing mannose found on the surface of foreign microbes. When mannose-binding lectin binds mannose, it undergoes a conformational change allowing it to bind a protein called MASP and form a complex which activates the complement system. Human cells are not bound by mannose-binding lectin because their surface sugars end in sialic acid rather than mannose.

C-reactive protein (CRP) binds to phosphorylcholine portions of lipopolysaccharides in bacterial and fungal cell walls, targeting them for phagocytosis by macrophages which express a receptor for CRP. Because CRP is the first acute phase protein to increase in response to inflammation, measurement of circulating levels of CRP is a simple and widely used biochemical test to assess the presence and severity of inflammation in patients (p. 532).

Complement

The **complement** system is a collection of circulating proteins that assist, or complement, other components of the immune system in killing microorganisms.

Complement may be activated on the surface of a microbe in three main ways. The **classical pathway** is triggered by antibodies which have bound the microbe. The **alternative pathway** is triggered automatically on some microbes simply because they lack a regulatory protein present on all host cells which prevents complement activation. The **lectin pathway** is mediated by mannose-binding lectin.

Activation of complement generates C3b, the key molecule of the complement system

Whichever way the complement system is activated, there then follows a sequential cascade in which the product of one reaction is the trigger for the next reaction, leading to the generation of **C3 convertase**, an enzyme complex capable of splitting many molecules of C3 to C3b. The net effect is that microbes become completely coated with C3b, stimulating destruction of the microbe (Fig. 4.2). Mechanisms of complement mediated destruction include the following:

- **Opsonization**. The C3b molecule is an **opsonin** which coats foreign organisms and 'flags' them for phagocytosis. The C5a fragment is a potent chemoattractant for phagocytes.

- **Lysis**. C5b binds and recruits C6, C7, and C8 to the microbial surface. The C5b678 complex catalyses the polymerization of the final complement component, C9, which forms a transmembrane pore known as the **membrane attack complex** which lyses the cell.

The complement system is tightly regulated to prevent uncontrolled activation

Clearly it is important that the complement system is only activated on foreign cells and not on host cells. To achieve this, all normal host cells of the body express proteins on their surface which inhibit complement activation. **Decay accelerating factor** (DAF) disrupts the binding of C3b to the cell surface, and **membrane cofactor protein** helps to break down C3b into inactive fragments.

INTERESTING TO KNOW

Paroxysmal nocturnal haemoglobinuria

Patients with a deficiency of an enzyme required to synthesize a glycoprotein that anchors the complement regulatory proteins DAF and monocyte chemoattractant protein (MCP) in the cell membrane suffer from uncontrolled complement activation on their red blood cells, a disease called **paroxysmal nocturnal haemoglobinuria**. As well as suffering from haemolytic anaemia, patients with this disease also have a tendency to venous thrombosis for reasons that are poorly understood.

Key points: Innate immunity

- The innate immune system functions as an immediate form of host defence and also serves to prime the adaptive immune response.

- The main components of innate immunity are the epithelial surfaces, phagocytes, and the complement system.

- Epithelial surfaces of the skin, respiratory tract, gastrointestinal tract, and genitourinary tract act as a physical barrier and have a number of other antimicrobial properties.

- Phagocytes recognize foreign motifs on microbes via pattern recognition receptors such as mannose receptors and Toll-like receptors, stimulating engulfment and destruction of the microorganism.

- Cytokines released by phagocytes encountering microbes stimulate production of acute phase proteins such as mannose-binding lectin and C-reactive protein which enhance killing of microbes.

- The complement system is a group of plasma proteins which are sequentially activated on contact with microbial surfaces or antibodies bound to microbes. Complement proteins aid the killing of microbes by targeting them for phagocytosis, stimulating inflammation, and directly lysing them.

- The innate and adaptive immune systems are linked such that even if the innate system is inadequate to eradicate invasion, it can delay spread of the infection whilst it summons help from the more discriminatory adaptive immune system.

Adaptive immunity

Although innate immunity can effectively combat many infections, microorganisms have evolved ways to resist it. Defence against these infections is the task of the adaptive immune system.

Adaptive immunity has two important properties that distinguish it from innate immunity: **specificity**

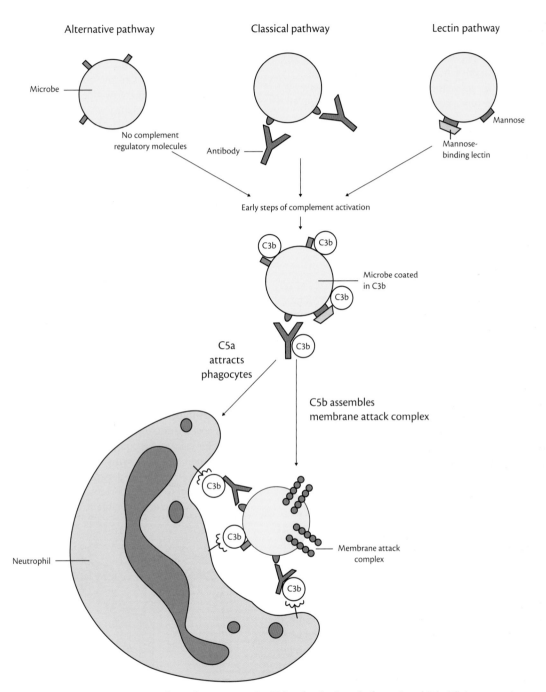

Fig. 4.2 Complement system. Activation of complement on a microbial surface leads to the formation of C3b. C3b is an opsonin, tagging the microbe for killing by phagocytes which are attracted to the site by C5a. The C5b fragment assembles the membrane attack complex which punches holes in the surface of the microbe.

and **memory**. Specificity refers to the fine discriminatory power of the adaptive immune system, being able to distinguish between at least 1 billion different antigens. The adaptive immune system also has memory, meaning that it mounts increasingly more powerful responses on repeated exposure to the same antigen.

Lymphocytes

The main cell of the adaptive immune system is the **lymphocyte**. There are two types of lymphocyte: **B lymphocytes** and **T lymphocytes**. B lymphocytes are the antibody-producing cells that mediate **humoral immunity**, whereas T lymphocytes are responsible for **cellular immunity**.

The high specificity of lymphocytes is due to their surface antigen receptors

Whereas the innate immune system recognizes structures shared by many different microbes, the receptors on lymphocytes only recognize one specific **antigen**. An antigen is a broad term for any substance that elicits an immune response. The antigen receptors are called the **B cell receptor** (BCR) on B lymphocytes and the **T cell receptor** (TCR) on T lymphocytes.

The great diversity of different antigen receptors in the lymphocyte repertoire is generated during lymphocyte development, which occurs in the *bone marrow* for B lymphocytes and in the *thymus* for T lymphocytes. The antigen receptors are generated by combining several different genes together through a recombination process during which variability in the nucleotide sequence of the genes is introduced. During their maturation, only cells with useful antigen receptors are preserved. Those that strongly recognize self-antigens are deleted by apoptosis to prevent autoimmunity.

Lymphocytes that meet their antigen rapidly proliferate and differentiate into effector cells

When lymphocytes encounter their specific antigen, they proliferate and differentiate into effector cells. B lymphocytes become **plasma cells** which secrete large quantities of antibody, whereas T lymphocytes upregulate machinery involved in destroying intracellular microbes. **Memory cells** are also generated when lymphocytes are stimulated by their antigen. These are long-lived lymphocytes which survive even in the absence of the antigen, but rapidly respond and proliferate if re-exposed to antigen.

Humoral immunity

Humoral immunity is mediated by proteins called **antibodies** or **immunoglobulins** and is important in protection against extracellular microorganisms.

Antibodies are made up of two identical heavy chains and two identical light chains which are connected to form a Y-shaped structure (Fig. 4.3). The 'arms' of the immunoglobulin together comprise the antigen-binding region (Fab) which has a variable structure. The 'tail' of the molecule is the constant region (Fc) which mediates the effector functions of the antibody via binding sites for phagocytes and components of the complement system. *Only once antibody has bound to antigen are the binding sites on the Fc portion exposed*, ensuring that the immune response is only activated when an antibody has bound its target antigen.

Antibodies work in four main ways (Fig. 4.4):

◆ **Neutralization**. Antibodies can prevent infection by blocking the biological activity of a target molecule required for infection, e.g. a toxin binding to its receptor, or a binding protein required for infection of host cells.

◆ **Opsonization**. Antibodies coating the surface of a microbe promote their ingestion by phagocytes.

◆ **Antibody-dependent cellular cytotoxicity**. Antibodies coating microbes also recruit cells such as natural killer cells and eosinophils and activate them to release their granules which contain proteins that kill the target. Antibody-dependent cellular cytotoxicity appears to be important in defence against organisms which are too large to phagocytose.

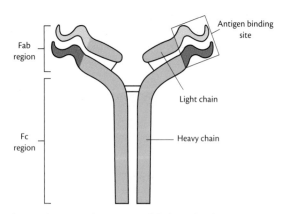

Fig. 4.3 Structure of an immunoglobulin molecule.

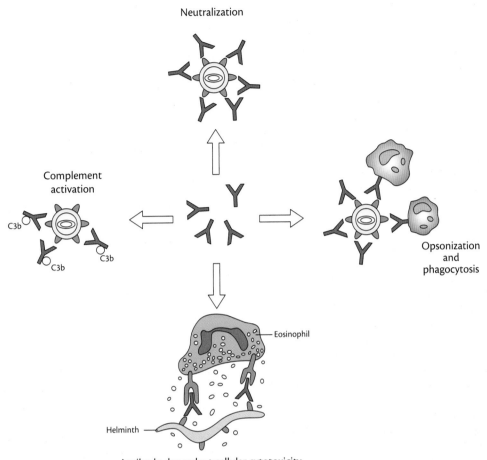

Fig. 4.4 Effector functions of antibodies.

- **Complement activation**. Antibodies bound to their antigen can activate the complement system and cause direct lysis of the organism.

Note how many of these mechanisms actually depend on components of the innate immune system. Here, the antibodies of the adaptive immune system act greatly to enhance the antimicrobial power of innate immunity. This is another example of the cooperation between innate and adaptive immunity.

Immunoglobulins can be divided into classes according to the heavy chain in the molecule

Immunoglobulins can be divided into classes depending on which heavy chain is used in the molecule.

Immunoglobulin G (IgG) is the major immunoglobulin in serum and is the most versatile immunoglobulin, capable of carrying out all the functions of immunoglobulin molecules. IgG is also the only class of immunoglobulin that crosses the placenta. IgG exists as a monomer.

Immunoglobulin A (IgA) is the second most common serum immunoglobulin where it exists as a monomer. Normally IgA does not fix complement but can bind to phagocytes and stimulate phagocytosis. IgA is also the major class of immunoglobulin found in secretions such as tears, saliva, and gastrointestinal juices. IgA in secretions exists as a dimer.

Immunoglobulin M (IgM) is the third most common serum immunoglobulin. It is the first type of immunoglobulin to be made by naïve B lymphocytes. IgM normally exists as a pentamer of five identical IgM molecules, making it extremely good at fixing complement and lysing microorganisms.

Immunoglobulin E (IgE) is the least common serum immunoglobulin. It binds tightly to IgE receptors on the surface of mast cells and eosinophils. IgE is involved in defence against large parasites; binding of eosinophils to IgE-coated parasites results in killing of the organism. IgE is also important in allergic diseases caused by immediate hypersensitivity reactions (see later).

B lymphocyte development begins in the bone marrow with production of naïve B lymphocytes

The production of B lymphocytes begins in the bone marrow, where precursor B lymphoblasts undergo immunoglobulin gene rearrangement and differentiate into naïve B lymphocytes. Naïve B cells are small lymphocytes that leave the bone marrow to circulate in the blood and occupy primary lymphoid follicles (mostly in lymph nodes).

B lymphocytes stimulated by antigen undergo class switching and somatic hypermutation

Naïve B lymphocytes that encounter their antigen and are successfully activated by CD4+ helper T lymphocytes undergo *blastic transformation*, forming larger cells called **centroblasts** which migrate into the centre of a lymphoid follicle and form a **germinal centre**.

In the germinal centre, two important events occur. Firstly the B lymphocytes stop producing IgM antibodies and instead produce other classes of immunoglobulin such as IgG and IgA. This is known as **class switching** and enables the humoral immune response to combat different microbes optimally. For instance,

an important defence against bacteria is opsonization by antibodies stimulating phagocytosis. This is best mediated by antibodies such as IgG that bind to high affinity receptors on phagocytes specific for the IgG heavy chain.

Secondly, the centroblasts proliferate very rapidly, during which the immunoglobulin genes become susceptible to point mutations, a process known as **somatic hypermutation**. This extensive mutation results in the generation of different immunoglobulin molecules which bind with widely varying affinities to the antigen that initiated the response.

The affinity of each immunoglobulin is tested by binding to antigen on follicular dendritic cells

Centroblasts that have completed somatic hypermutation mature into **centrocytes**. The new immunoglobulin molecule produced by each centrocyte is then tested by how strongly it binds to its antigen. This is achieved by cells in the germinal centre called **follicular dendritic cells** which hold numerous intact antigens on their cell surface in the form of antigen–antibody complexes.

Centrocytes with mutations that result in decreased affinity for antigen rapidly die by apoptosis, while centrocytes with mutations that result in increasing affinity are able to bind to antigen trapped on the processes of follicular dendritic cells. This rescues them from apoptosis, allowing them to differentiate into either memory B cells or antibody-producing plasma cells. Memory B cells reside at the edge of lymphoid follicles in lymph nodes in an area known as the marginal zone, whereas plasma cells home back to the bone marrow (Fig. 4.5).

Non-protein antigens do not require T cell help to produce antibodies

Non-protein antigens such as polysaccharides, lipids, and nucleic acids are invisible to T cells as they cannot be displayed in major histocompatibility complex (MHC) molecules. These antigens are still able to induce antibody responses without T cell help. It is thought that these T cell independent antigens are able to provide strong enough signals for B cell activation in the absence of T cell help because they contain multiple repeating epitopes that cross-link many of the surface immunoglobulin receptors on the B cell.

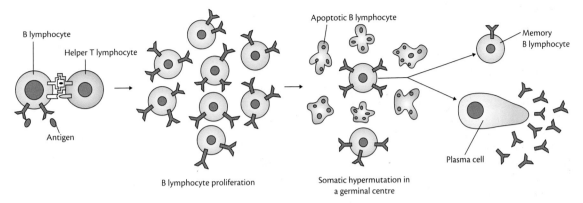

Fig. 4.5 Humoral immunity. Naïve B lymphocytes that encounter their antigen and receive appropriate T cell help enter a germinal centre where they proliferate and undergo somatic hypermutation of the immunoglobulin gene. Only B lymphocytes with the best fitting immunoglobulin are selected to survive and differentiate into memory cells or plasma cells. The remainder are doomed to die by apoptosis in the germinal centre.

Key points: Humoral immunity

- Humoral immunity is the arm of the adaptive immune system mediated by antibodies.

- Antibodies may operate through a number of mechanisms including neutralization, opsonization, antibody-dependent cellular cytotoxicity, and activation of complement.

- Antibody production is initiated following binding of antigen to its specific B cell receptor on the surface of naïve B lymphocytes.

- Successful activation of naïve B lymphocytes also requires an additional signal from CD4+ helper T lymphocytes.

- B lymphocytes that have bound antigen enter the germinal centre of a lymphoid follicle in a lymph node where they undergo class switching and somatic hypermutation to generate the best fitting IgG or IgA antibody.

- Non-protein antigens can also stimulate antibody production by B lymphocytes without the aid of CD4+ helper T lymphocytes by cross-linking many surface B cell receptors on the naïve B cell.

Cellular immunity

Antibodies do not have access to microorganisms that infect and proliferate within cells. Defence against intracellular microbes is mediated by cellular immunity led by T lymphocytes.

T lymphocytes differ from B lymphocytes in that they can only recognize small peptide antigens presented to them by MHC molecules. The MHC genes are highly polymorphic, meaning there are many different alleles of the genes within the population. With the exception of monozygotic twins, no two individuals have exactly the same set of MHC genes. Human MHC genes are also known as **human leukocyte antigens** (HLAs).

T lymphocyte development occurs in the bone marrow and thymus

T lymphocytes begin development in the bone marrow but then migrate to the thymus where they rearrange their TCR genes. In the thymus, T lymphocytes come into contact with dendritic cells and macrophages presenting self peptides bound to major histocompatibility molecules. The strength of the interaction between each T lymphocyte determines its fate. T lymphocytes binding too strongly are deleted by apoptosis as they are potentially autoreactive. T lymphocytes that bind very weakly are also deleted as they are unable to recognize self major histocompatibility molecules well enough to make them useful. The T lymphocytes that survive are therefore those which can recognize their own major histocompatibility molecules but do not bind strongly to self peptides. The end result is a repertoire of T lymphocytes that are self-*recognizing* but not self-*reactive*.

INTERESTING TO KNOW

Thymoma

A **thymoma** is a neoplasm of the thymus derived from thymic epithelial cells. Most thymomas are benign tumours which may present in a variety of ways. There may be symptoms related to compression of nearby tissues, or the neoplasm may be found incidentally on imaging or at cardiac surgery. In addition, there is an association between thymoma and the condition **myasthenia gravis** (p. 447). Fifteen per cent of people with myasthenia gravis have a thymoma at diagnosis, and up to half of patients diagnosed with a thymoma go on to develop myasthenia gravis.

T lymphocytes are divided into CD4+ helper and CD8+ cytotoxic T lymphocytes

T lymphocytes that survive thymic selection differentiate into two major subtypes according to whether they express **CD4** surface molecules or **CD8** surface molecules. CD4+ T lymphocytes are known as **helper T lymphocytes**, whereas CD8+ T lymphocytes are known as **cytotoxic T lymphocytes**.

CD4+ and CD8+ T lymphocytes are distinguished by their functions and by the type of MHC molecule they bind to. CD4+ helper T lymphocytes bind to class II MHC molecules expressed mainly by specialized **antigen-presenting cells** such as dendritic cells and macrophages. CD8+ cytotoxic T lymphocytes bind to class I MHC molecules expressed by all nucleated cells.

The origin of peptides displayed by MHC class I and II are different

Extracellular proteins are internalized by antigen-presenting cells into vesicles and are processed into peptides for display by class II MHC molecules, whereas intracellular proteins in the cytosol of nucleated cells are processed for display by class I MHC molecules.

The segregation of these two pathways allows sampling of proteins in the extracellular and intracellular environments, and also allows the immune system to respond optimally to extracellular and intracellular microorganisms. Extracellular microbes are phagocytosed by antigen-presenting cells, and peptides derived from the organism are presented to CD4+ helper T lymphocytes which then stimulate phagocytes and help B lymphocytes specific for the antigen to produce antibodies. Conversely, cells infected with intracellular organisms such as viruses will display foreign peptides on surface class I MHC molecules to the appropriate CD8+ cytotoxic T lymphocyte, which will kill the infected cell.

Binding of TCR to the correct antigen displayed by MHC leads to activation of the T lymphocyte

Binding of the TCR to its antigen provides the first signal for activation of the T lymphocyte. Full activation requires a second signal from a co-stimulator. The best defined co-stimulator molecules for T lymphocytes are two related proteins called B7.1 and B7.2, both of which are expressed on antigen-presenting cells. The B7 proteins are recognized by a receptor on the T lymphocyte called CD28. The requirement for both signals ensures T lymphocytes are activated appropriately.

In response to full stimulation, naïve T lymphocytes rapidly proliferate to produce a large pool of antigen-specific T cells. The proliferating T lymphocytes then begin to express genes appropriate to their function (Fig. 4.6).

CD4+ helper T lymphocytes orchestrate the function of other immune cells

Activated CD4+ helper T lymphocytes begin producing surface molecules and cytokines that function to

---

INTERESTING TO KNOW

CTLA4

T lymphocytes also have surface molecules that provide an inhibitory signal to the cell. One such molecule is **cytotoxic T lymphocyte-associated antigen 4** (CTLA4), an important regulatory protein that prevents proliferation of autoreactive T lymphocytes. CTLA4 is closely related to the CD28 protein; they both bind the same ligands B7.1 and B7.2. However, whilst binding to CD28 activates T lymphocytes, binding to CTLA4 inhibits T lymphocytes. CTLA4 is therefore important in regulating and maintaining self-tolerance. Trials using synthetic antibodies that bind to and activate CTLA4 are being carried out for autoimmune conditions such as rheumatoid arthritis.

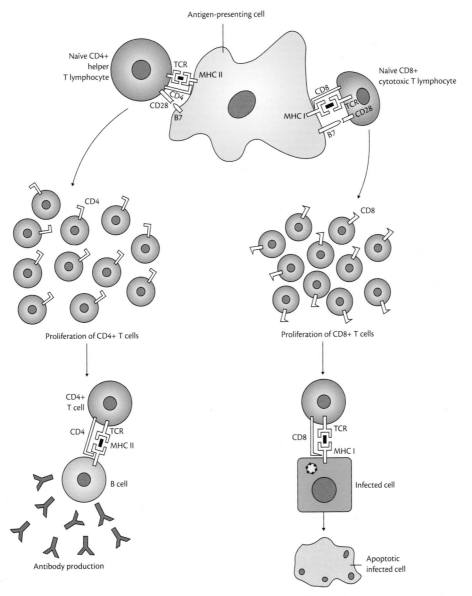

Fig. 4.6 Cellular immunity. T lymphocytes activated by antigen-presenting cells proliferate and express genes appropriate to their actions. Activated CD4+ helper T cells interact with other cells of the immune system such as B lymphocytes, whilst activated CD8+ cytotoxic T lymphocytes destroy infected host cells.

activate other immune cells such as macrophages and B lymphocytes. The most important surface molecule is CD40 ligand (CD40L). Engagement of CD40L on CD4+ helper T lymphocytes to CD40 on macrophages and B lymphocytes provides a powerful activation signal.

Activated CD4+ helper T lymphocytes can be divided into Th1 and Th2 subtypes

Activated CD4+ helper T lymphocytes can be divided into two main subsets according to the types of cytokines they produce: Th1 and Th2. The most important cytokine produced by Th1 helper T lymphocytes is interferon-γ (IFN-γ). IFN-γ is a powerful activator of macrophages and also stimulates the production of antibodies that opsonize organisms for phagocytosis. Th2 helper T lymphocytes produce cytokines such as IL-4, which stimulates production of IgE antibodies, and IL-5 which activates eosinophils.

The balance between Th1 and Th2 cells determines the outcome of many infections, with Th1 promoting and Th2 cells suppressing the response against intracellular organisms. In reality, the Th1 and Th2 model is a gross oversimplification of what is a dynamic and complex system; however, it serves to illustrate how the immune response is designed to respond in the most appropriate manner to each microbe.

CD8+ cytotoxic T lymphocytes kill infected host cells

CD8+ cytotoxic T lymphocytes recognizing infected host cells may kill the cell in two ways. One method involves the insertion of a transmembrane pore-forming molecule called **perforin** through which the T cell pours in proteolytic enzymes. The other method is by binding of **Fas ligand** (FasL) on the cytotoxic T lymphocyte to Fas on the infected host cell, generating a signal which instructs the host cell to undergo apoptosis.

Key points: Cellular immunity

- Cell-mediated immunity is the arm of the adaptive immune system that eradicates intracellular microbes.

- T lymphocytes are the main cells involved in cell-mediated immunity.

- T cells have surface T cell receptors which recognize specific peptide antigens displayed by MHC molecules.

- Activation of T lymphocytes requires antigen recognition by the TCR and a co-stimulatory signal via the CD28 signal, provided by the B7.1 and B7.2 proteins found on antigen-presenting cells.

- Successful T lymphocyte activation leads to marked proliferation of the T cell clone and expression of genes that mediate the effector functions of the T cells.

- CD4+ helper T cells secrete cytokines which orchestrate the actions of other cells of the immune system. Th1 helper T cells produce IFN-γ which activates macrophages to eliminate ingested microbes and stimulates the production of IgG antibodies to opsonize antigens. Th2 helper T cells produce IL-4 and IL-5 which stimulate IgE production and activate eosinophils.

- The balance between Th1 and Th2 helper T cells determines the outcome of many infections, with Th1 promoting and Th2 cells suppressing the response against intracellular organisms.

- CD8+ cytotoxic T lymphocytes kill infected cells via perforin or FasL.

How cytotoxic T lymphocytes decide which method of cell death to inflict upon their target is not clear.

Hypersensitivity reactions

Although the immune response is designed to protect the body against microbes, there are many diseases caused by the immune system. **Hypersensitivity reaction** is a broad term referring to a disease which is immune mediated. Often the immune reaction leads to cell injury and cell death, but sometimes there is a change in cell function rather than actual cell destruction.

A hypersensitivity reaction may be directed against an exogenous antigen from the environment (e.g. a microbe) or directed against a self-antigen, in which case the hypersensitivity reaction is a form of **autoimmunity**.

Hypersensitivity reactions are classified according to the dominant immunological mechanism that is responsible for the tissue damage (Fig. 4.7). Note that many immunological diseases may be mediated by more than one type of hypersensitivity reaction. For example, in the disease **hypersensitivity pneumonitis**, lung injury is caused by a mixture of type III and type IV hypersensitivity reactions to inhaled antigens (p. 128).

Immediate (type I) hypersensitivity

Immediate hypersensitivity is characterized by production of IgE antibodies in response to an antigen. The IgE antibodies bind to the surface of mast cells via IgE receptors. Cross-linking of IgE antibodies on mast cells

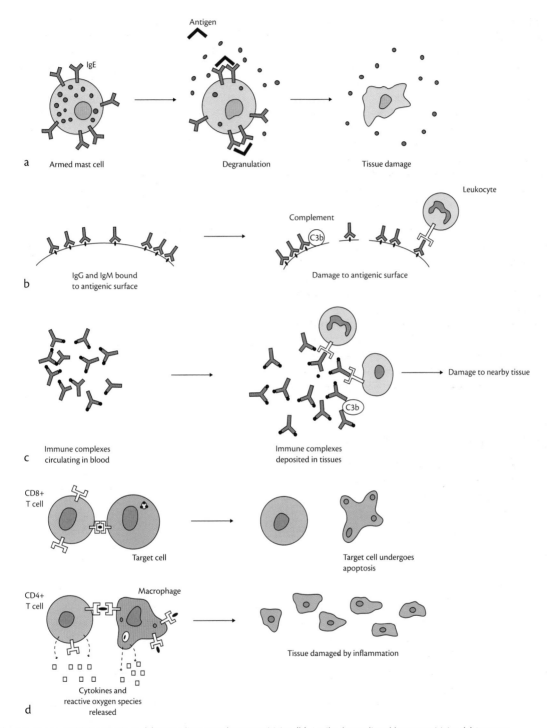

Fig. 4.7 Hypersensitivity reactions. (a) Immediate-type hypersensitivity. (b) Antibody-mediated hypersensitivity. (c) Immune complex-mediated hypersensitivity. (d) T cell-mediated hypersensitivity.

by antigen then causes degranulation. The immediate release of mast cell mediators such as histamine stimulates acute inflammation in the tissue.

Immediate hypersensitivity reactions are typical of people with **atopy**, a genetic predisposition to produce large quantities of IgE in response to environmental antigens such as pollen, house dust mites, and some foods. Diseases associated with atopy include asthma, allergic rhinitis, atopic dermatitis, and food allergies. **Anaphylaxis** represents a systemic form of immediate hypersensitivity in which there is widespread release of histamine throughout the body. In its most severe form, anaphylaxis leads to **anaphylactic shock**, which is life threatening.

Immediate hypersensitivity diseases affect over 20 per cent of people, and their incidence is rising. The reason for the recent increase in incidence of atopic diseases is not clear. A number of environmental factors have been shown to reduce the risk of developing atopic disease, for instance having older siblings and having more childhood infections. The hygiene hypothesis of atopy theorizes that changes in infant diets and a reduced exposure to infections in childhood alter the maturation of the immune system. Circulating T lymphocytes of children with atopy appear to be poor at producing IFN-γ, instead producing cytokines which favour the production of IgE from B lymphocytes.

JARGON BUSTER

Allergy

The term **allergy** was proposed in 1906 to refer to any altered state of immune reactivity. In Europe, the term allergy is generally used in its original sense for any form of hypersensitivity, whereas in the USA its use is restricted only to immediate (type I) hypersensitivity.

Antibody-mediated (type II) hypersensitivity

Antibody-mediated hypersensitivity is caused by IgG or IgM antibodies binding to a *fixed* antigen in a tissue. Most often the antigen is a protein on a cell surface, but it may also be part of the extracellular matrix. Binding of the antibody to the antigen activates complement, leading to cellular injury. Examples of antibody-mediated hypersensitivity include immune haemolytic anaemia and bullous pemphigoid.

Some antibody-mediated hypersensitivity reactions lead to disease without causing tissue destruction. For example, the thyroid-stimulating hormone (TSH) receptor-stimulating antibodies in Graves' disease cause hyperthyroidism by binding to, and activating, the TSH receptor on thyroid follicular epithelial cells, but there is no actual destruction of the thyroid.

Immune complex-mediated (type III) hypersensitivity

In **immune complex hypersensitivity**, IgG or IgM antibodies are also important, but here the antigen is circulating in the blood rather than fixed in a tissue. The antibodies bind to the antigen, forming **immune complexes** which circulate in the blood and become deposited in tissues, where they activate complement.

Circulating immune complexes may deposit at many different sites in the body but seem to have a predilection for small blood vessels, the kidneys, and joints. Immune complex-mediated diseases tend to be multisystem diseases in which vasculitis, arthritis, and glomerulonephritis are prominent features. A good example of a disease mediated largely by immune complex hypersensitivity is systemic lupus erythematosus.

T cell-mediated (type IV) hypersensitivity

T cell-mediated hypersensitivity tissue damage does not involve antibody formation. Instead, the disease is caused by activated T lymphocytes which cause tissue injury by direct cell killing and by releasing cytokines that activate macrophages. Because activation and proliferation of T lymphocytes takes 1–2 days, this type of hypersensitivity is also known as **delayed-type hypersensitivity**. Examples of diseases in which T cell-mediated hypersensitivity is important include contact dermatitis, Hashimoto's thyroiditis, primary biliary cirrhosis, and tuberculosis.

Key points: Hypersensitivity reactions

◆ Hypersensitivity reactions refer broadly to any disease which is immune mediated.

◆ Hypersensitivity reactions are classified according to the predominant immunological mechanism involved.

Key points: Hypersensitivity reactions—cont'd

- Immediate hypersensitivity reactions are due to cross-linking of surface IgE on mast cells by environmental antigens. Examples include asthma, allergic rhinitis, and atopic dermatitis. Anaphylaxis is a severe, generalized form of immediate hypersensitivity which can lead to life-threatening anaphylactic shock.

- Antibody-mediated hypersensitivity is due to IgM or IgG antibodies binding to a fixed tissue antigen. Usually complement activation leads to tissue destruction and disease. Sometimes the antibody causes disease by changing cell function rather than causing cell loss, e.g. Graves' disease.

- Immune complex-mediated hypersensitivity is due to antibodies binding to circulating antigens and forming immune complexes. Circulating immune complexes then deposit in a variety of tissues and activate complement, leading to cell injury. Diseases caused by immune complex hypersensitivity are often multisystem diseases that involve blood vessels, joints, and glomeruli, e.g. systemic lupus erythematosus.

- T cell-mediated hypersensitivity is caused by activated T lymphocytes and does not involve antibody production. Activated T lymphocytes bring about cell damage by producing cytokines that activate macrophages and by direct cell killing. Examples of diseases involving T cell-mediated hypersensitivity include Hashimoto's thyroiditis, and tuberculosis.

Autoimmune disease

When a hypersensitivity reaction is directed against a self-antigen, the disease is also known as an **autoimmune disease**. Autoimmunity occurs when there is failure of immunological **tolerance**, the ability to discriminate between self and non-self.

Autoimmune diseases are usually characterized by chronic inflammation leading to destruction of the involved tissue but without an obvious trigger. A number of diseases are known, or suspected, to be autoimmune (Table 4.1). Epidemiological studies show that developing one autoimmune disease tends to increase the chance of developing another.

We still know very little about the aetiology and pathogenesis of autoimmune diseases. One of the most popular theories is that some environmental agent, such as an infection, triggers the activation of self-reactive lymphocytes in a genetically susceptible individual. Infection may lead to increased expression of stimulatory molecules and production of proinflammatory cytokines, which may lead to the activation of self-reactive lymphocytes. Alternatively, if a microorganism has peptide antigens which are similar to self-antigens, then an immune response to the foreign antigen may cross-react with a self-antigen, a phenomenon termed **molecular mimicry**.

Although plausible in theory, there is no actual scientific evidence to support the role of infection in triggering autoimmunity. Another equally possible theory is that autoimmunity is in fact a spontaneous phenomenon that simply occurs by chance. Certainly the onset of most autoimmune diseases appears to be genuinely random rather than following an infection. Essentially, developing an autoimmune disease may simply be a case of bad luck!

Whatever triggers off the sequence of events leading to autoimmunity, it is likely that genetic variability

TABLE 4.1 Autoimmune diseases

Organ specific
Graves' disease
Hashimoto's thyroiditis
Multiple sclerosis
Autoimmune gastritis
Primary biliary cirrhosis
Type 1 diabetes mellitus
Addison's disease
Myasthenia gravis
Autoimmune hepatitis
Multisystem
Rheumatoid arthritis
Systemic lupus erythematosus
Systemic sclerosis

between individuals is also important in determining whether disease occurs or not. For instance, polymorphisms in the CTLA4 gene have been shown to be strongly associated with certain autoimmune diseases.

Immunodeficiency

A defect in the functioning of the immune system is known as an **immunodeficiency**, and may be congenital or acquired. The clinical picture resulting from immunodeficiency varies widely depending on the nature of the defect, ranging from a mild often asymptomatic state to a rapidly lethal condition due to overwhelming infection.

Congenital immunodeficiency

Congenital immunodeficiencies are caused by genetic defects that affect the normal function of some component of the immune system. The abnormality may affect the innate immune system, B lymphocytes, T lymphocytes, or multiple components.

Isolated IgA deficiency is the most common disorder of humoral immunity

IgA deficiency is the most common congenital immune disease, believed to affect as many as 1 in 700 people. In this condition, there is failure of B lymphocytes to terminally differentiate into IgA-secreting plasma cells. Serum IgA levels are markedly depressed whilst all other immunoglobulin types are normal. Most people with IgA deficiency are healthy with no significant clinical consequences, and the diagnosis is discovered by chance.

LINK BOX

IgA deficiency and gluten-sensitive enteropathy

The high incidence of IgA deficiency is important to remember when measuring IgA endomysial antibodies as a screening test for suspected gluten-sensitive enteropathy. Patients with gluten-sensitive enteropathy who also happen to be IgA deficient will test negative for IgA endomysial antibodies. For this reason, it is important to check total IgA levels at the same time (p. 154).

Common variable immunodeficiency causes reduced immunoglobulin production in adult life

Common variable immunodeficiency is an inherited immunodeficiency state affecting about 1 in 30 000 Caucasians, associated with markedly reduced serum levels of all immunoglobulin types. The underlying mechanism is complex and not well understood, but the fundamental abnormality appears to be a failure in generating the appropriate environment for B lymphocyte differentiation within lymphoid follicles. Most patients have a combination of molecular abnormalities rather than a single gene defect.

Patients typically present at about 30 years of age with recurrent pneumonia, diarrhoea due to *Giardia lamblia* infection, and recurrent attacks of herpes simplex. Autoimmune disorders causing anaemia, thrombocytopenia, and neutropenia are also common.

Hyper IgM syndrome is caused by a mutation in the CD40L gene

Hyper IgM syndrome is an inherited immunodeficiency condition in which there is a failure in class switching by activated B lymphocytes. Most cases are caused by an inherited mutation in the gene encoding **CD40 ligand**, the surface molecule expressed by activated helper T lymphocytes which stimulates B lymphocytes to produce IgG instead of IgM. Serum levels of IgG and IgA are low, but IgM levels are normal or high.

Hyper IgM syndrome usually presents in infancy with recurrent opportunistic infections, especially with *Pneumocystis carinii*, suggesting that failure to express CD40L has wider implications for T lymphocyte function beyond B lymphocyte activation. Rather like common variable immunodeficiency, there is also a tendency to develop autoimmune diseases against the cellular elements of the blood leading to severe autoimmune anaemia, thrombocytopenia, and neutropenia.

Acquired immunodeficiency

Acquired disorders of the immune system are much more common than congenital ones. Many of these are iatrogenic, such as treatment with immune suppressing drugs, chemotherapy treatment, and removal of the spleen. The most common diseases leading to severe immunosuppression are lymphoid malignancies and infection with human immunodeficiency virus (HIV).

Splenectomy

Most patients who lose their spleen do so following surgical removal. This may be performed as an emergency following trauma to the organ, or electively as part of the planned treatment of haematological disorders such as idiopathic thrombocytopenic purpura or autoimmune haemolytic anaemia.

Loss of splenic function places patients at risk of infection with encapsulated bacteria such as *Streptococcus pneumoniae*, *Haemophilus influenzae*, and *Neisseria meningitidis* as the spleen is the main site of phagocytosis of these organisms when they have been coated with antibodies to the capsule. The risk of infection is greatest in children and in the first 2 years following splenectomy. Patients without a spleen should therefore be vaccinated against *S. pneumoniae* and given long-term penicillin prophylaxis.

Lymphoid malignancies

Various types of lymphoid malignancy are associated with immunodeficiency, the two most common being chronic lymphocytic leukaemia and myeloma.

The majority of patients with chronic lymphocytic leukaemia develop hypogammaglobulinaemia (low levels of circulating immunoglobulins) during the course of the disease. Although this is mild in most patients, some patients develop severe hypogammaglobulinaemia and suffer from recurrent infections, particularly of the respiratory tract. The mechanism of the antibody deficiency is complex and seems to be due to a combination of production of inhibitory factors released by the malignant cells and also interference with normal trafficking of T and B lymphocytes through lymph nodes packed full of neoplastic lymphocytes.

Patients with myeloma often have antibody deficiency, and are particularly susceptible to pneumococcal pneumonia and septicaemia. The mechanism appears to be production of factors by the malignant plasma cells that inhibit normal antibody production.

HIV infection

HIV infection is a massive global health problem

HIV is a retrovirus which infects and destroys certain cells of the immune system, leading to a profound immunodeficiency state known as **acquired immune deficiency syndrome** (AIDS). HIV infection is a global pandemic, with over 40 million people currently infected with the virus. During 2004, 5 million people became newly infected with HIV and 3.1 million people died from AIDS. Sub-Saharan Africa is by far the worst affected area in the world, accounting for over 60 per cent of all people living with HIV.

Sexual transmission is the main mode of HIV infection

HIV is spread predominantly by sexual transmission. Intravenous drug abusers may also acquire HIV by direct inoculation of the virus into the blood through infected needles. Infected mothers may also transmit the infection to their newborn babies. Fortunately transmission of HIV in transfused blood products has now been virtually eliminated by stringent donor screening.

HIV infects and destroys CD4+ cells of the immune system

HIV infects cells of the immune system that express the CD4 molecule. The major cell type infected and destroyed by HIV is the CD4+ helper T lymphocyte, though other important cells such as macrophages and dendritic cells are also infected by the virus.

HIV infection follows a predictable natural history which terminates in AIDS

Following infection with HIV, there is widespread seeding of the lymphoid tissues by the virus. Activation of the immune response initially controls the infection, and the viral load declines substantially. Killing of infected cells by HIV-specific CD8+ cytotoxic T lymphocytes appears to be the main mechanism responsible for containment of the virus.

Despite activation of the immune system, the infection is not completely cleared. This is probably because the virus establishes a reservoir of infection within macrophages and dendritic cells in the spleen and lymph nodes. These infected cells are not recognized by the HIV-specific CD8+ cytotoxic T lymphocytes because the virus downregulates the MHC class I molecules on the macrophages and dendritic cells.

During this period of clinical latency, patients are usually asymptomatic though they may have minor abnormalities such as persistent lymphadenopathy or an isolated thrombocytopenia. Although the CD4+ T lymphocyte count remains normal, billions of CD4+ T cells are dying and being replaced every day.

Over a period of time, HIV escapes immune control by CD8+ cytotoxic T lymphocytes and the immune system can no longer control the infection. The main mechanism of viral escape is almost certainly related to the ability of the virus to vary the sequence of its genome. By continuously generating new antigenic variation, the virus eventually mutates into a form to which the host's T cell repertoire is weakly responsive. The viral load rapidly increases and renewal of CD4+ T cells cannot keep up with the rate of loss. The CD4+ T lymphocyte count falls precipitously and the patient is said to have AIDS.

Patients with AIDS are susceptible to opportunistic infections

Patients with AIDS become highly susceptible to infection by intracellular microbes normally contained by T cells (Fig. 4.8). Many of these infections are opportunistic as they are caused by organisms normally present in the environment that do not infect healthy people. Common sites of involvement include:

- Lungs. Pneumonia is a very common infection in patients with AIDS and is often what brings the diagnosis to light. Pneumonia may be caused by a number of organisms including *Pneumocystis carinii*, cytomegalovirus, *Mycobacterium tuberculosis*, and atypical mycobacteria.

- Gastrointestinal tract. Chronic persistent diarrhoea is a common symptom in patients with AIDS and may be due to a number of infections including the parasite *Cryptosporidium* and atypical mycobacteria such as *Mycobacterium avium intracellulare*. Oesophageal candidiasis is also common and should always raise the suspicion of immunosuppression as the oesophagus is normally resistant to infection.

- Central nervous system. The central nervous system is less commonly affected than the lungs and gastrointestinal tract in AIDS, but when affected may have devastating consequences such as multiple abscesses caused by the protozoan *Toxoplasma gondii* and a meningitis caused by the fungus *Cryptococcus neoformans*.

Virally driven neoplasms are also common in AIDS patients

Patients with AIDS are also susceptible to developing tumours caused by viral infection, e.g. cervical and anal carcinoma driven by human papillomavirus, B cell lymphomas driven by Epstein–Barr virus, and **Kaposi's sarcoma** driven by human herpes virus 8. Kaposi's sarcoma is a malignant vascular tumour that is normally rare, but is the most common neoplasm seen in AIDS patients.

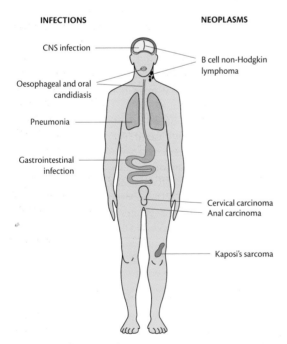

INFECTIONS

NEOPLASMS

CNS infection

B cell non-Hodgkin lymphoma

Oesophageal and oral candidiasis

Pneumonia

Gastrointestinal infection

Cervical carcinoma
Anal carcinoma

Kaposi's sarcoma

Fig. 4.8 Manifestations of AIDS.

Key points: Immunodeficiency

- Immunodeficiency may be congenital or acquired, and may affect any component of the immune system with a wide variety of manifestations.

- Common congenital immunodeficiencies include isolated IgA deficiency and common variable immunodeficiency.

- Acquired immunodeficiency is much more common than congenital immunodeficiency, and is often due to splenectomy, immunosuppressive drugs, lymphoid malignancies, and HIV.

- AIDS is the result of destruction of CD4+ cells of the immune system by HIV.

- Patients with AIDS are susceptible to a number of opportunistic infections such as *Pneumocystis carinii* pneumonia, and virally driven neoplasms such as B-cell lymphomas and Kaposi's sarcoma.

Neoplasia

Introduction

A **neoplasm** is an abnormal mass of tissue which shows uncoordinated growth and serves no useful purpose. The word neoplasm literally means 'new growth' and is often used synonymously with the word **tumour** which simply means 'swelling'.

Malignant neoplasms are also called **cancers**. Cancer is a major cause of morbidity and mortality across the world. Currently in the UK, one in three people will be diagnosed with cancer during their lifetime. One in five of these will die as a result of the cancer. As cancer is more common with increasing age, the ageing population means that cancer will become even more common.

Note that a **hamartoma** is a developmental abnormality which contains the same tissues as the organ in which it is found but in the wrong proportions. Although they are non-neoplastic, they may cause concern for a neoplasm because they give rise to a mass lesion.

Classification of neoplasms

Neoplasms are generally classified according to their behaviour into **benign** or **malignant** and by their **histogenesis** (cell of origin).

Benign neoplasms

Benign neoplasms remain confined to their site of origin

Benign tumours usually have a slow rate of growth, do not spread, and have a very good prognosis. Although benign neoplasms usually run an innocuous course, they can be dangerous if they compress vital nearby structures, or if the neoplasm has endocrine functions leading to uncontrolled secretion of a hormone.

Malignant neoplasms

Malignant neoplasms can spread to distant parts of the body

Malignant neoplasms are so abnormal that they show no respect for anatomical boundaries. Malignant neoplastic cells detach from their normal position and grow into the surrounding tissue in a destructive manner. This invasive behaviour is one of the defining features of a malignant neoplasm.

The most sinister property of malignant neoplasms is their ability to spread, or **metastasize**, to distant sites and produce secondary tumours called **metastases** which then grow independently from the primary tumour.

Tumour histogenesis

The **histogenesis** of a tumour refers to its presumed cell of origin. Although sometimes the macroscopic appearance of a tumour is highly characteristic of a particular histogenesis, definitive cell typing of a tumour can only be determined by microscopic examination of the tumour. Although tumours may arise from any of the nucleated cells of the body, the majority of tumours arise from epithelial cells.

Nomenclature of neoplasms

Armed with the knowledge about the cell of origin of a neoplasm and its behaviour, one is able to name it (Table 5.1).

Epithelial neoplasms

Epithelial cells line the internal and external surfaces of the body, such as the skin, respiratory tract, gastrointestinal tract, and urinary tract. The two most common types of epithelium are the multilayered squamous epithelium covering the skin and lining the oesophagus, and the single layered glandular epithelium lining the

TABLE 5.1	Examples of neoplasms	
	Benign	**Malignant**
Epithelial	Acanthoma/ papilloma	Squamous cell carcinoma
	Adenoma	Adenocarcinoma
Mesenchymal	Lipoma	Liposarcoma
	Leiomyoma	Leiomyosarcoma
	Haemangioma	Angiosarcoma
	Osteoma	Osteosarcoma

respiratory and gastrointestinal tracts. The urinary tract is lined by a type of epithelium intermediate between squamous and glandular epithelium, known as transitional epithelium or urothelium.

Benign neoplasms of squamous epithelium are called **acanthomas**, though if they appear branching they are often called **papillomas**, e.g. laryngeal papilloma. Benign neoplasms of glandular epithelium are called **adenomas**, e.g. follicular adenoma of the thyroid, or pleomorphic adenoma of a salivary gland.

Epithelial malignancies are called carcinomas

A carcinoma which contains cells which microscopically show features of squamous epithelium, such as intercellular bridges or keratin formation, is called a **squamous cell carcinoma** (Fig. 5.1). An epithelial malignancy which shows features of glandular differentiation, such as gland formation or mucin production, is called an **adenocarcinoma** (Fig. 5.2).

Carcinomas are often preceded by a phase of **dysplasia**, in which an area of epithelium contains neoplastic cells but without invasion. If the dysplastic cells completely replace the full thickness of the epithelium, the term **carcinoma in situ** may be used. Only once the basement membrane on which the epithelium sits is breached and the cells have invaded the underlying tissue is the term carcinoma used (Fig. 5.3). It is important to appreciate that whilst most carcinomas arise from epithelial dysplasia, not all areas of dysplastic epithelium progress into a carcinoma; many remain stable and some spontaneously regress.

Connective tissue neoplasms

Connective tissue is a biological tissue that supports and protects organs. Connective tissue includes adipose

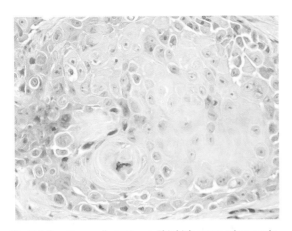

Fig. 5.1 Squamous cell carcinoma. This high power microscopic image shows a squamous cell carcinoma. If you look very closely between the neoplastic cells you may just be able to make out fine intercellular bridges between the cells, a key feature of a squamous cell carcinoma.

tissue, muscle, blood vessels, and bone. Connective tissue neoplasms may be benign or malignant.

Benign connective tissue neoplasms are named after the cell of origin followed by the suffix '-oma':

♦ **Lipoma**, a benign tumour of fat cells (adipocytes)

♦ **Leiomyoma**, a benign tumour of smooth muscle cells

♦ **Angioma**, a benign tumour of blood vessels

♦ **Osteoma**, a benign tumour of bone.

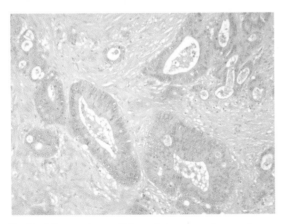

Fig. 5.2 Adenocarcinoma. This medium power microscopic image shows malignant epithelial cells forming glands with a central lumen, a defining feature of an adenocarcinoma.

Malignant mesenchymal neoplasms are named after the cell of origin but then followed by the suffix '-sarcoma':

♦ **Liposarcoma**, a malignant tumour of adipocytes

♦ **Leiomyosarcoma**, a malignant tumour of smooth muscle

♦ **Rhabdomyosarcoma**, a malignant tumour of skeletal muscle

♦ **Angiosarcoma**, a malignant tumour of blood vessels

♦ **Osteosarcoma**, a malignant tumour of bone.

Other types of neoplasm

There are a number of other neoplasms which do not fit readily into an epithelial or connective tissue category and so are given different names. Common examples include:

♦ **Lymphomas, leukaemias**, and **myeloma** are haematological malignancies derived from cells of the blood or bone marrow.

♦ **Malignant melanoma** is a highly malignant neoplasm derived from melanocytes.

♦ **Malignant mesothelioma** is a malignant tumour derived from mesothelial cells which usually arises from the pleura.

♦ **Germ cell tumours** are a diverse group of tumours derived from germ cells which usually arise in the gonads.

♦ **Embryonal tumours** are a group of malignant neoplasms seen predominantly in childhood composed of very primitive embryonic tissue, e.g. neuroblastoma or nephroblastoma.

> ## Key points: Classification of neoplasms
>
> ♦ Neoplasms are classified according to their behaviour and their cell of origin.
>
> ♦ Benign neoplasms remain confined to their site of origin and do not spread. If they are excised, they do not normally recur.

Continued

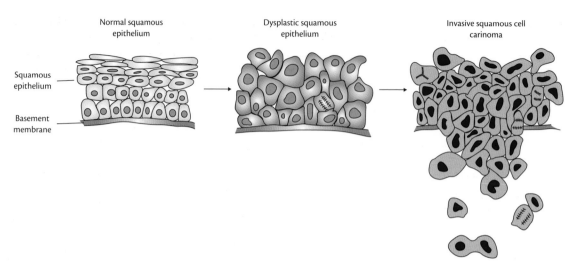

Fig. 5.3 Diagrammatic representation of development of a squamous cell carcinoma. The normal squamous epithelium first becomes dysplastic, meaning the epithelium becomes disorganized and the cells appear abnormal with large, dark nuclei. However, the neoplastic cells remain confined to the epithelium. Once the neoplastic squamous epithelial cells breach the basement membrane and invade the underlying tissue, the lesion is called a squamous cell carcinoma.

Key points: Classification of neoplasms—cont'd

♦ Malignant neoplasms show invasive behaviour, growing in a destructive manner into the surrounding tissues. Malignant neoplasms are also able to spread to distant sites, a property known as metastasis.

♦ Epithelial neoplasms are the most common type of neoplasm. Malignant epithelial neoplasms are called carcinomas.

♦ Connective tissue neoplasms may be benign or malignant. Benign connective tissue tumours have the suffix '-oma'. Malignant connective tissue tumours have the suffix '-sarcoma'.

Carcinogenesis

Carcinogenesis refers to the sequence of events leading to the development of a malignant neoplasm. Needless to say, there is a great deal of research directed at uncovering the precise molecular details of carcinogenesis in the hope that we can slow, halt, reverse, or prevent the process.

JARGON BUSTER

Transformation

The change from a normal cell into a malignant cell is sometimes referred to as **transformation**. The two absolute requirements for defining a cell as transformed are immortality and the ability to form malignant tumours when transplanted into a suitable host.

Carcinogenesis is the result of the accumulation of mutations in genes critical to the control of cell growth and division. Our knowledge of the genetic basis of many common cancers is increasing rapidly. New molecular genetic tools have been developed that allow the screening of large numbers of tumours for defects in specific genes. This is helping us to work out which particular genes are particularly important in the development of certain types of cancer.

The aetiology of many cancers remains unclear, although most potentially carcinogenic agents act either by directly damaging DNA or by stimulating cells to undergo mitosis (a cell is most susceptible to acquiring mutations when it is replicating its DNA). Well recognized risk factors for malignancy therefore include:

- Radiation and chemicals which damage DNA, e.g. sunlight and cigarette smoke.
- Chronic inflammatory diseases which stimulate persistent proliferation of cells, e.g. ulcerative colitis (which predisposes to colorectal carcinoma).
- High levels of hormones causing proliferation of a tissue, e.g. oestrogens predisposing to breast carcinoma and endometrial carcinoma.
- Certain viruses produce proteins which damage DNA, e.g. human papillomavirus.

The cell cycle

The central abnormality in neoplastic cells is loss of control over cell proliferation such that the cells continue to divide. Understanding the normal cell cycle is therefore essential to understanding carcinogenesis. The cell cycle has four phases (Fig. 5.4):

- G_1: gap 1, a preparation phase.
- S: synthesis of DNA.
- G_2: gap 2, during which assembly of the apparatus for chromosome distribution occurs.
- M: mitosis, when the cell actually divides.

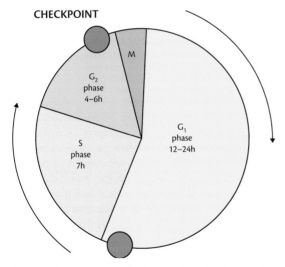

CHECKPOINT

Fig. 5.4 Cell cycle. The cell cycle is comprised of G_1, S, G_2, and M phases. The two main checkpoints occur at the transition from G_1 to S, and from G_2 to M.

Cells enter the cell cycle from a resting phase called G_0 which is non-proliferative. Cells in G_0 may re-enter the cell cycle at G_1 and regain proliferative ability. Cells which have undergone terminal differentiation cannot re-enter the cell cycle.

Control of the cell cycle is crucial to prevent uncontrolled growth of cells

The cell cycle operates under tight regulation. There are several checkpoints in the cell cycle which are regulated by **cyclins** and **cyclin-dependent kinases** (CDK). If no genetic defect in the cell is detected, then the cyclin and the CDK form a complex which activates transcription factors which then turn on the transcription of specific genes necessary for the next step of the cell cycle. If the cell detects DNA damage, formation of the cyclin–CDK complex is not completed and progression through the cell cycle is halted.

Genes controlling cell division can be divided into proto-oncogenes and tumour suppressor genes

Proto-oncogenes are human genes which code for proteins that promote division of cells under normal circumstances. If these genes become abnormally activated by mutation, they are called **oncogenes** to distinguish them from their normal counterparts. There are many different types of mutation that can result in excess activity of an oncogene, including point mutations, translocations, and deletions of genetic material. In some cases, the genetic sequence itself is normal but the gene becomes *amplified* such that the neoplastic cell contains many copies of the oncogene with resultant excessive production of the gene product.

LINK BOX

HER2 amplification in breast carcinoma

Some breast carcinomas are characterized by amplification of the HER2 gene such that the neoplastic cells become coated with numerous growth-stimulating receptors. HER2 positive breast carcinomas have a worse prognosis than HER2 negative breast carcinomas (p. 293).

Tumour suppressor genes code for proteins that inhibit cellular division. In this instance, it is inactivation of the activity of these genes that promotes the development of malignancy. To lose their effects in the cell, both gene copies must be rendered non-functional. Of interest, tumour suppressor genes are often 'silenced' due to methylation of their promoter regions rather than by mutation in the actual coding sequence of the gene.

Oncogenes

Oncogenes are mutated genes that promote cell division. Genetic mutations which lead to increased activity of oncogenes therefore increase the growth potential of a cell. Many different oncogenes have been identified, but all of them code for proteins playing some part in cellular signalling (Fig. 5.5) and include:

♦ Growth factor receptors

♦ Signal transducing proteins

♦ Transcription factors.

Activating mutations in growth factor receptors are oncogenic

Many growth factors stimulate cell proliferation by interacting with a transmembrane receptor that has tyrosine kinase activity. Binding of the growth factor to these receptors stimulates intrinsic kinase activity in the cytoplasmic part of the receptor, leading to phosphorylation and activation of intracellular signalling molecules. Mutations in the genes encoding these receptors may lead to persistent activation of the receptor, even in the absence of its normal ligand, and continuous stimulation of cell division.

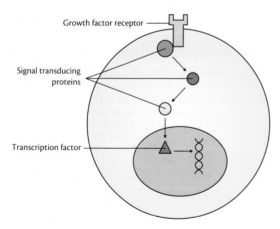

Fig. 5.5 Oncoproteins. Oncogenes code for proteins with key roles in growth-stimulating cell signalling pathways.

Growth factor receptor

Signal transducing proteins

Transcription factor

> **LINK BOX**
>
> ## Growth factor receptors and human malignancies
>
> Examples of growth factor receptors in which mutations are commonly identified include RET in medullary thyroid carcinoma (p. 320), MET in papillary renal cell carcinomas (p. 234), and KIT in gastrointestinal stromal tumours (p. 150).

RAS is the best known example of an oncogene encoding a signal transducing protein

RAS is one of the molecules involved in the signalling cascade following activation of growth factor receptors. The RAS gene encodes a protein called p21 which promotes entry into the cell cycle. Activating mutations in the RAS gene, which lock p21 in an 'on' position, are one of the most frequent mutations found in human malignancies.

Overexpression of transcription factors may also lead to uncontrolled cell growth

The final stage in the signalling process of a growth factor is the production of transcription factors which enter the nucleus and bind to DNA, stimulating the expression of genes involved in cell proliferation. Examples of such transcription factors include Myc, Jun, and Fos. Mutations in the genes encoding these transcription factors which lead to increased expression of the transcription factor are oncogenic. Myc gene mutations are commonly found in lung carcinomas and breast carcinomas.

Tumour suppressor genes

Tumour suppressor genes may be divided into **caretaker** genes responsible for repairing DNA damage, and **gatekeeper** genes which halt the proliferation of a cell with DNA damage and/or stimulate it to undergo apoptosis (Table 5.2). Three of the most important tumour suppressor genes in human malignancies are **P53**, **CDKN2A**, and **RB**, all of which code for proteins important in control of the cell cycle (Fig. 5.6)

P53 mutation is the most common genetic injury in cancers

The product of the P53 gene is a protein, p53, upregulated at times of DNA damage. p53 halts the cell from

TABLE 5.2	Tumour suppressor genes
Gatekeeper genes	
P53	
RB	
CDKN2A	
APC	
Caretaker genes	
BRCA1	
BRCA2	
MLH1	
MSH2	

dividing and then upregulates DNA repair proteins. If repair is not possible, the cell is forced to commit suicide by apoptosis. Loss of function of p53 is therefore a potentially catastrophic molecular event, as it allows genetic damage to survive and accumulate within each successive generation of cells.

CDKN2A codes for a protein called p16 which controls progression through the cell cycle

The cyclin-dependent kinase inhibitor-2A (CDKN2A) gene encodes a protein called p16 which inhibits the action of CDK4 kinase, halting progression of the cell

cycle in G_1. Mutations in CDKN2A lead to production of an abnormal p16 protein which loses its capacity to block cyclin–CDK activity and prevent phosphorylation of Rb during the cell cycle.

RB codes a protein which allows entry into the cell cycle

The Rb protein product of the RB gene also regulates cell cycle progression. The ability of Rb to regulate the cell cycle correlates to its state of phosphorylation. Unphosphorylated Rb forms a complex with the E2F family of transcription factors, rendering E2F inactive. When Rb is phosphorylated by cyclin–CDK complexes, it is released from E2F allowing E2F to activate genes that allow entry into the cell cycle.

Metastasis

The defining features of malignant neoplasms are invasion and metastasis. Metastasis is one of the major reasons for the morbidity and mortality related to malignancy, and so understanding the mechanism of metastasis may help us to develop treatments to prevent it.

Under normal circumstances, all cells are under strict regulation to prevent them surviving outside their normal environment. Neoplastic cells that are able to metastasize have become so abnormal they fail to respond to any of the signals that would normally terminate them if they detach from their normal location.

In order to metastasize, neoplastic cells must complete the metastatic cascade

Successful metastasis requires a sequence of events to be completed, often referred to as the **metastatic cascade**. The neoplastic cell needs to lose its adhesion to the neighbouring cells, erode through the extracellular matrix, penetrate the lumen of a vessel, survive the various defence systems of the blood whilst travelling to a distant site, exit the vessel, and successfully implant and multiply in the new site (Fig. 5.7).

In view of all these hurdles, it is not surprising that many tumour cells fail to metastasize. The metastatic process is a highly inefficient process; tumours may shed millions of cells every day into the blood, most of which fail to become metastases. Unfortunately, survival of just one cell is one too many, as the presence of metastatic disease usually renders the disease incurable.

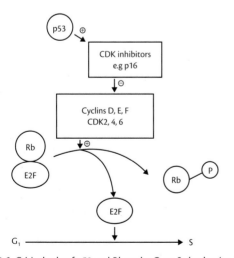

Fig. 5.6 Critical role of p53 and Rb at the G_1 to S checkpoint.

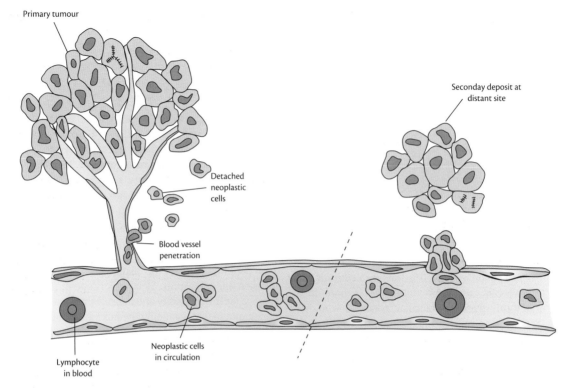

Fig. 5.7 Metastatic cascade. In order to metastasize, neoplastic cells must enter the circulation, travel to a distant site, leave the circulation, and successfully establish a new colony.

Malignant neoplasms metastasize by three principal routes

There are three ways in which malignant neoplasms can spread to distant sites:

- *Vascular spread*. Malignant cells entering veins draining the site of the neoplasm gain access to the circulation and may spread to distant sites. Commonly affected organs are the lungs, bone, brain, and adrenal glands. Gastrointestinal malignancies often spread to the liver which they can easily reach via the portal vein (Fig. 5.8).

- *Lymphatic spread*. Malignant cells often enter the lymphatic channels draining the site of the neoplasm and grow as secondary tumour deposits in the local lymph nodes. For instance, the axillary lymph nodes are commonly involved in cases of metastatic breast carcinoma.

- *Transcoelomic spread*. Malignant tumours growing near a body cavity such as the pleura or peritoneum can seed into these spaces and spread across them to other organs.

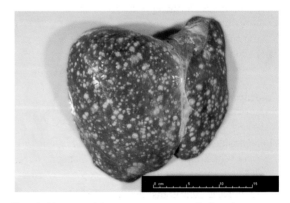

Fig. 5.8 Liver containing numerous metastatic deposits.

Key points: Carcinogenesis

- Carcinogenesis is the sequence of events leading to the development of a malignant neoplasm.

- Carcinogenesis is the result of accumulation of mutations in genes controlling cell proliferation.

- Genes that control cell proliferation are divided into proto-oncogenes and tumour suppressor genes.

- Proto-oncogenes code for proteins that normally stimulate cell growth. Mutations in these genes are usually activating mutations that lead to overexpression of the gene. Examples include KIT, RAS, and MYC.

- Tumour suppressor genes code for proteins that normally inhibit cell growth. Loss of the activity of both copies of these is therefore required for a tumour-promoting effect. Common examples include P53, CDKN2A, and RB.

- Metastasis is one of the defining features of a malignant neoplasm, allowing spread of the tumour to sites distant from its origin.

- Malignant neoplasms spread by three principal routes: vascular spread, lymphatic spread, and transcoelomic spread.

symptoms by some time. These include prolonged fever, weight loss, and loss of appetite.

- *Local* symptoms of a malignancy are related to tissue destruction at the site of the cancer. For instance, lung carcinomas may cause cough, haemoptysis, and chest wall pain. Rectal cancers often cause rectal bleeding and tenesmus.

- *Metastatic* symptoms are related to secondary deposits of the cancer in distant organs. Bony metastases cause persistent bony pain, and widespread pulmonary metastases cause breathlessness. Cerebral metastases may present with headaches or convulsions.

- *Paraneoplastic* symptoms are not directly related to a tumour deposit but are due to factors produced by the neoplastic cells such as growth factors or hormones (Table 5.3). A good example is hypercalcaemia caused by release of **parathyroid hormone-related peptide**.

Obtaining a tissue diagnosis in a patient with malignancy is vital

In many cases, patients suspected of having a malignancy on the basis of their symptoms undergo some form of imaging. For instance a smoker with a new persistent cough will have a chest radiograph, or an elderly man with obstructive jaundice will have a computed tomography (CT) scan looking especially at the

The patient with a malignancy

Cancer is a common disease, and you will come across many patients with cancer during your career. Further details about the important malignancies are set out in the relevant chapters of Part 2 of this book, but it is worthwhile here to consider some general principles relating to the effects of malignancy in the patient.

Symptoms related to a malignancy may be constitutional, local, metastatic, or paraneoplastic

When considering the possible symptoms of any malignancy, a useful approach is to categorize them into constitutional, local, metastatic, or paraneoplastic:

- *Constitutional* symptoms are common in patients with malignancies and these may precede localizing

TABLE 5.3 Examples of paraneoplastic syndromes and their cause

Syndrome	Cause
Finger clubbing	?
Deep venous thrombosis	Release of tumour procoagulants
Hypercalcaemia	Secretion of parathyroid hormone related peptide
Nephrotic syndrome	Immune complex deposition in glomeruli
Syndrome of inappropriate ADH secretion	Secretion of ADH
Cushing's syndrome	Secretion of ACTH
Polycythaemia	Secretion of erythropoietin

ADH, antidiuretic hormone; ACTH, adrenocorticotrophic hormone.

TABLE 5.4	Examples of biopsy methods for common tumours
Breast	Core biopsy or fine needle aspiration cytology
Lung	Transbronchial biopsy
Colorectal	Biopsy taken at colonoscopy or sigmoidoscopy
Prostate	Transrectal ultrasound-guided biopsies
Bladder	Biopsy taken at cystoscopy

pancreas. The radiological appearances may be strongly suggestive of a malignancy, especially if there is also evidence of secondary spread (e.g. if liver metastases are also seen).

Despite the almost certain diagnosis in a patient with a typical history and supportive radiological findings, it remains imperative in almost all cases to obtain a definitive diagnosis by removing part of the tumour for microscopic examination (Table 5.4). This is often called obtaining a 'tissue diagnosis'.

The two main methods of sampling are fine needle aspiration cytology (Fig. 5.9) or a needle core biopsy (Fig. 5.10). Sometimes it may be easier to access a suspected metastatic deposit (e.g. liver or lymph node) rather than the primary tumour.

Provided the biopsy is of good quality (and has not missed the tumour!), the pathologist examining the

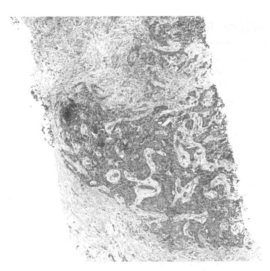

Fig. 5.10 This is a low power microscopic view of a needle core biopsy taken from a breast lump because an attempted fine needle aspiration was unsuccessful. The irregular dark purple islands of cells are part of a breast carcinoma. The background pink material is dense fibrotic tissue that has formed around the tumour. This is why breast carcinomas typically feel very firm on palpation.

biopsy should be able to define the precise type of malignancy, e.g. squamous cell carcinoma or adenocarcinoma. In cases where the primary site is uncertain, the pathologist may also be able to suggest likely primary sites based on the microscopic appearance of the tumour and its immunohistochemical profile (p. 536).

Tumour markers may also be helpful in the diagnosis and monitoring of malignancy

Tumour markers are proteins, enzymes, or hormones released by the tumour which can be measured in the blood (Table 5.5). Currently, tumour markers are not specific enough to be diagnostic of malignancy, but they can help support a clinical suspicion and are often useful in the follow up of patients with malignancy. For instance, measurement of serum **prostate specific antigen** is useful following treatment of prostate carcinoma to check for recurrence.

Determining the grade and stage of a tumour is required to plan treatment and predict prognosis

The **grade** of a neoplasm describes how closely it resembles normal tissue. The grade is determined by

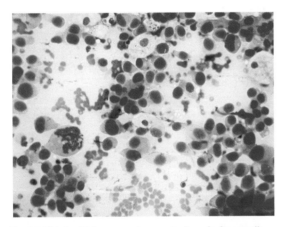

Fig. 5.9 This is a high power microscopic view of a fine needle aspiration cytology preparation from a breast lump. Some red blood cells are present in the background. Virtually all the other cells are discohesive malignant epithelial cells with nuclei of varying size and shape. A huge malignant cell on the left hand side is undergoing mitosis. This is a breast carcinoma.

TABLE 5.5 Tumour markers	
Markers	**Tumour**
Prostate specific antigen (PSA)	Prostatic carcinoma
α-Fetoprotein (AFP)	Hepatocellular carcinoma, germ cell tumours
Carcinoembryonic antigen (CEA)	Gastric, colorectal, and pancreatic carcinomas
Ca125	Ovarian carcinoma
Human chorionic gonadotropin (HCG)	Choriocarcinoma

scrutinizing the appearance of the tumour microscopically. Different tumours have their own grading systems, but usually the grade is given in the form of a number, and the lower the number the better the prognosis. Various parameters may be used to assign the grade, such as the degree of variation in size and shape of the tumour cells, and the number of mitotic figures.

The **stage** of a neoplasm refers to how far it has spread. Stage is a very important prognostic factor as generally the earlier a cancer is picked up, the better the outlook for the patient. A widely used staging scheme for most types of cancers is the **TNM system**. In this system, a malignant tumour is assigned a T (tumour) number related to the size and local spread of the tumour, an N (node) number related to the number and site of any lymph node involvement, and an M (metastasis) number for the presence of any distant metastases. The criteria for assigning each number depend on the organ involved. Cancers are expressed in the format Tx, Nx, Mx, e.g. T2, N1, M0. The higher the number in each group, the more extensive the spread.

Pneumonia and pulmonary thromboembolism are common causes of death in cancer patients

Patients with advanced malignancies may be predisposed to pneumonia for a number of reasons. Cancer causes a non-specific suppression of the immune system, and patients with advanced cancer are often too weak to cough effectively to keep their airways clean. Bedridden patients often aspirate food, and strong opiate pain killers suppress respiratory drive.

Pulmonary thromboembolism from venous thrombosis is a major cause of mortality in patients with malignancy. The risk of developing venous thrombosis varies with the type of cancer, being most common in colonic, lung, pancreatic, and breast carcinomas. The increased risk is due to the presence of molecules on the surface of malignant cells that activate coagulation ('tumour procoagulants'). Other important factors in cancer patients include immobility and dehydration.

JARGON BUSTER

Tumour differentiation

The grade of a tumour may also be expressed in terms of its **differentiation**, which is also related to how closely the microscopic appearance of the tumour resembles that of the normal tissue from which the tumour has arisen. Differentiation is therefore similar to grade. A well differentiated tumour closely resembles the normal tissue, whereas a poorly differentiated tumour has only a passing resemblance to the normal tissue. Moderately differentiated tumours are intermediate. Tumours which are so poorly differentiated that it is impossible to determine the origin of the tumour by microscopy alone are sometimes called **undifferentiated** or **anaplastic**.

Key points: The patient with a malignancy

- ◆ Malignant neoplasms may present with constitutional symptoms, local symptoms, metastatic symptoms, or paraneoplastic symptoms.

- ◆ Although imaging may strongly suggest malignancy, definitive diagnosis requires microscopic examination of a biopsy of the tumour.

- ◆ Knowledge of the precise tumour type allows appropriate treatment to be given and estimation of likely prognosis.

Continued

Key points: The patient with a malignancy—cont'd

- The grade and stage of a tumour are also important prognostic factors. The grade of a neoplasm describes how closely the tumour resembles normal tissue. The stage describes how far the tumour has spread and is often denoted using the TNM classification.

- Pneumonia and pulmonary embolism are common causes of death in patients with malignancy.

Further reading

http://info.cancerresearch.org.uk. In depth, up to date information on all major cancers.

PART II

Core diseases

CHAPTER 6

Cardiovascular disease

Chapter contents

Introduction

An adequate blood supply is vital for every organ and tissue in the body. The main role of the cardiovascular system is to continuously deliver oxygenated blood and remove deoxygenated blood from the tissues. Diseases of the cardiovascular system are the most common causes of death in the Western world, and most can be distilled down to two basic problems:

- *Localized* failure of the circulation due to narrowing (**stenosis**) or complete blockage (**occlusion**) of a blood vessel. Cell injury due to loss of blood supply to a tissue or impaired drainage of blood from a tissue is known as **ischaemia**.

- *Generalized* failure of the circulation (**shock**) due to either excessive loss of volume from the circulation or failure of the pumping action of the heart. The danger here is failure of multiple organs due to prolonged inadequate perfusion.

Before considering individual diseases of blood vessels and the heart, some important general concepts of circulatory pathology must first be discussed and understood.

General principles of circulatory pathology

Thrombosis

Thrombosis is a very common cause of vessel occlusion

The normal haemostatic system is a complex system which rapidly forms a localized plug at sites of vascular injury. Under normal circumstances, haemostasis is tightly regulated such that the clot is produced only at sites of injury. **Thrombosis** is a *pathological* event which occurs when the haemostatic system is abnormally activated, overwhelming the ability of the natural fibrinolytic system to control it. A solid mass of platelets, fibrin, and entrapped blood cells forms a **thrombus**, which may completely occlude the vessel.

Three general factors predispose to thrombus formation

Three factors increase the risk of thrombosis in a vessel, which may operate singly or in combination:

- *Changes in the vessel wall.* Under normal circumstances, the endothelial cells lining blood vessels prevent thrombosis by expressing antithrombotic proteins on their surface. Damaged endothelial cells, however, become prothrombotic and encourage the formation of a thrombus.

- *Changes in blood flow.* Under normal circumstances, flow in vessels keeps platelets away from the endothelial surface. Stasis allows platelets to come into contact with endothelium and allows the accumulation of coagulation components.

- *Changes in blood coagulability.* Blood can become more prone to clot under a number of circumstances. Women taking the oral contraceptive pill are at a slightly increased risk of thrombosis as the drug raises prothrombin levels. There are also a variety of inherited disorders associated with an increased risk of thrombosis due to mutations in key proteins that regulate coagulation.

These three factors were first noted by Virchow way back in 1845, and together form the famous **Virchow's triad** firmly rooted in pathological history (though Virchow himself never actually used the word 'triad' in any of his papers).

Thrombi can form in arteries, veins, and the heart

Thrombosis can occur anywhere in the circulatory system (veins, arteries, capillaries, and the heart), although the risk factors are often different between these sites. Venous thrombosis is usually related to stasis of blood and an increase in blood coagulability. Arterial thrombosis is usually related to changes in the vessel wall due to unstable atherosclerotic plaques. Cardiac thrombosis

is usually related to stasis of blood, due either to a myocardial infarction or atrial fibrillation.

LINK BOX

Thrombotic microangiopathies

Most thrombi form in the larger vessels of the circulatory system, but they can also form in the microcirculation. Diseases dominated by thrombus formation in small vessels are called **thrombotic microangiopathies** (p. 352).

Two important complications of thrombus formation are thromboembolism and infarction

Thrombi can completely resolve or undergo organization and recanalization, in which case they may remain clinically silent. Thrombi become significant if they cause *obstruction* of arteries or veins, or if they *embolize*.

An **embolus** is defined as a detached mass within the circulatory system that is carried in the blood to a site distant from its point of origin. Emboli are important because they can lodge in small vessels and block them off. Almost all emboli are fragments of dislodged thrombi, known as **thromboemboli**. Thromboemboli can cause a number of important problems depending on their site of origin (Fig. 6.1):

- Thromboemboli from systemic veins travel via the heart into the pulmonary arterial tree, causing pulmonary embolism.

- Thromboemboli originating in the heart enter the systemic arterial circulation where they may impact in cerebral arteries (causing stroke), the gut (causing small bowel infarction), and the lower limbs (causing acute limb ischaemia).

- Thromboemboli breaking off from complicated atherosclerotic plaques in the carotid arteries enter the cerebral circulation causing transient ischaemic attack and stroke.

Fat emboli, septic emboli, and amniotic fluid emboli are rarer types of emboli

Fat embolism may occur as a complication of severe bony trauma. Typically this follows fracture of long bones, but may also occur as a complication of orthopaedic procedures due to operative trauma. Fragments of the fatty

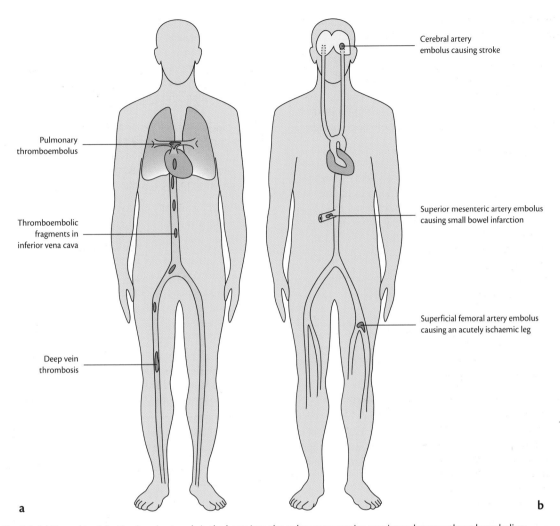

Fig. 6.1 (a) Thrombi originating in veins travel via the heart into the pulmonary arteries, causing pulmonary thromboembolism. (b) Thrombi in the systemic arterial system may embolize to the cerebral arteries causing stroke, to the superior mesenteric artery causing small bowel infarction, or to the femoral artery causing an acutely ischaemic leg.

bone marrow enter the circulation and can lodge in the pulmonary arteries in a similar way to pulmonary thromboemboli.

Septic emboli are fragments of infected material, usually derived from friable vegetations of infective endocarditis. Septic emboli can set up foci of infection in distant sites where they lodge, e.g. cerebral abscess (p. 431).

Amniotic fluid embolism is a rare but dreaded complication of pregnancy. During childbirth, amniotic fluid containing cells from fetal skin enter the mother's circulation leading to widespread endothelial cell damage. Amniotic fluid embolism is a cause of acute respiratory distress syndrome and acute disseminated intravascular coagulation, the combination of which is frequently lethal.

Key points: Thrombosis

♦ A thrombus is a solid mass of platelets and fibrin which can develop anywhere in the cardiovascular system.

♦ Thrombosis is predisposed to by changes in the vessel wall, changes in blood flow, and changes in blood coagulability.

♦ Thrombosis in arteries is usually associated with endothelial damage in association with a complicated atherosclerotic plaque. The most important complication of thrombosis in arteries is complete occlusion of the vessel by the thrombus, leading to death of the downstream tissue.

♦ In veins, stasis is the major contributing factor to thrombosis. The most feared complication of venous thrombosis is pulmonary thromboembolism.

Infarction

Necrosis due to ischaemia is called infarction

Complete occlusion of a vessel from any cause results in ischaemic cell damage to the downstream tissue. If this is prolonged, these cells will undergo necrosis. Necrosis as a result of ischaemia is called **infarction**.

The vast majority of infarcts are due to obstruction of an artery

Common types of infarcts include myocardial infarction ('heart attack'), cerebral infarction ('stroke'), and small bowel infarction. These are caused either by thrombosis overlying a complicated atherosclerotic plaque or by embolic impaction of thrombotic fragments in the vessel.

Infarcts can also be caused by blockage of venous drainage

Complete blockage of venous drainage from a tissue leading to infarction ('venous infarction') is less common than arterial infarction. Venous blockage causes the tissue to become massively suffused with blood, which continues to be pumped in but is unable to drain out.

Affected areas are deeply congested and appear dark purple or even black.

The usual cause of venous infarction is twisting ('torsion') or compression of the vascular pedicle of an organ. Examples include strangulation of the bowel, sigmoid volvulus, and torsion of the testis.

Key points: Infarction

♦ Infarction is death of tissue due to an abrupt cessation of blood supply.

♦ Infarction is usually due to blockage of an artery, either by a thrombus over a complicated atherosclerotic plaque or by thromboembolus.

♦ Venous infarction due to sudden blockage of venous drainage is also important.

Shock

Shock is a clinical term associated with generalized failure of tissue perfusion

The term **shock** can be used to denote various conditions. These include the response to passage of electric current through the body; the state that follows immediately after damage to the spinal cord; and the stunned reaction to bad news. In the clinical context, however, shock refers to a *systemic reduction in blood flow to all tissues*. This is in contrast to local failure of blood flow which may cause ischaemia of an individual organ, but not shock. Patients with severe shock are unwell and need urgent treatment to prevent failure of multiple organ systems and death (Fig. 6.2).

There are four broad categories of shock

There are many possible causes of shock. To help organize your thoughts, these causes are best divided into the following four categories:

♦ **Hypovolaemic shock**

♦ **Distributive shock**

♦ **Cardiogenic shock**

♦ **Obstructive shock.**

The basis of all of these is poor tissue perfusion.

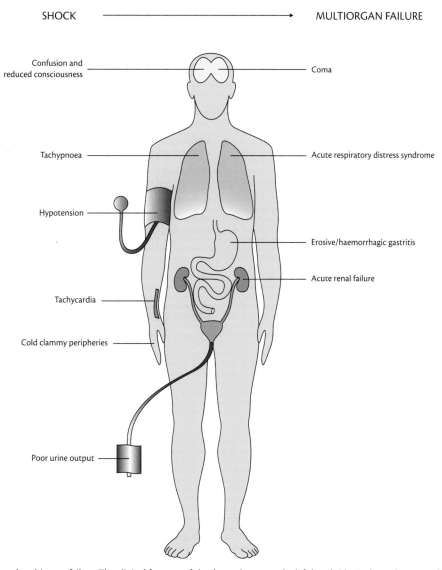

SHOCK ⟶ MULTIORGAN FAILURE

Confusion and reduced consciousness — Coma

Tachypnoea — Acute respiratory distress syndrome

Hypotension

Erosive/haemorrhagic gastritis

Acute renal failure

Tachycardia

Cold clammy peripheries

Poor urine output

Fig. 6.2 Shock and multiorgan failure. The clinical features of shock are shown on the left hand side. Prolonged untreated shock leads to the development of multiorgan failure, shown on the right hand side.

The patient with overt shock is usually clinically obvious

Shocked patients look unwell, even to the untrained eye. They are pale and their skin feels cold and clammy, particularly over the hands and feet. Often they are drowsy and appear confused. Their blood pressure is low and there is tachycardia. The underlying cause is often evident, e.g. a road traffic accident victim with significant trauma, or a patient who has suffered a massive haematemesis.

The early signs of developing shock may be subtle

In the early stages of shock, there are few clinical signs. *Up to 15% of circulating blood volume can be lost without any change in heart rate or blood pressure.* With increasing *abnormally rapid heart rate*

loss of volume, there is an increased sympathetic drive leading to tachycardia. Urine output declines, although this is often not immediately apparent unless the patient is catheterized and urine output is being measured. The blood pressure may appear normal at this stage; however, if blood pressure is measured with the patient lying down and standing up, a fall in pressure may be demonstrated (a 'postural drop').

Hypovolaemic shock is caused by a decrease in circulating volume

Hypovolaemia is a very common cause of shock. It is caused by loss of circulating blood volume, through either haemorrhage or loss of fluid from other sources.

External bleeding is usually clinically apparent, e.g. following trauma, or a large upper gastrointestinal bleed. Internal bleeding is not so immediately apparent and should be considered in patients with unexplained hypotension. Possible causes include a leaking aortic aneurysm, a ruptured ectopic pregnancy, or a torn internal organ following blunt trauma.

Loss of circulating fluid may also occur through extensive burns, in the urine of an uncontrolled diabetic, or through sequestration at a site within the body. For instance, an obstructed bowel can accumulate many litres of fluid within it.

In distributive shock, there is marked dilation of blood vessels

Unlike hypovolaemic shock, where the poor tissue perfusion is due to actual loss of circulating blood volume, distributive shock is due to widespread dilation of blood vessels. The 'size' of the vascular system exceeds the amount of blood within it. Thus even though blood volume is normal, blood pressure falls and tissue perfusion becomes inadequate. The two most common types of distributive shock are septic shock and anaphylactic shock.

Septic shock is the most common form of distributive shock and is a very common cause of death in hospitalized patients. It is the result of an overwhelming infection leading to widespread activation of the inflammatory response. There is profound vasodilation with a fall in blood pressure and tissue perfusion.

Although less common, **anaphylactic shock** is also an important cause of distributive shock. Here the marked vasodilation is caused by the release of large amounts of histamine from mast cells following an intense allergic reaction.

LINK BOX

Anaphylaxis

Anaphylactic shock is the most extreme manifestation of an immediate (type I) hypersensitivity reaction (p. 46).

Cardiogenic shock occurs when the pumping action of the heart is severely impaired

If the heart becomes so damaged that it fails to maintain the flow of the circulatory system, blood flow becomes inadequate, leading to shock. Such severe loss of cardiac function is most commonly due to extensive infarction of the left ventricle. In addition to the normal features of shock, there is severe congestion of the lungs and pulmonary oedema, which causes distressing breathlessness.

LINK BOX

Cardiogenic shock

About 10% of myocardial infarctions are complicated by the development of cardiogenic shock which is difficult to treat and carries a high mortality (p. 91).

Obstructive shock occurs if there is a massive blockage to the flow of blood

If there is significant obstruction or compression affecting a major vessel or the heart itself, then the whole cardiovascular system rapidly collapses, leading to shock.

Key points: Shock

+ Shock is the term for a generalized reduction in perfusion of all tissues.

+ There are four main groups of shock: hypovolaemic, distributive, cardiogenic, and obstructive.

+ Hypovolaemic shock and septic shock are the most common causes of shock.

+ The initial response to poor perfusion is tachycardia and a reduced urine output.

+ Without treatment, blood pressure falls, leading to failure of multiple organ systems.

This mechanism is responsible for the sudden death associated with conditions such as a large pulmonary embolus, a tension pneumothorax (which kinks the great veins), and bleeding into the pericardial sac with external pressure on the heart (cardiac tamponade). Prompt treatment of the latter two can prevent death.

Diseases of arteries

Normal arteries contain three distinct anatomical layers: the intima, media, and adventitia. The **intima** is the innermost layer and consists of a layer of endothelial cells supported by loose underlying connective tissue. An **internal elastic lamina** separates the intima from the middle layer, the **media**, which contains a mixture of smooth muscle cells and elastic fibres in variable proportions. The outermost layer, the **adventitia**, contains fibrous tissue. In large and medium sized arteries, the adventitia contains small blood vessels known as the **vasa vasorum** which supply blood to the outer half of the vessel.

Arteries are divided into four types according to their size and structure (Fig. 6.3):

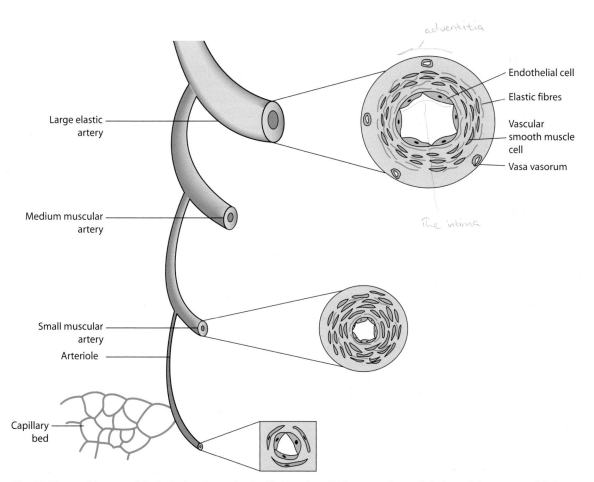

Fig. 6.3 The arterial system of the body. Arteries can be classified into four divisions according to their size and the structure of their walls. The capillary bed is derived from the arterioles.

- **Large elastic arteries**, e.g. the aorta and its major branches. These arteries have a large number of elastic fibres in the media, allowing them to expand during systole and then recoil during diastole to help blood flow through them.

- **Medium muscular arteries**, e.g. the coronary and renal arteries. Muscular arteries have a media rich in smooth muscle cells.

- **Small muscular arteries**. These have a similar structure to the medium sized muscular arteries but are smaller (<2 mm diameter).

- **Arterioles**. Arterioles are tiny vessels (just 20–100 µm diameter) within the substance of tissues and organs which give rise to capillaries. Arterioles consist of endothelial cells surrounded by just one or two layers of smooth muscle cells and no elastic layer.

Many of the important diseases of arteries selectively affect particular sized arteries. For instance, atherosclerosis affects large and medium sized arteries, whereas hypertension affects small arteries and arterioles.

Hypertension

Hypertension is an extremely common and important condition

Systemic arterial hypertension affects nearly a quarter of the adult population and is the most widely recognized treatable risk factor for a variety of important cardiovascular diseases including stroke and myocardial infarction. Despite this, many patients with hypertension remain undiagnosed and even when diagnosed are often untreated or undertreated.

Defining hypertension is a difficult task

To understand the problem of defining hypertension, one has to see its relevance to the population as a whole. Figure 6.4 shows how within a population blood pressure is a continuous variable with a normal distribution (blue curve), i.e. there is no obvious distinction between a normal blood pressure and a high blood pressure, with the majority of people falling somewhere in the middle. The risk of developing complications for a given blood pressure is also shown (red curve). The final curve is derived from the first two and shows the number of people at each level of blood pressure developing complications (green curve).

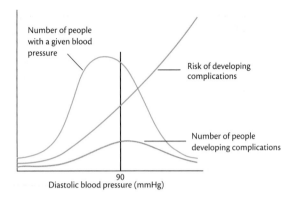

Fig. 6.4 Graph showing variation in blood pressure within a population.

You can see that although those people with very high blood pressures are individually at high risk of complications, the total number of them is low. Just treating these people would have little impact on the number of complications occurring in the population as a whole. Conversely, reducing the blood pressure of the whole population would significantly cut the number of complications, but a large number of people who would never have developed a complication would be needlessly taking drugs for the rest of their lives.

Making a cut-off to decide who is hypertensive and should be treated is a balance between these two extremes. Indeed, the definition of hypertension has changed over the years, and continues to do so with emerging evidence. Currently, hypertension is defined on the basis of clinical trials as the level of blood pressure above which treatment does more good than harm, which is currently set at 140/90 mmHg (black line in Fig. 6.4).

Over 95% of hypertensive patients have primary hypertension

In primary (or 'essential') hypertension, a single cause cannot be identified to explain the persistently elevated blood pressure. Obviously there must be a cause, but currently we do not know what it is. It has been hypothesized that, whatever the underlying cause, the ultimate mechanism which finally maintains elevated blood pressure is resetting of the renal handling of sodium such that a higher perfusion pressure is required for the kidneys to eliminate the daily sodium load.

Attempting to work out the initial alteration leading to hypertension is extremely difficult because by the time a patient is diagnosed with hypertension, the fundamental abnormalities which led to the hypertension may no longer be identifiable. This has made research into the aetiology of hypertension extremely difficult.

Only 5 per cent of hypertensive patients have a specific underlying cause

Although only a small proportion of hypertensive patients have a secondary cause, the possibility should always be considered (Table 6.1). Most of the causes of secondary hypertension can be excluded on the basis of simple physical and biochemical investigations. Note that a variety of other conditions may have hypertension as a feature, e.g. Cushing's syndrome and acromegaly, but these rarely *present* with hypertension.

Chronic renal disease is the most common cause of secondary hypertension

Patients with chronic renal disease develop hypertension early in the course of their disease, even before the glomerular filtration rate decreases. Over 90 per cent of patients with end-stage renal failure are hypertensive, and this is important as it has a major impact on the rate of progression of the renal disease and on their risk of cardiovascular disease.

As we shall see in Chapter 10, aggressive control of blood pressure in patients with chronic renal failure is a crucial part of their management. Not only is this known to slow their decline towards end-stage renal failure, but it also significantly lowers their risk of cardiovascular disease which is often what these patients die from.

Hypertension causes thickening of small arteries and arterioles

The principal lesion associated with chronic hypertension is thickening of small arteries and arterioles, known as **arteriosclerosis** and **arteriolosclerosis,** respectively.

TABLE 6.1   Secondary causes of hypertension
Chronic renal disease
Renal artery stenosis
Phaeochromocytoma
Primary hyperaldosteronism (Conn's syndrome)

Neither arteriosclerosis nor arteriolosclerosis are diagnostic of hypertension as identical changes can be seen as part of normal ageing in the absence of hypertension, and also in diabetic patients.

Small arteries in hypertension show thickening of the intimal layer due to increased amounts of connective tissue, as well as disruption and reduplication of the internal elastic lamina. Arterioles in hypertension are thickened due to the accumulation of plasma proteins and the deposition of basement membrane material in the wall. Because this gives the wall a glassy appearance down the microscope, these changes are also called 'hyaline arteriolosclerosis'.

Collectively, *these changes lead to a reduction in the size of the lumen of small arteries and arterioles causing low grade persistent ischaemia of the downstream tissue.* Although the wall is thickened, the fixed rigidity appears to make the vessels more likely to crack or rupture, leading to haemorrhage.

Hypertension also accelerates atherosclerosis in large and medium sized arteries

In addition to its effects on small arteries and arterioles, hypertension is also a risk factor for the development of atherosclerosis in large and medium sized arteries. Presumably the effect is mediated by a damaging effect on endothelial cells.

Hypertension leads to disease in the heart, brain, kidneys, and aorta

The effect of hypertension on blood vessels has pathological consequences in various organs (Fig. 6.5). Such damage is often referred to as 'end-organ damage' or 'target organ damage'.

- ◆ Heart. Hypertension imposes a persistent increased workload on the left ventricle which has to pump against the high systemic pressure. In response, the left ventricular myocardium undergoes pathological hypertrophy to maintain the cardiac output. Unfortunately, hypertrophy cannot be sustained forever in the face of hypertension, and eventually the left ventricle dilates and fails. *Chronic left ventricular failure is a common consequence of hypertension and the most common cause of death in untreated hypertensive patients.* This is often exacerbated by co-existing coronary artery atherosclerosis which is itself accelerated by hypertension. In the presence of left ventricular hypertrophy, the left atrium undergoes dilation and

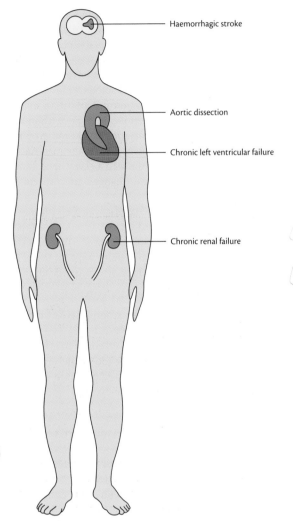

Fig. 6.5 Common conditions caused by hypertension.

Labels in figure:
- Haemorrhagic stroke
- Aortic dissection
- Chronic left ventricular failure
- Chronic renal failure

(handwritten marginal note, left side): weakening of the vessel wall leading to excessive enlargement of the blood vessel.

(handwritten marginal note, bottom): muscular twitching / muscle fibres acting without coordination.

stretching, which favours the development of atrial fibrillation. Hypertension is one of the common causes of atrial fibrillation.

- Brain. Hypertension causes the formation of small aneurysms (Charcot–Bouchard aneurysms) in arterioles within the substance of the brain. If these rupture, the intracerebral haemorrhage causes a stroke. *Hypertension is the most common cause of spontaneous intracerebral haemorrhage.*

- Kidney. Narrowing of small arteries and arterioles within the kidneys leads to ischaemic atrophy

of nephrons. The gradual irreversible loss of nephrons leads to chronic renal failure.

- Aorta. Hypertension predisposes to the development of abdominal aortic aneurysm (by accelerating atherosclerosis) and thoracic aortic dissection. Aortic dissection occurs when the intimal surface of the thoracic aorta develops a tear which allows the entry of blood into the arterial wall and extension along its length. Most patients with aortic dissection have a history of hypertension, though precisely how hypertension causes aortic dissection is controversial. It has been proposed that the initiating event is haemorrhage from a vasa vasorum into the media of the aorta, placing stress on the intima which then tears. Patients typically present with sudden severe 'tearing' chest pain which can closely mimic acute myocardial infarction. The most common cause of death is rupture of the dissection into the pericardial cavity, pleural cavity, or peritoneal cavity (Fig. 6.6).

Most hypertensive patients are asymptomatic

Unless a complication occurs, hypertension is almost always clinically silent. Sometimes patients may present with headaches or nose bleeds, but the diagnosis is usually made in an asymptomatic person when blood pressure is taken as part of a routine examination.

Patients newly diagnosed with hypertension should be screened for evidence of organ damage with simple tests such as an electrocardiogram (ECG) for evidence of left ventricular hypertrophy, a urine dipstick for proteinuria or haematuria, measurement of plasma urea and creatinine concentration for renal damage, and fundoscopy to visualize the retinal vessels. Although visual symptoms are rare in hypertension, inspection of the retina provides a simple way of assessing the effects of hypertension on blood vessels. Retinal changes can help determine if treatment is needed or if it is adequate.

Primary hypertension cannot be cured

Although primary hypertension cannot be cured, it can usually be controlled with a combination of lifestyle modifications and lifelong medication. Most patients will have readily identifiable lifestyle factors that contribute to the development of high blood pressure, such as lack of exercise and excessive consumption of salt and alcohol. These should be addressed first before

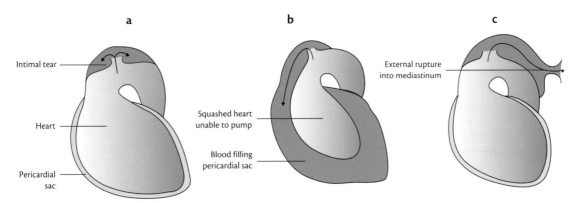

Fig. 6.6 Aortic dissection. (a) Containment of the dissection leads to tearing chest pain but does not cause immediate death. (b) Retrograde spread of a dissection into the pericardial cavity leads to massive haemopericardium, cardiac tamponade, and death. (c) External rupture of a dissection into the mediastinum leads to massive haemorrhage and death.

drug therapy is introduced. The objective is to decrease blood pressure sufficiently to reduce the risk of end-organ damage.

Hypertensive crisis is defined as a severe elevation in blood pressure

A **hypertensive crisis** occurs if the blood pressure reaches very high levels, typically above 200 mmHg systolic or above 120 mmHg diastolic. The danger associated with a very high blood pressure, particularly when the rate of rise is very rapid, is the development of destructive changes in small arteries and arterioles. A very useful and quick method of assessing for microvascular damage is to perform fundoscopy to visualize the vessels of the retina to examine for retinal haemorrhages, exudates, and papilloedema.

The brain and kidneys are particularly susceptible in hypertensive crises

If a hypertensive crisis is complicated by evidence of organ dysfunction due to microvascular injury, the episode is known as a **hypertensive emergency**. Two common hypertensive emergencies are hypertensive encephalopathy and acute renal failure. Hypertensive encephalopathy occurs because cerebral vessels are unable to autoregulate in the face of the very high blood pressure, resulting in cerebral underperfusion and cerebral oedema. Typical symptoms include headache, drowsiness, and visual disturbance. Necrosis of arterioles in the kidneys may also lead to acute renal failure.

> ### Key points: Hypertension
>
> ◆ Hypertension refers to the presence of a persistently elevated systemic blood pressure.
>
> ◆ Hypertension is very common and often undertreated.
>
> ◆ The vast majority of cases of hypertension are primary, with no clear underlying cause. The most common cause of secondary hypertension is chronic renal disease.
>
> ◆ Hypertension thickens and narrows small arteries and arterioles leading to chronic ischaemia of affected organs. Hypertension also promotes the development of atherosclerosis in large and medium sized arteries. Hypertension also weakens the wall of arterioles, risking rupture and haemorrhage.
>
> ◆ Hypertension is a common cause of chronic left ventricular failure, haemorrhagic stroke, chronic renal failure, and aortic dissection.

Atherosclerosis

There is no other single disease that has such a potent impact on health in the Western world as atherosclerosis. Atherosclerosis is responsible for a number of very common diseases (Fig. 6.7). In particular, coronary

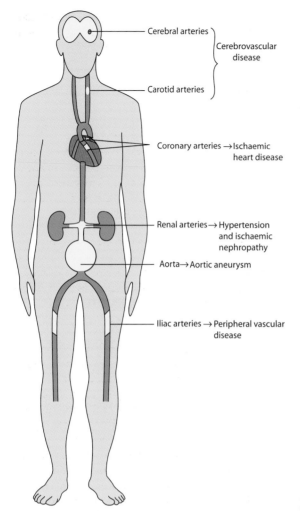

Fig. 6.7 Common diseases caused by atherosclerosis.

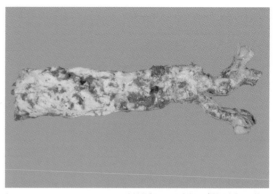

Fig. 6.8 Atherosclerotic plaques. This abdominal aorta has been opened up to reveal numerous complicated atherosclerotic plaques covering the intimal surface of the artery.

arteries or the pulmonary arteries is rare, because they are lower pressure systems.

Atherosclerosis is now recognized to be a chronic inflammatory disorder which develops in response to episodes of repeated vascular wall injury by a variety of well known risk factors (Table 6.2). Men who smoke a packet of cigarettes a day have a 70 per cent increase in death rate from ischaemic heart disease compared with non-smokers.

JARGON BUSTER

Atherosclerosis and vasculitis

Although inflammation in blood vessel walls is seen in both atherosclerosis and vasculitis, the two entities are quite different. In atherosclerosis, the inflammation is in response to injury to the intima of the artery. Although the chronic inflammation is important in driving the disease process, the inflammation is 'appropriate'. In vasculitis, however, the primary problem is an *inappropriate* inflammatory attack on blood vessels with destruction of the vessel wall (p. 485).

artery disease, cerebrovascular disease, and peripheral vascular disease together account for about 40 per cent of male and 30 per cent of female deaths in those under 75 years of age. It is therefore worth considering in some detail.

Atherosclerosis is an inflammatory disease of large and medium sized systemic arteries

Atherosclerosis is a disease of arteries which leads to the formation of lipid-laden lesions called atherosclerotic, or atheromatous, plaques in the vessel wall. It predominantly affects large and medium sized vessels of the systemic circulation, such as the aorta and coronary arteries (Fig. 6.8). Involvement of smaller systemic

Atherosclerotic plaques produce disease in three main ways

There are three ways in which atherosclerotic plaques lead to symptomatic disease:

* *Gradual narrowing of the vessel.* If a plaque grows large enough to limit blood flow through the vessel, then

TABLE 6.2	Risk factors for atherosclerosis
Age	
Male sex	
Obesity	
Diabetes mellitus	
Hypertension	
Smoking	

symptoms resulting from ischaemia of the supplied tissue may result, especially in situations when oxygen demand is increased (e.g. exercise), a situation known as 'inducible ischaemia'.

• *Sudden occlusion of the vessel*. Unstable advanced plaques are prone to developing complications such as ulceration, cracking, or rupture. Such 'complicated' atherosclerotic plaques stimulate overlying platelet aggregation which may evolve into an occlusive thrombus. Prolonged occlusion of an artery by a thrombus causes infarction of the tissue supplied by that artery.

• *Erosion of the vessel wall and aneurysmal change*. The mechanism by which atherosclerosis leads to the formation of an aneurysm is uncertain. Evidence suggests that the thickening of the intima by the plaque reduces diffusion of nutrients from the lumen to the media, leading to degeneration of the media with progressive replacement by collagen. Collagen is non-contractile and inelastic, and therefore poor at supporting vessel walls under high pressure, leading to aneurysmal change. The abdominal aorta is the most common site for atherosclerotic aneurysms.

Endothelial cell injury is the earliest event in atheroma formation

The precise mechanisms early in the evolution of an atherosclerotic plaque are not entirely clear; however, endothelial cell injury and activation is thought to be central. Activated endothelial cells undergo switches in gene expression, leading to the production of adhesion molecules and cytokines, which attract inflammatory cells, and various prothrombotic molecules.

Endothelial cell activation also leads to the accumulation of lipid just underneath the endothelial cells where it is taken up by macrophages. Collections of lipid-laden macrophages sitting in the intimal layer

may be visible as yellow elevations called **fatty streaks**. The fatty streak has no clinical significance, but is important because it can progress to an atherosclerotic plaque.

Oxidized lipid drives an ongoing inflammatory response in the vessel wall

Lipid accumulating in the intima of the artery can become oxidized by the action of inflammatory cells recruited into the vessel by activated endothelial cells. Oxidized lipid is instrumental in the development of atherosclerotic plaques by stimulating the recruitment of further inflammatory cells into the lesion and driving a persistent inflammatory process.

Vascular smooth muscle cells have a protective role in atherosclerotic plaques

In response to ongoing inflammation in the intima of the artery, vascular smooth muscle cells in the media of the vessel migrate into the intima where they become incorporated into the developing atherosclerotic lesion.

During the process of migration, vascular smooth muscle cells completely change their phenotype. Rather than making contractile proteins, they adopt a repair phenotype which allows them to proliferate and secrete extracellular matrix proteins. A thick fibrous cap forms over the lipid core which is essential in isolating the inflammatory process from the circulation.

The final result is a **stable atherosclerotic plaque**, which is an intimal lesion composed of oxidized lipid and an inflammatory cell infiltrate in its core, covered by a fibrous cap consisting of vascular smooth muscle cells and their extracellular matrix (Fig. 6.9).

The stability of an atherosclerotic plaque is determined by its cellular composition, not its size

It was thought for many years that atherosclerotic plaques were fairly static lesions and that most clinical problems were related to their size. The traditional understanding was that larger plaques encroached more on the lumen of the artery and therefore caused more restriction of blood flow and were also more likely to rupture. More recent work on the biology of plaques has revolutionized this concept. We now know that, in fact, plaques are extremely *dynamic* structures which are constantly changing in response to the behaviour of the different cell types within them.

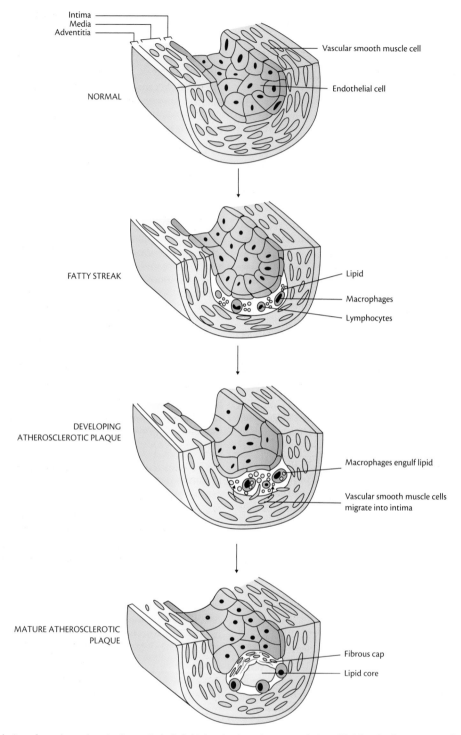

Fig. 6.9 Evolution of an atherosclerotic plaque. Endothelial injury leads to the accumulation of lipid and inflammatory cells in the intima of large and medium sized arteries. In response to ongoing inflammation in the intima, vascular smooth muscle cells migrate from the media into the intima where they secrete collagen, forming a thick fibrous cap over the lipid-rich core.

The most important determinant of plaque stability is the balance between the number of inflammatory cells (the 'bad guys') versus the number of protective vascular smooth muscle cells in the fibrous cap (the 'good guys'). Smooth muscle cells are protective because they produce the fibrous cap that stabilizes the plaque. Inflammatory cells, on the other hand, destabilize plaques by digesting the fibrous cap and killing smooth muscle cells.

Stable atherosclerotic plaques therefore characteristically contain few inflammatory cells and large numbers of smooth muscle cells, and have a thick fibrous cap that is resistant to rupture. These stable lesions may grow large enough to cause symptoms of inducible ischaemia, but are less likely to cause acute vascular events as their thick fibrous cap protects them from rupture. In contrast, unstable plaques contain more inflammatory cells and have a thinner fibrous cap that is more prone to rupture under haemodynamic stress, causing acute events (Fig. 6.10).

INTERESTING TO KNOW

Statins and atherosclerosis

The **statins** are a group of drugs which inhibit hydroxymethylglutaryl-coenzyme A (HMG-CoA) reductase, a key enzyme required for the synthesis of cholesterol. Statins have been shown to be effective in reducing the number of acute vascular events caused by atherosclerosis. It is thought that statins work by stabilizing atherosclerotic plaques due to their effects on reducing circulating lipid levels and through anti-inflammatory properties.

What determines the rate of progression and outcome of an atherosclerotic plaque in an individual is yet to be established. One of the most puzzling features of atherosclerosis is the wide variation in severity and location of lesions between individuals, even those with similar risk factors. It is thought that subtle, genetically determined differences in the production and activity of inflammatory mediators may play a vital role.

Atherosclerosis is usually widespread within an individual

Remember that a patient with evidence of atherosclerotic disease in one organ system will almost certainly have disease in other systems. These patients are often called 'vasculopaths' to emphasize that they invariably have widespread atherosclerosis affecting most of their major arteries. Vasculopaths are often smokers with significant respiratory disease too. Awareness of such co-morbidity is important, as a patient undergoing surgical treatment for peripheral vascular disease or an aortic aneurysm is also likely to have impaired cardiac and respiratory function, both of which will impact on their fitness for surgery and the outcome.

Public education is extremely important in reducing the incidence of atherosclerotic diseases

Modifying the various risk factors for atherosclerosis is by far the most powerful tool for preventing atherosclerosis. The importance of smoking cessation, weight reduction, regular exercise, and dietary modifications

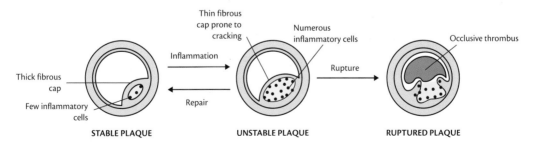

Fig. 6.10 Plaque stability. Stable plaques have few inflammatory cells with a thick fibrous cap. Increased inflammatory activity within an atherosclerotic plaque results in thinning of the fibrous cap, making it unstable and more liable to complications such as rupture.

cannot be overemphasized to the public, and especially to 'vasculopathic' patients.

Key points: Atherosclerosis

- Atherosclerosis is a very common chronic inflammatory disorder of large and medium sized systemic arteries.

- Atherosclerosis occurs in response to persistent injury to endothelial cells by factors such as smoking, diabetes, and hypertension.

- The end result is the formation of mature atheromatous plaques which protrude into the vessel lumen.

- Plaques may be stable or unstable depending on their cellular constituents.

- Stable plaques cause disease by encroaching on the lumen and causing symptoms of reversible ischaemia in the organ supplied.

- Unstable plaques are prone to complications such as erosion, cracking, or rupture which stimulate thrombosis and total vessel occlusion.

- Plaques can also weaken the vessel wall, predisposing to aneurysmal change.

Peripheral vascular disease

Peripheral vascular disease refers to a group of conditions caused by compromise of the arterial circulation to the lower limbs. Almost all cases are related to narrowing by atherosclerosis. The severity of the symptoms is related to the degree of the obstruction.

Chronic limb ischaemia usually presents with intermittent claudication

Chronic arterial insufficiency of the lower limbs manifests initially as **intermittent claudication**. Intermittent claudication is pain in the calf and thigh which occurs during exercise, and rapidly relieves upon resting. It is a good example of a symptom of inducible ischaemia caused by inadequate perfusion of the skeletal muscle of the leg during exercise.

Severe obstruction of arterial flow to the leg causes critical leg ischaemia

With progression of peripheral vascular disease, patients may develop **critical leg ischaemia**. Critical leg ischaemia is defined as gangrenous change, ulceration, or rest pain lasting for 2 weeks.

Rest pain is distinct from intermittent claudication as the pain involves the *foot* due to ischaemia of the skin and subcutaneous tissue, and the pain is present at *rest* and often at night (when gravity no longer aids arterial flow).

The progression from claudication to rest pain reflects severe arterial occlusive disease. Usually there is widespread atherosclerosis affecting proximal and distal arteries, making treatment with stenting or bypass grafting difficult. Usually some attempt at reconstruction is made, but often the only treatment option for patients with severe rest pain or non-healing ulceration is amputation.

JARGON BUSTER

Gangrene

Gangrene is an ancient clinical term that refers to necrotic tissues modified by exposure to air resulting in drying (dry gangrene) or by infection (wet gangrene). Dry gangrene is preferable to wet gangrene because bacteria cannot grow in dry tissue. Toes deprived of blood in critical leg ischaemia usually show dry gangrene. Wet gangrene is an ominous development as there is rapid spread of bacteria in the devitalized tissue with spread into the blood stream.

Acute limb ischaemia is an emergency

Sudden occlusion of an artery to the lower limb causes acute leg ischaemia. The most common cause is thrombosis associated with a complicated atherosclerotic plaque, but emboli should also be considered. Traumatic damage to an artery in the leg is also a common cause of acute leg ischaemia, e.g. following a road traffic accident. The acutely ischaemic leg is painful, cold, pale, and pulseless. Urgent surgical intervention is required to restore the circulation, else the limb will be lost.

Key points: Peripheral vascular disease

- Peripheral vascular disease refers to symptoms and signs in the lower limbs caused by an inadequate blood supply.

- Most cases of peripheral vascular disease are related to atherosclerosis.

- Chronic limb ischaemia typically presents with intermittent claudication.

- Intermittent claudication responds well to measures such as stopping smoking and participating in supervised exercise regimes. Patients with persistent symptoms may require reconstructive surgery to bypass the areas of narrowing.

- Patients with very widespread atherosclerosis may go on to develop critical leg ischaemia. Reconstruction is less likely to provide a good outcome and amputation may be necessary.

- Acute limb ischaemia occurs due to thrombosis or embolism occluding the arteries supplying the leg. The leg is painful, cold, pale, and pulseless. An acutely ischaemic leg is a surgical emergency requiring urgent treatment to save the leg.

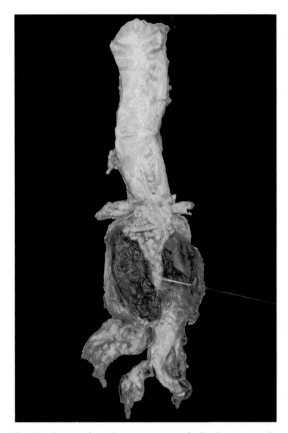

Fig. 6.11 Ruptured aortic aneurysm. A probe has been inserted through the point of rupture.

Abdominal aortic aneurysm

An aneurysm is an abnormal localized permanent dilation of a blood vessel

The most commonly encountered site for an aneurysm is the aorta. Aortic aneurysms usually occur in the abdominal portion of the artery and atherosclerosis is almost always the cause. Usually the abdominal aorta is the only site involved, but patients can also have aneurysms in other arteries such as the femoral or popliteal arteries.

Most abdominal aortic aneurysms are clinically silent, but they progressively enlarge until the aortic wall becomes so thin that there is a high risk of rupture (Fig. 6.11). Rupture of an aortic aneurysm into the peritoneal cavity causes massive intraperitoneal haemorrhage, hypovolaemic shock, and death. These patients rarely reach hospital alive.

If an aortic aneurysm ruptures into the retroperitoneal tissues, a retroperitoneal haematoma forms as the resistance of the tissues stops further bleeding. These patients have severe abdominal pain and are hypotensive, but they remain conscious and often make it into hospital. Without surgical repair of the aorta, death is inevitable. Even with attempted repair, operative mortality is very high, with about half of all patients dying either during or shortly after surgery.

Elective repair of an unruptured aortic aneurysm is comparatively safe. For this reason, there are current studies examining the benefit of screening at-risk populations for asymptomatic aneurysms using ultrasound and offering surgery to those with aneurysms larger than 6 cm diameter with the greatest risk of rupturing.

LINK BOX

Aneurysms

As well as atherosclerotic abdominal aortic aneurysms, other important aneurysms are **berry aneurysms** which cause subarachnoid haemorrhage if they rupture, and **Charcot–Bouchard aneurysms** which cause intracerebral haemorrhage if they rupture (p. 425).

Diseases of the heart

Heart failure

Heart failure is characterized by impairment of the heart's function as a pump

The term **heart failure** is a very non-specific term which refers to the presence of *symptoms due to inadequate pumping action of the heart*. Heart failure is not a diagnosis, it is a clinical syndrome that has many different causes. Patients should therefore not be labelled as simply having 'heart failure' but should be investigated to determine the underlying cause.

There are a wide variety of classifications of heart failure that have been proposed over the years. The most conceptually and clinically useful classifications are those that divide heart failure into **acute** or **chronic** (depending on the clinical presentation) and also into **left** or **right** to specify where the dominant site of injury is.

Left-sided heart failure is the more common type of heart failure, because the most frequent causes of cardiac injury primarily affect the left ventricle. Although failure of the right side of the heart commonly complicates left-sided failure resulting in failure of both sides of the heart ('biventricular' or 'congestive' cardiac failure), the term 'right heart failure' is usually reserved for cases developing independently of left-sided heart disease.

Acute heart failure has a dramatic presentation

Acute heart failure occurs if there is a sudden major insult to one of the chambers of the heart, catastrophically impairing cardiac function. There is no scope for compensation, and cardiac output suddenly cannot be maintained.

Acute heart failure is almost always due to sudden failure of the left ventricle as a complication of a myocardial infarction. This may occur either when an extensive infarct renders a large volume of the left ventricle non-functional, or when infarction causes one of the papillary muscles of the mitral valve to rupture completely. Instant failure of the left ventricle leads to severe congestion in the pulmonary venous system and the rapid accumulation of fluid within the alveolar spaces. The patient suffers severe breathlessness and hypoxia. In the worst cases, there is underperfusion of organs and the development of cardiogenic shock.

Acute *right*-sided heart failure does occur, but less frequently. Unlike acute left-sided failure, acute failure of the right heart is rarely ischaemic in origin. The most common cause of acute right failure is a massive pulmonary embolus causing sudden blockage of a major pulmonary artery. The pressure in the pulmonary arterial system rises dramatically and the right heart cannot generate enough force to maintain an output. The inevitable result is acute failure of the right heart and instantaneous death.

JARGON BUSTER

Acute cardiac failure and cardiogenic shock

Acute cardiac failure is often confused with cardiogenic shock. They are similar conditions, but there is one crucial difference between them: the blood pressure. When acute cardiac failure is so severe that blood pressure cannot be maintained, the condition is called cardiogenic shock. This is a grave condition which is difficult to manage and carries a high mortality.

Chronic heart failure is a slowly progressive disorder

Chronic heart failure occurs when one or more of the heart chambers are damaged slowly over a longer period of time. In contrast to acute heart failure, the loss of function occurs gradually, allowing compensatory mechanisms to maintain cardiac output. Compensation is seen in the form of **myocardial hypertrophy** of the stressed chamber(s).

In the short term, myocardial hypertrophy is a useful mechanism to sustain cardiac output and prevent

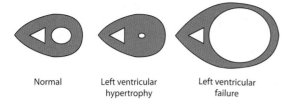

Fig. 6.12 Comparison of a normal heart, a heart with left ventricular hypertrophy, and a heart with left ventricular failure.

symptoms of heart failure, but it cannot be sustained in the face of persistent stress. Eventually the myocardium becomes irreversibly damaged and the chamber dilates (Fig. 6.12). Cardiac output cannot be maintained, and symptoms of heart failure gradually appear.

Pathological hypertrophy involves a switch from adult to fetal gene expression

Cardiac hypertrophy in response to injury (pathological hypertrophy) is quite different from that which develops in athletes (physiological hypertrophy). Myocytes undergoing pathological hypertrophy undergo major switches in the pattern of gene expression. Rather than expressing the genes of the adult heart, stressed myocytes revert to expressing genes that are normally transcribed in the fetal heart.

One interesting change that occurs in the failing heart is a reversion to a fetal method of energy metabolism. The fetal heart primarily metabolizes maternal glucose via glycolysis. After birth, however, glycolytic enzymes are downregulated and the adult heart primarily relies on β-oxidation of fatty acids as an energy source. The failing heart recapitulates fetal energy metabolism by re-expressing glycolytic enzymes and using glucose as a source of energy. Because the glycolytic pathway requires less oxygen, it is thought that this may be an adaptive response to reduce oxygen demand by the heart.

Chronic right heart failure is usually a consequence of lung disease

Chronic right heart failure refers to predominant dysfunction of the right side of the heart. It should not be used to refer to cases where the right heart fails as a result of primary left heart failure. Chronic right heart failure is much less common than chronic left heart failure. Right-sided failure occurs as a complication of pulmonary hypertension due to persistent lung disease such as chronic obstructive pulmonary disease, pulmonary fibrosis, and recurrent pulmonary emboli.

Chronic left heart failure is by far the most common form of heart failure

Chronic failure of the left side of the heart is far and away the most common type of heart failure you will come across. Almost all cases of chronic left heart failure are more specifically due to chronic left *ventricular* failure. In fact, you will find that very often when the term 'heart failure' or 'chronic heart failure' is used unqualified, it is usually meant to mean chronic left ventricular failure.

LINK BOX

Mitral stenosis and chronic left heart failure

Of all the common causes of chronic left-sided heart failure, the only major cause which does not affect the left ventricle is pure mitral stenosis where there is failure of the left atrium (p. 95).

Chronic left ventricular failure

Chronic left ventricular failure (LVF) is one of the most common and most important problems in clinical medicine. Most patients die within 3 years of diagnosis, making the prognosis of chronic LVF worse than many cancers. Despite this, making a confident clinical diagnosis can be difficult especially in cases of early compensated heart failure.

Chronic LVF is a progressive disorder

Chronic LVF tends to be a progressive disorder in which a vicious circle becomes established which escalates cardiac workload and worsens the degree of LVF (Fig. 6.13). Because poor cardiac output reduces tissue perfusion, the body responds by increasing sympathetic drive and activating the renin–angiotensin–aldosterone system. The end result is retention of sodium and water by the kidneys, which leads to increasing myocardial stress and declining cardiac function.

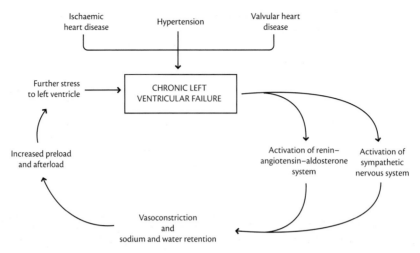

Fig. 6.13 The neurohormonal response in chronic left ventricular failure.

Neurohormonal response in chronic LVF

Because the compensatory mechanisms in chronic LVF involve activation of sympathetic nerves and hormonal systems, it is often referred to as the **neurohormonal response**.

Chronic LVF may be divided into systolic or diastolic failure

In most patients with chronic LVF, the underlying problem is failure of the pumping action of the ventricle during systole. The ventricle is usually dilated and fails to contract normally such that the proportion of blood ejected in each beat (normally 50–70 per cent), the **ejection fraction**, is reduced.

In some patients with symptoms of chronic LVF, systolic function is found not to be impaired. Instead, there is failure of the ventricle to fill adequately due to increased stiffness of the wall. Patients with this finding are said to have *diastolic* chronic LVF. Diastolic cases form the minority of cases of heart failure, but is increasingly recognized in older patients with hypertension. Diastolic dysfunction appears to carry a better prognosis.

Coronary artery atherosclerosis, hypertension, and valve disease account for most cases of chronic LVF

Chronic LVF is best thought of as the end result of any form of persistent heart disease affecting the left ventricle. The most common causes of chronic LVF are:

- **Coronary artery atherosclerosis**, due to episodes of myocardial infarction leading to numerous areas of scarred myocardium with poor contractile function.

- **Hypertension**, by increasing the resistance against which the left ventricle has to pump.

- **Mitral or aortic valve disease**, by increasing the resistance against which the left ventricle has to pump, or by constant refilling of the left ventricle with blood previously pumped out.

Note that very often more than one cause may exist, such as hypertension and ischaemic heart disease. Only once coronary artery atherosclerosis, hypertension, and valvular disease have been rigorously excluded should other causes of chronic LVF be considered.

Patients with chronic LVF feel tired and debilitated

Patients with chronic LVF generally feel pretty rotten due to generalized lethargy and tiredness. Much of this is probably due to effects of poor perfusion of muscle.

Patients with chronic LVF often have a substantial reduction in muscle bulk and early fatiguability.

Congestion in the pulmonary venous system causes breathlessness

Breathlessness is common in chronic LVF due to congestion in the pulmonary veins (Fig. 6.14). Poor function of the respiratory musculature may also play a role. In mild cases, this may only occur on exercise or lying flat (orthopnoea). Paroxysmal nocturnal dyspnoea is a related symptom, where the build up of fluid when lying flat causes sudden onset of breathlessness in the night. As left ventricular function worsens, the breathlessness also worsens until patients are breathless at rest.

Peripheral oedema is also a common manifestation of heart failure

Oedema in heart failure is seen initially in the lower limb extremities, but can progress to quite florid truncal oedema and ascites. It was once attributed to the rise in venous pressure leading to a parallel rise in

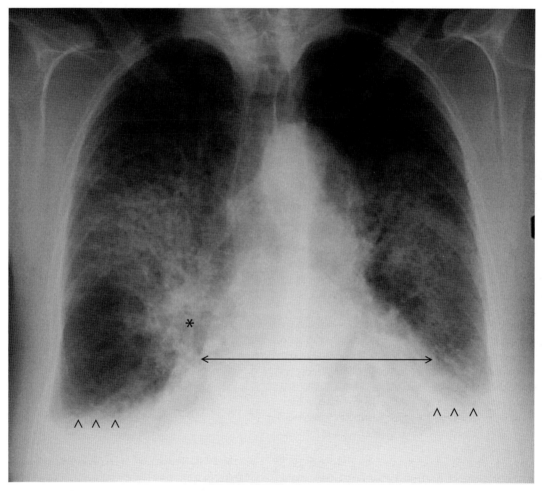

Fig. 6.14 Chest radiograph in severe chronic left ventricular failure. The heart is enlarged, reflecting the dilated chambers (double arrow). The alveolar shadowing represents pulmonary oedema from high pulmonary venous pressure (asterisk). The hemidiaphragms are not visible because of pleural effusions (arrowheads).

ary pressure and oedema (the 'damming back' y). This concept is now known to be untenable, as oedema can precede any demonstrable rise in central venous pressure. Although still very poorly understood, it is widely agreed that the pivotal cause of oedema in chronic LVF is retention of sodium and water by the kidneys in response to activation of the renin–angiotensin–aldosterone system by renal underperfusion.

Arrhythmias are common in heart failure

Disturbances of cardiac rhythm are common consequences of heart failure, regardless of the underlying aetiology. Atrial fibrillation is seen in about one-quarter of patients with heart failure at presentation, and up to half of all patients with established disease. As the disease progresses, ventricular arrhythmias such as ventricular ectopic beats and ventricular tachycardia become increasingly common. Indeed, frequent ventricular arrhythmias recorded on ambulatory ECG monitoring are one of the poor prognostic indicators in patients with heart failure and is a common cause of sudden death.

Echocardiography plays a critical role in the diagnosis of heart failure

Although the diagnosis of chronic LVF may be strongly suspected from a combination of the history, physical examination, chest radiograph, and ECG, all patients should undergo echocardiography. Echocardiography can supply several useful pieces of information. First it can confirm the presence of left ventricular impairment, and determine whether it is systolic or diastolic. Secondly, it can assess the status of the heart valves as they might be the underlying cause of the LVF.

Measurement of BNP is becoming a very useful tool in heart failure

B type natriuretic peptide (BNP) is a hormone secreted by ventricular myocytes in response to volume and pressure overload in the heart. Plasma levels of BNP are raised in patients with poor ventricular function, a finding which is very useful to help distinguish between cardiac and pulmonary causes of shortness of breath. BNP has also been shown to be a powerful prognostic marker for heart failure; higher levels of BNP are associated with a higher relative risk of death. The main drawback of BNP is financial. With each assay costing £15–20, the total cost of testing everyone suspected of having cardiac failure would be extremely high.

Treatment of heart failure aims to relieve symptoms and improve prognosis

Management of chronic LVF is essentially twofold: to relieve symptoms and to improve prognosis. The most commonly used agents for symptomatic relief are loop diuretics, together with agents such as angiotensin-converting enzyme (ACE) inhibitors and β-blockers to improve prognosis. ACE inhibitors in particular have been shown to reduce the rate of progression of heart failure and reduce mortality in all grades of heart failure.

Patients with chronic heart failure may decompensate if their heart is stressed

Patients with chronic heart failure frequently experience episodes of acute worsening in their symptoms. This is often described as 'acute decompensation' and is very commonly seen in routine clinical practice when a concurrent illness (often only a trivial infection) places additional burden on a critically failing heart and pushes the patient into acute failure.

Key points: Heart failure

+ Heart failure refers to a constellation of symptoms and signs which occur when the pumping action of the heart is inadequate for the needs of the body.

+ Heart failure is not a diagnosis; it reflects the end stage of a variety of cardiac diseases which have damaged the heart.

+ Acute heart failure presents dramatically with severe breathlessness due to massive pulmonary oedema. Acute heart failure is most commonly seen following a large myocardial infarction.

+ Chronic heart failure presents insidiously with gradually worsening shortness of breath.

+ Most cases of chronic heart failure are due to chronic LVF.

+ The most common causes of chronic LVF are coronary artery disease, hypertension, and valvular disease.

+ Initially the left ventricle compensates by undergoing hypertrophy but eventually dilates and fails, leading to progressively worsening symptoms of fatigue, breathlessness, and peripheral oedema.

Most patients with chronic heart failure experience a relapsing and remitting course, with periods of stability interspersed with episodes of decompensation, leading to worsening of symptoms which may necessitate hospitalization.

Ischaemic heart disease

Ischaemic heart disease is a very general term for any condition resulting from inadequate blood supply to the heart. In the vast majority of cases, this is due to coronary artery atherosclerosis, and you will find that the terms 'ischaemic heart disease', 'coronary artery disease', and 'coronary heart disease' are all used interchangeably.

The coronary arteries originate from the root of the aorta. The **right coronary artery** supplies most of the right ventricle. The left coronary artery has two main branches, the **left anterior descending artery** and the **circumflex artery,** which together supply the interventricular septum and most of the left ventricle.

Coronary flow depends on a pressure gradient between the aorta and the intramyocardial coronary arterioles. During systole, there is little gradient as the intramyocardial arteries are compressed. Coronary flow is therefore almost entirely diastolic.

The main disorders categorized under ischaemic heart disease are chronic stable angina, the acute coronary syndromes, and acute myocardial infarction. Ischaemic heart disease is also a common cause of disturbances in cardiac rhythm. As we have already seen, ischaemic heart disease is also the most common cause of chronic heart failure.

Chronic stable angina

Stable angina is characterized by episodes of ischaemic chest pain

Stable angina is a clinical picture characterized by recurrent episodes of ischaemic chest pain. Ischaemic chest pain is typically a central, substernal pain which is frequently described using terms such as pressure, gnawing, tightness, and heaviness. The pain may radiate up to the jaw and down the arms, particularly the left arm. Sometimes it may present only as jaw or arm pain.

Symptoms of angina occur when oxygen supply to the myocardium is insufficient

The symptoms of angina are the result of transient episodes of myocardial ischaemia which occur if myocardial oxygen demand outstrips supply. In almost all cases, the underlying cause is a critical stenosis of one or more coronary arteries by large atherosclerotic plaques. Typically the pain is brought on by a predictable level of exercise and is rapidly relieved by rest.

The severity of the symptoms depends on a complex interplay between many factors affecting myocardial oxygen demand and supply. For instance, the development of left ventricular hypertrophy (a common occurrence in elderly people with hypertension or aortic stenosis) will increase myocardial oxygen demand and exacerbate the symptoms.

INTERESTING TO KNOW

Angina with normal coronary arteries

Occasionally, angina can be seen in patients without significant coronary artery atherosclerosis. A common cause is severe aortic stenosis which can lead to angina by increasing myocardial oxygen demand (it causes left ventricular hypertrophy) and reducing coronary blood supply. Coronary blood supply is reduced because the gradient between the aorta and left ventricular diastolic pressure is insufficient to generate adequate flow (remember most coronary artery flow occurs during diastole).

Acute coronary syndromes

Acute coronary syndromes are a spectrum of clinical conditions which occur when there is a sudden severe reduction in myocardial perfusion, resulting in symptoms of severe myocardial ischaemia. An acute coronary syndrome is a medical emergency which if untreated will progress to a full thickness acute myocardial infarction in over 10% of cases. Timely and accurate clinical recognition of an acute coronary syndrome is essential to allow for the rapid and appropriate treatment of this potentially life-threatening condition.

Acute coronary syndromes are due to an acute change in an unstable atherosclerotic plaque

Acute coronary syndromes are almost always due to an abrupt change in an unstable atherosclerotic plaque in a coronary artery. Typically there is erosion or cracking of the plaque, stimulating overlying platelet aggregation, often accompanied by marked spasm of the vessel. Distal embolization of platelet clumps also contributes to the ischaemia.

Acute coronary syndromes cause prolonged ischaemic chest pain

The hallmark of an acute coronary syndrome is persistent ischaemic chest pain. Unlike stable angina, *it does not resolve with rest or pharmacological intervention.* The pain frequently waxes and wanes, lasting from a few minutes to as long as 20–30 min. The precise clinical picture depends on the severity of obstruction, how prolonged it is, and how much myocardium is involved.

Acute coronary syndromes encompass the terms unstable angina and NSTEMI

Included within the spectrum of acute coronary syndromes are the entities known as **unstable angina** and **non-ST elevation myocardial infarction** (NSTEMI). Unstable angina and NSTEMI differ primarily in the severity of myocardial ischaemia (Fig. 6.15). In NSTEMI, the ischaemia is severe enough to result in the release of specific biochemical markers of myocardial necrosis, such as troponin, into the blood.

Blood levels of troponin are therefore used to distinguish between patients with unstable angina and NSTEMI. At the time of presentation, before the results of blood tests are known, unstable angina and NSTEMI are usually indistinguishable.

Troponins are very sensitive and specific markers of myocardial necrosis

Troponins are molecules that regulate the interaction of actin and myosin in muscle. Troponins are released into the blood from damaged muscle. Because cardiac troponins are distinct from skeletal muscle troponins, cardiac troponins are highly sensitive and specific markers of myocardial necrosis, and the level of the rise correlates with the amount of myocyte damage.

The troponin level allows risk stratification in patients with acute coronary syndromes as the more myocardial necrosis there has been, the higher the risk to the patient. The main drawback of troponins are that they may not rise until 12 h after the myocardial damage, meaning that the test cannot be used as an immediate test to rule out a significant cardiac cause of chest pain in A&E.

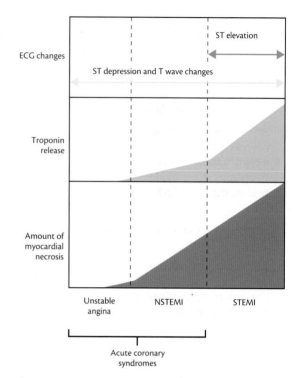

Fig. 6.15 Acute coronary syndromes. The acute coronary syndromes are a continuous spectrum of disease which merge into ST elevation acute myocardial infarction depending on the extent of myocardial necrosis.

Treatment of acute coronary syndrome aims to dissolve the platelet-rich aggregation

The developing mass that forms in cases of acute coronary syndromes tends to be platelet rich. Treatment options include **antiplatelet drugs** such as aspirin, clopidogrel, and glycoprotein IIb/IIIa antagonists, together with **antithrombin drugs** such as low molecular weight heparin.

The number of agents used and the level of aggression of the treatment will depend on how severe the episode is gauged to be. Severity can be gauged according to the extent of the ischaemic changes on the ECG, the level of troponin rise (if any), and the persistence of chest pain. Note that thrombolytic agents such as streptokinase as used for acute myocardial infarction have not been shown to be of benefit in patients with an acute coronary syndrome.

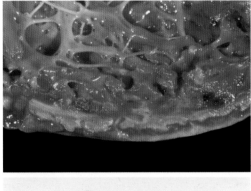

a

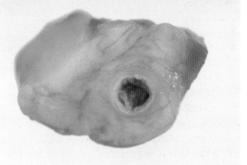

b

Fig. 6.16 (a) Typical appearances of an acute myocardial infarction after 3–4 days due to an occlusive thrombus overlying a ruptured atherosclerotic plaque in the left anterior descending coronary artery (b).

Acute myocardial infarction

Acute myocardial infarction, or 'heart attack', occurs when there is ischaemic death of the full thickness of an area of myocardium. When this occurs, the ECG shows ST elevation in the leads reading the affected areas of the heart. Acute myocardial infarctions are therefore often called **ST elevation myocardial infarctions** (STEMIs) to distinguish them from smaller infarctions which are not full thickness (NSTEMIs).

STEMI is caused by rupture of an unstable atherosclerotic plaque

A full thickness acute myocardial infarction is almost always caused by complete occlusion of a coronary artery by a fibrin-rich thrombus (Fig. 6.16). The thrombus typically forms because an unstable atherosclerotic plaque ruptures, exposing the highly thrombogenic lipid core to the blood.

The site of the infarction is determined by which coronary artery is involved

The extent and distribution of the myocardial infarct depend on which coronary artery is occluded (Fig. 6.17). Most myocardial infarctions affect the left ventricle. Infarction of the right ventricle is less common, but about one half of patients with inferior myocardial infarctions show evidence of right ventricular ischaemia or infarction on ECG. Recognizing these patients is important as their prognosis tends to be worse than those with an isolated inferior left ventricular infarct.

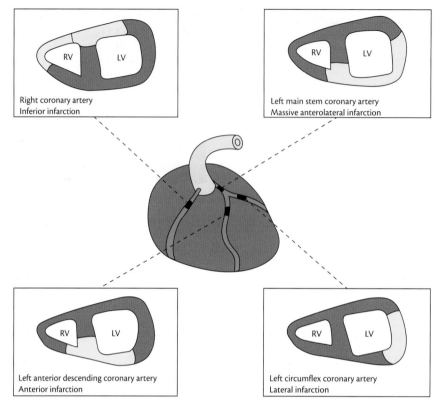

Fig. 6.17 Territories of myocardial infarction according to the coronary artery involved.

STEMI usually presents with severe ischaemic chest pain

Patients with STEMI typically present with severe ischaemic chest pain, which may be indistinguishable from an acute coronary syndrome. The pain is usually sudden, often occurring at rest, and persists until diamorphine is administered. There is often accompanying breathlessness, sweating, and nausea. Patients are very aware that something serious is happening, and often describe a terrifying sense of impending death.

As always in medicine, the classical picture can vary considerably. Whilst the pain is usually very severe, it can be less severe or even absent. So-called 'silent' infarctions are particularly common in diabetics and the elderly. Often the only clue to the infarction is the presence of breathlessness, sweating, or nausea.

Conventional treatment of myocardial infarction includes aspirin to prevent further platelet aggregation and a fibrinolytic drug such as streptokinase to lyse

the occluding thrombus. In centres that can offer the service, primary coronary angioplasty gives the best survival results.

There are many possible complications of ST elevation myocardial infarction

Acute myocardial infarctions have a number of well recognized complications (Table 6.3). These are best divided into short-term complications which are likely to be seen whilst the patient is recovering in hospital, and long-term complications which may surface after the patient has been discharged from hospital.

Acute myocardial infarction is associated with a proarrhythmic environment

Patients with acute myocardial infarction are very prone to developing ventricular arrhythmias. This is probably related to the flood of potassium released from the necrotic myocytes which induces arrhythmias

TABLE 6.3 Complications of acute myocardial infarction

Short term
Rhythm disturbances
Acute left ventricular failure
Rupture of the ventricular wall
Mural thrombus formation
Acute pericarditis
Long term
Chronic cardiac failure
Ventricular aneurysm formation

in the hyperexcitable tissue around the infarct. There are no specific features to help identify those at risk for sustained ventricular arrhythmias, so all patients should be placed on a cardiac monitor.

Ventricular fibrillation is the most feared myocardial infarction-related arrhythmia, leading to instant cardiac arrest and death unless immediate defibrillation is delivered. Ventricular fibrillation is an important cause of death within the first 24 h after infarction.

Ventricular tachycardia is very common in the early post-infarct period. Most cases are self-limiting, without haemodynamic compromise, and do not require treatment.

Accelerated idioventricular rhythm is a type of ventricular arrhythmia which frequently occurs in the first 12 h after infarction, particularly after reperfusion. It is an ectopic rhythm diagnosed on the ECG by the presence of more than three consecutive premature ventricular beats *which has a rate faster than the normal ventricular escape rhythm, but slower than ventricular tachycardia.* It is generally benign, brief (<1 min), and asymptomatic, and thus requires no specific treatment.

Bradycardia may also occur if the infarct affects the function of the sinus node or the atrioventricular node.

Infarction of a large area of the left ventricle may cause acute left ventricular failure

Remember from earlier that the most common cause of sudden acute cardiac failure is a large myocardial infarction. Infarction of a large volume of myocardium produces a heart with inadequate pumping action to sustain cardiac output. The patient with acute LVF is very unwell, with distressing breathlessness from alveolar oedema and signs of cardiovascular insufficiency such as a low blood pressure and tachycardia.

Acute pump failure with the development of shock is known as **cardiogenic shock** and is the most common cause of in-hospital death from acute myocardial infarction.

Rupture of the ventricular wall is a catastrophic event which is often fatal

Rupture of the ventricular wall is a potentially disastrous complication of acute myocardial infarction. Rupture only occurs in full thickness infarcts, as surviving myocardium overlying smaller subendocardial infarcts prevents rupture.

Most ruptures occur 3–5 days after the infarction, a critical window of time during which the infarct is very soft because the extracellular matrix has been degraded by inflammatory cells, but the new matrix has not yet been laid down.

Rupture can also occur sooner after the infarct, although the mechanism is different. Early ruptures tend to occur at the interface between infarcted myocardium and normal myocardium. The kinetic myocardium shears against the akinetic infarcted myocardium and tears through the ventricular wall.

The outcome of ventricular rupture depends on the site. Rupture of the free wall of the left ventricle is the most common site, resulting in haemopericardium and rapid death due to cardiac tamponade. Rupture of the ventricular septum leads to a septal defect with a left-to-right shunt and the onset of acute LVF. Rupture of a papillary muscle of the mitral valve is the least common, causing acute LVF due to acute mitral regurgitation.

Thrombus can form over the akinetic area of myocardium

Inflammation of the endocardium overlying an infarct promotes platelet adhesion and fibrin deposition. Moreover, the poor contractility of the infarcted myocardium allows the early thrombus to continue to grow. Particles of thrombus can detach and cause systemic emboli, risking stroke.

Myocardial infarction is one of the most common causes of acute pericarditis

Pericarditis refers to inflammation of the pericardium. A full thickness acute myocardial infarction is the most common cause of acute pericarditis. Symptoms related to pericarditis usually develop 1–3 days after the myocardial infarction, and may lead to dull chest pain which is distinct from ischaemic chest pain. There is no specific treatment and the pericarditis usually resolves spontaneously.

Chronic LVF and ventricular aneurysm are common long-term complications of STEMI

Patients who have suffered a myocardial infarction are at high risk of developing chronic LVF later in life. These patients have a number of factors which contribute to cardiac failure, including coronary artery atherosclerosis and an element of mitral regurgitation due to poor contractility and shortening of the papillary muscles.

Key points: Acute myocardial infarction

- Acute ST elevation myocardial infarction (STEMI) occurs when there is full thickness infarction of an area of myocardium.

- STEMI is due to rupture of an unstable atherosclerotic plaque stimulating the evolution of an overlying fibrin-rich thrombus which completely occludes a coronary artery.

- STEMI is diagnosed on the basis of appropriate ECG changes together with a compatible history.

- The territory of the infarct depends on which coronary artery is involved, and this can be reliably predicted from the ECG changes.

- Sudden death due to STEMI is usually due to a ventricular arrhythmia.

- Short-term complications of myocardial infarction include acute left ventricular failure, rupture of the ventricular wall, thrombus formation, and acute pericarditis.

- Long-term complications of myocardial infarction include chronic left ventricular failure and ventricular aneurysm formation.

Remodelling of the ventricular wall after the infarct may lead to profound thinning and dilation of the chamber with aneurysmal change. Patients are at increased risk of developing ventricular tachycardia due to re-entry circuits forming along the periphery of the aneurysm. Mural thrombi also often develop within aneurysms and are a source of systemic emboli.

Arrhythmias

Coronary artery disease is the most common cause of cardiac arrhythmias

A cardiac arrhythmia is an abnormality in the timing of the sequence of cardiac depolarization. The mechanism underlying most cardiac arrhythmias is an abnormality in impulse conduction caused by structural heart disease. Damage as a result of ischaemic heart disease leads to areas of slow conduction and provides portals for the generation of abnormal rhythms. Other structural heart disease such as valve disease may also cause arrhythmias.

Most arrhythmias occur transiently, usually as a complication of an ischaemic episode. They usually terminate either spontaneously or with specific treatment. The most important and common arrhythmia that persists in patients and is often an incidental finding is atrial fibrillation.

Atrial fibrillation is the most common sustained cardiac arrhythmia

Atrial fibrillation (AF) results from the presence of multiple small electrical circuits that propagate simultaneously throughout the atria. These chaotic circuits replace the normal sinus rhythm leading to an irregular, fast heart rhythm. On the ECG, AF causes an irregular heart rate and loss of the P wave (the P wave results from coordinated atrial systolic electrical activity).

AF is usually due to an underlying heart disease which stresses the atrial myocardium (Table 6.4). Coronary artery disease, mitral valve disease, and hypertension account

TABLE 6.4   Causes of atrial fibrillation

Coronary artery disease
Hypertension
Mitral valve disease
Hyperthyroidism
Lone AF

for most cases of AF. Some non-cardiac problems such as high alcohol intake and hyperthyroidism are also known to be associated with AF. Sometimes, particularly in younger patients under 60, no clear underlying cause can be found ('lone' AF).

AF causes loss of atrial systole and stasis of blood in the left atrium

AF has two important knock-on effects:

◆ *Loss of atrial systole*. In the normal heart, atrial systolic contraction contributes about 10% of the stroke volume. With advancing age, atrial systole has a greater contribution towards stroke volume (up to 30 per cent), especially if there is co-existing dysfunction of the left ventricle (as there often is in patients with AF). Loss of atrial systole due to AF often causes breathlessness, especially during exercise.

◆ *Stasis of blood within the left atrium*. Stasis of blood is a major risk factor for promoting thrombus formation. Stasis of blood caused by AF renders the left atrium, particularly the left atrial appendage, susceptible to thrombus formation with risk of systemic embolism. Stroke due to cerebral infarction as a result of thromboembolism from the left atrium is a potentially devastating complication of AF.

AF may come to light in a variety of ways

Many cases of AF are picked up incidentally without any obvious symptoms from the arrhythmia in the patient. The irregular pulse may be picked up on physical examination or a routine ECG will show AF. Patients presenting with symptoms may do so with palpitations, a reduced exercise tolerance, or more dramatically with an embolic event such as a transient ischaemic attack or stroke. Remember that the underlying disorder causing the AF may also lead to symptoms.

AF can be classified to help guide treatment

AF is often divided into three categories:

◆ Paroxysmal (spontaneous return to sinus rhythm)

◆ Persistent (sinus rhythm achievable with intervention)

◆ Permanent (sinus rhythm not achievable even with intervention).

Generally speaking, paroxysmal and persistent AF will eventually progress to permanent AF, especially where there is underlying heart disease. This classification is useful clinically as it guides appropriate management strategies.

In paroxysmal and persistent AF, the aim is to restore and maintain sinus rhythm. This improves symptoms by reinstating atrial systolic contribution to stroke volume and removes the risk of thrombosis. In permanent AF, however, sinus rhythm cannot be restored, so the aim of treatment is to control the heart rate and prevent thrombosis with anticoagulants.

Key points: Atrial fibrillation

◆ AF is common in the elderly and is an important cause of stroke.

◆ The most common causes of AF are coronary artery disease, hypertension, and mitral valve disease. AF therefore often co-exists with other types of heart disease.

◆ AF is often asymptomatic, the diagnosis being made incidentally on physical examination or ECG.

◆ AF can be divided into paroxysmal, persistent, and permanent.

◆ The aim of treating paroxysmal and persistent AF is restoration of sinus rhythm.

◆ Permanent AF is treated with drugs to control the heart rate and anticoagulation to prevent thromboembolic stroke in high risk patients.

Valvular heart disease

The cardiac valves are thin flexible membranes which close tightly to prevent backward flow of blood in the heart. A variety of inflammatory, infectious, and degenerative diseases can damage cardiac valves and impair their function. The most commonly affected valves are left sided, i.e. the mitral and aortic valves.

The normal aortic valve has three leaflets which are attached to the aortic wall at a tough fibrous structure called the **annulus**. The shape of the leaflets allows blood to leave the left ventricle during systole but prevents its regurgitation during diastole.

The mitral valve is a bicuspid valve. The two leaflets, like the aortic valve, are attached to an annulus. Unlike the aortic valve, however, the mitral valve leaflets are also supported by an apparatus consisting of **chordae tendinae** which connect the leaflets to **papillary muscles**. The annulus acts as an anchor against which the papillary muscles contract during systole, pulling the cusps together and holding blood within the ventricle. The proper functioning of the mitral valve therefore depends on the integrity not only of the valve leaflets, but also of the chordae and the papillary muscles.

Diseased valves may become stenosed and/or regurgitant

When a valve becomes damaged, the leaflets may become thickened or fused enough to narrow the aperture and obstruct blood flow. This is called valvular stenosis. Stenosis of a valve leads to pressure overload of the heart chamber trying to pump blood through the narrowed valve orifice. Similar to the effects of hypertension, this leads to pathological hypertrophy of the heart in an attempt to compensate. Eventually, however, the chamber is unable to maintain adequate output in the face of the increased burden: the chamber dilates and fails.

Diseases that destroy the valve tissue may allow retrograde blood flow. This is called valvular regurgitation or insufficiency. Valvular regurgitation also increases the work of the heart because a large proportion of blood pumped out of a chamber spills back in through the incompetent valve.

The clinical effects of regurgitation depend on the speed with which it develops

Unlike valvular *stenosis* which usually develops slowly over time, *regurgitation* may develop suddenly or slowly. If the regurgitation develops slowly, the volume load increases gradually allowing the heart chambers to accommodate the increased workload by undergoing hypertrophy to maintain cardiac output. The patient initially remains asymptomatic until the heart can no longer cope and the chambers dilate, leading to the development of symptoms of chronic heart failure, i.e. fatigue, breathlessness on exertion, and orthopnoea.

In contrast, if a valve becomes *suddenly* regurgitant, the affected heart chambers cannot accommodate the sudden increase in volume. The heart instantly fails to maintain cardiac output, resulting in acute heart failure with sudden cardiovascular compromise. These patients become acutely very unwell.

Valvular disease has a number of consequences on the function of the heart

We have just seen how valvular diseases, by increasing the work of the heart, are a common cause of chronic heart failure. A number of other cardiac conditions are also related to valvular diseases, illustrating how the impact of disease in one part of the heart can lead to disease of other parts.

◆ By destroying valve tissue, infective endocarditis may cause valvular disease. However, valvular disease of any kind is also a risk factor for developing endocarditis.

◆ Chamber dilation and remodelling in response to volume or pressure overload predisposes to the development of arrhythmias. This is particularly seen with mitral valve disease and atrial fibrillation.

Having considered some general principles of valvular disease, we now move on to consider the common individual valve diseases in more detail.

Mitral stenosis

Chronic rheumatic valvular disease is the most common cause of mitral stenosis

Acute rheumatic fever is an immunologically mediated inflammatory disease which occasionally occurs a few weeks after an episode of Group A streptococcal pharyngitis. The precise mechanisms underlying the disease remain elusive; however, it is strongly suspected that acute rheumatic fever is due to antibodies against certain Group A streptococci cross-reacting with native tissues in the body, including the joints, skin, and the heart. Involvement of the heart is known as acute rheumatic heart disease or acute rheumatic carditis.

Acute rheumatic carditis is a *pancarditis*, i.e. it involves all three layers of the heart (endocardium, myocardium, and pericardium). The myocardial and pericardial components of rheumatic pancarditis typically resolve without permanent sequelae. In contrast, the acute valvulitis may progress to **chronic rheumatic valvular disease**. During the healing phase, the valve leaflets develop diffuse fibrosis causing them to become deformed, thickened, and less pliable. Adhesions develop between the leaflets, resulting in a stenotic valve that does not open freely. Symptoms from mitral stenosis do not usually develop until more than 10 years after the acute episode.

Although the incidence of overt acute rheumatic disease in the developed world has fallen, chronic rheumatic valvular disease remains by far the most common cause of mitral stenosis. Other causes are rare.

A stenosed mitral valve slows the movement of blood from the left atrium into the left ventricle

The main disturbance in mitral stenosis is slow filling of the left ventricle during diastole. This does not matter too much at rest when the heart rate is slow because the filling period is relatively long. However, when the heart rate increases upon exercising, adequate flow from the left atrium to the left ventricle can only be maintained by increasing left atrial pressure through left atrial hypertrophy. Eventually the left atrium fails, leading to pulmonary venous congestion.

The main symptom of mitral stenosis is progressive breathlessness

Patients with mitral stenosis usually present with the gradual onset of breathlessness as the left atrium enlarges and fails. Sometimes the onset of breathlessness occurs more abruptly; this is often due to the onset of AF. Because patients with mitral stenosis rely on atrial systole to fill their left ventricle, the development of AF can lead to a significant reduction in cardiac output. The development of AF also predisposes patients to developing thrombosis in the left atrium, with risk of systemic embolization.

Unlike mitral regurgitation and aortic valve disease, in mitral stenosis the left ventricle is usually not enlarged or dilated as it is not overloaded. *Mitral stenosis is therefore one of only a few causes of chronic left-sided heart failure due to failure of the left atrium rather than the left ventricle.*

Mitral regurgitation

Mitral regurgitation may be acute or chronic. Chronic mitral regurgitation has many causes, but the most common are ischaemic heart disease, mitral valve prolapse, and infective endocarditis. It is important to appreciate that a degree of physiological mitral regurgitation is often present in young fit people and has no pathological significance.

Ischaemic heart disease is the most common cause of chronic mitral regurgitation

Ischaemic heart disease leads to chronic incompetence of the mitral valve by impairing contraction of the papillary muscles. The papillary muscles are particularly vulnerable to ischaemia because they are supplied by terminal branches of the coronary arteries. Patients with ischaemic heart disease also often have co-existent LVF associated with ventricular dilation. Dilation of the ventricle widens the valve annulus, drawing the cusps of the valve apart and further contributing to the regurgitation.

In mitral valve prolapse the valve cusps become thinned and floppy

Mitral valve prolapse or 'floppy mitral valve' is a condition in which the mitral valve leaflets accumulate large amounts of mucoid material causing them to stretch and billow into the left atrium during ventricular systole. The reason behind the accumulation of mucoid material is unclear but is thought to be due to an inherited defect affecting extracellular matrix metabolism.

In most cases, mitral valve prolapse is an isolated finding but may also be found as part of a variety of other conditions, such as Marfan's syndrome and autosomal dominant polycystic kidney disease. Although the condition is common, only a minority of patients have severe enough mitral regurgitation to warrant surgical treatment.

Chronic mitral regurgitation causes volume overload of the left ventricle

In the presence of mitral regurgitation, much of the output of the left ventricle in systole is back into the left atrium rather than into the aorta. The backward movement begins almost immediately after the start of left ventricular contraction when the aortic valve is still closed. This is not surprising given the lower pressure in the left atrium. By the time the aortic valve opens, up to a quarter of the stroke volume may have already entered the left atrium.

In chronic mitral regurgitation, the process develops sufficiently slowly to allow the left atrium to stretch and accommodate the regurgitant blood without any significant rise in pressure. This protects the pulmonary circulation from a rise in pressure, so the patient is initially asymptomatic. As the disease advances and the left atrium can no longer cope, left atrial pressure begins to rise, leading to progressive congestion in the pulmonary venous system. The patient then develops symptoms of heart failure.

Many patients with chronic mitral regurgitation can be managed medically with drugs to enhance emptying of the left ventricle. However, patients with significant disease should be considered for surgical intervention. Repair of the valve is increasingly favoured in mitral regurgitation and has excellent results, but replacement may be the best option if there is severe disease.

The most common cause of acute mitral incompetence is papillary muscle rupture

In acute mitral regurgitation, the valve becomes suddenly incompetent. The most common cause is rupture of a papillary muscle as a complication of a left ventricular myocardial infarction. A sudden volume load is imposed on the left atrium during ventricular systole. Left atrial pressure abruptly rises leading to a rise in pulmonary venous pressure. The patient develops acute heart failure and becomes very unwell with severe breathlessness.

Aortic stenosis

Aortic stenosis is the most common valve disease

Aortic stenosis is a narrowing of the aortic valve orifice commonly seen in elderly people. Aortic stenosis is usually caused by calcification in the valve cusps related to the cumulative effects of years of trauma from turbulent blood flow across the valve (Fig. 6.18).

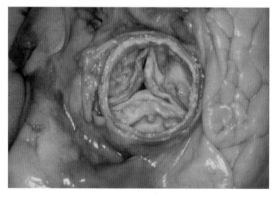

Fig. 6.18 Calcific aortic stenosis. This aortic valve is studded with nodules of calcium causing significant narrowing of the valve orifice.

This would explain why aortic stenosis in younger people is invariably related to the presence of a congenitally bicuspid valve whose shape promotes turbulent flow through the valve.

Aortic stenosis may also be caused by rheumatic aortic valve disease. Rheumatic changes are characterized by diffuse fibrous thickening and scarring of the cusps. Like degenerative aortic stenosis there may be calcification, but unique to rheumatic disease is actual fusion of the commissures. Rheumatic aortic valve disease almost always occurs with co-involvement of the mitral valve.

There is a long asymptomatic period in aortic stenosis

Aortic stenosis may be present for many years and produce few, if any, clinical symptoms. Sometimes the condition may be diagnosed if the harsh ejection systolic murmur is picked up during a routine examination. The typical symptoms are chest pain, syncope, and breathlessness, which usually develop in that order and reflect worsening prognosis. Once symptoms due to aortic stenosis appear, urgent surgical valve replacement is indicated as the risk of sudden death increases dramatically with the onset of symptoms. Asymptomatic patients, even with severe stenosis, are usually just kept under regular review.

JARGON BUSTER

Aortic sclerosis

Do not confuse aortic *sclerosis* with aortic *stenosis*, as the two are different. **Aortic sclerosis** refers to mild thickening of the aortic valve but *without obstruction to outflow from the left ventricle*, and occurs in up to a quarter of elderly people. An ejection systolic murmur may also be present, but no significant pressure gradient can be demonstrated across the valve at echocardiography. Aortic sclerosis can progress to aortic stenosis.

Aortic regurgitation

Aortic regurgitation may present acutely or chronically

Acute aortic regurgitation is most commonly seen as a complication of aortic valve endocarditis or an aortic dissection that has extended proximally to involve the aortic valve ring. Acute aortic regurgitation presents suddenly with acute heart failure or cardiogenic shock, together with symptoms related to the underlying cause, i.e. tearing chest pain in aortic dissection, and fever in endocarditis. Acute aortic regurgitation is an emergency, requiring prompt surgical intervention.

Chronic aortic regurgitation is caused by diseases that slowly dilate the aortic root (such as Marfan's syndrome or ankylosing spondylitis) or by abnormalities of the valve leaflets, which are usually congenital. The regurgitation leads to chronic overload of the left ventricle with compensatory changes so that cardiac output remains normal. Patients experience a long asymptomatic period as the left ventricle gradually dilates until symptoms of chronic heart failure occur. Treatment is indicated once symptoms begin or once there is evidence of left ventricular dysfunction. Patients should therefore be reviewed every year to check for symptoms and to undergo echocardiography to assess the function of their left ventricle.

Key points: Valvular heart disease

- Valvular heart disease may result in stenosis or regurgitation of the valve.

- Stenosis always develops slowly and usually presents with the onset of chronic heart failure.

- Regurgitation may occur acutely or chronically. Acute valve regurgitation results in acute heart failure necessitating urgent treatment. Chronic valve regurgitation develops slowly, causing symptoms of chronic heart failure.

- Aortic stenosis and mitral regurgitation are the two most common valve diseases.

- Aortic stenosis is usually due to degenerative calcification of the valve as a result of ageing. Symptomatic aortic stenosis demands urgent valve replacement.

- Mitral regurgitation is usually due to either ischaemic heart disease or mitral valve prolapse. Medical management with drugs can be sufficient, but, in patients with significant disease, surgery should be considered.

Infective endocarditis

Infective endocarditis is an infection of the interior surface of the heart

Infective endocarditis is a serious disease caused by infection of part of the interior surface of the heart. In most cases, a heart valve is affected, but the process can involve the endocardial surface of the atrium or ventricle.

Infective endocarditis arises through the following sequence of events:

- Bacteria are delivered to the heart during an episode of bacteraemia. This may be due to an event as trivial as tooth brushing, or associated with a more invasive procedure such as surgery.

- The organisms adhere to, and invade, the valve. The endocardium is normally very resistant to infection, so for infection to occur either there must be an abnormality of the endocardium which allows colonization by weakly pathogenic organisms, or, if the endocardium is normal, the organisms must be highly pathogenic.

- Multiplication of the bacteria. As the bacteria replicate, they become enmeshed within layers of platelets and fibrin on the valve surface, which protect them from host defences. As the infection continues, bulky friable masses called **vegetations** form which destroy the underlying valve (Fig. 6.19). The destruction is thought to be due to valvular softening caused by release of enzymes from activated neutrophils recruited to the site of infection.

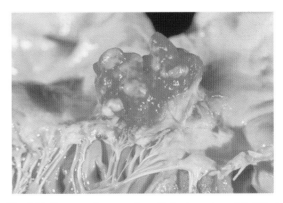

Fig. 6.19 Close-up of a vegetation of infective endocarditis. This is on the mitral valve; you can see the chordae tendinae attached to the valve leaflets.

Features common to all types of infective endocarditis include fever and constitutional symptoms due to the persisting infection, symptoms and signs related to valve damage, and a risk of septic emboli if the friable vegetations fragment. The degree of symptoms and the speed with which they develop vary markedly, depending on the virulence of the organism causing the endocarditis.

INTERESTING TO KNOW

Non-bacterial thrombotic endocarditis

Non-bacterial thrombotic endocarditis ('marantic endocarditis') refers to the presence of *sterile* vegetations on normal cardiac valves. It is commonly seen as a paraneoplastic condition complicating adenocarcinomas, particularly of pancreatic and gastrointestinal origin.

The cause of non-bacterial thrombotic endocarditis is not clear, but is thought to be related to a combination of immune complex deposition and increased blood coagulability. Unlike infective endocarditis, the vegetations of non-bacterial thrombotic endocarditis do not destroy the affected valve and there is no inflammation. As such, they do not cause cardiac complications, the main risk being embolization and infarction of distant organs.

Acute endocarditis is usually caused by S. aureus and may involve normal valves

Acute endocarditis is a fulminant illness in which symptoms of breathlessness and fatigue develop within days due to acute heart failure. There is rapid progression and a high risk of death.

The most common organism causing acute endocarditis is *Staphylococcus aureus*, a common skin commensal which gains access to the blood during invasive procedures. Two particularly common routes of inoculation which account for its prevalence are through indwelling intravascular lines and intravenous drug use.

Staphylococcus aureus has a particular affinity for establishing infection in the endocardium. It can directly colonize and invade the endocardium, even over entirely normal native valves. The infection is extremely destructive, and early valve replacement is needed more often

for *S. aureus* endocarditis than for other microbial causes.

Left-sided *S. aureus* endocarditis presents acutely with fever and signs of valve damage. Major systemic embolic events are commonly encountered: the most serious site of involvement is the central nervous system where emboli can cause brain abscesses. The mortality is high.

Right-sided *S. aureus* endocarditis, which usually involves the tricuspid valve, is primarily a disease of intravenous drug abusers. The disease presents acutely with fever and chills. A very important clue to the diagnosis is the presence of prominent pulmonary symptoms which are the result of numerous septic emboli lodging in the lungs.

Subacute endocarditis occurs in people with a structural abnormality of the heart

Subacute endocarditis is a less fulminant disease which occurs in people who are predisposed to valve infection by a structural abnormality of the heart. Patients with prosthetic heart valves are also included in this group.

The clinical picture is dominated by fever and constitutional symptoms rather than the effects of rapid valve destruction. The diagnosis may be difficult and is often overlooked. Because of its more prolonged clinical course, subacute endocarditis may be associated with a number of well described immunological manifestations due to the effects of persisting low grade inflammation. These include skin petechiae, retinal haemorrhages, and glomerulonephritis as a result of immune complex deposition within these tissues.

Many of the more exotic clinical manifestations of endocarditis that most textbooks describe in all their glory (Janeway lesions, Osler's nodes, Roth spots, clubbing, etc.) are all features of advanced untreated disease and are actually very rarely encountered in routine practice.

The most common organisms implicated in subacute endocarditis are streptococci

Most cases of subacute endocarditis are caused by *Streptococcus viridans*, a group of α-haemolytic streptococci which usually colonize the oropharynx and gain access to the heart during trivial episodes of bacteraemia, often associated with tooth brushing.

Streptococcus viridans are weakly pathogenic organisms which cannot directly infect the endocardium unless there is an underlying abnormality in the heart. The defects with the highest risk of endocarditis are those that form high velocity jets of blood between a high pressure system and a low pressure system, e.g. small ventricular septal defects and aortic regurgitation. If these damage an area of endocardium they lead to the formation of a small sterile lesion composed of platelets, fibrin, and macrophages which is then secondarily infected by the streptococci during episodes of bacteraemia.

Blood cultures and echocardiography are essential investigations in endocarditis

Any patient suspected of having infective endocarditis must have two essential investigations: **echocardiography** and **blood cultures**. Echocardiography allows imaging of the heart valves to identify the presence of vegetations and to assess valve function. Blood cultures are required to isolate the organism responsible for the endocarditis. At least three samples of blood from three different sites should be taken for culture over a 24 h period. A strict aseptic procedure is essential to prevent contamination of the sample. Distinguishing a genuine bacteraemia from contamination can be difficult; however, any organism isolated from at least two different sets of blood cultures is usually significant.

Infective endocarditis requires long-term treatment with antibiotics

Eradication of infection in endocarditis requires several weeks of treatment with high doses of intravenous antibiotics. Such intense treatment is required because the vegetations have a poor blood supply, and prolonged treatment is needed to eradicate the infection.

Key points: Infective endocarditis

- Infective endocarditis is an infection of the interior surface of the heart, which most commonly occurs on valve surfaces.

- Acute endocarditis is a fulminant illness caused by infection of native valves by pathogenic organisms such as *S. aureus*. Rapid valve destruction and acute heart failure occur, necessitating urgent valve replacement.

- Subacute endocarditis is a more protracted disease caused by weakly pathogenic organisms such as *S. viridans* infecting structurally abnormal valves. Fever is the dominant symptom, and most patients have a regurgitant murmur.

- Transthoracic echocardiography is needed to identify vegetations, and repeated blood cultures are necessary to identify the causative organism.

- Highly bactericidal antibiotics are needed intravenously for several weeks to eradicate infection.

Myocarditis

Myocarditis is usually caused by direct viral infection of the myocardium

Myocarditis refers to inflammation of the myocardium with necrosis of cardiac myocytes. The most common cause of myocarditis is viral infection of the myocardium, usually by coxsackie B virus.

An episode of acute myocarditis usually causes a non-specific flu-like illness with fatigue. Chest pain occurs in a minority of patients. It is very important to remember that necrosis of cardiac myocytes may lead to a rise in troponin levels in the blood, and in a patient with chest pain this may lead to an erroneous diagnosis of an acute coronary syndrome.

A small proportion of patients with viral myocarditis develop chronic heart failure

Myocarditis is usually a self-limiting illness which resolves with analgesia and rest. Occasionally patients suffer arrhythmias. The only important long-term complication is the small chance of developing chronic heart failure. Often the patient will not recall the original episode of myocarditis which was dismissed as 'flu'. Whenever a young patient or a patient with no evidence of ischaemic heart disease presents with heart failure, the possibility of previous myocarditis should be considered although causation is often difficult to prove. It has been suggested that many cases of dilated cardiomyopathy are the result of previous episodes of viral myocarditis.

Cardiomyopathy

Cardiomyopathy is a general term for a disease of heart muscle

The term **cardiomyopathy** was originally coined to describe a group of heart diseases resulting from a primary abnormality of the myocardium. They accounted for a small minority of patients with heart disease who did not have coronary artery disease, valvular disease, or hypertension.

Terminology has been an area of confusion here, as many clinicians use the term cardiomyopathy more generally for any disease of heart muscle. To clear up any confusion, the World Health Organization has recommended that cardiomyopathies be categorized into two groups: specific cardiomyopathies and primary cardiomyopathies.

Specific cardiomyopathies include ischaemic heart disease, valvular heart disease, and hypertensive heart disease, as well as involvement of heart muscle by a systemic problem such as sarcoidosis or alcohol.

Primary cardiomyopathies are diseases intrinsic to the myocardium. This group includes three main conditions: dilated cardiomyopathy, hypertrophic cardiomyopathy, and arrhythmogenic right ventricular cardiomyopathy (Fig. 6.20). It is becoming increasingly clear that there is a genetic basis to the primary cardiomyopathies, with mutations in genes coding for various proteins involved in the function of cardiac myocytes having been implicated.

Dilated cardiomyopathy is the most common of the primary cardiomyopathies

Dilated cardiomyopathy (DCM) is by far the most commonly encountered primary cardiomyopathy. The heart becomes enlarged and flabby due to dilation and thinning of all four cardiac chambers. As this pattern

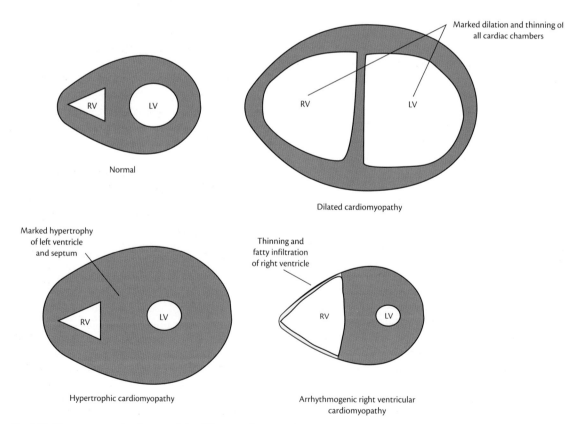

Fig. 6.20 Diagram comparing features of the different cardiomyopathies.

can be seen as the end result of any cause of heart disease, common causes of left ventricular failure *must* be excluded before making a diagnosis of DCM, in particular coronary artery disease, hypertension, and valvular disease. Valvular disease can be easily overlooked, especially calcific aortic stenosis producing only a soft or absent murmur. It has been suggested that many cases of dilated cardiomyopathy are the result of previous viral myocarditis.

Dilated cardiomyopathy usually presents with symptoms of cardiac failure. As we have seen, these include fatigue, breathlessness, and decreased exercise tolerance. Often clinical presentation is precipitated by an event such as upper respiratory tract infection or an extra fluid load, especially pregnancy. Sometimes the diagnosis may be made earlier in the course of the disease before symptoms of cardiac failure have begun, for instance due to an arrhythmia or a systemic embolus. Severe DCM is one of the most common reasons for heart transplantation.

Hypertrophic cardiomyopathy is defined by unexplained myocardial hypertrophy

In **hypertrophic cardiomyopathy** (HCM), the left ventricle and septum become enormously thickened for no apparent underlying reason. In order to make the diagnosis, any possible cause of left ventricular hypertrophy must be excluded. Making the diagnosis can often be extremely difficult, especially in athletes and in patients with mild hypertension in whom one has to decide whether the hypertrophy is greater than one would expect.

Fortunately the histological findings in HCM are, however, quite distinctive and provide the basis for a pathological diagnosis. The key feature is loss of the normal organization of myocytes and muscle bundles ('myocyte disarray').

HCM has a very wide spectrum of clinical presentation. Up to half of patients with HCM do not present with symptoms, but are diagnosed during family screening of an affected individual or as an unsuspected finding on physical, electrocardiographic, or echocardiographic examination. In adults presenting with symptoms, the most common symptoms are exertional chest pain and palpitations. Some patients may experience syncopal episodes, but the most worrying feature of HCM is its well recognized ability to cause sudden unexplained death on exertion, often in young adults. Thankfully this is a rare feature of HCM.

Arrhythmogenic right ventricular cardiomyopathy has only recently been described

Arrhythmogenic right ventricular cardiomyopathy (ARVC) is characterized by inflammation and thinning of the right ventricular wall associated with replacement of the myocardium with a mixture of fat and fibrous tissue. ARVC is thought to be due to mutations in cell adhesion genes which cause myocytes under mechanical stress to detach and die, with subsequent fibrofatty replacement.

The clinical presentation of ARVC is usually with an arrhythmia of right ventricular origin. The arrhythmia may be lethal, and sudden death related to exercise may be the initial manifestation of the disease. It is difficult to know how common ARVC is, as many patients probably remain asymptomatic.

Key points: Cardiomyopathy

- Cardiomyopathy refers to an intrinsic disorder of the myocardium.

- Cardiomyopathies may be specific or primary.

- Primary cardiomyopathies are thought to have a genetic basis.

- Dilated cardiomyopathy is the most common primary cardiomyopathy. It presents with symptoms of chronic heart failure with dilation of all four chambers of the heart but no clear underlying cause.

- Hypertrophic cardiomyopathy is characterized by unexplained hypertrophy of the left ventricle and septum. HCM can present in many ways, but the most important is sudden death due to a lethal arrhythmia.

- Arrhythmogenic right ventricular cardiomyopathy is the most recently described primary cardiomyopathy, characterized by thinning and fibrofatty replacement of the right ventricular wall. ARVC is also a cause of sudden death in young people due to a fatal arrhythmia.

Tumours of the heart

Tumours of the heart are extremely rare, presumably because most of the cells within the heart are terminally differentiated and so do not divide. The most common primary tumour is the **myxoma**, a benign tumour thought to arise from connective tissue cells which normally lie just underneath the endocardium.

Most myxomas arise in the left atrium as golfball-sized masses projecting into the left atrial cavity. Most present with breathlessness related to obstruction of the left ventricular inflow tract. The tumour is easily identified on echocardiography (Fig. 6.21).

Although the tumour is benign, excision is always performed urgently due to the risk of the friable tumour fragmenting and embolizing into the systemic circulation. At surgery, complete removal is ensured by excising the tumour at its base with a full thickness piece of atrial septum. The resulting defect in the atrial septum is repaired with a small patch.

Diseases of veins

Most important venous disease involves the veins of the leg. The limb veins can be divided into superficial

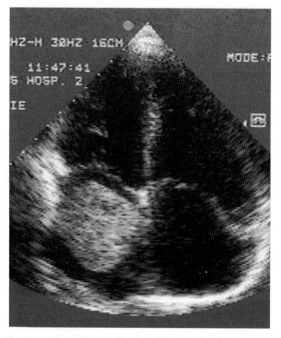

Fig. 6.21 Echocardiogram showing all four cardiac chambers with a myxoma filling most of the left atrium.

veins and deep veins according to their position relative to the deep fascia of the leg. The principal superficial veins of the lower limb are the long and short saphenous veins. Perforating veins connect the long saphenous vein with the deep veins; the valves of the perforating veins are arranged so as to prevent flow of blood back from the deep to the superficial veins.

Varicose veins

Varicose veins are caused by failure of the valves in superficial leg veins

Varicose veins are extremely common. They are tortuous dilated superficial leg veins, which come about when the superficial leg veins become engorged with blood due to failure of the valves. The mechanisms that cause the superficial vein valves to fail are still not known. What seems to happen is that the valve cusps degenerate and holes begin to develop in them. As each valve becomes progressively incompetent, there is increasing strain on the valve downstream. It is well recognized that occupations that require long periods of standing predispose to varicose veins, as in this position the pressure in the veins is elevated by up to 10 times. Since four-legged animals do not develop varicose veins, they appear to be the price we pay for our erect posture!

People with varicose veins usually present for cosmetic reasons

It is the unsightly appearance of varicose veins that most commonly leads to presentation. They can also lead to aching or discomfort in the legs, but uncomplicated varicose veins do not normally cause pain. Occasionally complications of varicose veins may develop. Thrombosis within them, known as **superficial thrombophlebitis**, can cause considerable discomfort, but fortunately significant embolism is rare. Trauma to a large varicose vein can lead to considerable haemorrhage, but this is easily controlled by elevating the leg and applying compression bandaging. The most serious problem is the development of venous ulceration in the leg, which is discussed below. Venous ulceration due entirely to superficial venous disease is known as **varicose ulceration**.

The deep veins of the leg can also become incompetent

Incompetence of the valves of the deep veins of the leg can also develop, probably in a similar way to varicose veins due to degeneration of the valve cusps.

In some patients, the valves of the deep veins are destroyed as a complication of a deep vein thrombosis. Although deep venous incompetence does not lead to visible tortuous veins, the development of skin complications (particularly venous ulceration) is a problem.

Venous hypertension in the lower limb

Venous hypertension leads to a range of skin problems of the lower limb

A proportion of patients with persistently elevated pressure in the veins of the leg develop skin complications as a result of effects on the microcirculation in the skin. An early sign of skin injury is brown pigmentation due to haemosiderin deposition in the skin which occurs because of bleeding from damaged skin capillaries. A later stage is **lipodermatosclerosis** which is a fibrotic process in which palpable induration develops in the skin and subcutaneous tissues. This particularly affects the area of the leg just above the malleoli, and may be the precursor of leg ulceration.

Venous disease is the most common cause of leg ulceration

Venous disease of the lower limb is the most common cause of leg ulceration in the Western world. However, other important causes to consider are atherosclerotic arterial disease (peripheral vascular disease) and diabetes.

Venous ulcers are usually located just above the medial or lateral malleolus and are almost always accompanied by the other skin changes of venous disease, i.e. haemosiderosis and lipodermatosclerosis (Fig. 6.22). If these are not present, then the ulcer is highly unlikely to be of venous origin.

Venous ulcers may be notoriously slow to heal and often require long-term regular application of compression bandaging, a task which is responsible for an enormous amount of work in the health service.

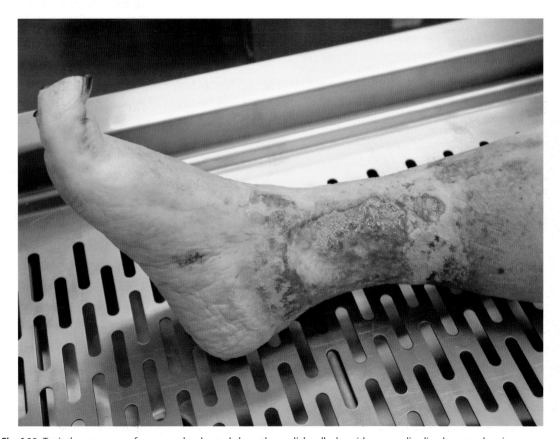

Fig. 6.22 Typical appearances of a venous ulcer located above the medial malleolus with surrounding lipodermatosclerosis.

TABLE 6.5 Risk factors for deep vein thrombosis
Long-haul flights
Immobility (bed rest >4 days)
Pregnancy
High dose oestrogen therapy
Recent surgery, particularly to the pelvis or lower limb
Malignancy
Congenital and acquired abnormalities of clotting

Deep vein thrombosis

Deep vein thrombosis is a common problem with potentially fatal complications

The great majority of venous thrombi occur in the deep veins of the leg. A number of risk factors are associated with the development of deep vein thrombosis (Table 6.5). Thrombi in the larger deep leg veins, especially those above the knee, are serious because they are much more likely to embolize. The most feared complication of venous thrombosis is embolism to the pulmonary arteries, causing a pulmonary embolism.

The effects of deep venous obstruction are often offset by collateral channels, meaning that deep venous thrombosis may be entirely asymptomatic in up to 50% of affected patients and may only come to light when the patient develops symptoms of a pulmonary embolism.

Key points: Venous disease

- The most common venous diseases involve the veins of the lower limbs.

- The veins in the legs can be divided into superficial and deep according to their position relative to the deep fascia of the leg.

- Varicose veins are visibly dilated tortuous superficial leg veins which occur due to failure of their valves. People usually present for cosmetic reasons.

- Failure of the valvular system of the deep leg veins may also occur. Although this does not lead to visibly dilated veins, the venous hypertension can lead to prominent changes in the skin of the lower limb.

- Venous hypertension in the leg causes a range of skin problems, the most important of which is venous ulceration of the lower limb.

- Deep vein thrombosis is the most important venous disease of the lower limb because of the risk of developing pulmonary embolism, a potentially fatal complication.

CHAPTER 7

Respiratory disease

Chapter contents

Introduction

The lungs are the organs of gas exchange. The process of gas exchange occurs in **alveoli** which are tiny (0.2 mm diameter) thin sacs where inhaled air comes into very close contact with capillaries of the lung, allowing diffusion of oxygen and carbon dioxide to and from the blood.

Each of the 300 million alveoli in the lungs must be connected to the environment if they are to participate in gas exchange. The connection is achieved by a large number of airways which all originate from successive branching of the trachea (Fig. 7.1). The first 16 generations of airways, which comprise the bronchi and bronchioles, are the conducting airways.

The functional unit of the lungs, the **acinus** (plural = **acini**), is that portion which is distal to the terminal bronchiole. The acinus comprises the respiratory bronchioles, the alveolar ducts, and the alveolar sacs, each of which give off increasing numbers of alveoli.

The entire respiratory tree from the nasal cavity to the respiratory bronchioles is lined by respiratory type epithelium, a pseudostratified epithelium consisting of a mixture of ciliated cells, mucus-secreting goblet cells, and neuroendocrine cells. These three epithelial cell types are all derived from the basal cells of the epithelium which function as precursor cells. As we shall see later, the basal cells are important as we think they are the cells that give rise to lung carcinomas.

Like many other organ systems, lung disease can be conveniently thought about by dividing up the organ into its constituent compartments, i.e. the airways, the lung parenchyma, the blood vessels, and the pleural surfaces. In this chapter, we will begin by discussing respiratory failure and bronchiectasis, both of which

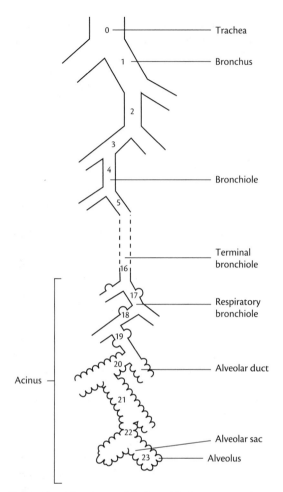

Fig. 7.1 Branching airways of the lungs. The first 16 generations contain no alveoli and are purely conducting airways. The next seven generations contain progressively more alveoli in the airway walls, and serve the dual purpose of conducting air to the alveolar sacs and also providing gas exchange.

may complicate a number of lung diseases, before going on to the core diseases affecting each of the four main components of the lung.

Hypoxia and respiratory failure

Hypoxia

Diseases of the lung which impair gas exchange cause hypoxia

There are two principal mechanisms by which pulmonary disease may lead to hypoxia: ventilation/perfusion mismatching and alveolar hypoventilation.

Ventilation/perfusion mismatching describes an area of lung in which there is an imbalance between ventilation and perfusion, such that blood leaving this part of the lung is poorly oxygenated. Ventilation/perfusion mismatching is the major mechanism by which most respiratory diseases lead to hypoxia.

Alveolar hypoventilation describes a situation in which there is a global reduction in the amount of oxygen delivered to the alveoli due to inadequate ventilation. Because both delivery of oxygen and removal of carbon dioxide are impaired, there is usually a combination of both hypoxia and hypercapnia.

Measuring arterial pO_2 and pCO_2 is a useful way to assess lung function

In order to establish that a patient is hypoxic, we need to measure the partial pressure of oxygen (pO_2) in arterial blood. This can be achieved by analysing a few millilitres of arterial blood following puncture of an accessible artery, usually the radial artery at the wrist or the femoral artery in the groin. As well as measuring oxygen, the partial pressure of carbon dioxide is also measured, a test known as an **arterial blood gas** (p. 532).

JARGON BUSTER

Lung function tests versus arterial blood gases

Although arterial blood gas analysis is a commonly performed way of assessing lung function in hospitalized patients, be careful not to confuse this with **lung function tests** which are an altogether different type of test. Lung function tests are geared more towards the assessment of the *mechanics* of breathing and are used to help diagnose conditions affecting airflow, such as chronic obstructive pulmonary disease and diffuse parenchymal lung diseases.

Respiratory failure

Respiratory failure is defined as an arterial pO_2 of less than 8 kPa

A patient is said to be in **respiratory failure** if they have pulmonary disease severe enough to cause dangerous hypoxia. Respiratory failure is therefore not a specific diagnosis, but rather a marker of the progression of an underlying lung disease, and is indeed dynamic, i.e. a patient can move in and out of respiratory failure

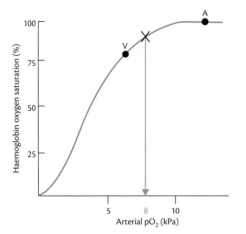

Fig. 7.2 Oxyhaemoglobin dissociation curve. This curve relates the percentage saturation of haemoglobin to pO_2. Points A and V represent typical values in arteries and veins respectively. Respiratory failure is defined as occurring if arterial pO_2 is 8 kPa or less (point X) because the percentage of haemoglobin saturation rapidly drops off below this level due to the sigmoid shape of the curve.

depending on therapy and the effects of the condition over time.

The reason why respiratory failure is defined as hypoxia less than 8 kPa is related to the oxyhaemoglobin dissociation curve. Most readers should be familiar with this sigmoid shaped curve, which relates pO_2 to the percentage saturation of haemoglobin with oxygen (Fig. 7.2). Note how once the pO_2 falls below 8 kPa, the percentage saturation of haemoglobin leaving the lungs falls precipitously.

There are two types of respiratory failure: type 1 and type 2

Respiratory failure is divided into two types, determined by the partial pressure of carbon dioxide (pCO_2) value. **Type 1 respiratory failure** is defined as a pO_2 less than 8 kPa together with a normal or low pCO_2. Type 1 respiratory failure tends to be caused by diseases which cause a ventilation/perfusion mismatch, e.g. pneumonia. Blood leaving alveoli with mismatched ventilation and perfusion will have a low pO_2 and a raised pCO_2. Increasing ventilation to normal areas of lung can remove the excess carbon dioxide but cannot compensate for the lowered pO_2 because the haemoglobin leaving these normal areas of lung will already be 100 per cent saturated with oxygen and thus the amount of oxygen carried cannot be increased further.

Type 2 respiratory failure is defined as a pO_2 less than 8 kPa together with a raised pCO_2. Type 2 respiratory failure tends to be caused by conditions leading to generalized alveolar hypoventilation and impaired transfer of both oxygen and carbon dioxide. Common conditions causing type 2 respiratory failure include chronic obstructive pulmonary disease (COPD) and neuromuscular disorders impairing the mechanics of breathing.

Patients can swing between the two types of respiratory failure

Differentiating between type 1 and type 2 respiratory failure is useful, but the distinction is by no means fixed. Many of the conditions causing type 1 respiratory failure can eventually progress to type 2 respiratory failure (Table 7.1).

For instance, an episode of acute asthma may be severe enough to impair oxygen exchange to cause severe hypoxia, but compensatory hyperventilation will keep carbon dioxide levels low, i.e. type 1 failure. If, however, the patient does not respond to treatment and they begin to tire from their raised respiratory rate, they will begin to hypoventilate. Widespread hypoventilation leads to accumulation of carbon dioxide as well as hypoxia, i.e. type 2 respiratory failure. This is why a *normal* carbon dioxide level in an acute asthmatic is an ominous sign of deterioration.

Respiratory failure may be acute or chronic

Like all other forms of organ failure, both acute and chronic forms of respiratory failure are recognized. Acute respiratory failure occurs when a person with previously healthy lungs suddenly develops respiratory

TABLE 7.1 Common causes of respiratory failure
Type 1
Severe pneumonia
Pulmonary embolism
Acute asthma
Pulmonary fibrosis
Acute left ventricular failure
Type 2
Chronic obstructive pulmonary disease
Neuromuscular disorders impairing ventilation
Severe acute asthma with tiring

failure. Common examples of diseases leading to acute respiratory failure include pneumonia, pulmonary embolus, and acute asthma. Following successful treatment, lung function typically returns to normal and the hypoxia resolves.

Chronic respiratory failure is a persistent problem which typically develops gradually in patients with chronic lung disease, most commonly COPD or pulmonary fibrosis. Neuromuscular disorders impairing the mechanics of breathing, such as muscular dystrophy and motor neurone disease, may also lead to chronic respiratory failure.

The clinical picture of chronic respiratory failure is often surprisingly undramatic with relatively few symptoms, but nonetheless the development of chronic respiratory failure is very significant, as the chronic hypoxia has important consequences.

Chronic hypoxia causes pulmonary hypertension and polycythaemia

Chronic hypoxia has some important knock-on effects, most notably the development of pulmonary hypertension and polycythaemia.

Pulmonary hypertension is thought to develop due to persistent constriction of pulmonary arteries. Pulmonary arteries are unusual because they *constrict* in response to hypoxia (rather than dilate). In the short term, this dynamic response is useful because it increases flow to areas of lung that are less hypoxic, thus maintaining ventilation/perfusion matching. Persistent constriction in response to chronic hypoxia, however, causes permanent changes in the walls of pulmonary arteries leading to pulmonary hypertension. Persistent pulmonary hypertension ultimately terminates in chronic right heart failure and death from a combination of cardiac and respiratory failure.

Polycythaemia is defined as an increase in red cell mass, and is the result of increased red blood cell production in response to hypoxia.

LINK BOX

Polycythaemia

Chronic hypoxia as a cause of polycythaemia is important to exclude before diagnosing patients with polycythaemia vera, a myeloproliferative disorder in which there is uncontrolled production of red blood cells (p. 361).

Key points: Hypoxia and respiratory failure

- If lung disease impairs gas exchange, then hypoxia may result.

- If hypoxia is severe enough to reduce the arterial pO_2 to below 8 kPa, then respiratory failure is said to have occurred.

- Respiratory failure may complicate any severe lung disease and can be acute or chronic.

- Type 1 respiratory failure is due to ventilation/perfusion mismatching and causes a low pO_2 but a normal or low pCO_2.

- Type 2 respiratory failure is due to widespread hypoventilation and causes a low pO_2 and a high pCO_2.

- Respiratory failure is dynamic. Patients may swing in and out of respiratory failure with treatment, and can move between types 1 and type 2.

Acute respiratory distress syndrome

Acute respiratory distress syndrome implies sudden very severe lung damage

Acute respiratory distress syndrome (ARDS) is a clinical term used to describe patients with an extremely severe, life-threatening form of acute respiratory failure. The basic principle is a sudden severe insult that causes widespread damage to previously healthy alveoli. *ARDS therefore loosely implies that something has catastrophically damaged the lungs.* ARDS enjoys a number of synonyms including 'acute lung injury' and 'shock lung', but they all mean the same thing.

Another term you will probably come across when reading about ARDS is **diffuse alveolar damage**. Diffuse alveolar damage is slightly different from ARDS in that it refers to the *histological* changes seen in the lungs of a patient with ARDS. Rather like the term ARDS, diffuse alveolar damage simply means severe lung damage without any specific reference to the underlying cause.

LINK BOX

Neonatal respiratory distress syndrome

ARDS is also sometimes known as *adult* respiratory distress syndrome to contrast it from *neonatal* respiratory distress syndrome. The neonatal form has a very similar pattern but is due to the inability of immature alveoli to produce surfactant (p. 492).

ARDS may be caused by a large number of unrelated disorders

ARDS may be caused by any condition which causes widespread damage to either pulmonary capillaries or alveolar epithelial cells (Table 7.2):

* **Sepsis** is the most common predisposing factor associated with the development of ARDS, probably due to toxic effects of neutrophil-derived inflammatory mediators in the lungs.

* **Severe traumatic injury**, especially multiple fractures and pulmonary contusion, is strongly associated with development of ARDS. Long bone fractures may give rise to ARDS through fat embolism. Pulmonary contusions cause ARDS through direct trauma to the lung.

* **Multiple blood transfusions** are another important risk factor for ARDS, independent of the reason for transfusion or the co-existence of trauma. The incidence of ARDS increases with the number of units transfused.

Whatever the underlying cause, the outcome is pretty much the same: there is widespread disruption of the alveolar–capillary barrier which has three main consequences (Fig. 7.3):

* Fluid leaks into the alveolar spaces, causing **pulmonary oedema**.

* Fibrin leaks into the alveoli, forming **hyaline membranes**.

TABLE 7.2 Causes of acute respiratory distress syndrome

Severe pneumonia
Septic shock
Severe trauma
Multiple transfusions
Near drowning

---

* Surfactant is lost, so **alveoli collapse**.

These three features all act to severely impair the transfer of gases in and out of the blood; hence patients with ARDS are *extremely breathless*. As the hyaline membranes become organized, the scarring causes the lungs to become stiff and non-compliant.

Mortality and morbidity is high in ARDS

The final outcome of ARDS depends on whether the patient can be adequately supported and the underlying problem successfully treated before fibrosis becomes too widespread. About 50 per cent of patients with ARDS die. The remainder who recover have a wide spectrum of residual disability depending on the degree of pulmonary fibrosis.

Key points: Acute respiratory distress syndrome

* Acute respiratory distress syndrome (ARDS) refers to a very severe acute respiratory failure due to sudden widespread lung injury.

* The most common causes of ARDS are sepsis and multiple trauma.

* The lung injury leads to severe pulmonary oedema, alveolar collapse, and the formation of hyaline membranes. These three features all act to impair gas exchange severely.

* Patients with ARDS are extremely breathless and severely hypoxic, requiring intensive ventilatory support.

* ARDS carries a high mortality, and those who survive often have residual respiratory disability as a result of scarring in the lungs.

Bronchiectasis

Bronchiectasis is abnormal permanent dilation of airways

Rather like respiratory failure, bronchiectasis is not a final diagnosis but rather a pattern of injury that may be seen as an end-stage complication of a variety of lung diseases. The defining feature of bronchiectasis

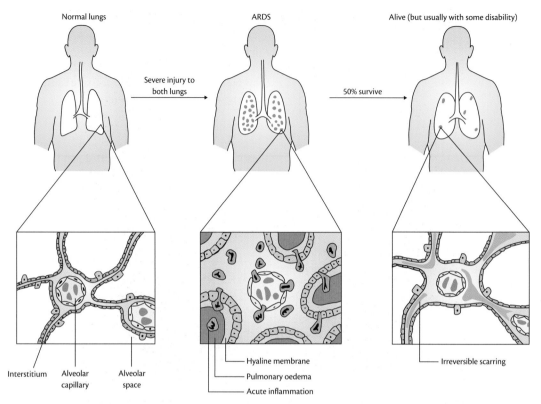

Fig. 7.3 Acute respiratory distress syndrome. In ARDS, severe injury to the lungs causes inflammatory widening of the interstitium with the formation of pulmonary oedema and hyaline membranes in the alveoli. Gas exchange by diffusion is severely impaired, leading to the severe hypoxia and breathlessness seen in ARDS.

is an *abnormal permanent dilation of airways.* The affected bronchi are most frequently those of the third and fourth generation. The larger first and second order bronchi are spared because their more substantial cartilage wall prevents dilation.

The abnormal dilation occurs because of destruction of the bronchial wall

Bronchiectasis develops in situations where a self-perpetuating cycle of obstruction and infection develops in the airways, leading to complete necrosis of the bronchial wall. Loss of supporting tissues such as smooth muscle and elastic fibres renders the airway susceptible to stretching

by the normal tractive forces operating on them by adjacent lung tissue. Over time, scarring leads to the permanent fixed dilation characteristic of the disease.

Bronchiectasis may be localized or diffuse

The abnormally dilated airways may be restricted to one part of a lung or diffusely affect both lungs. Localized bronchiectasis (Fig. 7.4) is most commonly seen as a complication of either *obstruction* to an area of the lung (e.g. by a tumour) or as a sequel to a focus of *severe pulmonary infection*, particularly one arising during childhood.

Diffuse bronchiectasis is almost always a result of inherited disorders which predispose the lungs to repeated

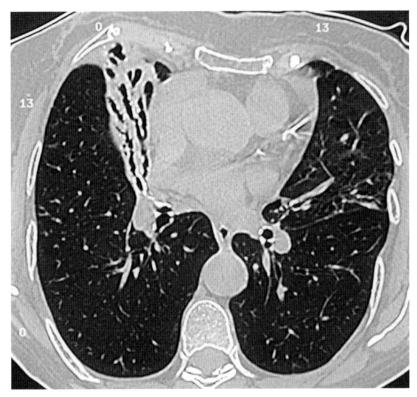

Fig. 7.4 This high resolution CT scan shows an area of localized bronchiectasis in the right lung next to the heart.

infections. The most common example is **cystic fibrosis**, but other well recognized causes include inherited disorders of ciliary clearance.

The main symptoms of bronchiectasis are persistent cough and sputum

The majority of patients with bronchiectasis have minimal symptoms of cough and sputum. Many patients go undiagnosed, merely seeing the cough and sputum production as no more than a nuisance. Bronchiectasis is usually suspected if the patient seeks help due to a long history of persistent cough and sputum production. In non-smokers, the diagnosis may be more easily considered, but in smokers it may be difficult to untangle it from smoking-related cough and sputum. It has been suggested that bronchiectasis may be more common than we think because many smokers with symptoms of cough and sputum put down to their smoking in fact have bronchiectasis.

Key points: Bronchiectasis

- Bronchiectasis is the irreversible abnormal dilation of bronchial walls.

- Bronchiectasis is the end result of a number of diseases leading to persistent destructive inflammation in the walls of the airways.

- Bronchiectasis may be localized or diffuse.

- The commonest cause of localized bronchiectasis is obstruction to a segment of lung.

- Cystic fibrosis is the commonest cause of diffuse bronchiectasis.

- The main manifestations of bronchiectasis are persistent cough and sputum production.

Diseases of pulmonary blood vessels

The lungs enjoy a dual blood supply from the bronchial arteries and the pulmonary arteries. The bronchial arteries are systemic arteries which supply the airways as far as the respiratory bronchioles, where they anastomose with branches of the pulmonary arteries. Capillaries derived from the pulmonary arteries form a meshwork around the alveoli and supply them with everything except oxygen, of which the alveoli have plenty.

The most important conditions affecting the pulmonary arteries are pulmonary thromboembolism and pulmonary hypertension.

Pulmonary embolism

Pulmonary embolism occurs when a pulmonary artery becomes occluded by an embolic thrombus derived from deep leg vein thrombosis (Fig. 7.5). Pulmonary embolism is an extremely common condition and an important cause of sudden death. There are two main consequences of pulmonary embolism:

♦ Respiratory compromise due to the area of non-perfused but ventilated segment of lung. Patients with pulmonary emboli are often hypoxic, which can be severe enough to cause type 1 respiratory failure.

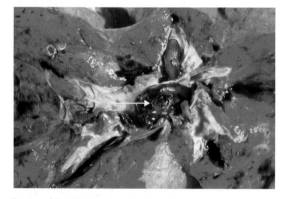

Fig. 7.5 This patient unexpectedly died in hospital. At post-mortem, when the pulmonary artery was opened up, this large thromboembolus was found impacted within the lumen (arrow). The source of this thromboembolus was a large propagating thrombus in the deep veins of the leg.

♦ Haemodynamic compromise due to the increased resistance to pulmonary blood flow caused by the embolic obstruction. This leads to an acute rise in pulmonary arterial blood pressure and puts a strain on the right side of the heart.

The clinical picture of pulmonary embolism depends on the extent of the pulmonary vasculature that is blocked, and the time scale involved.

Blockage of a major pulmonary artery causes sudden death

If a large embolus blocks the bifurcation of the pulmonary artery or one of the main pulmonary arteries, the pressure in the right side of the heart rises suddenly and dramatically. The right heart cannot match the pressure required to pump blood into the lungs, so it acutely fails with immediate cardiovascular arrest. The cardiac monitor attached during the resuscitation attempt usually shows pulseless electrical activity (PEA) as the electrical activity of the heart is intact but no output is achieved. Massive pulmonary embolism invariably causes virtually instantaneous death.

Blockage of medium sized pulmonary arteries causes acute breathlessness

Emboli lodging in a lobar or segmental pulmonary artery account for about 10 per cent of all cases of pulmonary embolism. There is breathlessness, but cardiovascular collapse does not occur. Infarction of an area of lung rarely occurs because the unaffected bronchial arteries can sustain the vitality of the lung. Pulmonary infarction only develops if there is pre-existing disease causing inadequacy of the bronchial arterial supply to the lungs. If an area of infarction does develop, there may be haemoptysis due to haemorrhage into the infarct and, if adjacent to the pleura, pleuritic-type chest pain.

Blockage of small peripheral vessels produces very vague symptoms

The vast majority of episodes of pulmonary embolism (some 85 per cent) affect small peripheral pulmonary arteries. *Unfortunately the symptomatology here can be very vague and difficult to characterize.* Patients may experience subtle degrees of breathlessness, chest discomfort, dizziness, or even palpitations. Often the only clinical sign is the presence of isolated tachypnoea and/or tachycardia. Because the diagnosis can be so difficult, one should always have a high index of suspicion for pulmonary embolism, especially in patients at risk of venous thrombosis.

Chronic recurrent pulmonary emboli cause pulmonary hypertension

A very small number of patients develop chronic recurrent minor pulmonary emboli. Most patients do not have an obvious history of venous thrombosis or pulmonary embolism. If the emboli do not resolve spontaneously, they undergo organization leading to blockage of numerous small vessels in the pulmonary vascular bed. Once sufficient vessels have been blocked, irreversible pulmonary hypertension develops and, ultimately, right ventricular failure.

Pulmonary hypertension

The pulmonary circulation is normally a low pressure system, operating at about one-eighth that of the systemic circulation. The normal systolic pulmonary arterial pressure is less than 20 mmHg at rest. **Pulmonary hypertension** is said to be present when the systolic pulmonary arterial pressure at rest is greater than 20 mmHg.

Unlike systemic hypertension, pulmonary hypertension is almost always secondary to underlying cardiac or pulmonary disease. The underlying mechanisms include:

- *Chronic hypoxia.* In the section on chronic respiratory failure, we have described the problem of chronic hypoxia causing pulmonary hypertension.

- *Obliteration of vascular beds.* Structural obliteration of the delicate pulmonary alveolar capillary network can also give rise to pulmonary hypertension.

- *Venous congestion.* Pulmonary venous congestion also leads to pulmonary arterial hypertension simply through the effects of back pressure.

The most common causes of pulmonary hypertension are COPD (chronic hypoxia and obliteration of vascular beds), recurrent pulmonary emboli (obliteration of vascular beds), and chronic left ventricular failure (venous congestion).

Pulmonary hypertension itself has further cardiovascular consequences. Just as prolonged systemic hypertension leads to left ventricular hypertrophy and eventually left ventricular failure, pulmonary hypertension causes *right* ventricular hypertrophy and *right*-sided heart failure.

INTERESTING TO KNOW

Primary pulmonary hypertension

Very occasionally, pulmonary hypertension occurs in the absence of underlying respiratory or cardiac disease. This is known as **primary pulmonary hypertension**. The typical presentation is the gradual onset of breathlessness on exertion, which progresses to breathlessness at rest. Other common symptoms are fatigue, angina (which, unusually, is due to *right* ventricular ischaemia), and episodes of syncope or near syncope. The prognosis in primary pulmonary hypertension is not good, with most patients dying within a few years of diagnosis due to right ventricular failure.

Diseases of the airways

Chronic obstructive pulmonary disease

COPD is characterized by persistent airflow obstruction

Chronic obstructive pulmonary disease (COPD) is a very common cause of breathlessness, due to airflow obstruction which is *poorly reversible* and usually *progressive*. The airflow obstruction is the result of damage to both small conducting airways and alveoli, which is almost always caused by smoking.

Only a minority of smokers develop COPD. The reason for this is unknown, but current evidence suggests that the inflammatory response is amplified in susceptible people.

COPD has replaced the old terms chronic bronchitis and emphysema

Historically, the terms chronic bronchitis and emphysema were used to describe the airway diseases associated with long-term heavy smoking. Chronic bronchitis was defined clinically as 'cough productive of sputum for three consecutive months for two consecutive years', whilst emphysema was defined as 'permanent dilatation of the airways distal to the terminal bronchiole'.

These terms are now being phased out, because they have very little relevance in the clinical setting. Many smokers have a persistent productive cough diagnostic for chronic bronchitis, but in the absence of any significant airway obstruction this is of no great clinical concern. The term emphysema is not particularly helpful either as the only way to make the diagnosis in its early stages is by close inspection of the cut surface of the lungs at autopsy (a situation not ideal for routine practice!). Even the best forms of imaging can only reliably detect emphysema once it is relatively severe.

COPD is instead defined as 'progressive airways obstruction which does not change markedly over several months'. Note that here the emphasis is on the obstructive element of the disease. This makes much better sense as it is the obstruction to airflow which causes the disabling symptoms of breathlessness and impairs quality of life. With this definition, establishing a diagnosis of COPD is made much easier because we can measure airflow by performing spirometry. The main downside of the definition is that it is quite non-specific and overlaps with other conditions, e.g. chronic incompletely reversible asthma.

Smoking has adverse effects throughout the lungs

All the airways throughout the respiratory tract are damaged by smoking, although the specific effects at each level are quite different (Fig. 7.6). In the bronchi, smoking causes an increase in the number of the mucus-producing glands in the submucosa and an increase in the number of goblet cells on the surface epithelium. Together these changes account for the increased sputum production characteristic of COPD

(and the old term chronic bronchitis). The irritant effect of smoke particles is also responsible for the chronic cough associated with smoking.

In the bronchioles, smoking causes a marked increase in inflammatory cells in the wall of the airway by a mechanism that is poorly understood. Eventually the smaller airways undergo fibrosis and narrow. *Stenosis of these small airways is thought to be the main source of airflow obstruction in COPD.*

In respiratory bronchioles there is destruction of the walls with loss of the elastic tissue. These airways dilate, giving rise to a pattern of emphysema known as centriacinar emphysema (this just describes its location within the acini). Loss of the elastic tissue of the terminal airways contributes to the reduction in airflow on expiration due to loss of the natural recoil of the lungs. Air trapping within the dilated terminal airways leads to the hyperinflated lungs characteristic of COPD.

The protease/antiprotease hypothesis may account for the lung destruction

The pathogenesis of the destructive effects in the terminal airways is complex. The currently favoured hypothesis is known as the **protease/antiprotease hypothesis**. Smoking causes sequestration of activated neutrophils in the lung where they release protease enzymes such as elastase. Because smoking inhibits the lung's natural antiprotease enzymes, large amounts of active elastase can enter the lung interstitium, bind to and degrade elastin, causing destruction and enlargement of the distal airspaces. This hypothesis is supported by the disease α_1-**antitrypsin deficiency** where an inherited deficiency of α_1-antitrypsin, a potent inhibitor of the enzyme elastase, leads to the premature onset of COPD due to widespread emphysematous change in the lungs.

The clinical effects of smoking vary between individuals

The cough and sputum from larger airway involvement and the breathlessness from small airways disease, although both caused by smoking, occur to different degrees in each individual. Some smokers may develop a smoker's cough and increased sputum production yet remain relatively free from obstruction and breathlessness. Other smokers, however, may develop quite profound breathlessness with minimal cough and sputum.

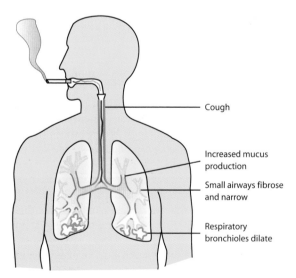

Cough

Increased mucus production

Small airways fibrose and narrow

Respiratory bronchioles dilate

Fig. 7.6 Effects of smoking on airways of different sizes.

Exertional breathlessness is the most common presenting symptom of COPD

The earliest symptom in the natural history of COPD is usually cough and sputum, which develop early in a smoking history. Initially it may occur after common colds, but usually increases in regularity and severity. Many patients simply put up with these symptoms without seeking medical attention.

If susceptible individuals continue to smoke, their small airways become increasingly obstructed until eventually the patient suddenly develops breathlessness on exertion. Because the small airways contribute very little to total airway resistance, widespread small airway disease must occur to cause breathlessness. As such, by the time a patient with COPD presents with breathlessness on exertion, *extensive irreversible damage has already been suffered in the lungs.*

With advanced disease, breathlessness occurs upon minimal exertion and then at rest. The patient becomes chronically hypoxic, causing pulmonary hypertension and eventually right-sided heart failure. Most patients die as a result of a combination of cardiac and respiratory failure.

Patients suspected of having COPD should undergo spirometry

In order to diagnose COPD, airflow obstruction must be demonstrated. This cannot be achieved using history or clinical examination, and even the chest radiograph may be normal in mild to moderate COPD.

Confirming airway obstruction requires **spirometry**, which measures the functional abilities of the lungs for conducting air. The characteristic feature of COPD is slowing of the rate of expiration, leading to a reduction in the volume of air expired in 1 s (FEV_1). Diagnosing COPD requires demonstration of a low FEV_1 and a low FEV_1/FVC ratio (Fig. 7.7). Spirometry is also helpful in assessing the severity of the disease.

Stopping smoking is the single most important action for patients with COPD

Current treatment options in COPD are purely symptomatic with inhaled bronchodilators. We are currently unable to prevent or reverse the decline in lung function. The only action that can slow the decline in lung function is to stop smoking. All patients with COPD who smoke should be encouraged to stop at every opportunity and be offered support programmes.

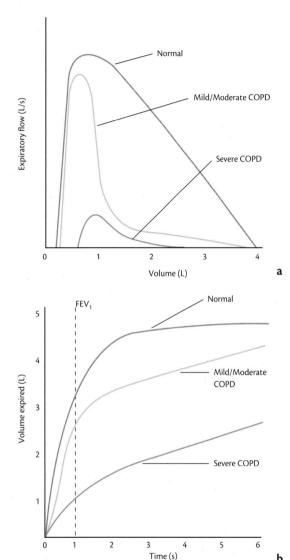

Fig. 7.7 (a) Flow–volume loops in a normal individual compared with patients with COPD. In mild to moderate COPD, immediate flow is relatively normal (this is why peak flow can be normal in patients with early COPD) but then airflow rapidly decreases. In severe COPD, airflow is very poor with prominent air trapping (note how at the start of expiration there is already nearly 1 l of air in the lungs). (b) Spirometry in a normal individual compared with patients with COPD. Note how in COPD the forced expiratory volume in 1 s (FEV_1) is reduced, but the final volume expired is relatively normal (they just take longer to get there!), hence the FEV_1 to FVC ratio is lowered.

An acute exacerbation of COPD is a very common clinical problem

An **acute exacerbation of COPD** is a sudden, sustained worsening in a patient's symptoms that is beyond their normal day to day variation. There is worsening breathlessness and cough, and increased sputum production. The patient may become drowsy or confused if the insult has pushed them into type 2 respiratory failure and they are retaining carbon dioxide.

Infection is the most common cause of an acute exacerbation of COPD

There are a number of possible causes of an acute exacerbation of COPD (Table 7.3), though infection is the most common. The most common bacterial causes of infection are *Streptococcus pneumoniae* and *Haemophilus influenzae*. Viral infections are probably responsible for a number of exacerbations; however, the exact proportion is unknown and antibiotics are usually administered as standard treatment if the sputum is purulent.

Key points: Chronic obstructive pulmonary disease

- COPD is characterized by progressive, poorly reversible airflow obstruction.

- The airflow obstruction is due to a combination of small airway narrowing and destructive changes in the terminal airways, which is virtually always the result of cigarette smoking.

- The earliest symptoms of COPD are persistent cough and sputum production. Later progressively worsening breathlessness develops.

- There is no single diagnostic test for COPD. Making the diagnosis relies on a combination of history and examination, and documentation of airflow obstruction on spirometry.

- Spirometry in COPD reveals a low FEV_1 and a low FEV_1/FVC ratio.

- Acute exacerbations of COPD are common and are usually due to infection.

- The chronic hypoxia associated with COPD leads to pulmonary hypertension and the development of right ventricular failure.

- Most patients eventually die from a combination of respiratory and cardiac failure.

Asthma

Asthma is the most common chronic pulmonary disorder

Asthma is an extremely common disorder which is now estimated to affect more than 10 per cent of children and more than 5 per cent of adults. Asthma is a chronic inflammatory disorder of large airways which causes bronchial hyper-responsiveness to a variety of stimuli that do not affect normal airways. This manifests itself as a clinical picture characterized by intermittent episodes of shortness of breath, wheeze, chest tightness, and cough as a result of reversible airway narrowing.

Atopy is common in asthmatics and plays a role in the evolution of the disease

Half of those who develop asthma do so in childhood before the age of 10 years. Most children who are asthmatic are also atopic. Atopy refers to a genetic tendency of the immune system to make large amounts of IgE directed against common environmental allergens and a predisposition to diseases such as atopic dermatitis, allergic rhinitis, and asthma. In asthma, a major source of allergens is the house dust mite.

Asthmatics have early and late inflammatory responses to provocative stimuli

When asthmatic individuals inhale environmental allergens, an immediate (type I) hypersensitivity reaction occurs in their large airways. Degranulation of mast cells and the release of histamine rapidly induces

---

TABLE 7.3   Causes of acute exacerbation of COPD

Infection
Pneumothorax
Pulmonary embolus
Left ventricular failure
Lung carcinoma

smooth muscle contraction, oedema, and mucus hyper-secretion in the airways. The combination of these events leads to airway narrowing within minutes of allergen exposure, and symptoms of breathlessness and wheezing.

A critical process that accompanies these acute events is the recruitment of more inflammatory cells into the airways with perpetuation of airway inflammation several hours after the initial exposure. An important component of this late inflammatory response is the recruitment of the Th2 subtype of T helper lymphocytes. Th2 lymphocytes, through production of cytokines,

promote the activation of mast cells and eosinophils, and drive further IgE production by B cells (Fig. 7.8).

The late inflammatory response is crucial in the development of hyper-reactive airways

The persisting inflammatory activity in the airways set up by the late inflammatory response causes epithelial cell injury and denudation of the airway, resulting in exposure of sensory nerve endings and increased smooth muscle responsiveness. The airways become hyper-reactive, meaning *that they also become liable to narrowing in response to a whole host of other stimuli,*

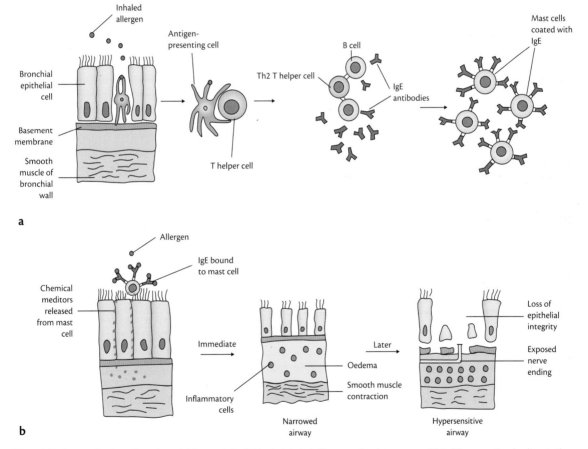

Fig. 7.8 Pathogenesis of atopic asthma. (a) In atopic individuals, inhaled allergens stimulate a strong Th2-driven reaction leading to the production of IgE antibodies against the allergen. Specific IgE antibodies against the allergen become bound to the surface of mast cells. (b) On re-exposure to the allergen, IgE on the mast cells become cross-linked, stimulating degranulation of the mast cell. The chemical mediators stimulate a rapid inflammatory response in the airway, leading to bronchospasm and symptoms of airway obstruction. Hours later, a further bout of persistent inflammation is set up in the airways which renders them hypersensitive.

TABLE 7.4 Common provocative factors in asthma
Dust mites
Particles shed from animal skin or fur
Exercise
Air pollutants, especially cigarette smoke
Viral upper respiratory tract infections
Drugs, e.g. β-blockers, aspirin

e.g. exercise, cold air, cigarette smoke, and viral respiratory infections (Table 7.4).

The response of the airways to persistent inflammation is the laying down of fibrous tissue, which explains the well recognized component of relatively fixed airway obstruction seen in some asthmatics.

The importance of the late inflammatory component of asthma in driving the disease process has encouraged a shift in the management of asthma, with earlier introduction of regular inhaled steroids to treatment regimes in an attempt to reduce bronchial hyper-reactivity and prevent airway fibrosis.

Non-atopic asthma may be related to gastro-oesophageal reflux disease

A number of asthmatics do not appear to be atopic. These patients tend not to have a positive family history of asthma, do not suffer from other allergies, and have normal IgE levels.

It has been suggested that gastro-oesophageal reflux and aspiration may play a role in non-atopic asthma. Reflux symptoms are reported in nearly 50 per cent of all patients with asthma compared with 10 per cent of the general population. There is also some evidence that treatment for reflux improves symptoms of asthma.

The clinical picture of asthma is of variable airflow obstruction

Symptoms of asthma include wheeze, breathlessness, cough, and chest tightness. These symptoms occurring with a variability in pattern and timing is classical of asthma. Nocturnal worsening is common, with symptoms disturbing sleep in the early hours of the morning (3–5 a.m.).

Making a certain diagnosis of asthma can be difficult

A diagnosis of asthma is usually reached on the basis of a compatible history together with objective demonstration of airflow obstruction that varies spontaneously over short periods of time. Serial measurements of peak flow rate in most patients with asthma show a characteristic pattern, with airflow limitation most severe on waking in the morning with improvement occurring during the morning. The most commonly used means to diagnose asthma in clinical practice is an increase of 20 per cent or more from baseline peak expiratory flow rate (PEFR) following inhalation of a bronchodilator, usually a short-acting β-adrenoreceptor agonist such as salbutamol.

Management of asthma should aim to eradicate symptoms completely

Asthma is not usually curable, but treatment should aim to prevent troublesome symptoms. Drug treatment is essentially twofold. Inhaled bronchodilators are given to alleviate the symptoms of asthma, and inhaled glucocorticoids dampen the inflammation in the airways. Glucocorticoids are the most effective treatment for asthma. They do not cure the disease but suppress the chronic inflammation in the airways by inhibiting the formation of cytokines such as interleukin-4 (IL-4), IL-5, and IL-13 which drive airway inflammation.

Key points: Asthma

- Asthma is the most common chronic pulmonary disease.

- Asthma is characterized by persistent inflammatory activity in the bronchial walls initiated by an immediate hypersensitivity response to inhaled allergens.

- The persistent inflammation makes the bronchi hyper-responsive to a number of provocative stimuli such as cold air and exercise.

- Clinically this manifests with intermittent symptoms of airway obstruction such as cough, wheeze, and breathlessness.

- Dampening the inflammation in the bronchial walls with inhaled glucocorticoids is a crucial part of the management of asthma.

Diseases of lung parenchyma

Pneumonia

Pneumonia refers to an inflammatory condition affecting the lung parenchyma

Strictly speaking, the terms 'pneumonia', 'pneumonitis' and 'alveolitis' mean the same thing, i.e. inflammation of the lung parenchyma. In practice, however, these terms have come to carry certain connotations. **Pneumonia** usually implies inflammation within the alveolar spaces due to an infective agent, whereas **pneumonitis** or **alveolitis** is reserved for inflammation within the alveolar walls without an infective aetiology. As is often the case in medical terminology, these definitions are by no means rigid, and you will no doubt discover that people use the terms pneumonia, pneumonitis, and alveolitis interchangeably.

The normal lung is sterile below the level of the larynx

The respiratory tract has a number of potent defence mechanisms which keep microorganisms out of the lungs. These include:

♦ *Nasal clearance.* Inhaled droplets containing microorganisms are either sneezed or blown out of the nose, or swept by ciliated epithelium down into the nasopharynx where they are swallowed

♦ *Tracheobronchial clearance.* This is achieved by the mucociliary escalator. Particles become trapped in the thin film of mucus lining the respiratory tree and the beating action of cilia continuously moves them up to the oropharynx where they are swallowed.

♦ *Alveolar clearance.* Organisms reaching the distal airways are phagocytosed by resident alveolar macrophages.

If these local defences become impaired, or the resistance of the host generally is lowered, microorganisms may colonize the lung. Either organisms which already colonize the upper respiratory system spread further down into the lungs, or infective organisms are inhaled into the lower respiratory tree by direct droplet spread. The presence of microorganisms and the tissue damage they cause incites an acute inflammatory response called pneumonia.

LINK BOX

Recurrent pneumonia

If a pneumonia is recurrent or slow to resolve, it may be the result of an underlying disease such as a lung cancer (p. 132) or myeloma (p. 368).

Pneumonia can be categorized in a number of different ways

Many pathology textbooks describe an anatomical pattern of pneumonia reflecting how infection spreads within the lung. Classically the distribution of visible consolidation was divided into 'bronchopneumonia' with widespread patchy involvement and 'lobar pneumonia' affecting the whole of a lobe. This distinction was largely based on macroscopic examination of lungs at autopsy in patients with florid pneumonias in a pre-antibiotic era. The problem with this classification is that it is difficult to apply in most cases as the patterns often overlap and the classical picture is extremely blurred by modern-day antibiotic therapy.

A more clinically relevant classification is based on the circumstances surrounding the development of the pneumonia:

♦ Community-acquired pneumonia

♦ Hospital-acquired pneumonia

♦ Aspiration pneumonia

♦ Immunosuppression pneumonia.

These subdivisions are much more useful because each type of pneumonia is associated with a particular group of likely pathogens. Patients can be easily placed into a category and the relevant antimicrobial therapy to target the most likely pathogens can be prescribed.

Community-acquired pneumonia is usually caused by *S. pneumoniae*

Community-acquired pneumonia can affect previously healthy people or those with underlying disease, especially a chronic lung disease. Although many different microbes may be the cause, only a few are common (Table 7.5). Of these the pneumococcus (*S. pneumoniae*) is overwhelmingly the most common. Pneumococcal pneumonia is an acute illness with the sudden onset of fever and cough productive of sputum which is purulent and

TABLE 7.5 Common organisms causing community-acquired pneumonia

Streptococcus pneumoniae
Mycoplasma pneumoniae
Haemophilus influenzae
Chlamydia pneumoniae
Legionella pneumophila
Viruses

often tinged with blood. Pleuritic type chest pain is often seen due to pleural involvement.

Mycoplasma and *Chlamydia* typically cause a mild pneumonia in young adults

Pneumonia caused by *Mycoplasma* and *Chlamydia* is similar in many ways. They both affect young adults, causing cough and shortness of breath with surprisingly little to find on clinical examination of the chest. Chest radiography is usually more dramatic, with diffuse patchy bilateral shadowing.

The organisms are often suspected, but harder to prove as culturing the organism requires tissue culture (they are both intracellular pathogens) and few laboratories offer the test. Blood can be taken in order to look for a rise in antibody titres over the following days; whilst this is a helpful retrospective diagnosis, it cannot be used when the patient presents. In practice, acquiring definite proof of the organisms is a somewhat academic exercise as they are easily treated empirically when suspected.

Legionnaire's disease is a much more serious infection

Although Legionnaire's disease is often grouped with *Mycoplasma* and *Chlamydia* as an 'atypical pneumonia', Legionnaire's disease is quite different in many respects. The infection typically involves older adults, and is a serious, often fatal, form of pneumonia. As well as the usual features of pneumonia, there is a profound systemic illness with high fever, muscle pains, and gastrointestinal upset.

Most cases of Legionnaire's disease are caused by the organism *Legionella pneumophila*. The infection is picked up by environmental exposure, and not by patient to patient transmission. Infection is typically through contamination of drinking water or air-conditioning units.

JARGON BUSTER

Atypical pneumonia

The term **atypical pneumonia** is still quite widely used and can be confusing. The name was originally used to describe pneumonias that were different because they did not respond to penicillin, and the inflammation tended to be within the alveolar wall ('interstitial') rather than the more usual intra-alveolar pattern.

The term is now best used to describe those community acquired infections caused by intracellular pathogens, e.g. a virus, *Mycoplasma pneumoniae*, *Chlamydia pneumoniae*, or *Legionella pneumophila*. With the obvious exception of the viruses, these organisms tend to respond to macrolide antibiotics such as erythromycin.

Hospital-acquired pneumonia occurs 2 days or more after admission to hospital

Hospital-acquired pneumonia is an extremely important cause of death or prolonged stay in hospitalized patients. The microbiology is very different from that of community-acquired pneumonias, as Gram negative bacteria are responsible for up to 60 per cent of cases. The organisms causing community-acquired pneumonia do feature, but with a much reduced frequency (pneumococcus in only about 5 per cent of cases).

The reason for the switch in causative organisms is related to the well recognized observation that patients with serious illnesses commonly have abnormal colonization of their upper respiratory tract by Gram negative bacteria such as *Klebsiella*, *Escherichia coli*, and *Pseudomonas*. If these organisms manage to colonize the lower respiratory tract when host resistance is lowered, pneumonia will occur.

Aspiration pneumonia is a risk in patients with an impairment of airway protection

Most pneumonias are probably caused by aspiration of organisms into the lower airways; however, the term aspiration pneumonia is reserved for patients in whom relatively large volumes of material are aspirated. Patients particularly predisposed to significant aspiration are those with an altered level of consciousness or abnormal swallowing reflexes. Common clinical scenarios where aspiration pneumonia is a risk include intoxicated patients, acute stroke patients with impaired swallowing, and septic patients with reduced consciousness.

Aspiration pneumonias are often mixed infections. They involve not only the aerobic bacteria implicated in conventional community-acquired or hospital-acquired pneumonias, but also anaerobic bacteria. Anaerobic bacterial infections can be quite destructive to the lung, and patients who aspirate large numbers of these organisms may be at risk of abscess formation unless appropriate treatment is started. Antibiotic regimes for a pneumonia where aspiration is a possible risk should therefore always include metronidazole, which has activity against anaerobic bacteria.

Immunosuppression pneumonia may be caused by a variety of organisms

Pneumonia in immunosuppressed individuals is becoming increasingly important with the growing incidence of human immunodeficiency virus (HIV) and iatrogenic immunosuppression. Pneumonia can progress extremely quickly in immunocompromised people and is the most common infective cause of death in this group of patients.

Conventional respiratory pathogens remain common culprits in immunosuppressed individuals, but generally the infection is more severe. In addition, more exotic organisms may be implicated (Table 7.6) and it is important to remember that multiple simultaneous infections may occur.

A key priority in an immunosuppressed patient is to determine whether or not there is *Pneumocystis carinii* pneumonia (PCP). *Pneumocystis carinii* is an atypical fungus which can lead to severe pneumonia in immunosuppressed patients. The risk of PCP relates well to the degree of immunosuppression, and in HIV patients is unlikely if the CD4 count is greater than 200 cells/µl.

TABLE 7.6 Common organisms causing immunosuppression pneumonia

Conventional respiratory pathogens
Mycobacterial infection, either *M. tuberculosis* or atypical mycobacteria
Viruses, e.g. cytomegalovirus and herpes simplex virus
Fungi, e.g. *Pneumocystis, Candida, Aspergillus*

Patients present with progressively worsening breathlessness, and a chest radiograph typically reveals fine bilateral infiltrates. High resolution computed tomography (HRCT) scanning shows a 'ground glass' pattern of alveolar consolidation.

Imaging is not diagnostic, and obtaining a definite microbiological diagnosis is crucial. There is no or little sputum production in PCP, so induced sputum production with nebulized saline is usually required to obtain a diagnostic specimen. If induced sputum specimens are negative for *P. carinii*, then bronchoscopy to obtain bronchoalveolar lavage fluid should be performed. The organism may be detected either with a silver stain or using a monoclonal antibody which binds the organism.

There are many possible complications of pneumonia

If a patient with pneumonia is particularly unwell or the treatment seems slow to take effect, one should always consider the development of a complication such as:

♦ **Respiratory failure**. A severe pneumonia can impair gas exchange to such an extent that there is inadequate oxygenation of the blood. If the pO_2 on an arterial blood gas measurement falls below 8 kPa, respiratory failure has occurred. Respiratory failure is one of the most important causes of death in pneumonia.

♦ **Septicaemia**. This is a common complication of pneumococcal pneumonia. Although the infection rarely spreads to other sites, the effect of the bacteraemia can be a problem by causing hypotension and septic shock.

♦ **Pleural effusion**. Accumulation of fluid within the pleural space occurs in about one-fifth of patients who are hospitalized for pneumonia. In most cases, the fluid is sterile, i.e. it is a reaction to the underlying infection rather than extension of the infection into the pleural cavity. Occasionally the fluid does become infected and in severe cases the pleural space becomes filled with pus, a condition called **empyema**.

♦ **Lung abscess**. An abscess is a pus-filled cavity which forms if infection destroys an area of tissue. In the lung, an abscess is typically a complication of a pneumonia caused by virulent organisms that are capable of destroying large volumes of lung parenchyma, such as *Staphylococcus aureus* and anaerobic organisms, especially if there is a large inoculum of organisms. Fortunately, the use of specific antibiotics that target these bacteria has significantly reduced the frequency of abscesses, and their danger of causing septicaemia and death.

Key points: Pneumonia

- Pneumonia refers to inflammation of the lung parenchyma due to infection.

- Pneumonia is one of the most common infectious diseases and is a common cause of death in debilitated people.

- The most useful classification of pneumonia is according to the circumstances in which the person develops it.

- Community-acquired pneumonia is most commonly due to *Streptococcus pneumoniae*.

- Hospital-acquired pneumonia is a very common cause of prolonged stay or death in hospitalized patients. Most of these cases are due to Gram negative bacteria.

- Aspiration pneumonia occurs in people with impaired airway protection. The infections are often mixed and include anaerobic organisms.

- Immunosuppressed patients can develop rapidly progressive pneumonia which may involve multiple organisms including opportunistic ones. *Pneumocystis carinii* pneumonia is a common cause of death in patients with HIV.

- Complications of pneumonia include respiratory failure, septicaemia, pleural effusion, and lung abscess.

Tuberculosis

Tuberculosis is the most common infectious disease in the world, and its incidence is rising. Much of this new epidemic is due to HIV infection; however, other factors include increased immigration from high risk areas, increased life expectancy of the elderly, social deprivation, and the emergence of drug-resistant strains (Table 7.7).

TABLE 7.7   People at risk of active tuberculosis

Immigrants from countries with high rates of tuberculosis
Elderly people
Immunocompromised individuals, particularly AIDS patients
Alcoholics

Tuberculosis is caused by the organism *Mycobacterium tuberculosis*

Mycobacterium tuberculosis, like all mycobacteria, is a small rod-shaped bacillus with a thick lipid-rich cell wall. The cell wall renders the organism resistant to decolorization by acid following staining, hence the term 'acid-fast bacilli'. The organisms are remarkably slow growing and are able to persist in a latent form within cells for many years, allowing reactivation of disease many years after infection is first acquired.

Infection is spread by inhalation of contaminated respiratory secretions

Tuberculosis is spread almost exclusively by the respiratory route from an infectious patient with 'open' or 'smear-positive' active pulmonary tuberculosis. The intact respiratory mucosa is very resistant to invasion by microorganisms. For infection to occur, the bacilli must be delivered to the terminal air spaces of the lung where they can avoid removal by the mucociliary elevator. Infection therefore begins right at the periphery of the lungs, usually just beneath the pleural surface.

Alveolar macrophages are unable to destroy the mycobacteria

Bacilli inhaled into the terminal airways are engulfed by resident alveolar macrophages. However, the organism can survive within the macrophages because they block the recruitment and assembly of proteins that mediate phagolysosome fusion within the macrophage, and their thick cell walls resist attack. Survival of the organism allows it to multiply within macrophages, eventually leading to cell death and release of more organisms.

Over a period of weeks, mycobacteria spread in macrophages via the blood to the apices of the lungs and multiple other organs such as the kidneys, adrenals, bones, and meninges. The strictly aerobic organism favours these sites because they have high oxygen levels. In the majority of infected individuals this dissemination remains entirely asymptomatic.

After a few weeks, T cell mediated immunity kicks in

Later on, specific immunity to the organism develops. Macrophages, acting as antigen-presenting cells, activate mycobacteria-specific CD4+ T helper cells via major histocompatibility complex (MHC) class II. For the majority of people acquiring a new tuberculous infection, the development of cell-mediated immunity is protective and holds the bacilli in check. Of particular importance are the Th1 subset of T helper cells which produce the cytokine interferon-γ. This cytokine is a powerful activator of macrophages, promoting increased levels of intracellular killing.

Activated macrophages aggregate around mycobacteria to form granulomas

Macrophages activated by cytokines from T cells enlarge into cells called **epithelioid macrophages**. Clusters of epithelioid macrophages surround the mycobacteria, forming granulomas which serve to wall off viable organisms in an anoxic and acidic environment which does not favour mycobacterial survival. The centre of the lesion becomes necrotic with an appearance like soft cheese (caseous necrosis), and most of the bacteria die. The lesion eventually becomes quiescent and sealed off by fibrous scar tissue which may calcify. A few bacilli may, however, survive in a dormant form and cause reactivation of tuberculosis months or years later.

In most cases the infection is contained and remains latent

In over 95 per cent of cases, development of specific cellular immunity against the organism contains the infection and the ultimate result is a calcified scar in the lung parenchyma and the draining hilar lymph node. Together this is referred to as the Ghon complex. Many people will have asymptomatic latent disease throughout their life.

A small minority of people are unable to contain the initial infection due to an inadequate T cell immune response, and progress immediately to active tuberculosis. Early progression to active disease is associated with severe immunosuppression (particularly HIV related) or a higher inoculum of more virulent organisms.

Active disease may be due to reactivation of latent disease or new infection

Often the underlying cause for reactivation is clear, e.g. immunosuppression. In many cases, there is no obvious immunodeficiency and the underlying reason for reactivation is unclear. Presumably there is some kind of subtle disruption in immune regulation, perhaps as a result of the immune system's response to other stimuli.

Active disease is related to an inappropriate T helper cell response

The development of active disease seems to depend critically on the subset of T helper cells. As we have already seen, a strong Th1 response is associated with protective immunity resulting in granuloma formation which contain the infection. If, however, the T helper cell response is more Th2 driven, an inappropriate repertoire of immune cells are recruited to the scene. There is an intense, but totally ineffective immune response to the organism's cell wall proteins leading to extensive tissue destruction and survival of the organism.

Active tuberculosis is best divided into pulmonary and extrapulmonary

Historically, active tuberculosis was classified as either 'primary' or 'post-primary' to reflect whether the disease is due to reactivation or newly acquired infection. More recent evidence has suggested that this distinction is unreliable as many patients presumed to have reactivation in fact are shown by DNA studies to have a newly acquired infection. The terms primary and post-primary, despite still featuring in many books, really mean very little and have no clinical value. For practical purposes, active tuberculosis should be simply divided into **pulmonary** and **extrapulmonary** (Fig. 7.9).

Active pulmonary tuberculosis presents as a chronic pneumonia

Patients with active pulmonary tuberculosis usually present after feeling unwell for weeks or months. The most common symptoms are a persistent cough together with prominent constitutional symptoms such as fever and night sweats. Loss of appetite and weight loss out of proportion to the reduced intake of food is also very common.

If the enlarging focus in a patient with active pulmonary disease erodes into an airway, the bacilli can enter the sputum and the patient is said to have 'open' tuberculosis. If a major airway is involved, the necrotic material drains away and the focus transforms into a

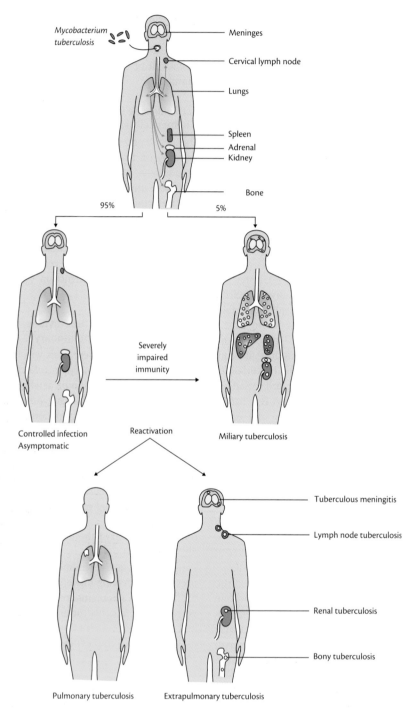

Fig. 7.9 Tuberculosis. The majority of patients infected with *M. tuberculosis* control the infection and remain asymptomatic. Reinfection or reactivation of disease in patients with impaired immunity leads to active tuberculosis which is usually pulmonary, but can involve extrapulmonary organs. Miliary tuberculosis is only seen in patients with very profound immunosuppression.

cavity containing enormous numbers of organisms in the cavity wall. Patients with cavitatory tuberculosis are particularly infectious because their sputum contains large numbers of mycobacteria and they cough frequently.

The diagnosis of pulmonary tuberculosis is based on a combination of findings

Making a diagnosis of pulmonary tuberculosis is usually achieved by a combination of radiological and laboratory features in a patient with a compatible history. Plain chest radiography is extremely useful, although the findings are usually only suggestive, but not diagnostic, of tuberculosis. The typical changes of tuberculosis are infiltrates involving the upper lobes that may show cavitation.

Laboratory tests for pulmonary tuberculosis rely on the microscopic examination and culture of sputum. Microscopic examination of sputum samples spread on to a slide (a sputum smear) reveals acid-fast bacilli in about 60 per cent of samples. Smear positivity correlates with a high burden of infection and infectivity.

Because other non-tuberculous mycobacteria can be found in sputum and are acid fast, culture remains the gold standard to confirm definitively that the isolate is *M. tuberculosis*. The problem with culture is that the results take 3–6 weeks due to the slow-growing nature of the organism. Very often patients are therefore assumed to have tuberculosis and so are started on appropriate therapy pending confirmation from culture.

Patients with severely impaired immunity may develop rapidly progressive disease

Patients with HIV infection or other forms of severe immunosuppression are at risk of developing rapidly progressive disease which may promptly lead to death if not recognized and treated. If infection spreads via the airways throughout large areas of lung parenchyma, a diffuse tuberculous bronchopneumonia develops. Such overwhelming infection was once known as 'galloping consumption'. If host resistance is severely impaired, the disease becomes widely disseminated resulting in numerous small foci of infection developing in many organs, a condition known as **miliary tuberculosis**.

Extrapulmonary tuberculosis commonly affects cervical lymph nodes and the kidneys

Of all cases of active tuberculosis, about 15 per cent involve organs other than the lungs. Remember how

TABLE 7.8   Common sites of extrapulmonary tuberculosis

Lymph nodes (mainly cervical and supraclavicular)
Kidneys
Bone and joints
Meninges

during the initial seeding of infection with *M. tuberculosis*, haematogenous dissemination of bacilli to a number of organs can occur. These localized infections, as in the lung, usually become walled off in small granulomas where mycobacteria remain dormant. If they reactivate at a later time, then extrapulmonary tuberculosis may result.

Extrapulmonary tuberculosis is particularly common in children and immunocompromised adults. In patients with HIV, pulmonary and extrapulmonary disease often co-exist. A number of organs may be involved (Table 7.8), the most common being cervical lymph nodes and the kidneys.

Tuberculosis requires compulsory treatment with multiple drugs and contact tracing

Treatment of tuberculosis requires multiple antituberculous drugs to be taken for 6 months. Treatment, except in exceptional cases, is compulsory, and patient compliance should be checked routinely.

Tuberculosis is a notifiable disease under public health regulations, and contact tracing is an integral part of managing patients with tuberculosis. About 10% of all cases of tuberculosis are diagnosed by contact tracing. Close contacts of patients with smear-positive pulmonary disease are at highest risk of infection. Contact tracing of people with extrapulmonary tuberculosis is not usually necessary.

Key points: Tuberculosis

- Tuberculosis is an infectious disease caused by the organism *Mycobacterium tuberculosis*.

- Most people infected with tuberculosis contain the infection and remain asymptomatic throughout life.

Continued

Key points: Tuberculosis—cont'd

- Some people reactivate the disease and develop active disease due to an immune problem which causes an inappropriate T helper cell response to the organism.

- Active tuberculosis may be pulmonary or extrapulmonary.

- Pulmonary tuberculosis typically presents with symptoms of a chronic pneumonia.

- Extrapulmonary tuberculosis commonly affects cervical lymph nodes and the kidneys.

- Treatment regimes require multiple drugs to be taken for 6 months.

- Compliance with treatment and completing the full course is essential to ensure eradication of the infection and prevent the development of multidrug-resistant strains.

Diffuse parenchymal lung diseases

Diffuse parenchymal lung diseases are characterized by interstitial inflammation

Diffuse parenchymal lung diseases (DPLDs) are a large group of conditions which share the characteristic feature of inflammation centred on the **interstitium** of the alveolar walls. The interstitium is the tissue lying between alveoli, in which pulmonary artery capillaries run. The previous term for these diseases was **interstitial lung diseases** and this is still commonly used. The term diffuse parenchymal lung diseases is more accurate because, although the inflammation is centred on the interstitium, there is also usually co-existing involvement of the alveoli and terminal airways.

Inflammation in the interstitium impairs gas exchange

Normally the interstitium is a thin layer, allowing the alveoli and capillaries to lie very close to one another for optimal diffusion between them. In a DPLD, the widespread recruitment of inflammatory cells expands and distorts the interstitium which impairs gas diffusion and causes breathlessness.

The danger with a DPLD is the development of permanent lung scarring

Episodes of alveolitis may be followed by complete resolution without residual damage to alveoli. In some instances, however, inflammation in the lung parenchyma due to a DPLD is followed by the laying down of scar tissue in the alveolar walls. The thickened alveolar walls are ineffective at gas exchange, resulting in worsening hypoxia and eventually chronic respiratory failure.

The final common pathway leading to lung fibrosis seems to be activation of macrophages, which release fibrogenic cytokines and stimulate fibroblasts in the interstitium to secrete large quantities of collagen (Fig. 7.10). Over time, scarring destroys the functional units of the lung and the end result is conversion of the lungs into a mass of cystic air spaces separated by dense scarring ('honeycomb lungs'). The chronic hypoxia causes pulmonary hypertension and right-sided heart failure (cor pulmonale). Prognosis is often poor in DPLD, with death occurring within 3 years of diagnosis from

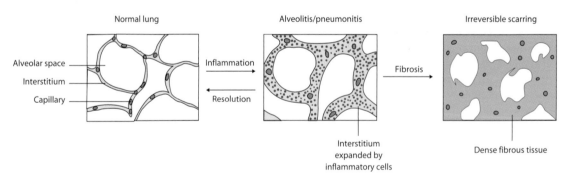

Fig. 7.10 Evolution of a diffuse parenchymal lung disease (DPLD). The normal interstitium is thin and contains pulmonary artery capillaries. In DPLD, the interstitium becomes expanded by an inflammatory cell infiltrate ('pneumonitis' or 'alveolitis'), impairing gas exchange. Complete resolution can occur, but the danger is development of fibrosis which permanently destroys the lung parenchyma.

a combination of respiratory and cardiac failure, even with attempted treatment.

There are a huge number of diffuse parenchymal lung diseases

DPLD may be caused by anything which sets up persistent inflammation within alveolar walls. The exhaustive list of all known causes is huge (>200 entities long!), but fortunately they can be divided into five basic categories (Fig. 7.11):

♦ Unknown cause (idiopathic interstitial lung diseases)

♦ Inhaled inorganic/mineral dusts (pneumoconioses)

♦ Inhaled organic particles (hypersensitivity pneumonitis)

♦ Side effects of treatment, particularly therapeutic radiation and certain drugs

♦ Involvement of the lung interstitium by multisystem diseases.

Patients with DPLD present with progressive breathlessness and a dry cough

Most patients with DPLD present with slowly progressive breathlessness and a dry cough. Other respiratory symptoms are uncommon. The most important job of the physician suspecting DPLD is to determine its nature quickly before more of the lung is irreversibly damaged. In particular, the past medical history, occupational history, and domestic environment can provide crucial diagnostic information.

Spirometry in DPLD shows a restrictive ventilatory defect

Despite the very large number of causes of DPLD, they all show a characteristic feature on spirometry known as a restrictive pattern, with a reduction in both FEV_1 and FVC (Fig. 7.12). The FEV_1/FVC ratio is therefore *preserved* in restrictive diseases, in contrast to the obstructive pattern where both FEV_1 and the FEV_1/FVC ratio are low. Spirometry is a useful preliminary investigation to perform in a patient suspected of having a DPLD. Although the test cannot provide a precise diagnosis, it is very helpful in corroborating a suspicion of a DPLD and provides an easy way of monitoring disease progression.

High resolution CT scanning of the chest is a very useful investigation in DPLD

High resolution CT scanning of the chest takes very thin (1–2 mm) sections through the lungs. Examining such thin slices enables a much more accurate assessment of the lung parenchyma, not only allowing the confirmation of the presence of a DPLD but very often even providing a precise diagnosis. If, following a panel of investigations, there is still doubt over the diagnosis then a lung biopsy should be considered.

Having considered the general principles of DPLDs, we now move on to discuss some of the common individual causes in more detail.

Idiopathic interstitial lung diseases

DPLDs with no clear underlying cause are known as idiopathic interstitial lung diseases

Very often no clear underlying cause can be found in a patient who has the features of a DPLD. All we can speculate is that some unidentified agent has caused

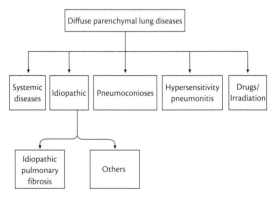

Fig. 7.11 Categories of diffuse parenchymal lung diseases.

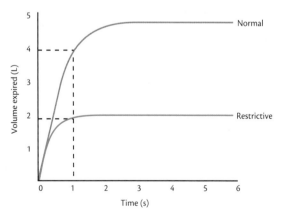

Fig. 7.12 Spirometry in diffuse parenchymal lung disease. The typical spirometric features of a DPLD is a restrictive pattern, with a reduction in both FEV_1 and FVC such that the FEV_1 to FVC ratio is preserved.

repeated cycles of alveolar injury and that the healing response has led to widespread lung fibrosis. Based on a variety of factors including the clinical picture, the imaging studies and the microscopic appearances of the lungs, several types of idiopathic interstitial lung disease have been described.

The most common idiopathic interstitial lung disease is idiopathic pulmonary fibrosis

Idiopathic pulmonary fibrosis (previously known as 'cryptogenic fibrosing alveolitis') is the most common idiopathic interstitial lung disease. Be careful not to confuse the *disease* idiopathic pulmonary fibrosis with the *term* idiopathic interstitial lung disease which refers generally to any DPLD of unknown cause.

Patients with idiopathic pulmonary fibrosis gradually develop worsening breathlessness and cough over a period of 5–10 years. Investigations such as imaging and lung function tests indicate a diffuse parenchymal lung disease; however, no clear cause can be found.

Before making a diagnosis of idiopathic pulmonary fibrosis, it is important rigorously to exclude other possible causes of lung fibrosis, particularly asbestosis which can be clinically indistinguishable. Taking a detailed thorough history is paramount in this respect.

If a lung biopsy from a patient with idiopathic pulmonary fibrosis is scrutinized, the histological pattern that one sees is known as **usual interstitial pneumonia** (UIP). Be careful not to equate the histological term UIP with the clinical entity of idiopathic pulmonary fibrosis. They are not the same thing. Although the UIP pattern must be seen on biopsy to diagnose idiopathic pulmonary fibrosis, UIP can also be seen with other types of DPLD that do have a clear cause, e.g. lung involvement by a multisystem autoimmune disease.

Unfortunately the prognosis of idiopathic pulmonary fibrosis is not good. Most patients follow a downhill course which leads to death just a few years from diagnosis.

Pneumoconioses

Pneumoconioses are DPLDs caused by inhaled inorganic dusts

Inhalation of large quantities of harmful inorganic dust particles can lead to interstitial inflammation and fibrosis. The dangerous particles are those that are small enough to reach the smallest airways and alveoli. Macrophages activated by the toxic particles secrete fibrogenic cytokines which stimulate the laying down of scar tissue.

Most cases of pneumoconioses are associated with occupational exposure, e.g. mining or tunnelling. The most well recognized inorganic dusts causing lung fibrosis are coal dust ('coal worker's pneumoconiosis'), silica ('silicosis'), and asbestos ('asbestosis'). The incidence of pneumoconiosis has dramatically declined as a result of dust control in mines and the fall in traditional trades associated with exposure. Fewer than 100 new cases each of coal-, silica-, and asbestos-related lung fibrosis are now seen each year in the UK.

JARGON BUSTER

Asbestosis

Note that asbestosis refers strictly to diffuse fibrosis of the lung parenchyma due to high levels of asbestos exposure. The term should not be used for the *pleural* changes associated with asbestos, which are much more common manifestations of asbestos exposure (p. 135).

Hypersensitivity pneumonitis

Hypersensitivity pneumonitis is a diffuse parenchymal lung disease caused by an excessive immune response to inhaled organic antigens. The mechanism of lung damage is therefore quite different from the pneumoconioses which are the result of a direct toxic effect of inorganic dusts.

Hypersensitivity pneumonitis may be caused by a wide variety of materials. Most of the offending agents are derived either from microorganisms (particularly fungal spores) or from animals such as birds. The types of antigen recognized to cause hypersensitivity pneumonitis are extremely diverse, creating an amusing list of diseases such as bird fancier's lung, farmer's lung, sewage worker's lung, and even paprika splitter's lung!

JARGON BUSTER

Extrinsic allergic alveolitis

Hypersensitivity pneumonitis is also sometimes called **extrinsic allergic alveolitis** in the UK. This term tends not to be used in the USA, where the term allergic is restricted only to diseases associated with immediate (type I) hypersensitivity reactions.

Exposure to high levels of antigen causes a type III hypersensitivity reaction

In hypersensitivity pneumonitis, exposure to high levels of antigen results in an immune reaction leading to the production of antibodies to the antigen. On repeat exposure, there is an abnormal immune response whereby the pre-formed antibodies bind to the antigen in the airways and form immune complexes which stimulate an acute inflammatory response (type III hypersensitivity reaction). The greater the antigen exposure, the greater the reaction and the worse the symptoms will be.

Note that type III hypersensitivity reactions do not lead to the widespread activation of macrophages, so patients with intermittent acute exposure to antigen are unlikely to develop fibrosis.

Persistent low level exposure to antigen leads to a type IV hypersensitivity reaction

If antigen exposure is low grade, a type III reaction does not occur, presumably because antigen levels are too low. Instead, macrophages take up the antigen and present it to CD4+ helper T lymphocytes, leading to a type IV hypersensitivity reaction with activated macrophages. Because numerous macrophages are activated, the development of progressive fibrosis becomes a risk.

Patients with intermittent high levels of antigen exposure usually present early

Patients with high levels of antigen exposure suffer disabling attacks of breathlessness due to the widespread inflammation from a type III reaction. Well recognized examples are the farmer who disturbs large amounts of hay or compost containing microbial antigens, or the pigeon keeper exposed to large amounts of antigen from the birds' feathers or excrement. These patients usually seek medical attention early, and the diagnosis of hypersensitivity pneumonitis can be made before a significant amount of irreversible fibrosis has occurred in the lung.

Patients with continuous low grade antigen exposure present much later

Hypersensitivity pneumonitis may also present in a more insidious way. This pattern is typically seen in patients with a very low grade but continuous exposure to the antigen. Typical examples include the housewife who keeps a single budgerigar at home. The chronic form is potentially much more serious because low grade inflammation leads to the slow development of irreversible lung fibrosis over many years, during which time the patient may be completely asymptomatic. By the time symptoms of breathlessness appear, much of the lung has been completely replaced by scar tissue.

Lung involvement by multisystem diseases

Sarcoidosis is the most common multisystem disease to cause DPLD

The development of lung fibrosis as part of a multisystem disease is well recognized. The most common multisystem disease to cause lung fibrosis is sarcoidosis, a disease characterized by the appearance of numerous non-caseating granulomas in multiple tissues and organs.

Other important diseases known to cause diffuse parenchymal lung disease include rheumatoid arthritis, systemic sclerosis, systemic lupus erythematosus, ankylosing spondylitis, and polymyositis.

Iatrogenic DPLD

Irradiation of the lungs and certain drugs can cause pulmonary fibrosis

Inflammation and fibrosis of the lung parenchyma is well recognized as a complication of irradiation of the lungs during treatment of primary lung tumours, metastatic lung deposits, and breast carcinoma.

Many drugs have also been implicated in causing pneumonitis, which may or may not be followed by fibrosis. Patients may present acutely with cough and shortness of breath, or insidiously due to progressive fibrosis. The most common culprits are antineoplastic drugs such as bleomycin, and the antiarrhythmic drug amiodarone. Most drug-induced DPLD is reversible if it is recognized early and the offending drug is discontinued.

Key points: Diffuse parenchymal lung diseases

- DPLDs are a large group of diseases characterized by inflammation centred on the interstitium of the alveolar walls.

- The concern in DPLDs is the development of fibrosis in response to the inflammation which irreversibly damages the lungs.

Continued

> ## Key points: Diffuse parenchymal lung diseases—cont'd
>
> - Patients usually present with gradually worsening breathlessness which terminates in chronic respiratory failure.
> - Idiopathic interstitial lung diseases are DPLDs with no obvious cause. The most common idiopathic interstitial lung disease is idiopathic pulmonary fibrosis, which has a poor prognosis.
> - Pneumoconioses due to inorganic mineral dusts such as coal, silica, or asbestos exposure are now rare.
> - Hypersensitivity pneumonitis is due to an abnormal immune reaction to inhaled organic antigens.
> - DPLD may be seen as part of a multisystem disease such as sarcoidosis, systemic lupus erythematosus, and rheumatoid arthritis.
> - DPLD may also be iatrogenic following radiotherapy to the chest or as a side effect of certain drugs.

Tumours of the lung

Tumours of the lung may be benign or malignant. The most common benign pulmonary tumour is the pulmonary hamartoma. The commonest primary malignant tumour of the lung is lung carcinoma. The lungs are also very common sites of metastases from malignant neoplasms arising at other sites.

Pulmonary hamartoma

Pulmonary hamartoma is the most common benign tumour of the lung

Pulmonary hamartoma is a relatively common benign lung lesion composed of a disorganized mixture of tissues normally present in the lung, such as cartilage, fibrous tissue, fat, and respiratory type epithelium. Ninety per cent of pulmonary hamartomas arise in the periphery of the lungs. It remains controversial as to whether it is actually a hamartoma or a genuine benign neoplasm. Although completely benign, pulmonary hamartomas are clinically significant

because they present as a solitary nodule on a chest radiograph and need to be distinguished from a malignant lung lesion.

Lung carcinoma

Lung carcinoma is the second most common cancer in the UK

Lung carcinoma is the second most common cancer in the UK (behind breast cancer), but is the most frequent cause of cancer death in both men and women. The outlook for patients diagnosed with lung cancer is therefore poor, with less than 10 per cent of people remaining alive 5 years from diagnosis.

Ninety per cent of cases of lung carcinoma can be attributed to smoking

There is very strong evidence that smoking is the most powerful risk factor for the development of lung cancer. There is a strong dose–response relationship, i.e. the heavier the smoker the more likely the development of lung cancer, and stopping smoking reduces the risk of developing lung cancer. Cigarette smoke has also been shown to contain a large number of compounds which are potentially carcinogenic. *It should therefore be appreciated that the most effective way to reduce the incidence of lung cancer is primary prevention by stopping smoking or never starting.*

Microscopy distinguishes four common types of lung carcinoma

Although a wide variety of different types of carcinoma have been reported in the lung, only four are commonly seen. In order of frequency, they are:

- **Squamous cell carcinoma**
- **Adenocarcinoma**
- **Small cell carcinoma**
- **Large cell carcinoma.**

Defining the precise type of carcinoma is only possible by microscopic examination of a sample of the tumour. Although we do not know for certain, it is highly likely that all lung carcinomas arise from the pluripotent bronchial precursor cell. The specific type of lung carcinoma that results depends on the differentiation pathway that the transformed precursor cell takes.

Because all lung carcinomas except for small cell carcinoma are currently managed in the same way, clinicians often divide lung carcinomas into just two groups for the purposes of management: small cell lung carcinoma (SCLC) or non-small cell lung carcinoma (NSCLC) which includes all the other types.

Squamous cell carcinomas arise from larger central airways

Squamous cell carcinoma of the lung is a malignant epithelial tumour arising in the lung which shows features of squamous differentiation, i.e. keratin formation and/or intercellular bridges.

The sequence of events that lead to the development of squamous cell carcinomas is well recognized: they derive from bronchial epithelium that has undergone metaplastic change to squamous epithelium in response to chronic damage from smoking. Continued carcinogenic assault results in dysplasia, followed by carcinoma in situ, and eventually invasive squamous cell carcinoma.

Squamous cell carcinomas tend to arise in the larger airways near the hilum of the lung. Tumours growing into the lumen can cause obstruction to the distal lung and predispose to pneumonia or the development of focal bronchiectasis (Fig. 7.13).

Adenocarcinomas of the lung arise from smaller airways deeper in the lungs

Adenocarcinoma of the lung is a malignant epithelial tumour arising in the lung which shows microscopic evidence of glandular differentiation by the neoplastic cells, i.e. gland formation or mucin production.

The sequence of events leading to the development of lung adenocarcinoma is not as well defined as for squamous cell carcinoma. A multistep sequence of events has been proposed for adenocarcinoma from a lesion called **atypical adenomatous hyperplasia** to

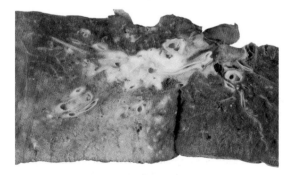

Fig. 7.13 A central lung carcinoma. Note how the lung tissue distal to the tumour shows flecks of yellow consolidation due to an obstructive pneumonia. The tumour was found to be a squamous cell carcinoma when examined microscopically.

invasive adenocarcinoma through a non-invasive lesion called a **bronchioloalveolar carcinoma**.

The incidence of lung adenocarcinoma has been rising, and now accounts for the same number of cases as squamous cell carcinoma. It is thought that this is due to a change in smoking patterns associated with newer types of cigarettes. Prior to the 1950s, smoke from cigarettes was too irritating to be inhaled deeply, and most of the carcinogens were deposited in the larger airways. Since then, the popularity of filters and new 'light' blends allows smokers to inhale more deeply. This smoking pattern deposits carcinogens in smaller peripheral airways where adenocarcinomas form.

Small cell carcinoma is a highly aggressive lung tumour which spreads rapidly

Small cell carcinoma is a malignant epithelial tumour consisting of small cells with little cytoplasm and ill defined cell borders. The tumour is typically extensively necrotic and the mitotic count is high. The old term 'oat cell carcinoma' which surfaces on occasion is no longer recognized and should not be used.

Small cell carcinomas are usually centrally located and are notorious for their rapid rate of growth and early spread. Extensive metastases are often already present at the time of diagnosis. Surgery is almost always futile and therefore rarely performed. Small cell carcinomas arise from bronchial epithelium but show differentiation into neuroendocrine cells containing neurosecretory granules. They are therefore the most common tumour type associated with ectopic hormone production.

Large cell carcinomas are undifferentiated tumours that cannot be otherwise categorized

Large cell carcinoma is a term applied to epithelial tumours that are so undifferentiated that they cannot be categorized. They almost certainly represent cases of squamous cell carcinoma or adenocarcinoma that have become so undifferentiated that they can no longer be distinguished by light microscopy. Large cell carcinomas tend to be bulky peripheral tumours which invade locally and disseminate widely. About half the patients have widespread disease at presentation.

There are many different ways in which lung cancer may present

Symptoms related to lung cancer can be divided into local, metastatic, systemic, and paraneoplastic. Local signs and symptoms are those due to the growth of the primary tumour mass or involved regional lymph nodes. These include:

- *Cough.* This is the most common initial presenting symptom. Patients with a persistent cough or a change in cough habit should be investigated if they are over 40 and are smokers.

- *Haemoptysis.* An ulcerating tumour mass will often bleed, causing blood-stained sputum production. It is uncommon as the sole presenting symptom but occurs at some stage in the disease in most patients.

- *Stridor/wheeze.* Localized persistent wheeze even after coughing is a significant observation suggestive of obstruction of a larger airway.

- *Hoarseness.* Invasion of the recurrent laryngeal nerve by the tumour leads to a persistently hoarse voice.

- *Breathlessness.* Dyspnoea is the presenting symptom in only a small number of patients, but becomes inevitable with disease progression. This is due to a combination of parenchymal destruction by the tumour, obstruction of airways with distal collapse, and other secondary effects such as a pleural effusion. Remember that heavy smokers will often have co-existing chronic airways disease which will also contribute to the overall picture.

- *Chest wall pain.* This is a common, though ill-defined, symptom at diagnosis and usually implies invasion of ribs or pleura by tumour.

- *Non-resolving pneumonia.* Infections are common in lung distal to airways blocked by tumour. Always consider an underlying malignancy in a patient with a pneumonia, especially if it is slow to resolve or recurs in the same location.

- *Superior vena cava obstruction.* Very large nodal masses may grow sufficiently to compress and obstruct blood flow down the superior vena cava. This presents with swelling of the head and neck region with prominent veins. The jugular venous pulse appears raised and fixed.

Lung cancer may metastasize to any organ of the body and produce symptoms that may form the presenting complaint. Commonly involved distant sites include the central nervous system, bones, and the liver.

Systemic symptoms refer to the general effects of the tumour mass on the body, giving rise to non-specific constitutional symptoms. Weight loss is a very common symptom and there is often a vague sense of ill health with a lack of energy and lack of interest in normal pursuits.

Paraneoplastic manifestations can be fairly common in lung tumours, and may pre-date symptoms from the primary tumour mass. They often produce quite non-specific symptoms:

- *Syndrome of inappropriate ADH secretion (SIADH).* Secretion of excess antidiuretic hormone (ADH) by tumour cells causes excess reabsorption of water from the collecting ducts of nephrons, leading to overhydration. The patient is usually asymptomatic until plasma sodium concentration falls below 120 mmol/l (normal range 135–145 mmol/l) due to dilution. Eventually symptoms related to cerebral oedema due to water intoxication occur. Initially there is clumsiness and tiredness which progresses to increasing drowsiness and confusion. Peripheral oedema is rare because the retained water is shared between the intracellular and extracellular compartments.

- *Ectopic ACTH.* This is typically associated with small cell carcinomas. Secretion of adenocorticotrophic hormone (ACTH) leads to bilateral hyperplasia of the adrenal cortex with secretion of large amounts of cortisol. The chief manifestations are thirst and polyuria. The typical features of Cushing's syndrome are rarely seen, as death often occurs before the features fully develop.

- *Hypercalcaemia.* This is more common with squamous cell carcinomas. As a paraneoplastic effect, it is due to the elaboration of a parathyroid hormone-related peptide by tumour cells which mimics the effect of parathyroid hormone leading to release of calcium from bone. Bear in mind that hypercalcaemia in the setting of lung cancer is usually not paraneoplastic, but rather the result of bony metastases.

In order to make the diagnosis, a sample of the tumour must be obtained

Like most cancers, treatment should not begin until the diagnosis of a lung tumour is confirmed by microscopic examination. As well as confirming the diagnosis of a lung carcinoma, the precise type of tumour can usually be identified. This is important as there is a distinction in the treatment for small cell carcinoma from the remainder.

One of the most common ways to sample a tumour for diagnosis is at bronchoscopy. Bronchoscopy involves the passing of a flexible fibreoptic tube into the respiratory tree via the nose, allowing visualization of the airways. Any suspicious lesion or mucosal abnormality can be biopsied for histological examination, and brushings and washings can be taken for cytological examination for malignant cells. Because of their central location, squamous cell carcinomas and small cell carcinomas are particularly readily sampled by bronchoscopy. Smaller peripheral lesions are often amenable to CT-guided fine needle aspiration for cytology.

Key points: Lung carcinoma

- Lung carcinoma is the second most common malignancy and the leading cause of cancer deaths.

- Almost all lung carcinomas are attributable to smoking.

- Lung carcinomas are derived from bronchial epithelium.

- There are four common lung carcinomas: squamous cell carcinoma, adenocarcinoma, small cell carcinoma, and large cell carcinoma.

- Lung carcinoma may present in many different ways and one should have a high index of suspicion in a long-term heavy smoker.

Pulmonary metastases

The lungs are very common sites for metastases. Common malignancies that spread to the lungs include breast carcinoma, colorectal carcinoma, renal cell carcinoma, and germ cell tumours of the testis.

Malignant tumours may reach the lungs via the blood stream or the lymphatic system, and typically cause numerous deposits scattered throughout the parenchyma of both lungs (so-called 'cannonball' metastases). Sometimes the lymphatic channels of the lungs become diffusely permeated by tumour deposits, causing the rapidly fatal condition **lymphangitis carcinomatosa**.

Pleural diseases

The pleural surfaces form the interface between the lungs and the chest wall. Like other mesothelial-lined cavities in the body, the pleura is a continuous sheet that is conveniently divided into two portions. The parietal pleura is closely applied to the chest wall and rib surfaces, and the visceral pleura covers the surfaces of the lungs. Between the two layers is a potential space which contains a small amount (~ 20 ml) of serous fluid for lubrication. The visceral pleura is innervated only by autonomic nerves and is insensitive to pain. The parietal pleura, however, is extensively supplied by sensory nerves derived from branches of the nerve supply to underlying structures, e.g. the intercostal and phrenic nerves.

The two main symptoms of pleural disease are pleuritic pain and breathlessness

Pleuritic pain (colloquially known as 'pleurisy') is a very sharp, stabbing pain triggered by inspiration or coughing, due to inflammation of *parietal* pleura. It typically arises when an inflammatory process in the periphery of a lung (e.g. pneumonia) involving the visceral pleura extends to involve the parietal pleura which invokes pleuritic pain via its somatic innervation.

Breathlessness due to pleural disease is usually due to accumulation of fluid in the pleural space (pleural effusion). Pleuritic pain is unusual with a large pleural effusion because the fluid prevents the inflamed visceral pleural surface from irritating the parietal pleura from which the sharp pain arises.

Pleural effusion

A pleural effusion results from the accumulation of fluid in the pleural space

Accumulation of excess fluid in the pleural space is known as a pleural effusion. If the amount of fluid is small, there may be no symptoms at all unless the underlying cause gives rise to symptoms. A large pleural effusion is an important cause of breathlessness.

The most common causes of a pleural effusion are:

- **Cardiac failure**. Small bilateral effusions are commonly seen in patients with congestive cardiac failure. Often the diagnosis is clear as the chest X-ray will also show other features of heart failure (e.g. an enlarged heart and prominent upper lobe vessels) in addition to the pleural effusions.

◆ **Pneumonia** (including tuberculosis). A sterile para-pneumonic effusion is often seen adjacent to an area of pneumonia.

◆ **Pulmonary embolism**. A pleural effusion may form as a complication of a pulmonary embolus, pre-sumably as a reaction to an area of infarction. The presence of pleuritic chest pain in a patient with a unilateral effusion and no other evidence of infection should raise the possibility of a pulmonary embolism.

◆ **Malignancy**. A primary lung cancer infiltrating the pleura may give rise to a pleural effusion. These are usually adenocarcinomas because they arise peripherally and are therefore more likely to involve the pleural surface. Other carcinomas which have metastasized to the pleura can also cause a pleural effusion, particularly breast carcinoma. Although less common, the possibility of malignant mesothelioma should be also considered as this often presents with a pleural effusion (see below).

◆ **Multisystem autoimmune diseases**. We have seen how these diseases (systemic lupus erythematosus, rheumatoid arthritis, etc.) can cause pulmonary fibro-sis. They can also involve the pleura and give rise to an isolated pleural effusion.

Sampling a pleural effusion for laboratory tests can be helpful

If the cause of a pleural effusion is not apparent, then very often a sample of the fluid can be drawn off using a needle inserted between the ribs into the pleural space, a technique known as pleural aspiration or a pleural 'tap'. Samples of the fluid can be sent to various divisions of the pathology laboratory for investigation.

If malignancy is suspected, then a fresh sample should be sent without delay for cytology. Cytology involves microscopic examination of the cells shed into the pleural fluid. This is particularly helpful for picking up a malignant effusion, as malignant cells shed into the fluid can be seen down the microscope.

If infection is suspected, a sample should be sent to microbiology for Gram staining and culture of the fluid. If tuberculosis is a possibility (tuberculosis often involves the pleura and causes a pleural effusion), this should be stated on the request form so that the fluid will also be specifically stained and cultured for mycobacteria.

Pneumothorax

A pneumothorax results from gas entering the pleural space

If gas enters and fills the pleural space, the adjacent lung collapses leading to breathlessness and pleu-ritic chest pain, a condition known as pneumothorax. There are two main ways gas may enter the pleural space:

◆ *Rupture of underlying lung through the visceral pleura*. If a diseased area of lung ruptures and breaches the visceral pleura, alveolar gas will enter the pleural space, causing pneumothorax. This occurs because pleural pressure is less than alveolar pressure due to the natural elastic recoil of the lungs.

◆ *External penetrating trauma or iatrogenic injury*. Here, the pneumothorax results from atmospheric air entering the pleural space through the wound.

A pneumothorax may be spontaneous, traumatic, or iatrogenic

In the clinical setting, it is helpful to divide pneumoth-oraces into either spontaneous, traumatic, or iatrogenic. Spontaneous pneumothoraces, which occur without any warning, may also be subdivided into primary or secondary (Table 7.9).

TABLE 7.9	Causes of pneumothorax
Spontaneous	
Primary	
Thin young men	
Secondary	
COPD	
Asthma	
Severe pneumonia	
Traumatic	
Penetrating chest wound	
Rib fractures	
Iatrogenic	
Subclavian vein cannulation	
Lung biopsy	

Primary spontaneous pneumothorax occurs in individuals with apparently healthy lungs. It is a relatively common condition which mostly afflicts young tall thin men. The pneumothorax is thought to be due to rupture of small delicate apical 'blebs' of lung tissue which result from stretching of the lungs in tall people. About a quarter of patients will have recurrences.

A secondary spontaneous pneumothorax occurs in people with underlying lung disease. The most common associations are COPD and asthma. Sometimes pneumothoraces can result from lung malignancy and severe infections if a necrotic area of lung ruptures into the pleural space.

Traumatic pneumothoraces occur due to injury to the chest wall and may be seen in victims of trauma, e.g. road traffic accidents.

Iatrogenic pneumothoraces occur due to accidental puncture of the pleural space during medical procedures. The most common procedure associated with a risk of pneumothorax is attempted central line insertion, particularly via the subclavian vein. A chest radiograph should always be performed after central line insertion to ensure a pneumothorax has not occurred (and to check correct positioning of the central line).

Asbestos-related pleural disease

Asbestos is a general term for a group of mineral fibres which are very resistant to heat, electricity, chemicals, and sound. These properties gave asbestos great commercial value and it was used extensively from the 1950s through to the mid-1980s for a variety of purposes, particularly insulation around steam pipes and boilers.

Unfortunately, asbestos is now known to be a hazard to health, and for this reason its use has declined considerably in recent years. However, the incidence of asbestos-related disease continues to increase, as there is a time lag of many years between exposure and the development of disease. Although some of the asbestos has been removed over the years, there are many thousands of tonnes of asbestos still present in buildings. Asbestos-related disease only occurs in people working regularly with asbestos for many years. There is no evidence that disease occurs simply by being in a building with asbestos in it.

We have already seen how lung fibrosis due to asbestos (asbestosis) requires very high levels of asbestos exposure. Much more commonly seen in patients exposed to asbestos is pleural disease, which can occur at quite

low levels of asbestos exposure—well below those needed to produce asbestosis. Four pleural conditions are known to result from asbestos exposure:

♦ **Pleural plaques**
♦ **Reactive pleural effusion**
♦ **Diffuse pleural fibrosis**
♦ **Malignant mesothelioma.**

The gradient of diseases with increasing exposure to asbestos is: pleural plaques and reactive pleural effusion (little exposure), diffuse pleural fibrosis, mesothelioma, and asbestosis (very high exposure).

Pleural plaques are benign lesions of the parietal pleura which cause no symptoms

Pleural plaques are lesions which develop on the parietal surface of the pleura, particularly on the diaphragmatic surfaces (Fig. 7.14). They are smooth raised plaques which are frequently associated with asbestos exposure especially when large, numerous, and bilateral. They are not pathognomic for asbestos as there are other causes such as trauma, and some pleural plaques appear to be idiopathic. Those that are associated with asbestos are markers of asbestos exposure only and do not indicate an increased risk of malignant mesothelioma.

Diffuse pleural fibrosis is thickening of the visceral pleura

Diffuse pleural fibrosis predominantly affects the visceral pleura. It can be associated with quite low

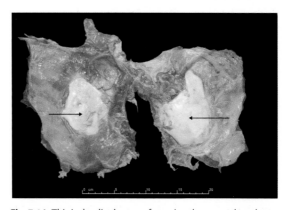

Fig. 7.14 This is the diaphragm of a patient known to have been exposed to asbestos. There are well circumscribed pleural plaques (arrows) on the parietal pleura of the domes of the diaphragm.

levels of asbestos exposure and most cases are asymptomatic. Occasionally, the fibrosis can be bilateral and extensive (surrounding the lung completely), in which case symptoms may result.

Malignant mesothelioma is a highly aggressive tumour of the pleura

Malignant mesothelioma is a malignant neoplasm derived from mesothelial cells which line the body cavities. Cases of mesotheliomas involving the peritoneum and pericardium have been described, but these are exceedingly rare. By far the most common site of malignant mesothelioma is the pleura, almost all of which are associated with asbestos exposure.

Mesotheliomas usually involve the parietal and visceral pleura in a diffuse fashion. As the tumour progresses, it gradually encases the lung and extends into adjacent structures such as the chest wall and pericardium (Fig. 7.15).

Most patients are men who present between the ages of 50 and 70 years with breathlessness and chest pain. The pain is usually a dull ache, due to invasion of the chest wall, rather than pleuritic. A pleural effusion is very often present. The diagnosis may be made on cytological examination of pleural fluid or on histological examination of a pleural biopsy.

The clinical course of malignant mesothelioma is dismal. The tumour relentlessly spreads locally within the thorax. Although chemotherapy may be of some benefit, there is no curative treatment and the mean survival is 18 months from diagnosis.

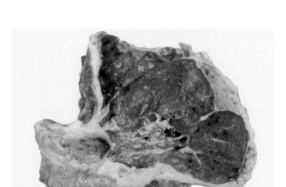

Fig. 7.15 Typical macroscopic appearance of malignant mesothelioma. Note how the tumour encases and compresses the lung.

> ## Key points: Asbestos-related pleural disease
>
> ◆ Asbestos causes pleural disease at lower levels of exposure than that needed to produce lung disease.
>
> ◆ Pleural plaques are highly suggestive of previous asbestos exposure. They are not in themselves precursors of malignancy.
>
> ◆ Malignant mesothelioma is a highly aggressive tumour of the pleura associated with asbestos exposure which spreads extensively within the chest wall, encasing the entire lung. The prognosis is dismal.

Gastrointestinal disease

Introduction

This chapter concerns itself with diseases of the oesophagus, stomach, small intestine, large intestine, and anus managed by gastroenterologists and gastrointestinal surgeons. Diseases of the accessory organs of the gastrointestinal tract such as salivary glands, liver, gallbladder, and pancreas come under the remit of other specialties and are dealt with in Chapters 9 and 19.

Oesophagus

The oesophagus is a muscular tube lined by squamous epithelium which connects the pharynx to the stomach. Its function is to transport food and liquid to the stomach, and to ensure that gastric contents do not regurgitate back up. This is achieved through a complex mechanism which coordinates peristaltic contractions with intermittent relaxation of the lower oesophageal sphincter.

Gastro-oesophageal reflux disease

Gastro-oesophageal reflux disease is the commonest oesophageal disorder

Gastro-oesophageal reflux disease (GORD), or **reflux oesophagitis**, is a disease caused by reflux of gastric contents from the stomach into the lower oesophagus. The squamous epithelium lining the oesophagus is not designed to resist the acidity of gastric juices and so may become inflamed (oesophagitis), leading to symptoms of GORD.

A degree of gastric reflux occurs in everyone but usually without symptoms. The reason why some people with reflux develop GORD is not clear, but probably depends on a number of factors such as the volume and acidity of the refluxed material and the resistance of the oesophagus to injury.

A sliding hiatus hernia is one major predisposing factor for reflux

Numerous factors have been implicated in episodes of reflux. These are mostly conditions associated with increased intra-abdominal pressure such as pregnancy or postural effects (e.g. lying flat). One well recognized major predisposing factor for reflux is the presence of a **sliding hiatus hernia**. This occurs when the gastro-oesophageal junction is drawn upwards such that a pouch of proximal stomach is abnormally located in the thorax.

Herniation of the gastro-oesophageal junction impairs its function as an antireflux barrier by removing the normal diaphragmatic compression around the lower oesophagus. Most patients with moderate to severe GORD will have a hiatus hernia, but it should be noted that hiatus hernia is a common condition and most patients with a hiatus hernia do not have GORD.

The classical symptom of GORD is burning retrosternal pain or 'heartburn'

Although heartburn is quite characteristic of GORD, in practice any kind of upper abdominal symptom may occur. Based on the prevalence of heartburn, GORD is very common. Although only a minority of sufferers develop complications, they can be serious. The two major complications, peptic stricture and Barrett's oesophagus, are typically only seen in patients with severe oesophagitis.

LINK BOX

GORD and non-atopic asthma

It has been suggested that extra-oesophageal reflux and aspiration into the respiratory tree may be important in the pathogenesis of non-atopic asthma (p. 118).

Peptic stricture is a benign narrowing of the distal oesophagus

A **peptic stricture** is a benign narrowing of the oesophagus caused by scarring and deformation of the distal oesophagus in response to persistent severe reflux oesophagitis. Peptic strictures are important because they can mimic the symptoms and appearances of a narrowing due to an oesophageal carcinoma (malignant stricture).

JARGON BUSTER

Peptic

The adjective **peptic** is used to describe a condition caused by the damaging effects of gastric secretions which contain the enzyme pepsin (among other things!).

Barrett's oesophagus is defined by columnar metaplasia of the lower oesophagus

Barrett's oesophagus is defined as *'an oesophagus in which any portion of the normal squamous lining has been replaced by a metaplastic columnar epithelium which is visible macroscopically.'* It is thought to represent an adaptive response of the oesophageal epithelium to the damaging effects of refluxed gastric material. Studies suggest that about 10 per cent of patients with GORD develop Barrett's oesophagus. It is not clear why some people have a particular propensity to develop Barrett's oesophagus, whilst others will never demonstrate it despite evidence of long-term GORD.

Barrett's oesophagus can only be diagnosed at endoscopy and confirmed with biopsy

There is no way of knowing if patients with GORD have developed Barrett's oesophagus based on their symptoms alone. In fact, many patients developing Barrett's oesophagus find their symptoms improve because the columnar epithelium is less sensitive to reflux. Barrett's oesophagus can therefore only be diagnosed at endoscopy, where the area of metaplastic epithelium is visible as a red velvety area. An endoscopic diagnosis of Barrett's oesophagus *must* be corroborated by taking biopsies from the area to confirm the presence of columnar epithelium microscopically (Fig. 8.1).

Barrett's oesophagus is a precursor lesion of oesophageal adenocarcinoma

Barrett's oesophagus is extremely important because in some (*not* all) patients the metaplastic columnar epithelium undergoes neoplastic transformation and develops into an invasive adenocarcinoma. The risk for developing adenocarcinoma of the oesophagus is some 50 times greater in patients with Barrett's oesophagus compared with the general population.

The development of an invasive adenocarcinoma in an area of Barrett's oesophagus is preceded by a phase of dysplasia of the columnar epithelium, in which the glandular epithelial cells appear neoplastic microscopically but invasion through the basement membrane has not yet occurred. Dysplasia can only be diagnosed microscopically; *there is no reliable endoscopic appearance of dysplasia*. Ruling out the presence of dysplasia is another important reason to biopsy areas of Barrett's oesophagus at endoscopy.

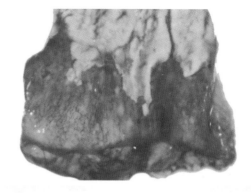
a

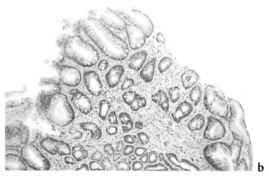
b

Fig. 8.1 Barrett's oesophagus. (a) This segment from the lower oesophagus shows the white keratinized squamous epithelium at the top. The red area at the bottom represents an area of Barrett's oesophagus. (b) An oesophageal biopsy taken from an area of endoscopic Barrett's oesophagus, confirming the presence of glandular epithelium.

Patients newly diagnosed with Barrett's oesophagus should be considered for entry into a surveillance programme

Because the development of oesophageal adenocarcinoma is preceded by a phase of dysplasia, it may be of benefit to some patients to enter into a surveillance programme involving endoscopy every 2 years with multiple biopsies taken from the area of Barrett's oesophagus to look for dysplasia.

It must be emphasized that not all patients are suitable for entry into such a programme and the actual individual risk of death from adenocarcinoma in a patient with Barrett's oesophagus remains small. Furthermore, unless the patient would be fit for the treatment (i.e. oesophagectomy), there is no point in putting them into such a programme.

If dysplasia is seen microscopically, it is graded into low grade or high grade

If dysplasia is seen by the pathologist examining a biopsy from an area of Barrett's oesophagus, they will grade it into either low grade or high grade. Patients diagnosed with low grade dysplasia undergo more frequent surveillance every 6 months with rebiopsy.

The presence of high grade dysplasia on a biopsy is a much more worrying feature. An invasive adenocarcinoma is either imminent or, worse, already present at an early stage somewhere else in the area of Barrett's change. For this reason, the tendency is to recommend that otherwise fit patients with evidence of high grade dysplasia undergo oesophagectomy as a curative procedure.

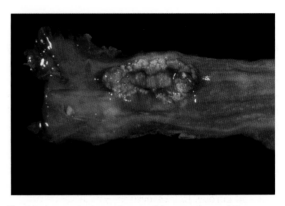

Fig. 8.2 An exophytic carcinoma of the oesophagus. Microscopy showed this to be a squamous cell carcinoma.

> ## Key points: Gastro-oesophageal reflux disease
>
> ◆ Gastro-oesophageal reflux disease is the most common oesophageal disorder in which burning retrosternal pain results from reflux of gastric contents into the lower oesophagus.
>
> ◆ A small number of patients with severe GORD develop complications such as a peptic stricture or Barrett's oesophagus.
>
> ◆ Barrett's oesophagus refers to an oesophagus in which part of the normal squamous epithelium has been replaced by metaplastic columnar type epithelium which is visible macroscopically at endoscopy. Barrett's oesophagus diagnosed at endoscopy must be confirmed histologically by taking biopsies from the area.
>
> ◆ Barrett's oesophagus is important because it is a precursor lesion of oesophageal adenocarcinoma.
>
> ◆ Although most patients with Barrett's oesophagus will not develop adenocarcinoma, it is recommended for some patients to enter a surveillance programme with regular endoscopy and biopsy of the area of Barrett's oesophagus to look for dysplasia.
>
> ◆ Low grade dysplasia should be managed with intense antiacid treatment and more frequent endoscopy and biopsy.
>
> ◆ High grade dysplasia is much more worrying and is a strong indication for oesophagectomy.

Oesophageal carcinoma

Oesophageal carcinomas are malignant epithelial tumours arising from the epithelial lining of the oesophagus (Fig. 8.2). Oesophageal carcinomas are about equally divided into squamous cell carcinomas and adenocarcinomas.

Squamous cell carcinoma of the oesophagus is related to heavy smoking and alcohol intake

Squamous cell carcinomas are malignant epithelial neoplasms showing evidence of squamous differentiation, such as keratin formation or intercellular bridges between the neoplastic cells. Squamous cell carcinomas of the oesophagus can develop anywhere in the oesophagus, but the middle third is the most common site. The two strongest risk factors are heavy alcohol intake (especially spirits) and smoking. The motility disorder achalasia is also associated with an increased risk of oesophageal squamous cell carcinoma (see later).

> ### LINK BOX
>
> ## Smoking and alcohol-related malignancies
>
> Heavy smokers and alcohol abusers are also prone to squamous cell carcinomas of the oral cavity (p. 451), hypopharynx (p. 460), and larynx (p. 461).

Adenocarcinoma of the oesophagus is related to Barrett's oesophagus

Adenocarcinomas are malignant epithelial neoplasms showing evidence of glandular differentiation, such as gland formation or mucin production by the neoplastic cells. Adenocarcinomas of the oesophagus arise from areas of high grade dysplasia on a background of Barrett's oesophagus due to GORD. They therefore arise principally in the lower oesophagus.

There is currently a lot of interest in oesophageal adenocarcinomas due to the very large increase in reported cases in recent decades, particularly in the USA and Europe. In fact, oesophageal adenocarcinoma currently has the most rapidly increasing incidence of any solid tumour in the Western world. This may be related to the increase in acid secretion and reflux disease associated with *Helicobacter pylori* eradication from the stomach.

Oesophageal carcinomas usually present late with rapidly progressive dysphagia for solids

The most common symptom of oesophageal carcinoma is **dysphagia**. The difficulty in swallowing is a result of narrowing of the oesophageal lumen by the tumour (malignant stricture). Patients describe the sensation of food getting stuck, and many make an alteration in their diet, opting for softer food. Patients often have marked loss of appetite and weight loss due to the fact that they have advanced cancer and their nutrition has been impaired for some time. Patients with these symptoms must undergo urgent upper gastrointestinal endoscopy to look for a tumour. Any suspicious areas or masses should be biopsied to prove or exclude carcinoma.

The prognosis of oesophageal carcinoma is poor

Fewer than 10 per cent of patients with an oesophageal carcinoma remain alive 5 years from diagnosis. This is related to the fact that when patients present with symptoms, the tumour has already spread through the oesophageal wall into the surrounding tissues and to regional lymph nodes. At this stage, surgical resection is not possible due to the high chance of recurrence.

Many patients will also have distant metastases from blood-borne spread, most commonly in the liver, lungs, and adrenal glands. Patients who for one reason or another are not candidates for curative surgery undergo palliative treatment to relieve their symptoms. Dysphagia is a very distressing symptom and a priority is to alleviate this by placing a stent across the malignant stricture at endoscopy.

The minority of patients with a potentially resectable tumour can be considered for oesophagectomy

The only potentially curative treatment for oesophageal carcinoma is removal of the oesophagus and part of the proximal stomach, a procedure known as an **oesophagectomy**. This is a major operation and the decision to proceed is only made after careful consideration. Patients are usually old and many will have co-existing lung and heart disease, especially those with squamous carcinomas who are usually heavy smokers.

> ### Key points: Oesophageal carcinoma
>
> - Oesophageal carcinomas are about equally divided into squamous cell carcinomas and adenocarcinomas.
> - Squamous cell carcinoma of the oesophagus is associated with heavy smoking and alcohol abuse, and tends to arise in the middle part of the oesophagus.
> - Adenocarcinoma of the oesophagus is associated with Barrett's oesophagus and tends to arise in the lower oesophagus.
> - Oesophageal carcinomas typically present with dysphagia and weight loss, by which time the tumours are often advanced and incurable.
> - The minority of patients with a potentially curable tumour may be offered an oesophagectomy if they are medically fit enough for the operation.

Infections of the oesophagus

In the immune competent, the oesophagus is very resistant to infection. Most individuals with infections of the oesophagus have impaired immunity, e.g. elderly debilitated patients, patients with HIV or a malignancy, or those taking immune-suppressing drugs.

Candidal oesophagitis is the most common infection of the oesophagus

The fungus *Candida albicans* is the most common organism that infects the oesophagus. The organism multiplies in the squamous epithelium, creating white patches on the oesophageal mucosal surface which may be visible at endoscopy.

Herpes simplex virus oesophagitis causes painful ulceration of the oesophagus

Herpes simplex virus oesophagitis arises due to reactivation of latent virus and spreads down sensory axons to the oesophagus. Numerous vesicles form in the oesophageal epithelium which, in severe cases, coalesce to form multiple ulcers in the oesophageal mucosa.

Drug-induced oesophagitis

A number of swallowed drugs can cause inflammation and ulceration of the oesophagus due to a local irritative effect. Drug-induced oesophagitis is a common problem in patients, particularly the elderly, who take their medication poorly, e.g. while lying down or with too little liquid. Common offenders are non-steroidal anti-inflammatory drugs (NSAIDs) and bisphosphonates. Avoidance of oesophagitis is the reason why bisphosphonates should always be taken first thing in the morning with a large amount of water whilst standing up!

Radiation oesophagitis

Radiation oesophagitis is inflammation of the oesophagus caused by radiation damage. It is mostly seen in patients with cancer receiving radiotherapy to the chest. The oesophagitis is usually mild, but can be severe with ulceration particularly if concomitant chemotherapy has been administered. Many patients find swallowing a liquid preparation of morphine helpful until their radiotherapy course is finished.

Achalasia

Achalasia is a motility disorder of the oesophagus in which the lower oesophageal sphincter fails to relax in response to swallowing and the smooth muscle of the oesophageal wall fails to propagate the peristaltic wave successfully. In response, the smooth muscle undergoes considerable hypertrophy and the oesophagus becomes markedly dilated and filled with stagnant fluid and food.

The cause of achalasia remains uncertain. Microscopic examination of the oesophageal wall shows significant loss of nerve fibres, associated with an inflammatory infiltrate of the myenteric plexus. This suggests that the pathogenesis of achalasia is related to immune-mediated destruction of the myenteric plexus; what causes this is not known.

The typical presentation of achalasia is slowly progressive dysphagia to both liquids and solids occurring in a middle-aged adult. There may be chest pain related to aborted attempts at peristalsis. Heartburn is not a feature as the tight lower oesophageal sphincter prevents reflux of gastric acid. A barium swallow shows narrowing of the distal oesophagus with proximal dilation. Endoscopy should always be performed, as these appearances may also be produced by an oesophageal carcinoma.

The most serious complication of achalasia is the development of squamous cell carcinoma.

Stomach

The stomach is a dilatable chamber which mechanically and chemically breaks up food into a semisolid consistency and stores it for controlled onward transmission. The stomach is divided into four compartments: cardia, fundus, body (corpus), and antrum (Fig. 8.3). Understanding this basic topography is important in understanding the major diseases.

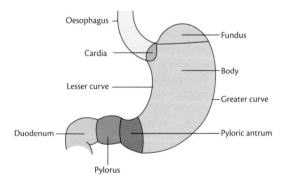

Fig. 8.3 Zones of the stomach. The acid-secreting glands are restricted to the mucosa of the body and fundus. The antrum contains the majority of the endocrine cells that secrete gastrin and somatostatin.

The stomach has evolved a formidable set of defences to protect itself

Chemical digestion in the stomach is largely achieved through the actions of secreted acid and the enzyme pepsin. These powerful agents pose a continuous threat of autodigestion, so the stomach requires mechanisms to defend itself.

The surface mucus barrier is the first line of defence against acid attack. The efficacy of this protective layer is enhanced by secretion of bicarbonate ions into the mucus by surface epithelial cells. This alkalinizes the mucus and protects against luminal acid.

Blood flow through the mucosa is also critical in defence by enabling disposal of hydrogen ions diffusing in from the gastric lumen. Furthermore, if surface epithelial cells are damaged, the gastric mucosa has the ability to proliferate and replace them very quickly.

NSAIDs and *Helicobacter pylori* are extremely important in gastric disease

Like the oesophagus, inflammation (and its consequences) and tumours are the most important conditions of the stomach. The underlying aetiologies in the stomach, however, are quite different from those in the oesophagus. *In the stomach, the role of* Helicobacter pylori *infection and the use of NSAIDs cannot be overemphasized.*

NSAIDs are gastric irritants and their use is extremely widespread. Well over 20 million prescriptions for NSAIDs are made every year in the UK and large amounts are also bought 'over the counter' for self-medication. Admittedly, in comparison with the vast number of people taking the drugs, the number of complications is relatively small, but many people who regularly take NSAIDs are not aware of the risk of complications. The problem is compounded by the fact that there are often no preceding gastrointestinal symptoms before a serious complication occurs.

Helicobacter pylori is a Gram negative bacterium that colonizes the stomach and is believed to infect over half the world's population. Since its initial discovery in 1983, a huge volume of work related to it has been published, and its causative role in a variety of gastric diseases has been universally accepted (Table 8.1).

Gastritis

Gastritis is a very ill defined term. Strictly speaking, it means inflammation in the stomach and thus should only be used by a pathologist examining a gastric biopsy.

TABLE 8.1	Outcome following infection with *H. pylori*
>80%	Asymptomatic gastritis
5–15%	Peptic ulcer disease
0–10%	Symptomatic gastritis
1–3%	Gastric carcinoma
0.5%	Gastric lymphoma

In everyday practice, however, the term gastritis is used very loosely, particularly by endoscopists who tend to describe any redness of the gastric mucosa as 'gastritis'.

Helicobacter pylori-associated gastritis

Helicobacter pylori infection is by far the most common cause of gastritis. The most likely mode of transmission is from person to person, by either the oral–oral route (through vomit or possibly saliva) or perhaps the faecal–oral route. Water-borne transmission due to faecal contamination may also be an important source of infection, especially in parts of the world where water is untreated.

Helicobacter pylori survives the hostile environment of the stomach by using its flagella to move to the antrum which is the least acidic area of the stomach (the antrum has few acid-producing parietal cells). The bacteria live in the thick mucus layer, taking advantage of the stomach's own protection. Any gastric acid that does reach the bacteria is neutralized by ammonia generated from urea by a urease enzyme synthesized by the bacteria.

The inflammation *H. pylori* sets up leads to an **antral-predominant gastritis**. It seems that from this initial point, there can be a variety of different outcomes (Fig. 8.4). What determines which of these pathways is followed is largely unknown. It almost certainly involves the interaction of a number of factors relating to both the virulence of the particular strain of *Helicobacter* and the individual's own defences. One thing has become clear: *the effect that the organism has on acid secretion is a critical factor in determining the outcome of the infection.*

Most patients subsequently develop an asymptomatic pangastritis

In the great majority of patients, acid secretion is slightly reduced allowing the bacteria to spread proximally into the stomach and set up a mild pangastritis

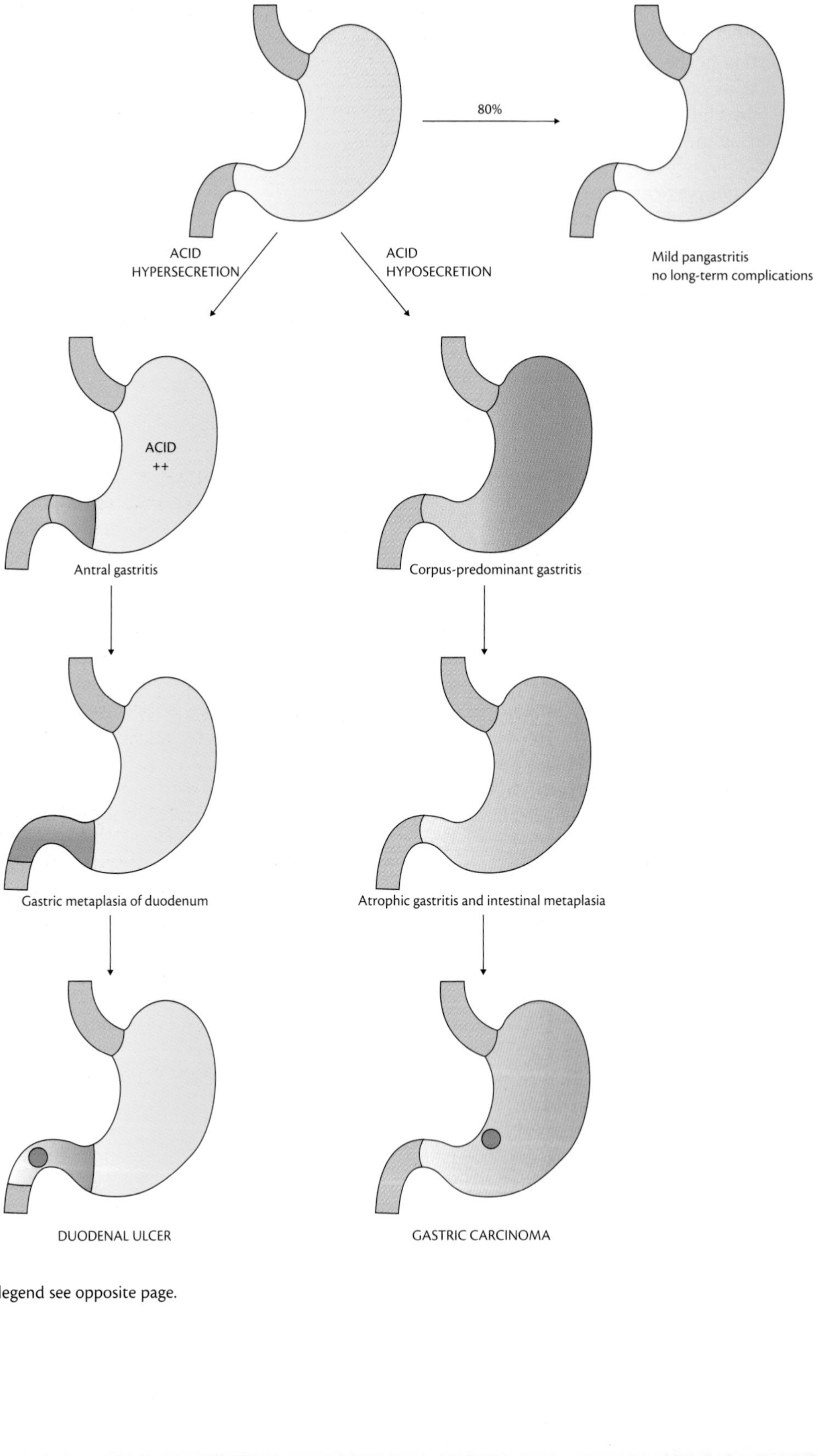

Fig. 8.4
For figure legend see opposite page.

Fig. 8.4 Possible outcomes of *H. pylori* infection. Most people infected with *H. pylori* develop an asymptomatic pangastritis with no long-term complications. Those with acid hypersecretion develop antral-predominant gastritis and risk duodenal ulceration. Those with acid hyposecretion develop a corpus-predominant gastritis and risk gastric carcinoma. *British Medical Journal* 2001, 323: 980–982, amended with permission from the BMJ publishing group.

(inflammation of the whole stomach). This seems to represent a balanced outcome of infection: a mild chronic gastritis is set up, the patient is asymptomatic, and there appears to be no significant risk of gastric complications.

> ### INTERESTING TO KNOW
>
> ## *H. pylori* and oesophageal adenocarcinoma
>
> An asymptomatic *H. pylori* pangastritis appears to be protective against oesophageal adenocarcinoma because of the slight reduction in the amount of acid secreted by the stomach. The sudden and alarming rise in incidence in oesophageal adenocarcinoma may be due to overenthusiastic use of *Helicobacter* eradication regimes in an attempt to treat patients with dyspepsia.

Patients with a persistent antral gastritis have a risk of duodenal ulceration

In some patients, *Helicobacter* infection causes an increase in acid secretion. This is thought to be due to a negative effect on the somatostatin-secreting cells located in the antrum. Somatostatin normally inhibits gastrin secretion, so loss of this negative feedback leads to hypergastrinaemia and increased acid production.

Excess acid passing into the duodenum causes inflammation of the first part of the duodenum. What happens next is critical in the evolution of duodenal ulcers. In response to the increased acid, *the epithelium of the first part of the duodenum undergoes gastric metaplasia* (i.e. the normal intestinal epithelium of the duodenum switches to a gastric type of epithelium). Although presumably an attempt at protecting itself, gastric metaplasia seems to be a deleterious response as it allows the first part of the duodenum to be colonized

by *Helicobacter* and become more inflamed, leading eventually to peptic ulceration.

Patients with a corpus-predominant gastritis have a risk of gastric carcinoma

In the remainder of patients, there is a marked decrease in acid production. This could be accounted for by an inhibitory effect on gastrin-secreting cells in the antrum leading to reduced stimulation to acid secretion from the corpus. Very low acidity allows the bacteria to heavily colonize the body of the stomach, causing a **corpus-predominant gastritis**. This situation is self-perpetuating because the corpus gastritis further depresses acid secretion. Over time, destruction of the acid-secreting glands leads to a **chronic atrophic gastritis**. Patients with a chronic atrophic gastritis may have areas of the stomach where the gastric epithelium undergoes metaplasia into an intestinal type of epithelium (intestinal metaplasia). The presence of intestinal metaplasia is important as a marker for the risk of the development of gastric carcinoma.

> ### INTERESTING TO KNOW
>
> ### Outcomes with *Helicobacter* infection
>
> The existence of these pathways is supported by two well recognized facts. First, patients with chronic duodenal ulcer have a very low incidence of gastric cancer because they have antral-predominant disease and avoid the pathway of chronic atrophic gastritis which leads to cancer. Secondly, the falling incidence of gastric cancer is believed to be due to increased treatment and eradication of *H. pylori*.

Autoimmune gastritis

Autoimmune gastritis is an organ-specific autoimmune disease associated with destruction of gastric parietal cells. Parietal cells generate the acid environment of the stomach and are found predominantly in the gastric glands located in the body and fundus of the stomach. The inflammation in autoimmune gastritis is therefore concentrated in the body and fundus of the stomach. This distribution distinguishes it from the pattern seen in *Helicobacter* gastritis where inflammation in the antrum is dominant.

Over time, autoimmune gastritis leads to extensive destruction and atrophy of the acid-secreting glands accompanied by intestinal metaplasia. This is a risk factor for the development of gastric carcinoma. Some patients also develop antibodies to **intrinsic factor**, the other product of parietal cells. Intrinsic factor binds to vitamin B12 and is required for its absorption in the terminal ileum. Depletion of vitamin B12 leads to a megaloblastic anaemia. Patients with anaemia due to lack of vitamin B12 as a result of autoimmune gastritis are said to have **pernicious anaemia** (p. 336).

Reactive gastritis

A reactive or chemical gastritis is a very common cause of redness of the gastric mucosa seen at endoscopy. It is the result of minor damage to the gastric mucosa by gastric irritants such as NSAIDs and alcohol. In the antrum, it is often due to reflux of bile from the duodenum into the stomach.

Although it causes non-specific erythema at endoscopy, there are typical microscopic features allowing the diagnosis to be made on a biopsy.

Erosive/haemorrhagic gastritis

An **erosive** or **haemorrhagic gastritis** refers to the appearance of a large number of defects in the gastric mucosa from which bleeding occurs. Bleeding can range from minor oozing to profuse bleeding leading to haematemesis. Profuse bleeding is more likely if deep defects expose large submucosal vessels.

An erosive/haemorrhagic gastritis occurs in two major settings:

- *Following ingestion of large quantities of NSAIDs, aspirin, or alcohol.* NSAID ingestion is the most common cause of erosive gastritis. Although in many cases there are no significant clinical manifestations, there is a risk of haemorrhage. This is a particular problem in elderly patients who have less robust gastric mucosal defence systems. Prescribing long-term NSAIDs in the elderly should be done with extreme caution.

- *The acutely unwell patient.* The incidence of erosive gastritis is very high (approaching 100 per cent) in seriously ill patients, especially those with sepsis, after major surgery, trauma, or burns. The risk of significant gastric haemorrhage is therefore of particular concern on the intensive therapy unit where all patients should be considered for prophylactic therapy with a proton pump inhibitor.

Acute erosions and ulcers causing an erosive/haemorrhagic gastritis usually heal rapidly and seldom recur if the underlying cause is removed or treated.

Key points: Gastritis

- Gastritis is a poorly defined term which strictly refers to inflammation in the stomach, but is often used to describe any redness of the gastric mucosa seen at endoscopy.

- Infection with *H. pylori* is the most common cause of gastritis. Although most patients infected with *H. pylori* remain asymptomatic, some develop complications including peptic ulceration, gastric carcinoma, and gastric lymphoma.

- Autoimmune gastritis is due to immune attack on the gastric parietal cells in the body of the stomach. These patients often present with a megaloblastic anaemia due to lack of intrinsic factor secretion (pernicious anaemia). Autoimmune gastritis is a risk factor for the development of gastric carcinoma.

- Reactive gastritis is a common cause of erythema of the gastric mucosa seen at endoscopy as a result of mild damage caused by gastric irritants such as NSAIDs, aspirin, and bile.

- Erosive/haemorrhagic gastritis describes a situation in which multiple defects form in the gastric mucosa from which bleeding occurs. Erosive/haemorrhagic gastritis may occur following the ingestion of large quantities of gastric irritants or in severely ill patients, e.g. those with sepsis or following major surgery.

Peptic ulcer disease

A **peptic ulcer** is a full thickness breach in the mucosa of the lower oesophagus, stomach, or duodenum which fails to heal over a reasonable period of time. What precisely constitutes 'reasonable' has not been defined. Attempts at repair lead to scarring at the base of the ulcer, such that restoration of the overlying submucosa and mucosa is no longer possible.

Peptic ulcers are usually solitary and located in the antrum of the stomach or the first part of the duodenum. The vast majority are seen in patients with an antral-predominant gastritis caused by our old friend *H. pylori*. Most of the remainder are probably due to NSAID use.

Peptic ulcers have a sharply defined punched out appearance

Knowing the typical appearance of peptic ulcers is important, particularly for the endoscopist. They have a characteristic 'punched out' appearance with clean edges, which are not raised or rolled, and a grey base (Fig. 8.5). Sometimes differentiating between a gastric peptic ulcer and an ulcerated gastric carcinoma can be difficult at endoscopy so multiple biopsies should be taken from any ulcerated lesion. Even if malignancy is not seen on the biopsies, multiple repeat biopsies should continue to be taken at regular intervals until the ulcer has healed.

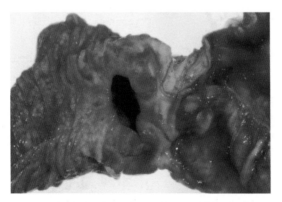

Fig. 8.5 A peptic ulcer located in the first part of the duodenum. Note the sharply defined edges, giving it a 'punched out' appearance.

Peptic ulcers may bleed, perforate, or form an obstructing stricture

Peptic ulcers have some important complications, many of which may be triggered by NSAID use:

- **Haemorrhage**. This is particularly seen as a complication of ulcers on the posterior wall of the duodenum which erode into the gastroduodenal artery. This is a common cause of haematemesis.

- **Perforation**. This causes acute abdominal pain and the rapid development of generalized peritonitis.

- **Fibrous stricture**. In the stomach this may cause gastric outflow obstruction with persistent vomiting and abdominal distension.

Note that malignant change in a peptic ulcer is extremely uncommon.

Key points: Peptic ulcer disease

- A peptic ulcer is a full thickness breach in the mucosa of the lower oesophagus, stomach, or duodenum which does not heal over time.

- Most peptic ulcers in the stomach and duodenum are caused by infection with *Helicobacter pylori*, though concomitant NSAID use exacerbates the condition.

- Peptic ulcers may present with dyspepsia or with a complication such as haemorrhage, perforation, or stricture formation.

- At upper gastrointestinal endoscopy, peptic ulcers have a typical punched out appearance.

- Multiple biopsies should be taken from any ulcerated gastric lesion to rule out gastric carcinoma, even if the appearances are typical of a peptic ulcer.

Gastric carcinoma

Gastric carcinoma is a malignant epithelial neoplasm arising from the epithelium of the gastric mucosa. Gastric carcinoma is a fairly common malignancy, although its incidence in the West is falling. Most gastric carcinomas develop on a background of chronic atrophic gastritis and intestinal metaplasia due to either *H. pylori* infection or autoimmune gastritis.

A small number of gastric carcinomas are believed to develop from adenomatous polyps of the stomach; however, this pathway is much less common than in the large bowel where the adenoma–carcinoma sequence is responsible for most colorectal carcinomas.

Virtually all gastric carcinomas are adenocarcinomas, i.e. the neoplastic cells show evidence of gland formation or mucin production. Microscopically, two types of gastric adenocarcinoma are recognized: the intestinal type and the diffuse type.

Intestinal type gastric adenocarcinoma is associated with atrophic gastritis and intestinal metaplasia

The intestinal type of gastric adenocarcinoma (Fig. 8.6) arises from a sequence of chronic atrophic gastritis, intestinal metaplasia, and dysplasia. Once dysplastic cells invade through the basement membrane of the epithelium, the lesion is called an adenocarcinoma. Atrophic gastritis is thought to promote the acquisition of mutations leading to dysplasia and carcinoma through a number of mechanisms including:

- Increased cell turnover due to damage caused by chronic gastritis.
- High levels of reactive oxygen species produced by inflammatory cells.
- Production of carcinogenic compounds from certain foods by opportunistic bacteria able to proliferate in the stomach due to low acid levels.

The falling incidence of gastric cancer is largely due to a reduction in intestinal type cancers. This is almost certainly due to decreasing rates of *H. pylori* infection. *Helicobacter pylori* infection is therefore a double edged sword—it protects against oesophageal adenocarcinoma but increases your risk of gastric carcinoma!

Diffuse type gastric adenocarcinoma arises from normal gastric mucosa

The diffuse type of gastric carcinoma is made up of poorly cohesive widely infiltrative malignant cells (Fig. 8.7). Signet ring cells, in which large amounts of intracytoplasmic mucin push the nucleus to one side, are commonly seen. The diffuse type of carcinoma develops from pathways independent of atrophic gastritis and intestinal metaplasia. It is usually widely infiltrative and may encase the entire stomach wall with tumour, producing the so-called 'leather bottle stomach' or **linitis plastica**. This type of adenocarcinoma is very aggressive and its incidence is remaining constant.

LINK BOX

Krukenberg tumour

Diffuse type gastric adenocarcinoma is the most common tumour to metastasize to both ovaries and give rise to the so-called **Krukenberg tumour** (p. 278).

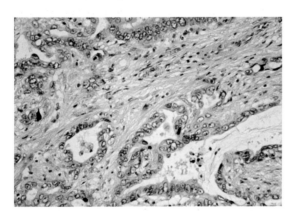

Fig. 8.6 Intestinal type of gastric carcinoma. Note the gland formation by the malignant cells.

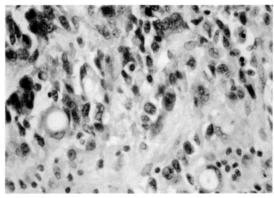

Fig. 8.7 Diffuse type of gastric carcinoma. Note the poorly cohesive malignant cells which tend to infiltrate surrounding tissues widely.

Gastric cancers are divided into early gastric cancer and advanced gastric cancer

Early gastric cancer refers to a gastric carcinoma which is confined to the mucosa or submucosa, irrespective of lymph node involvement. This type of cancer has a good chance of cure, with a 5 year survival rate of 90 per cent following surgical resection. Unfortunately, fewer than 1 per cent of all gastric cancers are picked up this early in the UK as the disease is usually asymptomatic and so patients never come to endoscopy. Even those who do come to endoscopy may have the diagnosis missed as many endoscopists are not familiar with the appearances of early gastric cancer. In Japan, where mass population screening for gastric cancer is performed using endoscopy, about one-third of gastric cancers are diagnosed as early gastric cancers.

Advanced gastric cancer refers to a gastric carcinoma that has infiltrated into the muscularis propria of the stomach or beyond. Most gastric carcinomas are advanced by the time patients present with symptoms of dyspepsia and weight loss.

- Early gastric cancer refers to a gastric carcinoma confined to the mucosa or submucosa, irrespective of lymph node involvement. The cure rate is excellent, but only a very small percentage of gastric carcinomas are diagnosed at this stage.

- Advanced gastric cancers have infiltrated into the muscularis propria or beyond. Most gastric carcinomas are advanced by the time the patient presents.

Gastric lymphoma

Gastric lymphoma can also be caused by *H. pylori* infection

A lymphoma is a neoplasm derived from mature B lymphocytes that have left the bone marrow and taken up residence in other organs (p. 363). The stomach normally has no lymphoid tissue within its walls; immune surveillance is not needed because the acidic environment kills most organisms. Infection with *H. pylori*, however, induces inflammation and lymphocytes are recruited into the stomach wall.

In a small minority (0.5 per cent) of patients infected with *H. pylori*, continued stimulation of B lymphocytes can lead to emergence of a neoplastic clone of B lymphocytes. The lymphoma is typically a low grade type of B cell lymphoma known as a **marginal zone lymphoma**. The lymphoma can form a large tumour mass which can mimic a gastric carcinoma, but distant spread of the lymphoma is unusual.

Interestingly, there is now compelling evidence that most gastric marginal zone lymphomas will regress in response to antibiotic therapy for *H. pylori*. What is not known for certain is whether all cases that show remission will stay in remission. Some argue that it is a disease from which one is never completely cured.

Key points: Gastric carcinoma

- Gastric carcinomas are malignant epithelial neoplasms arising from the epithelium of the gastric mucosa.

- Virtually all gastric carcinomas are adenocarcinomas which are divided according to their microscopic appearance into intestinal types and diffuse types.

- The intestinal type of gastric adenocarcinoma arises from a background of chronic atrophic gastritis, intestinal metaplasia, and dysplasia as a result of either *H. pylori* infection or autoimmune gastritis.

- The diffuse type of gastric adenocarcinoma develops from normal gastric mucosa through unclear mechanisms. This is a widely infiltrative and aggressive tumour.

LINK BOX

Chronic inflammation and marginal zone lymphomas

Chronic inflammation in other organs can lead to a marginal zone lymphoma, e.g. the thyroid in Hashimoto's thyroiditis (p. 317) and the salivary gland in Sjögren's syndrome (p. 455).

Gastrointestinal stromal tumour

Gastrointestinal stromal tumour is an uncommon neoplasm most often found in the stomach

Gastrointestinal stromal tumour (GIST) is a connective tissue neoplasm arising in the wall of the gastrointestinal tract. Sixty per cent of them occur in the stomach. It is thought that they are derived from the pacemaker cells of the bowel, the cells responsible for controlling the peristaltic wave. One of the defining features of a GIST is overexpression of a mutated form of the tyrosine kinase KIT which is permanently activated.

Rather than considering these tumours as simply benign or malignant, there is a gradual move to consider them as having low risk, intermediate risk, or high risk for recurrence/metastasis. Assessment of the mitotic activity of the neoplastic cells at microscopy is the best method of predicting how they will behave.

GISTs are usually exophytic tumours that often have central deep ulceration. Ulceration and bleeding of the tumour accounts for the way in which they may present, namely with abdominal pain or haematemesis. Most GISTs are treated with surgical resection. Interestingly, unresectable or metastatic cases have been found to be very sensitive to treatment with the tyrosine kinase inhibitor **imatinib**.

LINK BOX

Imatinib

Imatinib has also found success in the treatment of other malignancies associated with uncontrolled tyrosine kinase activity, such as chronic myeloid leukaemia (p. 361).

Small intestine

The main functions of the small intestine are to digest food and absorb the breakdown products. It also has vital immunological functions. The small intestine is exposed to a constant stream of antigenic material including food and microorganisms. The immune system of the bowel needs to be able to avoid constant inappropriate inflammatory over-reaction by recognizing which antigens to tolerate. This requires a complex and dynamic mucosal immune system. Dysregulation of this system can lead to inflammation and damage to the absorptive surface.

The most important conditions of the small intestine are obstruction, infection, and inflammatory disorders, of which the two most important in the UK are gluten-sensitive enteropathy and Crohn's disease. Tumours are exceedingly rare in the small intestine in comparison with the large bowel.

Small bowel obstruction

When the term 'bowel obstruction' is used, it usually refers to *mechanical* obstruction due to a physical blockage of the bowel. When there is a blockage anywhere in the intestine, there are a number of knock-on effects which explain the symptoms and signs, notably:

◆ The intestine above the level of obstruction endeavours to overcome the blockage by vigorous peristalsis. This causes *severe pain* that comes and goes in waves ('colicky' pain).

◆ The intestine proximal to the obstruction also becomes distended as it fills with gas and large quantities of fluid made up of the various digestive juices (~ 8 l in 24 h!). This leads to *persistent vomiting*.

◆ The intestine below the point of obstruction exhibits normal peristalsis allowing any residual content to be passed out. The bowel gas is then all absorbed, leaving an empty intestine. This leads to *absolute constipation*, meaning neither flatus nor faeces are passed.

With this in mind, the features of *small* bowel obstruction can be easily inferred:

◆ Acute onset of colicky abdominal pain.

◆ Abdominal distension. A good way to assess this is to ask if the patient has noticed more difficulty with their trousers!

◆ Early onset of vomiting. This is because the level of the obstruction is relatively high.

Note that constipation occurs *late* in small bowel obstruction and so may not be evident when the patient first arrives in hospital. Dehydration is common due to a combination of the repeated vomiting and sequestration of large amounts of fluid in the bowel. Very often, the picture is not completely clear cut. There might be episodic vomiting or diarrhoea due to intermittent release of the fluid contents collecting behind the blockage. This is called incomplete (or subacute) obstruction, and occurs when the blockage is intermittent or not complete.

Adhesions, hernias, intussusception, and volvulus account for most cases of small bowel obstruction

There are four common causes of small bowel obstruction, all of which are due to compression from outside the wall.

Adhesions are fibrous bridges that develop between viscera as a result of healing from areas of localized peritoneal inflammation. An important cause of localized peritoneal inflammation is handling and manipulation of the bowel during surgery. Previous abdominal surgery is therefore a risk factor for the development of adhesions and future small bowel obstruction.

Abdominal hernias are abnormal protrusions of peritoneal-lined sacs through defects in the abdominal wall. The typical sites of weakness are the inguinal and femoral canals, the umbilicus, and in surgical scars. Often the content of the hernia sac is just omental fat. If, however, a short segment of small bowel protrudes into the sac and becomes trapped in it, it may lead to small bowel obstruction. This is particularly dangerous if the hernia has a narrow orifice and blocks off the blood supply to the bowel (strangulation).

Intussusception occurs when a segment of small bowel telescopes into a distal segment. It is often seen in young children in whom often no cause is found. In adults, intussusception is usually associated with a lesion in the bowel such as the base of a Meckel's diverticulum or a large polyp. If these become trapped in the immediately distal segment of bowel, peristalsis may drive the invaginated bowel further into the distal bowel, leading to obstruction.

Volvulus occurs when a loop of bowel twists on its mesentery. This produces obstruction and infarction. Volvulus is most commonly seen in the large bowel, particularly the sigmoid colon and caecum (see later); however, it can also occur in the small bowel.

Strangulation may complicate any cause of mechanical small bowel obstruction

Strangulation occurs when a segment of bowel is trapped in such a way that its blood supply is progressively compromised. It is a potentially dangerous condition and demands early intervention before the bowel irreversibly infarcts.

The first effect of strangulation is compression of the low pressure veins, causing the bowel and its mesentery to become blue and congested. If the constricting agent is very tight, complete venous occlusion occurs and the colour of the intestine turns purple and becomes swollen and oedematous. This further increases the pressure at the point of obstruction, which may be sufficient to jeopardize the arterial supply to the segment of small bowel. If this happens then the mucosa, which is most susceptible to hypoperfusion, becomes necrotic and ulcerated. When the wall of the intestine becomes devitalized, bacteria can pass through it and cause bacterial peritonitis.

It is of the highest importance to distinguish strangulating from non-strangulating intestinal obstruction, as the former needs urgent surgery. The distinction is made entirely on clinical grounds and often takes fine clinical judgement. The most important clues are the presence of signs of peritonism, such as rebound tenderness overlying the strangulated segment of bowel. It is somewhat easier where the strangulation occurs in an external hernia as the lump is tense, tender, irreducible, and there is no cough impulse; often the overlying skin will be red and warm.

Key points: Small bowel obstruction

- Small bowel obstruction is usually mechanical in origin. The most common causes are adhesions, hernias, intussusception, and volvulus.

- The cardinal symptoms of small bowel obstruction are colicky abdominal pain, vomiting, and abdominal distension. Absolute constipation is a late feature.

- Small bowel obstruction can usually be managed conservatively with intravenous fluids and placement of a nasogastric tube. If there is evidence of superadded strangulation, urgent surgery is required to prevent infarction of the segment of small bowel.

Paralytic ileus

Mechanical small bowel obstruction should be distinguished from the condition **paralytic ileus** (sometimes referred to as just 'ileus'). Paralytic ileus is a reaction of the bowel to any form of irritation around it and is characterized by cessation of the normal peristaltic movements of the bowel.

Paralytic ileus also causes abdominal distension with constipation and vomiting; it therefore mimics mechanical obstruction, but there is no physical blockage. Ileus itself does not cause pain; however, there is often pain due to the underlying disorder causing it (which is usually *not* colicky). An important distinguishing feature on clinical examination is the bowel sounds. In mechanical obstruction, these are high pitched 'tinkling' sounds, whereas in paralytic ileus bowel sounds are absent. Common causes of paralytic ileus are:

◆ Postoperative. Any handling of the bowel at surgery will cause a reactive ileus. This is the most common type of ileus you will see and is the main reason why patients are kept nil by mouth after abdominal surgery until the bowel regains function.

◆ Any cause of a generalized peritonitis, e.g. perforation, small bowel infarction, or severe acute pancreatitis.

In both settings, the presence of electrolyte disturbances, particularly hypokalaemia, may exacerbate or prolong the ileus. Electrolyte levels are particularly likely to be deranged in the postoperative setting and in any severe condition leading to generalized peritonitis, so careful monitoring and control of electrolytes is important in these patients.

Infections of the small bowel

Large numbers of organisms are being continuously delivered to the gastrointestinal tract by swallowing. Most of them are wiped out in the stomach, such that organisms rarely reach the small intestine in sufficient numbers to cause infection. Small bowel infection therefore requires either a large infective load, or infection with small numbers of virulent organisms able to survive passage through the stomach (Table 8.2).

The hallmark of infections of the small intestine is diarrhoea. **Diarrhoea** refers to an abnormal increase in stool frequency and/or fluidity, and is the result of increased fluid and electrolyte loss in response to the infection.

Most cases of small bowel infection do not come to the attention of hospital doctors, or indeed general practitioners. The main worry is dehydration and electrolyte imbalance from profuse diarrhoea. This is mainly of concern in children and the elderly who have less reserve

TABLE 8.2	Important infections of the small intestine
Campylobacter jejuni	
Salmonella enterica	
Escherichia coli	
Noroviruses	
Giardia lamblia	

for compensation. In these situations, hospital admission for intravenous rehydration may be necessary.

JARGON BUSTER

Gastroenteritis

Gastroenteritis is a non-specific term for an illness characterized by diarrhoea, abdominal pain, nausea, and vomiting.

Campylobacter and *Salmonella* are the most common causes of infectious diarrhoea

The Gram negative bacteria *Campylobacter jejuni* and *Salmonella enterica* are the most common causes of infective diarrhoea in the UK. Infection is acquired by consuming contaminated food, particularly poultry and milk.

The bacteria invade epithelial cells in the terminal small intestine, leading to ulceration of the mucosal surface. The typical presentation is bloody diarrhoea, abdominal cramping, and fever. The diarrhoea is usually self-limiting and resolves without treatment. Hospitalization for fluid replacement may be required in the very young and the elderly. Antibiotics should not normally be used as they do not reduce or alter the course of the disease.

Both *Salmonella* and *Campylobacter* can be cultured from a faecal sample, though *Campylobacter* requires specific media and conditions to grow.

LINK BOX

Reactive arthritis

Reactive arthritis may follow a gastrointestinal infection caused by *Campylobacter* or *Salmonella*, usually in HLA-B27 positive patients (p. 413).

Enterotoxigenic *E. coli* is the most common cause of traveller's diarrhoea

Enterotoxigenic *Escherichia coli* (ETEC) is a strain of *E. coli* which is the most common cause of diarrhoea in travellers to foreign countries. ETEC possess fimbriae which allow the bacteria to adhere to small intestine epithelial cells and produce powerful toxins which cause massive fluid loss into the bowel lumen.

Viruses are common causes of outbreaks of diarrhoea in hospitals

Viruses can also cause diarrhoea. In infants and young children, **rotavirus** infection is the most common cause. In adults, the most common cause is infection with **noroviruses** (previously known as 'small round structured viruses'). Infections with noroviruses cause diarrhoea and vomiting which is highly infectious and spreads rapidly. They are very important causes of outbreaks of diarrhoea in hospital wards.

Giardia lamblia is a protozoan that can cause diarrhoea

Giardia lamblia is a protozoan transmitted by drinking water contaminated with cysts of the organism. The mature organism attaches to the brush border of the epithelial cells of the upper small bowel and the inflammatory response to the organism causes a mild diarrhoeal illness which lasts for about 7 days and then resolves. Immunocompromised individuals may develop chronic infection. *Giardia lamblia* is a common cause of chronic diarrhoea in patients with HIV.

Key points: Small bowel infections

- The hallmark of small bowel infection is diarrhoea.

- The most commonly implicated organisms are *Campylobacter jejuni* and *Salmonella enterica* which invade the small bowel wall causing bloody diarrhoea and abdominal cramping. Most cases are self-limiting and do not require specific treatment.

- Enterotoxigenic *E. coli* is the most common cause of traveller's diarrhoea.

- Norovirus infection is highly contagious and an important cause of outbreaks of hospital diarrhoea.

- *Giardia lamblia* is a protozoan that can cause a mild self-limiting diarrhoeal illness in healthy individuals or persistent diarrhoea in the immunocompromised.

Gluten-sensitive enteropathy

Gluten-sensitive enteropathy, or **coeliac disease**, is an inflammatory disease of the small intestine due to intolerance of dietary gluten which may affect absorption of important nutrients including iron, folate, and calcium.

Once thought to be a relatively rare disease, gluten-sensitive enteropathy is now recognized to be a common disorder, possibly affecting up to 1 in 300 people in the UK. This is due to the recognition that there are almost certainly a large number of adult patients with asymptomatic disease.

The mechanism through which gluten causes injury to the small bowel remains unknown. There is no doubt that the disease is closely linked with the possession of certain human leukocyte antigen (HLA) genes. What seems to be central to the disease process is inappropriate intestinal T cell activation triggered by dietary gluten in genetically susceptible individuals. The T cells drive a persistent chronic inflammation of the small bowel, leading to loss of the small bowel absorptive surface.

Many patients with gluten-sensitive enteropathy have minimal or no gastrointestinal symptoms

The diagnosis of gluten-sensitive enteropathy can be challenging. There are a wide variety of clinical manifestations, and gastrointestinal symptoms can be minimal. Most patients are diagnosed in adulthood and the most common presentation is with anaemia. The anaemia is usually due to iron deficiency, though folate deficiency may also contribute. Vitamin B12 deficiency is rare in gluten-sensitive enteropathy.

If intestinal symptoms do occur, they are variable and include discomfort, bloating, and altered bowel habit. Many patients are wrongly diagnosed with irritable bowel syndrome. In children, it is an important cause of failure to thrive and delayed puberty (p. 511).

LINK BOX

Gluten-sensitive enteropathy and dermatitis herpetiformis

Gluten-sensitive enteropathy may also present with the blistering skin condition dermatitis herpetiformis (p. 392).

Serology is a useful screening test for gluten-sensitive enteropathy

The first line of investigation of a patient with possible gluten-sensitive enteropathy is measurement of serum IgA **endomysial antibodies**. Endomysial antibodies bind to the connective tissue around smooth muscle and are measured by immunofluorescence. The test is reported as either positive or negative, as even low titres of endomysial antibodies are significant. Transglutaminase is the specific antigen to which the endomysial antibodies bind, and IgA tissue transglutaminase antibodies are measured using enzyme-linked immunosorbent assay (ELISA) techniques.

The presence of serum endomysial or transglutaminase antibodies is highly specific and sensitive for the presence of gluten-sensitive enteropathy, though the transglutaminase test is replacing endomysial antibody testing as the ELISA technique is cheaper and easier to perform.

The diagnosis of gluten-sensitive enteropathy requires small bowel biopsy

Although the presence of endomysial and tissue transglutaminase antibodies is strongly suggestive of gluten-sensitive enteropathy, guidelines still recommend taking small bowel biopsies to confirm the diagnosis. A diagnosis of gluten-sensitive enteropathy has lifelong implications for the patient, so it is sensible to be absolutely sure the diagnosis is correct. The distal duodenum is the usual site for biopsy, and multiple biopsies should be taken as the changes can be patchy.

Three key features are assessed on the biopsy (Fig. 8.8):

◆ The number of intraepithelial lymphocytes. An increase in intraepithelial lymphocyte density is the earliest and most sensitive indicator of gluten-sensitive enteropathy.

◆ The villous architecture. Damage to surface epithelial cells leads to loss of height of the villi.

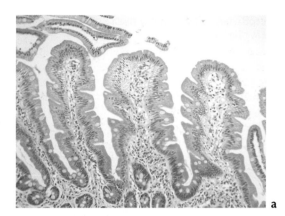

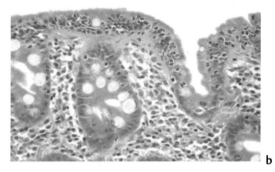

Fig. 8.8 (a) Normal duodenal mucosa. The villi have a normal height and shape, and there is no increase in intraepithelial lymphocytes. (b) Duodenal biopsy from a patient with gluten-sensitive enteropathy. The villi have completely disappeared and the surface epithelium contains many intraepithelial lymphocytes.

◆ The crypt length. The crypt zone is the proliferative compartment of the mucosa and it increases in length in an attempt to keep pace with the loss of surface cells.

The final component of the diagnosis is the improvement of symptoms upon withdrawal of gluten from the diet. This should be accompanied by a drop in the antibody titres and restoration of the normal villous architecture of the small bowel on a biopsy.

A lifelong gluten-free diet is the only treatment for gluten-sensitive enteropathy

The cornerstone of therapy for gluten-sensitive enteropathy is lifelong adherence to a gluten-free diet. This means the exclusion of foods containing wheat, rye, barley, and oats (although the toxicity of oats is still debated). The avoidance of these cereals is a formidable task as they are found in bread, biscuits, cakes, pastries, breakfast cereals, pasta, beer, and most soups, sauces, and puddings!

Most patients with gluten-sensitive enteropathy are osteopenic at diagnosis

Most patients with gluten-sensitive enteropathy have a reduced bone density. This is probably because they fail to reach their peak bone mass during young adult life due to malabsorption of calcium. The reduction in bone density is usually mild and most patients are only osteopenic. Some patients, however, may have a more profound reduction and actually be osteoporotic with an associated risk of fragility fracture. All patients diagnosed with gluten-sensitive enteropathy should therefore undergo bone densitometry to quantify their bone density.

Small bowel adenocarcinoma and EATL are rare complications of gluten-sensitive enteropathy

Patients with gluten-sensitive enteropathy are known to have a small risk of developing small bowel adenocarcinoma and a type of lymphoma known as **enteropathy-associated T cell lymphoma** (EATL). These should always be suspected if a patient with gluten-sensitive enteropathy suddenly deteriorates despite maintaining a gluten-free diet. Sometimes the underlying enteropathy is latent and only diagnosed when the segment of bowel is excised and the features of gluten-sensitive enteropathy are found microscopically.

EATL is believed to develop from intraepithelial T lymphocytes which become malignant due to prolonged stimulation. The lymphoma is extremely destructive, causing deep ulceration of the small bowel wall and formation of a mass lesion which can cause small bowel obstruction. Infiltration through the full thickness of the bowel wall can also lead to perforation. Patients often present acutely unwell with abdominal pain.

Key points: Gluten-sensitive enteropathy

- Gluten-sensitive enteropathy is a common inflammatory disorder of the small intestine due to intolerance to dietary gluten.

- The inflammation is associated with loss of the small bowel absorptive surface and malabsorption of important nutrients such as iron, folate, and calcium.

- Adults are often asymptomatic and present with an iron deficiency anaemia. Children usually present with failure to thrive and growth retardation. Gastrointestinal symptoms may be minimal.

- Measurement of serum IgA endomysial or transglutaminase antibodies are useful screening tests for gluten-sensitive enteropathy.

- The crucial diagnostic test is a distal duodenal biopsy showing an increase in intraepithelial lymphocytes, loss of villous height, and crypt hyperplasia.

- Treatment requires strict adherence to a lifelong gluten-free diet.

- Most patients with gluten-sensitive enteropathy have a reduced bone mass due to a failure to reach peak bone mass. Most patients are osteopenic at diagnosis, but some will have frank osteoporosis with risk of fracture.

- Small bowel adenocarcinoma and enteropathy-associated T cell lymphoma are rare but important complications of gluten-sensitive enteropathy.

Crohn's disease

Crohn's disease is one of the two idiopathic **inflammatory bowel diseases**. The second, ulcerative colitis, only affects the colon and is described later. Inflammatory bowel diseases are characterized by excess inflammatory activity in the wall of the bowel giving rise to chronic relapsing and remitting gastrointestinal symptoms.

The aetiology of inflammatory bowel disease remains an utter mystery. Experimental evidence using mouse models has provided compelling evidence that inflammatory bowel disease is the result of an inappropriate immune response to microorganisms. Mice with a gene knockout making them susceptible to developing inflammatory bowel disease do not develop the disease if they are reared in a germ-free environment.

Whether the organisms stimulating the disease are the bacteria of the normal intestinal flora or a genuine infective pathogen remains unknown; however, currently the former theory is favoured. Nevertheless, there are many strong proponents of the theory of a true infective cause for inflammatory bowel disease.

Crohn's disease and MAP

One of the great controversies in Crohn's disease is the possible aetiological role of *Mycobacterium avium* subspecies *paratuberculosis* (MAP). This organism is known to cause a disease similar to Crohn's disease in cattle, called Johne's disease. MAP is widely present in our food chain, and DNA of this organism has been recovered from resected intestines of Crohn's disease patients.

Despite these compelling data, the picture is far from clear. Finding MAP at the crime scene does not equate to a guilty verdict, as it may still be a mere contaminant that lodges easily in the ulcerated bowel. Another serious flaw in the MAP argument is the failure of Crohn's disease to worsen during immunosuppression. In patients with HIV, the activity of Crohn's disease *reduces* as their CD4+ T lymphocyte count falls. This is in stark comparison with the massive proliferation of other mycobacteria such as *M. tuberculosis* and *M. avium intracellulare* which thrive in the intestines of HIV patients.

Clearly, it is imperative to solve the question of MAP and Crohn's disease. If MAP is implicated in Crohn's disease, there will be massive public health measures needed to eliminate the organism from the food chain.

Crohn's disease typically affects the small bowel and colon

The main features of Crohn's disease that distinguish it from ulcerative colitis are:

+ Involvement of any part of the bowel, but most often the small bowel and colon.

+ Areas of diseased bowel are separated by areas of normal bowel.

+ The inflammation involves the full thickness of the bowel wall, leading to complications such as strictures and fistula formation.

The clinical manifestations of Crohn's disease are extremely variable. This is mostly due to the variety of locations that the disease may involve.

Ileal disease is usually associated with pain and obstructive symptoms. This is because Crohn's strictures are common in the small intestine. An inflammatory mass is often palpable in the right iliac fossa. Colonic disease is associated with diarrhoea and perianal disease. Pain is less of a feature in the large bowel as the lumen is wider and inflammatory thickening is less likely to cause obstructive symptoms. Rectal bleeding may occur but is not as severe as in ulcerative colitis.

Symptoms of anaemia are common and usually the result of iron deficiency from intestinal blood loss or less frequently from vitamin B12 or folate deficiency. Other features of malabsorption are infrequent unless there is very extensive small bowel disease.

Extraintestinal manifestations of Crohn's disease

Crohn's disease is also associated with a number of extraintestinal manifestations including enteropathic arthropathy (p. 413), anterior uveitis (p. 472), gallstones (p. 197), and erythema nodosum (p. 391).

Bowel affected by Crohn's disease is thickened, with fat wrapping and deep linear ulceration of the mucosa

One of the most useful and striking features of Crohn's disease, apparent immediately on examining the bowel, is **fat wrapping**. Fat wrapping, which is highly characteristic of Crohn's disease, refers to extension of subserosal and mesenteric fat around the circumferential aspect of the bowel and onto the antimesenteric border. Diseased areas of bowel also feel rubbery and thick, with stenosis and stricture formation. Affected areas of bowel may be adherent to adjacent loops of intestine or other structures.

If a diseased segment of bowel is opened up, the internal mucosal surface contains deep fissuring linear ulcers.

Coalescence of linear ulcers leads to the formation of numerous areas of mucosa lifted up by underlying heavy oedema. This is called **cobblestoning** of the mucosa (Fig. 8.9).

Microscopically, Crohn's disease shows patchy transmural inflammation of the bowel wall

It is not unreasonable for medical students and junior doctors to have a basic understanding of some of the microscopic features of Crohn's disease, if for no other reason than to appreciate why making the diagnosis can be very difficult. Indeed, what cannot be overemphasized is that Crohn's disease exhibits a very variable microscopic pattern, and some of the important features may be entirely absent in some cases.

The three microscopic features generally regarded as hallmarks of Crohn's disease are (Fig. 8.10):

- Patchy, full thickness inflammation of the bowel wall in the form of small lymphoid aggregates.
- Deep fissuring ulcers, often in the form of penetrating knife-like clefts through the bowel wall.
- The presence of granulomas, which may be found in any layer of the bowel wall.

Unfortunately, only rarely are all the characteristic features present in a single specimen. In particular, it is important to note that granulomas may be completely absent in up to half of all cases of Crohn's disease. Remember also that many samples submitted to pathologists are endoscopic biopsies that consist of the

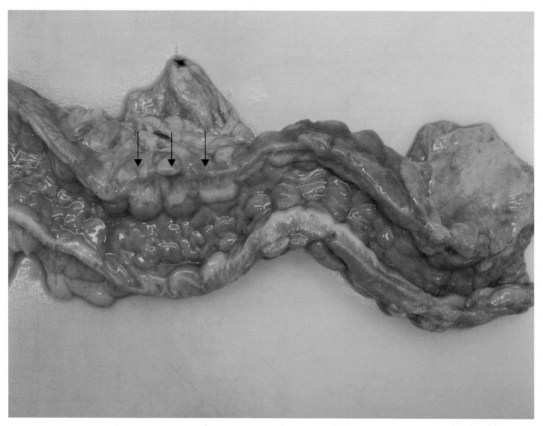

Fig. 8.9 Small intestinal Crohn's disease. This segment of small bowel resected for Crohn's disease has been opened fresh from the operating theatre and photographed before formalin fixation. Fat wrapping is seen where mesenteric fat is creeping over on to the antimesenteric surface of the small intestine (arrows). The bowel wall is also thickened. The mucosal surface shows coalescing linear ulceration, creating the characteristic cobblestone appearance.

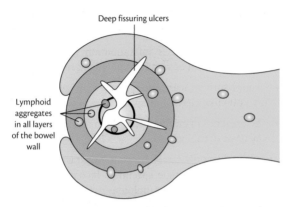

Fig. 8.10 Microscopic features of Crohn's disease. The typical features of Crohn's disease are patchy transmural inflammation in the form of lymphoid aggregates and deep knife-like ulceration.

mucosal layer only. This makes a confident diagnosis of Crohn's even more difficult as the most useful feature (inflammation in all layers of the bowel wall) cannot be assessed!

Most patients with Crohn's disease will require surgery at some point in their life

Most patients with Crohn's disease will require at least one operation during the course of their disease. Indications for surgery include failure to respond to medical therapy with immunosuppressive drugs, strictures causing mechanical obstruction, and fistula formation. Resections of segments of bowel should be kept as short as possible, and where possible, small intestinal strictures should be dealt with by incision and resuturing (stricturoplasty) rather than by excision.

Key points: Crohn's disease

- Crohn's disease is an inflammatory bowel disease which follows a relapsing and remitting course.
- The inflammation in the bowel wall is thought to be the result of an inappropriate immune response to bacteria of the intestinal flora.

- Crohn's disease may affect any part of the bowel, but most commonly involves the distal small bowel and colon. Perianal disease is also common.
- The most common presentation is diarrhoea, abdominal pain, and weight loss.
- Segments of bowel are affected in a discontinuous fashion with intervening areas of normal bowel.
- The main macroscopic features of Crohn's disease are fat wrapping, bowel wall thickening and stricturing, and linear ulceration of the mucosal surface.
- The typical microscopic features of Crohn's disease are patchy transmural inflammation with lymphoid aggregates, deep penetrating ulceration, and granulomas.
- Most patients come to surgery at some point in their lives, usually for treatment of strictures and fistulas. Resections should be as minimal as possible.

Small bowel infarction

We have already briefly alluded to infarction of the small bowel as a complication of a strangulated hernia. Usually this affects only the small segment of small bowel stuck in the tight orifice of the hernia sac. More extensive small bowel infarction may occur if the blood supply to the small bowel via the superior mesenteric artery is compromised (Fig. 8.11).

Superior mesenteric artery compromise may be caused by *in situ* thrombosis, embolism, or volvulus

Most cases of extensive small bowel infarction are caused by thrombosis of the superior mesenteric artery due to a complicated atherosclerotic plaque. Emboli originating from the heart in patients with atrial fibrillation or a left ventricular thrombus may also cause small bowel infarction. In elderly people, the small bowel mesentery becomes lax and may completely twist on itself, leading to extensive small bowel infarction.

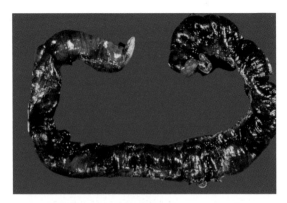

Fig. 8.11 Small bowel infarction. Typical appearance of an infarcted segment of small bowel. The dark colour is due to the intense congestion and haemorrhage within the intestine as a result of blockage to venous outflow.

Occlusion of the main trunk of the superior mesenteric artery leads to infarction of nearly the whole length of the small bowel, the caecum, and part of the ascending colon. More frequently, a branch of the superior mesenteric artery is implicated and the area of infarction is slightly less. Either way, a substantial area of small bowel is rendered rapidly ischaemic, leading to life-threatening complications.

Prolonged ischaemia leads to sloughing of the necrotic mucosa from the bowel wall

The mucosal layer of the small bowel is the most susceptible to ischaemia because the epithelial cells are very metabolically active. The mucosal layer undergoes necrosis and sloughs off into the bowel lumen. Loss of the integrity of the mucosal layer has two important complications:

* Large amounts of blood pour into the bowel lumen. Due to the large coil of intestine that is involved, this haemorrhage is sufficient to render the patient rapidly hypovolaemic and shocked.

* Gut bacteria rapidly permeate the devitalized intestinal wall and cause widespread peritonitis.

The classical presentation of acute small bowel infarction is therefore acute abdominal pain, bloody diarrhoea, and signs of hypovolaemia. Early recognition is crucial as there is rapid progression of peritonitis and septicaemia. Laparotomy must be performed as soon as possible to remove any dead bowel and to restore adequate blood flow to the gut. It is not too surprising that prognosis is universally poor, with a mortality of up to 90 per cent.

> ### Key points: Small bowel infarction
>
> * Small bowel infarction may be caused by thrombosis or embolus in the superior mesenteric artery, or volvulus of the entire small bowel mesentery.
>
> * Ischaemia of the small bowel leads to necrosis of the mucosal layer which sloughs off. Loss of the mucosal layer leads to massive haemorrhage into the bowel lumen and spread of bacteria across the bowel wall into the peritoneum.
>
> * Small bowel infarction presents with acute abdominal pain, bloody diarrhoea, and rapidly progressive peritonitis. The only chance of survival is early laparotomy, and overall survival is extremely poor.

Appendix

In humans, the appendix is not known to serve any definite purpose, though the presence of large amounts of lymphoid tissue in its wall suggests an immunological role. Acute inflammation of the appendix is the most common disease of the appendix. Tumours are occasionally found incidentally in appendices; these are usually carcinoid (endocrine cell) tumours.

Acute appendicitis

Acute appendicitis is the most common disease of the appendix and is by far the most frequent cause of an acute abdominal emergency. It may occur in people of any age.

The most common precipitating factor in acute appendicitis is obstruction of the appendiceal orifice. Impaction of solid faecal material and enlargement of lymphoid tissue are the most common culprits. Blockage of the appendix by numerous *Enterobius vermicularis* worms is also well recognized.

As mucoid secretions distend the obstructed appendix, the intraluminal pressure rises until it exceeds the venous pressure. Venous stasis then leads to ischaemia.

As a result, the mucosa ulcerates leading to secondary infection by luminal bacteria. The accumulation of neutrophils produces microabscesses and destruction of the wall.

The clinical picture of acute appendicitis may not follow the textbook descriptions!

Everyone is familiar with the classical presentation of acute appendicitis. The onset is acute, with the sudden development of central abdominal pain associated with nausea and vomiting. As the inflammation proceeds and involves the full thickness of the appendix, the parietal peritoneum in contact with it becomes involved. As this is innervated with somatic nerve endings, the pain then localizes to the right iliac fossa.

Difficulties in the diagnosis arise either from other conditions mimicking acute appendicitis (e.g. mesenteric adenitis, urinary tract infection, or gynaecological pathology) or from an atypical presentation of appendicitis because of the anatomical position of the appendix.

It is important to be able to recognize the appendix with acute appendicitis

Because the classical clinical picture is not always seen, the diagnosis of acute appendicitis is often not entirely secure until the appendix is inspected at surgery. A surgeon must therefore be able to distinguish the diseased appendix from a normal one.

In the early stages of appendicitis, the macroscopic changes may be quite subtle. The most helpful feature is dilation and congestion of the tiny vessels on the serosal surface. With progression, the appendix becomes much more congested, tense, dilated, and covered by a fibrinous exudate (Fig. 8.12). If the appendix looks normal, it is usually removed anyway, but this should prompt a further search in the abdominal cavity for alternative pathology.

Perforation of an acutely inflamed appendix is a serious complication

It is likely that spontaneous resolution occurs in some cases of early acute appendicitis, but once any significant amount of pus has formed there are likely to be complications unless the appendix is removed quickly. Perforation is the most common and serious complication. When associated with fulminating inflammation and massive wall necrosis, it commonly leads to generalized peritonitis and septicaemia which are dangerous complications.

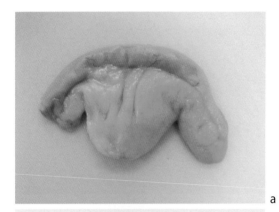

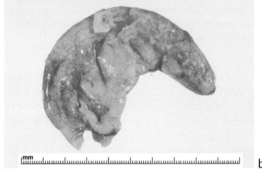

Fig. 8.12 Acute appendicitis. (a) A normal appendix. (b) Acute appendicitis. The inflamed appendix is dilated, heavily congested, and covered with fibrinous exudate.

Definitive diagnosis of acute appendicitis requires microscopic examination of the organ

Even when the diagnosis of acute appendicitis appears clear-cut at surgery, it remains critical to submit the organ for histological examination. The main reason for this is to confirm that the inflammation visible on the outside of the organ to the surgeon is indeed coming from the appendix. If under the microscope there is fibrinous exudate on the external surface of the appendix but none of the other features of acute appendicitis are present, it suggests that there has been extension of inflammation from elsewhere in the abdomen which was missed at surgery.

Carcinoid tumours of the appendix

Carcinoid tumours are derived from endocrine cells in the mucosal layer of the appendix. These cells are epithelial cells derived from the stem cells in the crypts but come to lie in small clusters in the lamina propria of the mucosa. They produce hormones that act locally to coordinate gut peristalsis.

Carcinoid tumours may arise throughout the gastrointestinal tract, though the appendix is the most common site. Most are small (<1 cm) tumours located at the tip of the appendix and are found incidentally in appendices removed for acute appendicitis or some other unrelated condition.

Although appendiceal carcinoids often show extensive local spread within the appendiceal wall, they rarely metastasize to lymph nodes or to distant sites, and excision of the appendix is usually curative.

Key points: Appendix

- Acute appendicitis is the most common disease of the appendix.

- Acute appendicitis arises due to obstruction of the appendiceal origin causing distension of the organ and ischaemia.

- Acute appendicitis typically causes central abdominal pain with nausea and vomiting, followed by localized right iliac fossa pain when the inflammation involves the parietal peritoneum.

- The acutely inflamed appendix can be recognized at surgery because it is dilated and covered with fibrinous exudate.

- Submitting the appendix for histological examination is important to confirm the diagnosis and to rule out other appendiceal pathology such as a carcinoid tumour.

Large intestine

The function of the large intestine is to convert the liquid material from the small bowel into well formed stools by absorbing water and electrolytes. The colon also salvages unabsorbed calories from incompletely digested carbohydrates by the action of anaerobic bacteria converting them to fatty acids. The rectum provides a storage function, enabling the elimination of stools at a socially acceptable time.

The most important types of disease affecting the large bowel are infections, inflammatory diseases, and tumours. Unlike the small bowel, tumours in the large bowel are extremely common and important. In order to understand these conditions, it is important to have a basic knowledge of large bowel anatomy (Fig. 8.13).

Large bowel obstruction

We have already seen how small bowel obstruction leads to colicky abdominal pain, vomiting, and abdominal distension. Mechanical obstruction of the large bowel gives rise to the same symptoms; however, the pattern is slightly different due to the level of the blockage. Constipation (which may be absolute) is an earlier more prominent feature in large bowel obstruction, whereas vomiting tends to occur later.

The most common causes of large bowel obstruction are:

- Tumours

- Sigmoid volvulus

- Diverticular strictures.

Large bowel obstruction due to tumours is generally bad news, as it usually implies advanced disease. An emergency operation to resect the tumour from an 'unprepped' colon in an unwell patient carries high morbidity and mortality. To help reduce this, there is a move towards placing a metal stent across the tumour in the acute setting rather than attempting full resection. This serves to relieve the obstruction, buying time to stabilize the patient and carry out proper staging investigations. Patients whose disease is too advanced for curative surgery can then be further palliated as required and avoid an unnecessary high risk resection. Those who turn out to have potentially curable disease can be properly prepared for definitive surgery which can be done as a one-stage elective resection.

Sigmoid volvulus occurs when the sigmoid colon twists on its mesentery. It is commonly seen in elderly patients and seems to be predisposed to by faecal overloading of the sigmoid together with laxity of the sigmoid mesocolon associated with age.

Infections of the large bowel

Infection of the large bowel (infectious colitis) typically causes **dysentery**, characterized by fever, abdominal

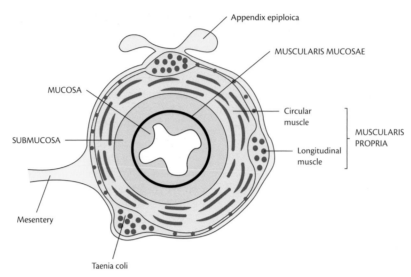

Fig. 8.13 Cross-section of normal large bowel showing important anatomical features. Note how the longitudinal muscle layer is very thin over most of the circumference of the colon, being mainly concentrated into three narrow bands, the taeniae coli.

cramping, and blood and pus in the faeces. If the inflammation extends as far as the rectum, passing stools may be painful and there may be a sensation of incomplete evacuation (tenesmus).

The most common cause of dysentery in the UK is infection with *Shigella* bacteria ('bacillary' dysentery). In tropical and subtropical countries, infection with the protozoan *Entamoeba histolytica* is also a common cause ('amoebic' dysentery). *Clostridium difficile* colitis is now a very common problem in patients treated with broad-spectrum antibiotics.

Shigellae invade the colonic mucosa and cause bloody diarrhoea

The *Shigella* species are Gram negative bacteria which are transmitted from person to person via the faecal–oral route. Only a small infectious load is needed to produce infection. *Shigellae* invade the epithelium of the colon, causing severe ulceration. There is severe lower abdominal cramping with watery diarrhoea which then becomes bloody.

Entamoeba histolytica can cause severe dysentery

Entamoeba histolytica infection is acquired through ingestion of contaminated food or drink. The parasite invades the mucosa of the large intestine, feeding off host tissues.

The infection may only cause mild diarrhoea, but can lead to very severe dysentery with bloody diarrhoea. The diagnosis can be made by visualizing parasite cysts in a stool sample by light microscopy.

Clostridium difficile diarrhoea follows broad-spectrum antibiotic treatment

Clostridium difficile is a common and important cause of profuse diarrhoea, especially in hospitalized elderly patients. The diarrhoea is caused by a toxin produced by the organism. In severe cases, there is ulceration of the colonic mucosa with the formation of solid plaques composed of mucus, pus, and cellular debris which adhere to the colonic wall (Fig. 8.14).

It is now well established that the underlying problem leading to *C. difficile* diarrhoea is treatment with broad-spectrum antibiotics, hence the alternative name **antibiotic-associated colitis**. Because *C. difficile* is a normal member of the commensal flora of the large bowel, it is thought that the antibiotic treatment inhibits other gut flora allowing overgrowth of *C. difficile*. It remains possible, however, that the infection is acquired by inhalation of *C. difficile* spores in patients with lowered resistance. Either way, the diagnosis is made by demonstrating the presence of the toxin in a stool sample. As the bacterium is anaerobic, treatment requires metronidazole.

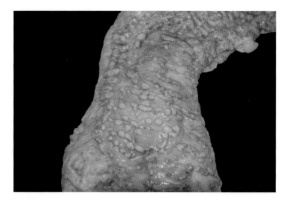

Fig. 8.14 *Clostridium difficile* colitis. This is a freshly opened colon from a patient with profuse diarrhoea following broad-spectrum antibiotic treatment. Note the large number of cream-coloured plaques studded across the mucosal surface, representing collections of neutrophils, fibrin, and cell debris.

Ulcerative colitis

Ulcerative colitis is one of the two inflammatory bowel diseases, the other being Crohn's disease. Like Crohn's disease, ulcerative colitis is also thought to be related to an inappropriate immune response to the bacteria of the colonic flora in genetically susceptible people.

Ulcerative colitis is distinguished from Crohn's disease by two main features:

- Only the large bowel is involved. The rectum is always affected and the disease extends proximally in a continuous fashion to involve a variable amount of the colon (Fig. 8.15). Minimal inflammation of the terminal ileum ('backwash ileitis') may occur in people with severe involvement of the whole colon, but significant small intestinal disease does not occur.

- The inflammation in ulcerative colitis involves the mucosal layer only. The remainder of the bowel wall is minimally involved. This means that patients with ulcerative colitis, unlike Crohn's disease, do not develop complications such as strictures or fistulas.

Bloody diarrhoea is the hallmark of active ulcerative colitis

Patients with ulcerative colitis usually present with a gradual onset of symptoms, often intermittent, which become more severe. The principal symptom is the passage of bloody diarrhoea. The diarrhoea is often preceded by symptoms of great urgency and followed after defecation by a sensation of incomplete evacuation (tenesmus). Patients with mild or moderate attacks usually look well and exhibit few physical signs.

In contrast, patients with a severe ulcerative colitis affecting most or all of the colon are obviously ill. They have severe diarrhoea which becomes a slurry of faecal material, pus, and blood. In addition they have systemic features such as anorexia, weight loss, fever, and tachycardia. These patients are at risk of developing dangerous

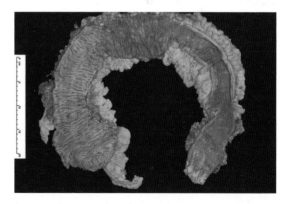

Fig. 8.15 Ulcerative colitis. This is a colectomy specimen from a patient with ulcerative colitis. The right colon is on the left of the picture (note the appendix) and the left colon and rectum are on the right side of the picture. The inflamed mucosa, which looks red, begins at the rectum and continuously affects the left colon until the transverse colon where there is a sharp transition into normal mucosa.

complications such as acute dilatation of the colon and perforation.

The main diagnostic problem is distinguishing ulcerative colitis from severe infective colitis or Crohn's disease of the colon. The diagnosis is made on the basis of history, the absence of faecal pathogens, and the endoscopic and histological appearances of the colon.

LINK BOX

Extraintestinal manifestations of ulcerative colitis

Extraintestinal manifestations of ulcerative colitis include primary sclerosing cholangitis (p. 189) and enteropathic arthropathy (p. 413).

Ulcerative colitis causes a range of macroscopic appearances depending on its severity

The earliest visible sign of ulcerative colitis on the mucosal surface is a blurring of the normal vascular pattern due to hyperaemia and oedema. With increasing severity, the mucosa assumes a granular velvety appearance. The mucosa becomes very friable and can be readily scraped away, exposing the underlying muscle coats. Full thickness ulceration leads to spontaneous bleeding into the bowel lumen.

Patients with long-standing disease often develop inflammatory polyps in the colon. They are the result of full thickness ulceration of the mucosa with undermining of the adjacent surviving mucosa, which is raised up by oedema and projects into the lumen. They have no malignant potential.

Ulcerative colitis is characterized microscopically by diffuse mucosal inflammation

The most typical feature of ulcerative colitis microscopically is *diffuse inflammation confined to the mucosal layer*. Contrast this with Crohn's disease where the inflammation is patchy and seen throughout all layers of the bowel wall. Other typical features of ulcerative colitis include collections of neutrophils sitting within crypt spaces ('crypt abscesses') and evidence of damage to the large bowel crypts which are distorted, shortened, and show abnormal branching (Fig. 8.16).

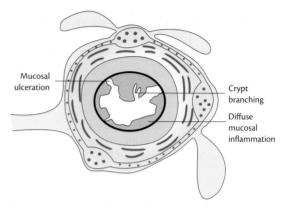

Fig. 8.16 Microscopic features of ulcerative colitis. Ulcerative colitis is characterized by diffuse mucosal inflammation with crypt architectural distortion.

Labels: Mucosal ulceration; Crypt branching; Diffuse mucosal inflammation

Fulminant ulcerative colitis can lead to dilation and perforation of the colon

In the most severe cases of ulcerative colitis, the inflammation may extend beyond the mucosa and into the muscle coat of the colon. This is known as **fulminant ulcerative colitis** and is the *only* context in ulcerative colitis where inflammation can be seen beyond the mucosa.

Involvement of the muscle coat causes toxic atrophy of muscle cells, leading to dilation of a segment of large bowel ('toxic megacolon'). In almost all cases, this complication occurs in the transverse colon. All the layers of the bowel wall become markedly thinned such that the colon has the consistency of wet filter paper. Early surgical intervention to remove the bowel before the development of multiple perforations is essential.

Perforation is the most feared complication of fulminant ulcerative colitis

Perforation, which carries significant mortality, is the most feared complication of severe ulcerative colitis. It usually complicates acute colonic dilation, but may occur in the absence of dilation. Like perforation anywhere in the bowel, there is a rapid onset of generalized peritonitis and a reactive paralytic ileus. Remember that the physical signs of peritonitis may be blunted by the anti-inflammatory effects of steroid therapy: *reduced or absent bowel sounds due to the paralytic ileus may be the only clinical feature*. An erect chest X-ray is usually diagnostic, by revealing the presence of air under both hemidiaphragms.

Patients with ulcerative colitis are at increased risk of colorectal carcinoma

Ulcerative colitis is a risk factor for the development of colorectal carcinoma. Those at maximum risk are patients with extensive colitis and with a long history of disease. Carcinomas developing in a background of ulcerative colitis are different from 'conventional' colorectal carcinomas in that they tend to be flat, ill defined tumours which arise from similarly ill defined areas of dysplasia rather than from adenomatous polyps.

Patients with long-standing extensive colitis should therefore undergo colonoscopic surveillance. The aim is to pick up patients with dysplasia before the development of an adenocarcinoma. Because the dysplastic lesions can be extremely subtle, the colonoscopist must be vigilant and biopsy any suspicious areas. If the pathologist examining the biopsy sees dysplasia in the epithelium, they will grade it into either low grade or high grade dysplasia.

Low grade dysplasia requires more frequent colonoscopic surveillance with the taking of multiple biopsies from the whole colon. The presence of high grade dysplasia is of great concern and should prompt immediate consideration of complete surgical removal of the whole colon and rectum (panproctocolectomy).

Key points: Ulcerative colitis

- Ulcerative colitis is a chronic inflammatory bowel disease of unknown aetiology which affects the rectum and a variable amount of colon in a continuous fashion.

- The course of the disease is characterized by acute attacks separated by periods of remission.

- Bloody diarrhoea is the hallmark of an acute attack of ulcerative colitis.

- Mucosa affected by ulcerative colitis becomes granular and friable, and bleeds spontaneously.

- Microscopically, there is diffuse inflammation involving the mucosal layer only with crypt abscess formation and crypt architectural distortion.

- In fulminant ulcerative colitis, the inflammation extends into the muscle coat of the colon. The colonic wall becomes markedly thinned with risk of dilation and/or perforation.

- Patients with ulcerative colitis of long duration need surveillance colonoscopy. The aim is to pick up dysplasia before the development of invasive adenocarcinoma.

Colorectal neoplasia

Colorectal adenocarcinoma, which develops from the glandular epithelium lining the large bowel, is the second most common cause of cancer death in the UK, being responsible for over 16 000 deaths per year. Colorectal adenocarcinomas may arise in any part of the large bowel, but the majority occur in the rectum and sigmoid colon.

The most important aetiological factor in colorectal carcinoma is diet

A typical Western high fat, high protein, low fibre diet is implicated in colorectal carcinoma. One theory is that carcinogens are produced by bacterial metabolism of products derived from animal fat. A low fibre diet contributes by slowing colonic transit which gives more time for carcinogen production and increased contact time between carcinogens and mucosal epithelial cells.

Most colorectal carcinomas develop from adenomas

Like cancers in other major organs, colorectal adenocarcinoma has a well recognized precursor lesion from which it usually develops: the **adenoma**. Despite their name, colorectal adenomas should not be thought of as benign growths. They are best considered as *dysplastic neoplasms with malignant potential*.

It is now well accepted on the basis of a series of genetic studies that adenomas can progress to invasive adenocarcinomas. The 'adenoma–carcinoma sequence' occurs over many years through successive accumulation of mutations in critical genes controlling cell replication (Fig. 8.17).

A crucial early event in the development of an adenoma is the acquisition of mutation(s) that leads to a spatial reorganization of the colonic crypt. Normal

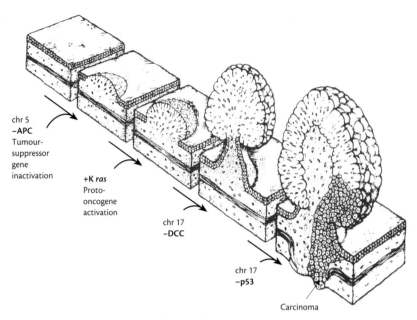

chr 5
−APC
Tumour-
suppressor
gene
inactivation

+K *ras*
Proto-
oncogene
activation

chr 17
−DCC

chr 17
−p53

Carcinoma

Fig. 8.17 The adenoma–carcinoma sequence. Postulated model of colorectal carcinogenesis showing progression from normal epithelium to adenoma to carcinoma as genetic mutations accumulate.

crypts maintain a polarity, with the proliferative compartment being sequestered at the base. In adenomas, one of the effects of the initial mutations is to allow proliferative cells to accumulate superficially. It is thought that exposure of the proliferating cells to luminal carcinogens increases the likelihood of further mutations and gradual progression towards invasive behaviour.

A key gene implicated in the early stage of adenoma formation is APC

APC (adenomatous polyposis coli) is a tumour suppressor gene which under normal circumstances binds to a molecule called β-catenin, and targets it for degradation. β-Catenin is a protein involved in a cellular signalling pathway that leads to the stimulation of cellular proliferation and inhibition of apoptosis. Mutations in the APC gene reduce the affinity of the APC protein for β-catenin, leading to accumulation of β-catenin with a resulting increase in cell proliferation. This is a major cause of the spatial reorganization of the colonic crypts mentioned earlier.

The role of APC has been discovered by studying families with the disease **familial adenomatous**

polyposis (FAP). This is an inherited condition characterized by a germline mutation in the APC gene. Affected individuals develop thousands of adenomatous polyps throughout their large bowel by the second decade of life. The risk that one or more of these will become malignant is 100%. All patients with FAP are therefore advised to undergo panproctocolectomy in early adulthood. Although rare, FAP has been an important model for the study of colorectal carcinogenesis. It has provided an opportunity to observe the very earliest stages in the formation of adenomas and the genetic changes associated with the adenoma–carcinoma sequence.

Most adenomas fail to become adenocarcinomas in a typical person's lifespan

It must be remembered that the great majority of adenomas fail to become adenocarcinomas in the course of a typical lifespan. However, there are certain features which are associated with a greater risk of transformation:

◆ *Size.* Larger adenomas are more likely to become malignant. Studies suggest that the prevalence of cancer in adenomas under 1 cm is about 1 per cent, in those between 1 and 2 cm it is about 10 per cent, and in those over 2 cm there is nearly a 50 per cent malignancy rate.

- *Histological type.* Based on their microscopic architecture, adenomas are classified as tubular, tubulovillous, or villous. Tubular adenomas are the most common subtype. Adenomas with a villous architecture have the highest malignant potential.

- *Degree of epithelial dysplasia.* All colorectal adenomas are by definition dysplastic. The changes can be graded into those showing mild, moderate, or severe dysplasia. Malignant potential increases with increasing degrees of dysplasia. Dysplasia is the most selective marker of increased malignant potential.

These three features are inter-related: as a general rule, the larger adenomas tend to be of villous type and have more severe epithelial dysplasia. Fortunately the majority of adenomas are small, tubular, and show low grade dysplasia (Fig. 8.18).

Invasion through the muscularis mucosae into the submucosa defines colorectal adenocarcinoma

At most sites in the body, an epithelial neoplasm is defined as malignant once the basement membrane has been breached. The situation in the colon and rectum is different; only once the neoplasm has penetrated through the muscularis mucosae into the submucosa is the tumour called an adenocarcinoma. This is because colorectal epithelial neoplasms appear to have no

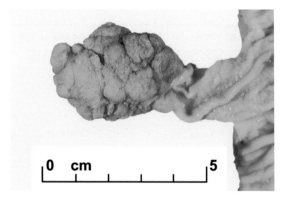

Fig. 8.18 This polyp was present in a colectomy specimen performed for colonic carcinoma, at a site distant from the carcinoma. Microscopy showed it to be a tubular adenoma with mild dysplasia.

potential for lymph node spread until they have invaded the submucosal layer, presumably due to the relative paucity of lymphatics within colorectal mucosa. *As long as neoplastic cells are confined within the mucosal layer, the nomenclature 'adenoma' or 'dysplasia' is still appropriate* (Fig. 8.19).

Symptoms of colorectal carcinoma do not usually occur until the tumour grows quite large

In its early stages, colorectal carcinoma is clinically silent. The symptoms that occur as the tumour grows depend on its location in the large bowel. In the right side of the colon where the diameter of the lumen is large and the faecal contents are liquid, tumours can grow large before any symptoms occur. The first indication of a right-sided colorectal cancer is often the finding of iron deficiency anaemia due to chronic blood loss from the tumour (Fig. 8.20).

In contrast, cancers on the left side of the colon, where the calibre of the lumen is small and faecal contents more solid, often constrict the lumen producing obstructive symptoms. These are manifested as changes in bowel habit and abdominal pain. Rectal tumours often give rise to the sensation of incomplete evacuation after defecation (tenesmus).

Some patients may present with acute large bowel obstruction due to a very advanced tumour. Perforation of the bowel due to a tumour is uncommon, but carries a very poor prognosis due to immediate peritonitis and dissemination of malignant cells into the peritoneal cavity.

The stage of a colorectal carcinoma is the most important prognostic factor

The main determinant of prognosis in colorectal carcinoma is the extent of spread of the tumour. Colorectal carcinomas spread by three main routes: local spread, lymphatic spread to regional lymph nodes, and haematogenous spread to distant organs.

Local spread of colonic carcinomas is through the bowel wall into the pericolic fat. The peritoneal surface is relatively resistant to tumour spread, but breach allows spread into adjacent organs such as bladder, or other loops of bowel. The lymph nodes involved by colorectal carcinomas are present in the pericolic/mesorectal fat surrounding the large bowel. Haematogenous spread of colorectal carcinoma is most commonly to the liver via the portal vein.

Two staging systems are widely used in colorectal carcinoma, Dukes and TNM (Table 8.3).

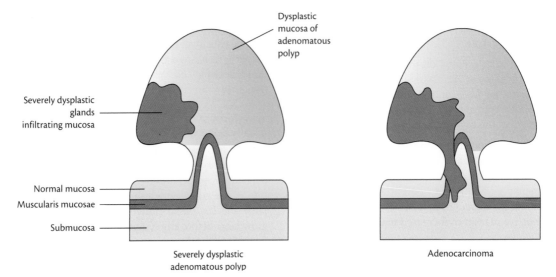

Fig. 8.19 On the left is a picture of a severely dysplastic adenomatous polyp. In one area (dark blue), severely dysplastic glands have breached the basement membrane and infiltrated the lamina propria of the large bowel mucosa within the polyp. However, because the muscularis mucosae has not been breached, this lesion is still called a severely dysplastic adenomatous polyp. Only once the muscularis mucosae has been infiltrated is the term adenocarcinoma used (right).

Spread of rectal tumours deserves special mention

Spread of rectal tumours is slightly different, as the anatomical margins of the rectum are unlike the rest of

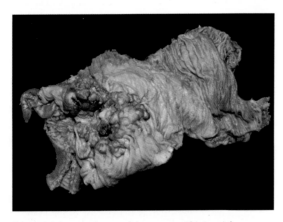

Fig. 8.20 Adenocarcinoma of the caecum. This is a right hemicolectomy specimen in which a small piece of terminal ileum, the caecum, the appendix, and ascending colon have been removed. A large tumour is seen in the caecum which was confirmed on microscopy to be an adenocarcinoma. This tumour was picked up at colonoscopy performed because the patient was found to have an unexplained iron deficiency anaemia.

the large bowel. Most of the large bowel is suspended in the abdominal cavity, invested in peritoneum. This is important from the perspective of tumour spread, as tumours tend not to breach peritoneal surfaces but rather spread down through the fatty tissue of the pericolic fat. When resecting a colonic tumour, the most important surgical margin is therefore the mesenteric margin from where the segment of bowel has been cut away from the posterior abdominal wall.

TABLE 8.3	Staging schemes for colorectal carcinoma	
Tumour spread	**Dukes**	**TNM**
Submucosa	A	T1
Muscle coat	A	T2
Beyond muscle coat	B	T3
Through peritoneum	B	T4
No lymph node spread	A/B	N0
1–3 lymph nodes involved	C1	N1
>3 lymph nodes involved	C1	N2
Apical node involved	C2	N1/N2
Distant metastases	D	M1

Dysplastic mucosa of adenomatous polyp

Severely dysplastic glands infiltrating mucosa

Normal mucosa

Muscularis mucosae

Submucosa

Severely dysplastic adenomatous polyp

Adenocarcinoma

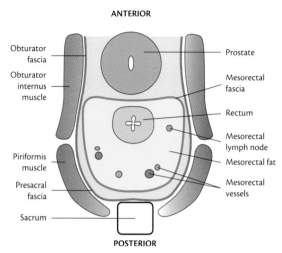

ANTERIOR

Obturator fascia

Obturator internus muscle

Piriformis muscle

Presacral fascia

Sacrum

Prostate

Mesorectal fascia

Rectum

Mesorectal lymph node

Mesorectal fat

Mesorectal vessels

POSTERIOR

Fig. 8.21 Transverse section of the midrectum in the male. At this level, the rectum lies below the peritoneal cavity completely surrounded by mesorectal fat. Rectal tumours have a potential for spread throughout the mesorectum, so it is vital that surgical resection of the rectum for rectal cancer includes the whole mesorectum with an intact mesorectal fascia.

Most of the rectum, however, lies outside of the peritoneal cavity surrounded entirely by mesorectal fat, or just 'mesorectum'. The mesorectum is a distinct compartment enclosed by the mesorectal fascia which contains fat through which vessels and nerves run to supply the rectum. The rectum by definition has no mesentery. As the rectum is completely surrounded by fat, and tumours spread more easily through fat, the surgeon must perform a much more careful circumferential excision to remove the entire mesorectum with the mesorectal fascia intact to minimize the chance of local recurrence of the rectal cancer (Fig. 8.21).

The NHS Bowel Screening Programme will be rolled out over the next 3 years

Funding has been secured to introduce a national screening programme for colorectal carcinoma, which should be fully rolled out by 2009. The screening programme targets men and women aged 60–69 and the screening test is **faecal occult blood** (FOB) which tests stool for small traces of blood in the stool.

The test is sent to the patient at their home address and they perform the test in the privacy of their own home. Patients with positive FOB testing are then invited for colonoscopy to examine their large bowel. One of the main difficulties of this screening programme is the high number of positive tests in people without colorectal carcinoma due to other common large bowel disorders causing bleeding, such as diverticular disease and haemorrhoids.

Key points: Colorectal neoplasia

- Colorectal carcinoma is the second most common cause of cancer death in the UK.

- Most colorectal carcinomas develop from precursor lesions called adenomatous polyps which are by definition dysplastic.

- The adenoma–carcinoma sequence is associated with the stepwise accumulation of genetic mutations resulting in cells with the ability to invade and metastasize.

- Epithelial neoplasms in the large bowel should only be defined as adenocarcinomas once they have invaded through the muscularis mucosae into the submucosa.

- Spread occurs locally, via lymphatics to regional lymph nodes, and via the blood to distant organs.

- The liver is a common site for colorectal adenocarcinoma metastases.

- Prognosis is related to the stage of the disease.

- National screening for colorectal carcinoma using faecal occult blood testing should be in place in the UK by 2009.

Other colorectal polyps

A polyp is a very general term for any growth that protrudes from a surface

A number of different colorectal polyps are recognized. Because it is impossible to distinguish each type with certainty at colonoscopy, all polyps should be removed for microscopic examination.

We have already discussed **adenomatous polyps** which are the most important type of polyp because of their potential to develop over time into an adenocarcinoma. **Inflammatory polyps** have also already been mentioned in association with ulcerative colitis.

The **hyperplastic polyp** is the other main type of colorectal polyp. The majority occur in the rectum and sigmoid colon. They are sometimes known as regenerative or metaplastic polyps. It was widely believed for a long time that these types of polyps were completely benign with no malignant potential. Recently, however, studies have challenged this view. It seems that some types of hyperplastic polyp may have the potential to develop into adenocarcinomas, particularly large hyperplastic polyps and ones that are located in the right side of the colon. For the time being at least, the general consensus is that most hyperplastic polyps have a very low risk of malignant change.

Diverticular disease

Diverticular disease is a common and important condition of the distal large bowel which is responsible for considerable morbidity and a small, but significant, mortality in the elderly. Of all the people with diverticula, only some 10 per cent have symptoms and around 1 per cent will come to surgery.

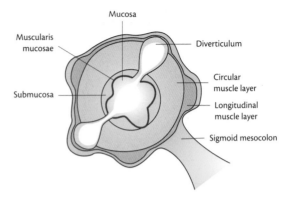

Fig. 8.22 Diverticular disease. Diverticula are outpouchings of mucosa that herniate through the circular muscle layer of the large bowel. Their tips are separated from the pericolic fat by only a thin layer of longitudinal muscle.

> ### JARGON BUSTER
>
> ## Diverticulosis versus diverticulitis
>
> Diverticulosis, or diverticular disease, merely refers to the presence of multiple diverticula. Diverticulitis means inflammation of a diverticulum.

Diverticula are pouches of mucosa that have herniated through weak points in the large bowel wall

Diverticula are pouches of colonic mucosa that herniate through the circular muscle layer of the muscularis propria and come to lie in the pericolic fat outside the bowel wall (Fig. 8.22). Two factors are required for this to happen: a *raised intraluminal pressure* and *areas of weakness in the colonic wall*.

Intraluminal pressure is raised due to insufficient dietary fibre. Fibre binds salt and water in the colon giving bulky moist faeces that are easily propelled through the colon. Propulsion of faeces from a low fibre diet requires increased muscular effort leading to muscular hypertrophy and a raised intraluminal pressure. People with diverticular disease consume less vegetables, brown bread, and potatoes, and more meat

and dairy products than those without. Vegetarians have a low level of diverticular disease.

The weakness in the colonic wall is a reflection of the normal anatomy of the large bowel. There are natural defects in the circular muscle layer where blood vessels pass through to supply the mucosal layers, and there is little additional support from the longitudinal muscle layer as this is only a very thin covering in those areas where it is not bunched into the taeniae coli.

These two factors explain why diverticula are most common in the sigmoid colon, as faeces become increasingly hard to propel in the distal large bowel. The rectum tends to be spared because it has a complete circumferential longitudinal muscle coat which provides extra support.

Diverticular disease may closely mimic colonic adenocarcinoma

Diverticular disease often leads to narrowing of the sigmoid colon due to a combination of muscular hypertrophy and the effect of numerous redundant mucosal folds filling the lumen. The narrowing leads to intermittent abdominal pain and altered bowel habit. Ongoing bleeding from diverticula may also lead to positive faecal occult blood tests and iron deficiency anaemia. All of these features are also typical of a colonic adenocarcinoma. Even the radiological appearances may cause confusion as a stricturing diverticular mass can closely mimic adenocarcinoma.

Acute diverticulitis is a common cause of acute abdominal pain in the elderly

Acute diverticulitis is caused by faecal matter impacting within the neck of a diverticulum, stimulating inflammation and symptoms of left iliac fossa pain. If the inflammation spreads into pericolic fat and involves the peritoneal surface, there will also be symptoms and signs of localized peritonitis.

Common complications of acute diverticulitis include pericolic abscess formation, perforation, and fistula formation into the bladder (colovesical fistula).

Diverticular disease is also a cause of acute lower gastrointestinal bleeding

Although, in most cases, blood loss from diverticula is small and occult, it may occasionally be massive. The cause of the haemorrhage is usually inflammatory erosion through the diverticular wall and into an adjacent artery which may be of considerable size.

Key points: Diverticular disease

- Diverticular disease is very common in the elderly population.

- Diverticula are outpouchings of mucosa that herniate through weak points in the colonic muscle coat in people with high intraluminal pressures.

- Virtually all cases of diverticular disease are confined to the sigmoid colon.

- Most people with diverticular disease remain free of symptoms.

- Diverticular disease can mimic colonic adenocarcinoma by causing symptoms of intermittent abdominal pain, a change in bowel habit, and iron deficiency anaemia.

- Acute diverticulitis is a common cause of acute left iliac fossa pain in the elderly. Complications of acute diverticulitis include pericolic abscess formation, perforation, and fistula formation.

- Diverticula are also sources of acute lower gastrointestinal bleeding.

Anal and perianal disease

The anal canal and perianal region give rise to some common conditions. Most are isolated conditions in patients with no underlying disease. However, it must be remembered that perianal disease, particularly fissures and multiple branching fistulae are often seen as a manifestation of Crohn's disease. Before continuing, it is worth refreshing one's memory about the relevant anatomy (Fig. 8.23).

Haemorrhoids

Haemorrhoids are prolapsed anal cushions

The anal cushions are specialized vascular structures made up of arterioles, venules, and arteriovenous communications. There are three main anal cushions situated in the upper anal canal in the left lateral, right anterior, and right posterior parts of the anal canal (the so-called 3, 7 and 11 o'clock positions). The cushions are held in the upper anal canal by muscular fibres from the conjoined longitudinal muscle in the intersphincteric plane.

The anal cushions are part of the normal anatomy within the anal canal and are believed to be important in maintaining continence. As an individual coughs, strains, or sneezes, the cushions engorge and maintain closure of the anal canal to prevent leakage of stool. They may also be important in sensation of the anal canal, specifically in differentiating liquid, solid, and gas.

Haemorrhoids exist when the suspensory mechanism holding the anal cushions in place is disrupted, allowing them to prolapse into the anal canal. Previous suggestions that haemorrhoids were simply dilated venous channels have been discounted and there is no evidence that they occur with increased frequency in portal hypertension.

Haemorrhoids may occur at any time during adult life. The factors leading to prolapse of the anal cushions and the development of haemorrhoids are not well understood. Many affected patients give a history of straining at defecation due to constipation. Chronic straining may be relevant by causing venous engorgement of the cushions and stretching and disruption of the surrounding supporting structures. Once haemorrhoids have prolapsed, the venous drainage from the anal cushions is impeded, so they become progressively engorged.

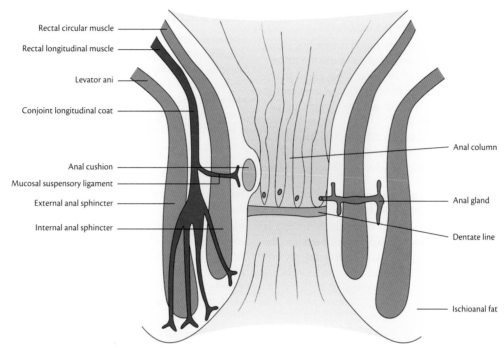

Fig. 8.23 Anatomy of the anal canal. Note the location of the submucosal anal cushions that give rise to haemorrhoids. Infection tracking down the anal glands can give rise to abscesses and perianal fistulas.

The most common symptom of haemorrhoids is painless bright red rectal bleeding. The blood is usually noticed on the toilet paper. Bleeding from haemorrhoids is rarely profuse and not normally severe enough to cause iron deficiency anaemia. An iron deficiency anaemia must never be ascribed to haemorrhoids without fully investigating the upper and lower gastrointestinal tract for malignancy.

Anal fissure

An anal fissure is a split in the squamous mucosa of the lower anal canal

Anal fissures are tears in the mucosa of the lower anal canal, which are almost always found posteriorly in the midline. The pathogenesis of anal fissures is not clear. Chronic infection may lead to loss of the normal elasticity and mobility of the mucosa and it is probable that trauma from the passage of hard faeces may be a precipitating factor. Anal fissures are exquisitely painful, and secondary constipation from fear of pain exacerbates the problem.

Anorectal fistula

An anorectal fistula or abscess usually begins with an infection of the anal glands

The anal glands are structures whose ducts drain mucus secretions into the rectal lumen. Most of these glands lie in the submucosa; however, some of these glands can lie deeper, either within or beyond the internal sphincter muscle. Infection arising at the opening of these deep glands can therefore track deeply into perirectal tissue, causing an **anorectal abscess**. If the infection tracks even further and reaches the external skin around the anus, an **anorectal fistula** results.

Anal cancer

Anal cancer is uncommon, seen most commonly in male homosexuals

Most anal cancers are squamous cell carcinomas related to sexually transmitted infection with high risk human papillomavirus (HPV). In a similar way to cervical squamous cancer caused by HPV, anal cancer arises through a series of dysplastic lesions known as anal intraepithelial neoplasia (AIN).

> ## Key points: Anal and perianal disease
>
> ◆ Haemorrhoids are prolapsed anal cushions which are a common cause of rectal bleeding and discomfort.
>
> ◆ An anal fissure is a split in the mucosa of the lower anal canal, found posteriorly in the midline.
>
> ◆ An anorectal abscess results from infection in an anal gland tracking deeply into the perirectal tissue.
>
> ◆ An anorectal fistula occurs if an anorectal abscess tracks right up to, and breaks through, the perianal skin.
>
> ◆ Anal cancers are mostly squamous cell carcinomas associated with human papillomavirus infection.

Peritoneal cavity

The **peritoneum** is a serous membrane that lines the abdominal cavity. It is a single continuous structure, but is more easily understood if divided into two portions: the parietal peritoneum and the visceral peritoneum.

Parietal peritoneum is the peritoneum which covers the anterior and posterior abdominal walls, the under surface of the diaphragm, and the pelvic cavity. This portion is richly supplied with nerves and when irritated causes severe pain accurately localized to the affected area.

Where the parietal peritoneum leaves the posterior abdominal wall or diaphragm to form a partial or complete investment for an organ it is called **visceral peritoneum**. Visceral peritoneum, which forms the serosal layer of abdominal organs, is poorly supplied with nerves and so pain arising from it is vague and poorly localized.

Ascites

In health, only a small amount of peritoneal fluid is present to allow smooth gliding of the viscera. Ascites is the accumulation of excess fluid in the peritoneal cavity. There are three common causes:

◆ Advanced cirrhosis

◆ Disseminated abdominal malignancy

◆ Severe right-sided, or biventricular, cardiac failure.

The mechanisms underlying malignant ascites are fairly well recognized. Malignant cells in the peritoneal cavity disrupt the barrier between the peritoneum and the interstitial space leading to increased leakage of fluid into the cavity.

The mechanisms leading to ascites in cirrhosis and cardiac failure are much more complex. No current theory can satisfactorily explain the pathogenesis and account for all the various observations that can be seen in these patients. What does seem certain is that two factors are necessary for the development of ascites: *portal hypertension* and *salt and water retention*.

The development of portal hypertension in cirrhosis is explained by vascular distortion from the diffuse fibrosis, and in severe heart failure by congestion in the venous system. How salt and water retention occurs is much harder to explain. One theory is that it is due to a reduction in effective renal blood flow stimulating increased renin release from the kidneys and consequent secondary hyperaldosteronism. The high aldosterone levels then stimulate salt and water retention by the kidneys. Whilst superficially attractive, this hypothesis fails to explain certain facts, in particular why many patients with cirrhosis develop salt retention with ascites in the presence of a normal aldosterone concentration.

Peritonitis

Peritonitis refers to inflammation of a peritoneal surface. Despite the views of many textbooks, peritonitis does not necessarily equate to infection of the peritoneum. Although infection commonly supervenes as a secondary phenomenon, it is not essential for peritoneal inflammation. Symptoms and signs of peritonitis, known as **peritonism**, only occur when *parietal* peritoneum becomes inflamed, and can be divided into localized and generalized peritonism.

Localized peritonism occurs when inflammation in an abdominal organ extends to the peritoneal surface

Localized peritonism occurs when a focal area of parietal peritoneum becomes inflamed. This usually occurs when an inflammatory process in an abdominal organ extends to the serosal surface and then involves the adjacent parietal peritoneum. This is often seen in the context of:

+ Acute appendicitis

+ Strangulation of a segment of small bowel

+ Acute diverticulitis.

In these settings, the clinical signs of localized peritonism are very useful in implicating that the underlying disorder is severe. The most important sign is **guarding** and **rigidity** of the abdominal wall over the area of the abdomen that is involved, with **rebound tenderness**. Rebound tenderness refers to a sudden severe pain when the palpating hand is released from the abdomen. It can be demonstrated more kindly by pain on percussion over the area of interest.

Generalized peritonism results from a catastrophic abdominal event

Generalized peritonism occurs when the whole peritoneal cavity becomes inflamed. This usually results from a catastrophic abdominal event such as:

+ Perforation of an abdominal organ. Most often, the perforation is at the site of a duodenal ulcer or acute diverticulitis. Spillage of the contents of the bowel causes a chemical peritonitis which is rapidly followed by secondary infection. Sometimes a perforation may be rapidly walled off by omentum, containing the spread and causing a localized peritonitis rather than a generalized peritonitis.

+ Small bowel infarction. Death of a large coil of intestine leads to massive transudation of toxins and bacteria across the necrotic bowel wall leading to widespread peritonitis.

+ Severe acute pancreatitis.

Diffuse or generalized peritonism causes severe abdominal pain made worse by anything that disturbs the peritoneum. The patient usually lies still to minimize the pain and takes very shallow breaths to avoid moving the abdomen. These simple visual signs are important clinical clues. Even in patients with severe diffuse abdominal pain, the point of maximal rebound tenderness roughly overlies the pathological process. Remember that generalized peritonitis usually causes a paralytic ileus, so there will also be superimposed vomiting and constipation with absent bowel sounds.

Functional gastrointestinal disorders

In clinical practice, many patients who present with chronic or recurrent gastrointestinal symptoms do not have a structural or biochemical explanation identified by routine diagnostic tests. These patients are labelled as having a **functional gastrointestinal disorder**. Functional does not imply a psychiatric disturbance or absence of disease but rather a known or suspected underlying disorder of gut function.

The most widely recognized functional gastrointestinal disorders are non-ulcer dyspepsia and irritable bowel syndrome. Together these account for some 40–60 per cent of all referrals to gastroenterology outpatient departments.

Non-ulcer dyspepsia

Dyspepsia is a broad term which encompasses a group of symptoms which alerts one to consider disease of the upper gastrointestinal tract. It includes symptoms of upper abdominal discomfort, nausea, vomiting, bloating, belching, and heartburn amongst others. 'Indigestion' is sometimes used by the public as a surrogate term.

Dyspepsia may be caused by many of the diseases we discussed at the start of this chapter (such as oesophagitis, peptic ulcers, and oesophageal and gastric malignancies) as well as diseases related to nearby anatomical organs, e.g. gallstones, myocardial ischaemia, or a leaking aortic aneurysm.

Despite the large number of possible causes for dyspepsia, in a large proportion of cases no clear cause for the symptoms can be determined. In fact, well over half of all patients with dyspepsia who undergo upper gastrointestinal endoscopy have no significant abnormality to account for the dyspepsia. This large group of people are labelled as having 'functional' or **non-ulcer dyspepsia**. The cause of the dyspepsia in these patients is unclear. Treatment is therefore aimed at alleviating the symptoms, but is often ineffective.

Irritable bowel syndrome

Irritable bowel syndrome is characterized by a host of gastrointestinal symptoms, most notably recurrent abdominal pain and an erratic disturbance of defecation. Bloating is also common. Rather frustratingly for doctor and patient alike, all investigations are normal.

Despite the benign nature of the disorder, the symptoms can be extremely disabling with a significant impact on quality of life. Many patients will avoid certain activities such as socializing and travelling as a result of their symptoms.

The cause of irritable bowel syndrome is unknown. It is likely that some patients have unrecognized gastrointestinal pathology, and popular theories include a disorder of neuromuscular function or that visceral sensation is somehow enhanced. However, strong evidence for either of these theories is lacking. There is, however, convincing evidence for a substantial psychological component to irritable bowel syndrome. Many patients have a history of adverse life advents, sexual abuse, and generally consult their doctors more than average for vague symptoms.

Like non-ulcer dyspepsia, treatment is symptomatic (e.g. antidiarrhoeal and antispasmodic drugs) but not always effective. About 30% of patients remain symptomatic after 5 years.

> ### Key points: Functional gastrointestinal disorders
>
> - Functional gastrointestinal disorders are characterized by persistent unexplained gastrointestinal symptoms.
>
> - The two most common functional gastrointestinal disorders are non-ulcer dyspepsia and irritable bowel syndrome. Together these account for over half of all referrals to gastroenterology outpatient clinics.
>
> - Non-ulcer dyspepsia refers to upper abdominal symptoms in which no clear cause can be found.
>
> - Irritable bowel syndrome refers to lower abdominal symptoms in which no clear cause can be found.
>
> - Treatment of functional gastrointestinal disorders is aimed at relieving symptoms, but is often ineffective.

Further reading

Sartor RB (2005). Does *Mycobacterium avium* subspecies *paratuberculosis* cause Crohn's disease? *Gut* 54: 896–898.
www.bsg.org.uk, British Society of Gastroenterology.

Hepatobiliary and pancreatic disease

Introduction

This chapter deals with diseases of the liver, gallbladder, bile ducts, and pancreas. Most of these conditions are managed by hepatologists and hepatobiliary surgeons.

Liver

The liver is the largest solid organ in the body and is composed predominantly of epithelial cells called hepatocytes. The hepatocytes perform all the major functions of the liver which are broadly:

- Metabolic. The liver is central to carbohydrate, protein, and fat metabolism.

- Synthetic. Many important proteins are synthesized in the liver, including albumin, clotting factors, and complement proteins.

- Storage. The liver is the main storage site for glycogen, triglycerides, iron, copper, and fat-soluble vitamins.

- Detoxification. The liver is the principal site for detoxification of endogenous substances (e.g. ammonia) and foreign compounds such as drugs.

- Production of bile. Bile is a fluid which has two fundamental functions: it contains bile acids which are critical for the digestion and absorption of fat, and it allows the elimination of many waste products from the body, e.g. cholesterol and bilirubin.

In order to carry out these diverse functions, hepatocytes must be well perfused with blood, and the structure of the liver reflects this. Hepatocytes are arranged in a complex network of interconnecting cords or 'plates' which are one cell thick. Between the liver cell plates lie vascular sinusoids containing blood mixed from the portal venous and hepatic arterial systems. Hepatocytes are therefore immersed in blood on two sides. The liver is, in essence, like a large sponge where the holes represent vascular sinusoids filled with blood flowing from portal tracts towards central veins (Fig. 9.1).

The liver is vulnerable to a variety of insults. Agents which commonly damage the liver include:

+ Infections, particularly the hepatitis viruses.

+ Alcohol, which remains the most common cause of liver disease.

+ Drugs. Therapeutic medication is also a very common cause of liver disease.

+ Autoimmune disease, which may target hepatocytes or the biliary system.

+ Accumulation of metabolic products in hepatocytes, often due to inherited disorders of metabolism.

Like many organ systems, liver disease is best considered as 'acute liver disease' or 'chronic liver disease'. Often the same agents can produce either acute or chronic illness, depending on the length of exposure and the host response. Jaundice is the main manifestation of acute liver disease, usually in association with systemic upset. Chronic liver disease, however, is often asymptomatic until advanced. Very severe damage to the liver leading to loss of most of its function causes the syndrome of hepatic failure.

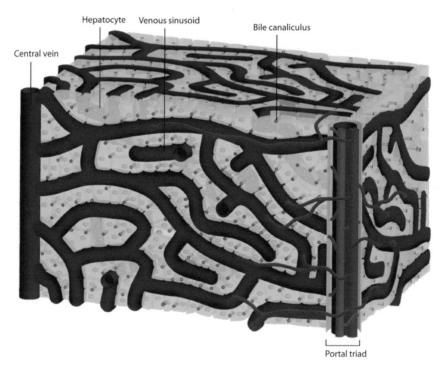

Fig. 9.1 Microanatomy of the liver. The liver is composed of one cell thick liver cell plates surrounded by venous sinusoids. Blood flows from the portal veins and hepatic arteries towards the central veins. Bile formed from hepatocytes flows in the opposite direction in canaliculi to drain into bile ducts in the portal triads.

Measurements of liver function

Liver function tests measure bilirubin and a panel of liver enzymes

Liver function tests are one of the more common biochemical tests performed in routine clinical practice. Most laboratories measure **plasma bilirubin** together with a panel of **liver enzymes** including aspartate aminotransferase (AST), alanine aminotransferase (ALT), alkaline phosphatase (ALP), and γ-glutamyltransferase (GGT). Although these are called 'liver function tests', it is important to realize that they are really assessing liver damage rather than function.

The pattern of change in liver enzymes can give a clue to the type of underlying disease

If there is extensive *biliary* damage, ALP is usually disproportionately high compared with the aminotransferase enzymes. Conversely when *hepatocyte* necrosis predominates (e.g. in acute viral hepatitis), AST and ALT elevation predominates.

An isolated elevation of ALP when other enzymes are normal suggests bone disease (often Paget's disease) as ALP is produced by both bone and liver. ALP is also produced locally by the liver in infiltrative conditions, and its elevation is a useful early marker of liver metastases. Plasma ALP is therefore often raised in malignant disease and may be due to bony and/or hepatic deposits.

GGT provides a sensitive indicator of hepatobiliary disease but is of no value in distinguishing between hepatocellular or biliary damage. A raised plasma GGT in conjunction with a raised ALP is therefore useful to point towards a biliary cause for the high ALP rather than a bony cause. An isolated rise in GGT usually reflects *enzyme induction* rather than hepatocyte damage. Enzyme induction refers to an increase in enzyme production within liver cells such that a higher amount is released into the plasma as part of normal cell turnover. Induction of GGT is almost always due to either alcohol consumption or drugs.

Although liver function tests often indicate the nature of the liver disease, it is rarely possible to make a specific diagnosis on the basis of liver function test results alone. Nonetheless, they are cheap tests which are reliable at picking up liver disease and directing further diagnostic investigations such as imaging of the liver/biliary tract or a liver biopsy. Plasma enzyme levels can also be very useful in monitoring liver disease once the diagnosis has been made.

Bilirubin is a useless and toxic breakdown product of haemoglobin

In the time it takes you to read this sentence, about 20 million of your red blood cells will have died, generating some 5×10^{15} molecules of haemoglobin requiring disposal! The protein making up the globin chains and the iron in the haem portion are precious and are reused. The complex ring structure that remains when iron is removed from haem cannot be recycled and is converted to unconjugated bilirubin in macrophages.

Unconjugated bilirubin is transported in the blood bound to albumin to the liver. Hepatocytes take up the unconjugated bilirubin, and the enzyme **glucuronyl transferase** catalyses the binding of glucuronic acid to bilirubin, a process called **conjugation**. Conjugated bilirubin is water soluble and is secreted into bile, where it eventually reaches the duodenum via the biliary system and is eliminated in the faeces (Fig. 9.2).

Normally there is no conjugated bilirubin in the blood, as it is all secreted into bile. If liver or biliary disease impairs the passage of conjugated bilirubin in the bile, conjugated bilirubin accumulates in plasma and, because it is water soluble, it is filtered by the kidneys and appears in the urine (bilirubinuria), causing it to darken. Bilirubinuria is always pathological.

Jaundice

Jaundice is a sign resulting from hyperbilirubinaemia

If large amounts of bilirubin accumulate in the blood (hyperbilirubinaemia), the patient develops a yellow discoloration of the skin and sclerae known as **jaundice** or **icterus**. Jaundice is a well recognized feature of liver disease, though two important points should be emphasized:

◆ Many patients with significant liver disease are not jaundiced, and do not become jaundiced until they have very advanced liver disease.

◆ Liver and biliary diseases are not the only causes of jaundice.

Causes of jaundice can be divided into pre-hepatic, hepatocellular, and obstructive

Because there are many causes of jaundice, it is helpful to divide them into 'pre-hepatic', 'hepatocellular', and 'obstructive', depending on the main site of the problem leading to the jaundice (Table 9.1). A further

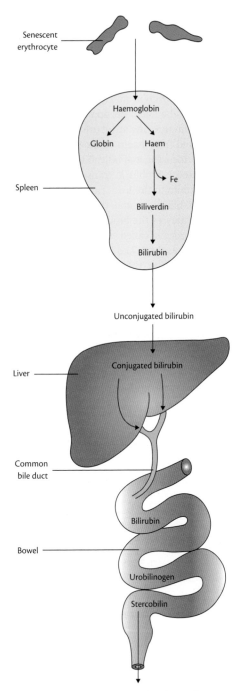

Fig. 9.2 Bilirubin metabolism. Haemoglobin derived from senescent erythrocytes is converted in the splenic macrophages to unconjugated bilirubin which travels in the blood to the liver where it is conjugated in hepatocytes and excreted in bile into the intestine.

TABLE 9.1	Causes of jaundice
Pre-hepatic	
Haemolysis	
Hepatocellular	
Acute hepatitis due to hepatitis virus, drugs, alcohol	
Advanced chronic liver disease	
Gilbert's syndrome	
Obstruction	
Gallstones in the common bile duct	
Pancreatic tumours	
Carcinoma of an extrahepatic bile duct	

distinction that is often made is whether the excess bilirubin is predominantly unconjugated or conjugated.

Pre-hepatic jaundice is due to increased production of bilirubin

The main cause of pre-hepatic jaundice is haemolysis, which leads to increased production of *unconjugated* bilirubin. Haemolysis itself has many causes including inherited red cell defects (such as hereditary spherocytosis) and autoimmune destruction. Because the excess bilirubin is unconjugated, it is not excreted by the kidneys and so the urine colour remains normal.

LINK BOX

Haemolysis

A further potential hepatobiliary complication of long-standing haemolysis is the development of pigment gallstones (p. 197).

Hepatocellular jaundice is due to impaired uptake or conjugation of bilirubin

Hepatocellular jaundice may occur as a feature of any disease which results in decreased uptake, conjugation, or export of bilirubin by hepatocytes. The excess bilirubin is usually a mixture of conjugated and unconjugated bilirubin, and so the urine may darken slightly.

The most common mechanism of hepatocellular jaundice is hepatocyte damage. Jaundice is a common symptom of acute liver disease (e.g. acute viral hepatitis or acute alcoholic hepatitis), and usually resolves completely. Jaundice may also occur in chronic liver disease; however, it is often a late feature and implies advanced disease.

Not all cases of hepatocellular jaundice are due to hepatocyte damage. A very common cause of hepatocellular jaundice is **Gilbert's syndrome**, an inherited condition whereby the activity of the glucuronyl transferase enzyme is reduced. Patients suffer from intermittent episodes of mild jaundice, particularly after long periods without food or during an intercurrent illness. Liver function tests confirm a raised bilirubin (which is unconjugated) with normal liver enzyme levels. The disease is entirely harmless.

Obstructive jaundice is due to blockage to the flow of bile

Obstruction to the flow of bile may occur at any level in the biliary tree, from the small interlobular bile ducts within the liver to the large extrahepatic ducts such as the common bile duct. The term **cholestasis** is often used to refer to an arrest or marked reduction in bile flow. Cholestasis essentially equates to biliary obstruction, but it is not synonymous with obstructive jaundice, as cholestasis may be present without jaundice (e.g. in the early stages of primary biliary cirrhosis).

The most common causes of obstructive jaundice are:

- Gallstones lodged in the common bile duct
- Carcinoma of the head of the pancreas
- Carcinoma of an extrahepatic bile duct.

Obstructive jaundice is almost entirely the result of a *conjugated* hyperbilirubinaemia, and so the urine turns particularly dark. Lack of bile excretion into the intestine leads to the formation of pale stools, as bilirubin derivatives normally give faeces their colour. Another very common and important symptom in obstructive jaundice is **pruritus** (itching). The mechanism of pruritus is not well understood but is presumed to be due to accumulation in the skin of components normally excreted in bile. Pruritus is often the earliest symptom noted and may precede the development of jaundice by quite some time.

Infection is a risk in an obstructed biliary system

The immediate problem with obstruction, especially in the larger bile ducts, is the risk of infection. As a general rule, obstruction plus infection in any small 'tube' in the body is bad news. In the biliary system, obstruction places the patient at risk of developing **ascending cholangitis** and sepsis.

The offending organisms are usually Gram negative gastrointestinal bacteria which gain entry to the biliary tree via the ampulla of Vater. Any patient with prolonged obstructive jaundice should therefore be prescribed a prophylactic antibiotic with good activity against Gram negative bacteria, the usual choice being ciprofloxacin.

Key points: Jaundice

- Jaundice is a yellow discoloration of the skin and eyes due to hyperbilirubinaemia.

- Jaundice is a common symptom of liver and biliary disease, which may occur early in the course of the disease (e.g. acute viral hepatitis) but often does not arise until disease is advanced (e.g. primary biliary cirrhosis).

- The causes of jaundice are divided into pre-hepatic, hepatocellular, and obstructive.

- Pre-hepatic jaundice is due to haemolysis.

- Hepatocellular jaundice may be due to hepatocyte damage or inherited defects of bilirubin handling by hepatocytes.

- Obstructive jaundice is characterized by jaundice plus symptoms of cholestasis such as pruritus, pale stools, and dark urine. Common causes include gallstones and carcinoma of the head of the pancreas.

Hepatic failure

Hepatic failure is a clinical syndrome which occurs when there is loss of over 90 per cent of the functional capacity of the liver. This may occur as a result of sudden massive damage to a normal liver (acute hepatic failure) or after a minor insult to an already chronically diseased liver (decompensated hepatic failure) (Fig. 9.3). Note that some people may refer to decompensated hepatic failure as chronic hepatic failure, a term which should not be confused with chronic liver *disease*.

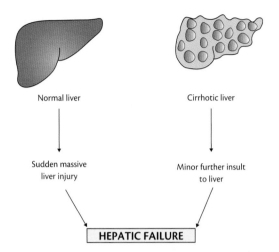

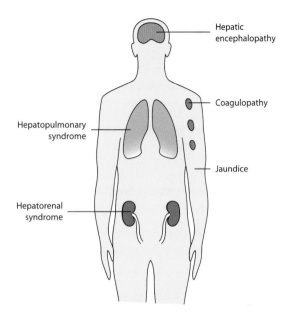

Fig. 9.3 Routes to hepatic failure. Hepatic failure may occur following massive damage to a normal liver (acute hepatic failure) or following a minor insult to a chronically damaged liver (decompensated hepatic failure).

Fig. 9.4 Cardinal features of hepatic failure.

Acute hepatic failure is caused by sudden massive hepatocyte necrosis

Acute hepatic failure occurs in a person with a previously normal liver following a sudden catastrophic insult to the liver. Typically there is a very severe acute hepatitis leading to massive hepatic necrosis, the most common causes being acute viral hepatitis, acute alcoholic hepatitis, or acute drug-related hepatitis (either as a severe abnormal reaction or due to overdose of a hepatotoxic drug such as paracetamol). Acute hepatic failure is, fortunately, uncommon.

Decompensated liver failure is much more common than acute hepatic failure

Decompensated hepatic failure occurs when a patient with pre-existing stable (compensated) cirrhosis 'decompensates' and develops symptoms and signs of hepatic failure. *Decompensation is the final terminal event in the evolution of a progressive chronic liver disease and often leads to death.* We discuss this in more detail later in the chapter in the section on cirrhosis.

The key features of hepatic failure are hepatic encephalopathy, severe coagulopathy, and jaundice

The onset of hepatic failure is heralded by the following combination of features (Fig. 9.4):

- **Hepatic encephalopathy.** This refers to a whole spectrum of neurological and behavioural symptoms attributed to the accumulation of toxic substances in the brain which the failing liver is unable to detoxify. In the early stages, its manifestations may be quite subtle, for example irritability and sleep disturbance. With worsening encephalopathy, there is increasing lethargy and disorientation, terminating in coma and death.

- **Severe coagulopathy.** The tendency to bleeding is principally caused by a reduction in the synthesis of clotting factors by hepatocytes. The best laboratory indicator of clotting abnormalities in hepatic failure is the prothrombin time, often expressed as the INR (international normalized ratio).

- **Jaundice.** The jaundice in hepatic failure is predominantly due to conjugated hyperbilirubinaemia.

These features are common to both acute and decompensated hepatic failure, although patients with decompensated failure will also have additional features related to the pre-existing cirrhosis such as palmar erythema, spider nevi, splenomegaly, and ascites.

Hepatic failure, regardless of cause, is a life-threatening disorder

The development of hepatic failure is a grave complication of a liver disease. Patients with hepatic failure are highly susceptible to the development of failure of other organs, particularly the lungs (**hepatopulmonary syndrome**) and the kidneys (**hepatorenal syndrome**). The association of liver failure with respiratory and renal failure is not well understood, but is thought to be related to widespread vasodilation in the lungs and kidneys. Abnormal shunting of blood in the lungs leads to hypoxia, and a reduction in effective perfusion of the kidneys leads to acute renal failure.

Infection is also a major problem in hepatic failure, and the development of sepsis with multiorgan failure is a common cause of death in patients with hepatic failure.

Acute liver disease

Acute liver disease is a general term for any episode of liver damage that completely resolves within 6 months. The most common causes of acute liver injury are **acute infection with a hepatitis virus, alcohol**, and **drugs**.

Most cases of acute liver disease are so mild that they never come to medical attention

In most instances, an episode of acute liver injury causes mild, transient symptoms of fatigue and nausea only. Because there is no jaundice, the symptoms are often dismissed by the patient as 'flu', and recovery occurs without any lasting consequences. As medical attention is not sought, the minor temporary derangements in liver function tests that would be seen on blood testing are never identified.

If acute liver injury is more severe, the patient suffers an episode of acute icteric hepatitis

Acute icteric hepatitis is the most common *clinically recognizable* presentation of acute liver injury. In a typical attack, there is an initial prodrome lasting several days comprising malaise, anorexia, mild fever, and upper abdominal discomfort. The prodrome is followed by the onset of jaundice, which is often what prompts the patient to seek help. The jaundice may last for any time between a few days to a few weeks, after which it slowly subsides. Pruritus may also occur if there is an element of cholestasis. Resolution of symptoms and normalization of liver function tests may take several weeks to a few months.

Very rarely, an episode of acute hepatitis may be so severe that extensive hepatocyte necrosis causes the development of acute hepatic failure.

Acute viral hepatitis

The hepatitis viruses are a group of unrelated viruses that are grouped together because they lead to liver damage without significant involvement of other organs. The most clinically important hepatitis viruses are **hepatitis A**, **B**, and **C**. Hepatitis D and E also exist but are much less commonly encountered.

Hepatitis A, B, and C are all non-cytopathic viruses, i.e. they do not destroy the hepatocytes they infect. The liver cell damage is caused by the immune system recognizing infected hepatocytes and destroying them. The outcomes of infection with the hepatitis viruses are compared in Fig. 9.5.

Acute hepatitis A infection is almost always followed by complete recovery

Hepatitis A virus (HAV) is transmitted faeco-orally, and can be passed on even if only a tiny amount of faeces from an infected person comes into contact with another person's mouth. Transmission in most people occurs through consumption of food or drinking water contaminated with faeces from an infected individual. Homosexual males may be at high risk of infection through direct oral–anal contact.

In almost all cases, the hepatitis A virus is cleared from the liver by a specific T lymphocyte response. Often the patient remains completely asymptomatic. If there are symptoms, then the typical presentation is with an episode of acute icteric hepatitis, and the diagnosis of acute hepatitis A can be made by the presence of hepatitis A IgM antibodies in the blood, confirming a recent infection. Nearly all patients recover completely. The development of chronic hepatitis A is extremely rare.

Acute hepatitis B infection is also usually followed by complete recovery

Hepatitis B virus (HBV) is a hardy virus which can survive in the blood of an infected person as well as other body fluids such as saliva, semen, and vaginal secretions. HBV can therefore be transmitted through a number of different routes including contaminated needles, sexual contact, and from an infected mother to her baby.

It is important to be aware of the four genes encoded by the HBV genome, as their products, and antibodies generated against them, are often used as markers of infection (Fig. 9.6).

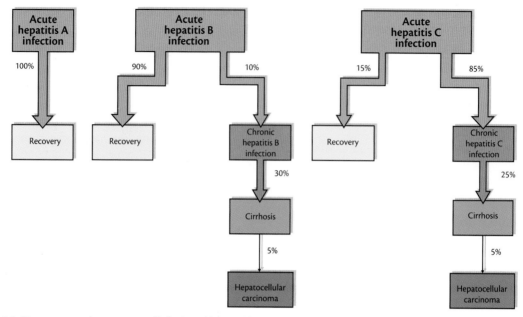

Fig. 9.5 Diagram comparing outcomes of infection with hepatitis A, B, and C viruses.

- **Core gene**. The core gene encodes two core proteins, the **core antigen** (HBcAg) and the **e antigen** (HBeAg).

- **Surface gene**. The core proteins are enclosed in a coat that contains the **hepatitis B surface antigen** (HBsAg). Large quantities of free HBsAg protein are manufactured by infected hepatocytes and released into the blood. Free HBsAg particles are not infectious, but they do stimulate the production of anti-HBsAg antibodies by the host. The presence of HBsAg in serum is a useful marker of current infection with HBV.

- **Polymerase gene**. This encodes the viral DNA polymerase enzyme.

- **X gene**. The small X protein product activates viral transcription and is also believed to be important in the pathogenesis of HBV-related hepatocellular carcinoma.

Like acute hepatitis A, many people with acute hepatitis B infection remain free of symptoms or have only a mild systemic upset. Only a minority of people develop a clinically recognizable attack of acute icteric hepatitis. In the great majority of cases, a strong T cell response to multiple viral antigens leads to eradication of the infection. Levels of HBsAg in the blood decline and anti-HBsAg antibodies appear.

Patients who mount a weak, ineffective T cell response fail to clear the virus and develop chronic viral hepatitis. This is seen more commonly than with hepatitis A, but still in only about 10 per cent of all patients. Chronic infection with HBV can be diagnosed by persistence of HBsAg in the serum. The presence of the e antigen (HBeAg) in serum indicates active viral replication, associated with a higher viral load and more severe liver damage.

Most patients are unable to eradicate the hepatitis C virus

Hepatitis C virus (HCV) is much more fragile than HBV. Because it survives poorly outside the blood, the principal mode of transmission is through infected blood. With the advent of screening of donated blood for hepatitis C, the incidence of transfusion-related hepatitis C thankfully has fallen dramatically. Currently, the dominant mode of HCV transmission is inoculation of infected blood from contaminated needles in intravenous drug abusers, followed by injuries in health

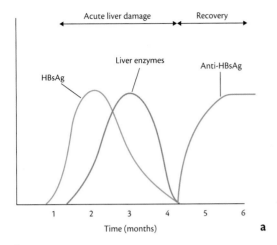

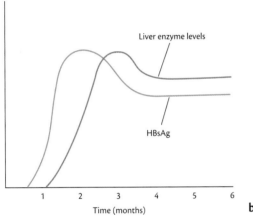

Fig. 9.6 Serology in hepatitis B virus infection. (a) Most patients with acute hepatitis B infection successfully clear the virus, with disappearance of HBsAg, resolution of abnormal liver enzyme levels, and appearance of serum anti-HBsAg antibodies. (b) Patients with a weak immune response to HBV develop chronic HBV infection. HBsAg levels remain high, and persistent liver cell damage results in persistently raised liver enzymes. Note that people vaccinated against HBV have anti-HBsAg antibodies but not HBsAg.

care workers. Sexual transmission of hepatitis C does not appear to be important.

Like acute hepatitis A and B, the initial acute infection with hepatitis C very often goes unrecognized. *Unlike hepatitis A and B, however, only 15 per cent of patients clear HCV.* Although HCV-specific T cells can be detected in people with hepatitis C infection, the T cells seem unable to clear the virus. Somehow, HCV escapes

immune elimination through mechanisms we do not understand.

As we shall shortly see, chronic hepatitis C infection is one of the most common causes of chronic liver disease and, because the acute infection is often unrecognized, patients may not even realize they are infected until considerable liver damage has occurred.

Other causes of acute liver disease

Acute icteric hepatitis may also be caused by drugs and alcohol

Drug-induced acute liver injury may have a very similar course to acute viral hepatitis, and should always be considered in the differential diagnosis, especially if hepatitis serology turns out to be negative. A full drug history should therefore be taken from any patient presenting with evidence of acute hepatitis. Although any drug could potentially be responsible, the most common culprits are antibiotics and non-steroidal anti-inflammatory drugs (NSAIDs).

Alcoholic hepatitis also presents in a similar way. The history may be helpful if the patient is forthcoming about their drinking habits. If not, there may be clues to an alcoholic aetiology in the blood tests: alcohol typically causes less marked elevations of serum aminotransferases than in viral hepatitis (AST usually <300 U/l in alcoholic hepatitis versus >1000 U/l in viral hepatitis), and the mean corpuscular volume (MCV) is often raised in alcoholics.

Occasionally an episode of acute hepatitis turns out to be the start of a chronic liver disease

It is always worth bearing in mind that sometimes a chronic liver disease initially presents with an episode of acute hepatitis which then fails to resolve. For instance, about one-third of patients with autoimmune hepatitis present with a clinical picture of acute hepatitis. Although uncommon, acute **Wilson's disease** is always an important diagnosis to consider (see later).

Chronic liver disease

Chronic liver disease refers to liver damage persisting for more than 6 months without resolution. Due to the large functional reserve and regenerative capacity of the liver, many patients with chronic liver disease are completely asymptomatic or minimally symptomatic.

The main concern in chronic liver disease is that some patients develop progressive liver *fibrosis* which over many years may lead to cirrhosis. Not all patients who develop liver fibrosis necessarily end up with cirrhosis, and the rate of progression is extremely variable, even in patients with the same underlying aetiology.

There are three main ways in which chronic liver disease may come to light

Patients with chronic liver disease may present in a number of ways:

• *The chance discovery of abnormal liver function tests persisting for at least 6 months in an asymptomatic person.* This mode of presentation accounts for 80 per cent of cases of chronic liver disease.

• *Symptoms of chronic liver disease or cirrhosis.* Patients with chronic liver disease may present complaining of feeling non-specifically unwell with tiredness and loss of libido. Physical examination may reveal signs of chronic liver disease (Fig. 9.7) and liver function tests are found to be abnormal. Patients with established cirrhosis may present with a complication related to portal hypertension such as ascites or a variceal bleed. Together these account for approximately 15 per cent of presentations.

• *An episode of acute hepatitis which fails to resolve.* The liver enzyme elevations persist for at least 6 months. This is the least frequent presentation and accounts for no more than 5 per cent of cases.

Chronic liver disease may be due to a number of conditions

There are a number of causes of chronic liver disease (Table 9.2). Working out the underlying cause in a patient suspected of having chronic liver disease involves a battery of tests designed to narrow down the list of likely causes. These range from simple blood tests, to imaging of the liver with ultrasound, to more invasive tests such as a liver biopsy.

Knowing the underlying cause is extremely important, as some conditions, such as autoimmune hepatitis and Wilson's disease, are amenable to treatment.

Liver biopsy establishes the activity of a chronic liver disease and the degree of liver fibrosis

A liver biopsy is a useful investigation in patients with chronic liver disease for three main reasons. First, it often helps in making the diagnosis of the cause of the chronic liver disease, although often this is strongly suspected from blood tests and imaging investigations that have already been carried out. Secondly, it allows an assessment of the degree of inflammatory activity within the liver which may help decide if and when treatment should be given. Thirdly, it allows an assessment of the degree of fibrosis in the liver.

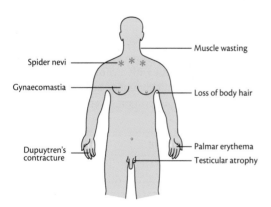

Fig. 9.7 Features of chronic liver disease. Patients with chronic liver disease may show a variety of clinical signs. Note that patients may exhibit some or all of these features, and that many patients with chronic liver disease may show none at all.

TABLE 9.2 Causes of chronic liver disease
Common
Alcoholic liver disease
Non-alcoholic liver disease
Chronic hepatitis C
Less common
Chronic hepatitis B
Drugs
Autoimmune hepatitis
Primary biliary cirrhosis
Rare
Primary sclerosing cholangitis
Wilson's disease
α_1-Antitrypsin deficiency
Haemochromatosis

Because liver function tests correlate poorly with the degree of fibrosis in the liver, a biopsy is the only method to stage a chronic liver disease accurately.

Chronic viral hepatitis

Chronic hepatitis B and C are common causes of chronic liver disease

As we saw earlier, *acute* infection with hepatitis B and C is often subclinical and so may go undiagnosed. In most patients with chronic infection, viral carriage in the liver persists over years or decades but progressive fibrosis does not occur. The diagnosis is usually only made if liver function tests are carried out and turn out to be abnormal.

However, a minority of patients with chronic hepatitis B or C develop progressive liver fibrosis over a period of 15–20 years leading eventually to symptoms and signs of chronic liver disease. The risk of developing fibrosis is higher in chronic hepatitis C than hepatitis B. Rapid progression to cirrhosis (5–10 years from infection) may occur in people co-infected with multiple hepatitis viruses and in people who also abuse alcohol.

The diagnosis of chronic viral hepatitis is established through serological markers of infection. Patients with chronic HBV are positive for HBsAg, and patients with chronic HCV have positive serum anti-HCV IgG antibodies. Liver biopsy is still required to corroborate the diagnosis and, importantly, to assess the activity of the disease and establish the degree of any fibrosis present.

Alcoholic liver disease

Alcohol is the most common cause of liver disease

Alcohol is a hepatotoxin, and liver damage is directly related to daily alcohol intake. Alcoholic liver disease encompasses three entities: **alcoholic fatty liver**, **alcoholic hepatitis**, and **alcoholic cirrhosis**. Contrary to popular belief, these three conditions are not part of a progressive continuum related to alcohol intake; they may co-exist in any combination and may well be quite separate entities.

Almost all excessive alcohol drinkers develop a fatty liver

Because cellular energy in hepatocytes is diverted away from fat metabolism to the metabolism of alcohol, fat accumulates in liver cells. The whole liver becomes enlarged, soft, yellow, and greasy. Despite these striking changes, patients with alcoholic fatty liver disease often have no symptoms and the fatty change is completely reversible if there is abstinence from alcohol.

Alcohol is an important cause of an episode of acute hepatitis

The defining features of alcoholic hepatitis are the presence of *inflammation* in the liver together with *hepatocyte necrosis*. The symptoms and prognosis of alcoholic hepatitis depend on how severe the inflammation and necrosis are. Mild cases may only cause malaise, anorexia, and right upper quadrant abdominal discomfort. More severe involvement may cause an episode of acute hepatitis with jaundice. If there is extensive hepatocyte necrosis, acute hepatic failure develops which carries a very high mortality.

Alcohol is the most common cause of cirrhosis

A smaller proportion of heavy drinkers (~ 10 per cent) develop irreversible liver fibrosis if they continue to drink. Classically liver fibrosis was thought to be a healing response to episodes of alcoholic hepatitis. In fact, alcoholic hepatitis is not a prerequisite for the development of liver fibrosis; byproducts of alcohol have been shown to activate hepatic stellate cells directly and lead to fibrosis.

Why some drinkers only develop fatty liver and others get alcoholic hepatitis or cirrhosis is not known at present, although undoubtedly the more one drinks the more likely one is to develop serious forms of liver disease.

LINK BOX

Alcohol

Although the liver is the organ most prone to developing alcohol-related problems, many other organs may develop alcohol-related disease, e.g. alcoholic cardiomyopathy, acute pancreatitis (p. 199), chronic pancreatitis (p. 201), erosive/haemorrhagic gastritis (p. 146), and squamous cell carcinomas of the oral cavity (p. 451) and oesophagus (p. 140).

Non-alcoholic liver disease

Non-alcoholic liver disease closely resembles alcoholic liver disease

The term **non-alcoholic liver disease**, rather confusingly, does not refer to any liver disease not due to alcohol, but rather a specific spectrum of liver diseases which are identical to those seen in alcoholic liver disease (i.e. fatty liver, hepatitis, and cirrhosis) but which occur in individuals consuming *little or no alcohol*.

Well recognized risk factors for the development of non-alcoholic liver disease include obesity, diabetes mellitus, and hyperlipidaemia. Given the high prevalence of these conditions, non-alcoholic liver disease is becoming an extremely common problem.

Non-alcoholic fatty liver disease is the earliest feature of non-alcoholic liver disease

The earliest stage in the evolution of non-alcoholic liver disease is the deposition of fat in the liver (**non-alcoholic fatty liver disease** or NAFLD). Patients with NAFLD are usually asymptomatic but may come to clinical attention due to abnormal liver function tests. Insulin resistance has been proposed to be central to the development of NAFLD. Resistance to the actions of insulin causes increased peripheral lipolysis and increases the delivery of free fatty acids to the liver.

Non-alcoholic steatohepatitis is now known to be a common cause of cirrhosis

A minority of patients with NAFLD develop inflammation within the liver in association with the fatty change, a condition known as **non-alcoholic steatohepatitis** (NASH). Previously regarded as a rare and harmless disorder, NASH has recently emerged as a common chronic liver disease which can lead to progressive liver fibrosis and cirrhosis in some patients. We now think that NASH may account for many cases of cirrhosis previously labelled as 'cryptogenic'.

The main difficulty in diagnosing non-alcoholic liver disease is excluding alcoholic liver disease

Because all of the ultrasound and histological findings are identical in both alcoholic and non-alcoholic disease, distinguishing between them can only be done through the patient's history. High alcohol consumption must be exhaustively excluded as a cause of liver disease before a diagnosis of NAFLD or NASH can be made. Unfortunately this may prove difficult if the patient is reluctant to disclose this information. Even in the genuine absence of alcohol abuse, many are still accused of having alcoholic liver disease!

Prognosis in NASH is generally good, except in the small proportion of those who develop cirrhosis. One of the main worries in patients with NASH is that they seem to be at a particular risk of developing hepatocellular carcinoma, even in the absence of cirrhosis. The most effective current treatment regimes are weight reduction, a low fat diet, and abstinence from alcohol.

INTERESTING TO KNOW

Thiazolidinediones and NASH

Thiazolidinediones, which act to increase insulin sensitivity, have shown promise in the treatment of NASH in pilot studies and await further assessment in larger trials.

Autoimmune hepatitis

Autoimmune hepatitis is caused by autoimmune destruction of hepatocytes

Autoimmune hepatitis is characterized by *clinically significant* liver disease attributed to an autoimmune response targeted against the liver. Our current thinking is that something first damages the liver (probably an episode of acute viral hepatitis or drug-related hepatitis), and then susceptible patients somehow become sensitized to their liver and start destroying it over time.

Like most autoimmune conditions, autoimmune hepatitis typically affects middle-aged women. Most patients present with non-specific symptoms related to chronic liver disease such as malaise or fever, and are subsequently found to have disordered liver function tests. By the time of presentation, many patients may already have cirrhosis. Features that characterize autoimmune hepatitis are high transaminase levels, markedly raised levels of IgG, and the presence of circulating autoantibodies, particularly **antinuclear antibodies** and **anti-smooth muscle antibodies**.

Most patients respond dramatically to immunosuppression with glucocorticoids, with a reduction in liver enzyme levels and inflammatory activity on the liver biopsy. Provided treatment is started before cirrhosis has developed, the prognosis is extremely good, with almost all patients remaining alive and well 10 years later. Patients with cirrhosis, or those who respond poorly to treatment, are good candidates for liver transplantation.

Primary biliary cirrhosis

Primary biliary cirrhosis is caused by autoimmune destruction of intrahepatic bile ducts

Primary biliary cirrhosis (PBC) is another autoimmune disease which can lead to chronic liver disease. Unlike autoimmune hepatitis where the target is hepatocytes, in primary biliary cirrhosis the immune system selectively destroys **cholangiocytes**. Cholangiocytes are the epithelial cells lining small interlobular bile ducts in the portal tracts within the substance of the liver. The term primary biliary cirrhosis is slightly unfortunate, as the disease may last for many years before cirrhosis is established.

Patients with PBC usually present with intractable pruritus and intense lethargy

In the early stages of the disease, patients may be asymptomatic or have non-specific symptoms such as fatigue and general malaise. Intractable pruritus is the most common symptom that leads the patient to seek medical attention, and this should always prompt consideration of cholestasis.

Liver function tests usually reveal raised ALP and GGT levels, corroborating the suspicion of biliary disease. The major marker of the disease is the presence of circulating **antimitochondrial autoantibodies**, which are found in over 95 per cent of patients. All patients with PBC also have high levels of circulating IgM, another important diagnostic feature which is found even in the small number of patients who do not have antimitochondrial antibodies.

Biliary destruction in PBC appears to be mediated by autoreactive T lymphocytes

The antimitochondrial antibodies in patients with PBC react against the pyruvate dehydrogenase E2 complex located in the inner mitochondrial matrix. Both T and B lymphocytes reactive against PDC-E2 are found in portal tracts in patients with PBC, but it is thought that the destruction of biliary epithelial cells is mediated by the autoreactive T lymphocytes.

One of the mysteries of PBC is why the autoimmune attack selectively destroys biliary epithelial cells when all nucleated cells contain the PDC-E2 complex in their mitochondria. A recent finding that could explain this dilemma is that processing of the PDC-E2 complex during apoptosis differs in biliary epithelial cells from other epithelial cells, such that the antigenic component of the complex remains immunologically intact in biliary epithelial cells but is destroyed in other cell types.

PBC progresses to cirrhosis and death over many years

The only effective treatment for PBC is ursodeoxycholic acid, a bile acid found in small quantities in normal bile. Ursodeoxycholic acid appears to slow the progression of the disease if given in the early stages of the disease. It is not effective in advanced disease.

Even with treatment, almost all patients develop progressive liver fibrosis which, over a period of about 20 years, terminates in cirrhosis and decompensated hepatic failure. The onset of jaundice in PBC is a late feature and usually heralds clinical deterioration. Rather like autoimmune hepatitis, patients with PBC are often young and without other significant diseases, so are good candidates for liver transplantation.

Key points: Primary biliary cirrhosis

- Primary biliary cirrhosis is a chronic liver disease associated with autoimmune destruction of small intrahepatic bile ducts.

- The disease affects mostly middle-aged women, and the cause remains enigmatic.

- Pruritus and lethargy are the most common presenting symptoms, and the presence of biliary disease is suggested by an elevated ALP and GGT.

- The presence of high levels of serum IgM antibodies and circulating antimitochondrial antibodies is strongly suggestive of the diagnosis.

- The natural history of the disease is progression to cirrhosis and death over a period of 15–20 years.

Primary sclerosing cholangitis

Primary sclerosing cholangitis causes narrowing of large bile ducts

Primary sclerosing cholangitis (PSC) is a chronic cholestatic disease caused by fibrosis in the wall of large bile ducts leading to areas of narrowing throughout the biliary tree. The disease usually affects the extrahepatic and large intrahepatic bile ducts.

Before making a diagnosis of PSC, it is important to exclude conditions known secondarily to cause narrowing of larger bile ducts such as bile duct gallstones, or previous surgery or instrumentation of the biliary tree.

The aetiology of primary sclerosing cholangitis is unknown, though there is a very strong association with ulcerative colitis. Up to 75% of cases of PSC develop in patients known to have ulcerative colitis and many patients are diagnosed early in the course of the disease when an isolated rise in ALP is found during routine follow-up of patients with known ulcerative colitis.

Imaging of the biliary tree is the most important diagnostic test for PSC

In contrast to PBC, where antimitochondrial antibodies are the most helpful diagnostic test, the most useful test in PSC is imaging of the biliary tree, looking for irregularity of the calibre of extrahepatic and intrahepatic ducts. Such changes can usually be identified non-invasively using magnetic resonance cholangiopancreatography (MRCP), though demonstrating minor intrahepatic abnormalities may require endoscopic retrograde cholangiopancreatography (ERCP) (Fig. 9.8).

Confirmation of the diagnosis of PSC requires liver biopsy

A clinical and radiological diagnosis of PSC can be confirmed if a liver biopsy shows inflammation around the intrahepatic bile ducts with surrounding fibrosis. The liver biopsy also permits an assessment of the degree of liver fibrosis, allowing the disease to be staged. Often, frustratingly, the patchy nature of the disease may mean the diagnosis cannot be confirmed if all of the bile ducts in the biopsy happen not to be involved.

Patients with PSC die either from hepatic failure or from bile duct carcinoma

PSC is a progressive disease which eventually leads to liver fibrosis and cirrhosis. Sooner or later decompensated hepatic failure develops, leading to death. There is no specific treatment that can arrest the progression of the disease, and transplantation provides the only opportunity for cure.

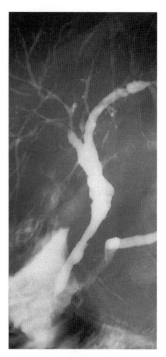

Fig. 9.8 Typical endoscopic retrograde cholangiographic findings in primary sclerosing cholangitis showing stricturing and dilation of the intra- and extrahepatic biliary tree.

About a quarter of patients with long-standing PSC die before the development of hepatic failure from **bile duct carcinoma**, an extremely aggressive malignancy with a mean survival of just 9 months. There is no reliable method of predicting which patients will develop this terrible complication.

Key points: Primary sclerosing cholangitis

♦ Primary sclerosing cholangitis is characterized by narrowing of large bile ducts, leading to progressive liver damage and eventual cirrhosis.

♦ The cause of PSC is unknown, though there is a very strong association with ulcerative colitis.

♦ Most cases of PSC are diagnosed when a patient being followed-up for known ulcerative colitis is found to have a persistent rise in ALP.

Drug-induced chronic liver disease

Drugs should always be considered as a possible cause of chronic liver disease

We have already seen that drugs are a common cause of acute liver injury and, in rare instances, full-blown acute hepatic failure. Drugs may also cause chronic liver disease (Table 9.3), which may be clinically and histologically identical to other chronic liver diseases. As removal of the drug is usually followed by recovery of liver function, it is important to consider any drug as a possible cause of unexplained chronic liver disease, especially when hepatitis serology is negative.

Inherited causes of chronic liver disease

Wilson's disease

Wilson's disease is an inherited disorder in which copper accumulates in the body

Wilson's disease is an inherited disorder of copper metabolism in which there is a genetic defect in a copper-transporting protein vital for the removal of copper into bile. Unable to dispose of excess body copper, the liver accumulates large quantities of copper.

TABLE 9.3	Drugs which can cause chronic liver disease
Amiodarone	
Chlorambucil	
Diclofenac	
Methotrexate	
Valproate	

When the storage capacity of the liver is exhausted, excess copper then becomes deposited in other organs such as the brain, kidneys, and cornea.

Excess copper in the liver leads to chronic liver injury, whilst accumulation in the brain leads to neurological symptoms, initially incoordination and tremor. Wilson's disease often leads to strange combinations of symptoms, making it difficult to diagnose.

When suspected, the diagnosis is usually easy to make by finding a low level of the copper-binding protein **caeruloplasmin** in the serum, together with the demonstration of excess copper in the liver by special staining of a liver biopsy. Often excess copper in the cornea can be seen as a brown ring at the periphery of the iris which is known as a Kayser–Fleischer ring.

Although rare, Wilson's disease is extremely important to remember as it is easily treated if diagnosed. Missing a diagnosis of Wilson's disease is disastrous, as left untreated the disease is lethal. You will not diagnose it unless you think of it in any patient with evidence of liver disease.

α_1-Antitrypsin deficiency

α_1-Antitrypsin deficiency causes chronic liver disease and emphysema

α_1-Antitrypsin is a protein made by the liver which keeps the body's tissues, particularly elastin, from being digested by enzymes released from neutrophils. Deficiency of α_1-antitrypsin is an inherited cause of chronic liver injury as well as predisposing to the development of emphysema in the lungs. In adult life, the disease may be diagnosed incidentally due to abnormal liver function tests, or at its end-stage with frank cirrhosis.

Hereditary haemochromatosis

Hereditary haemochromatosis causes excessive iron accumulation in the liver

Hereditary haemochromatosis is an inherited disease caused by a defect in a gene coding for a protein that controls iron handling in the gut. Patients with the disease absorb iron too easily from the gut, leading to accumulation of iron in a variety of tissues including the liver, pancreas, pituitary, heart, and skin. Typically the disease does not become manifest until at least age 40.

Liver disease is the most serious problem in haemochromatosis. Total liver iron reaches some 100 times above the normal level, leading to chronic hepatocellular injury and risk of fibrosis and cirrhosis. Patients with haemochromatosis are also at particular risk of developing hepatocellular carcinoma, even in the absence of cirrhosis.

Pathology in the other major tissues involved may give rise to secondary diabetes mellitus, pituitary failure, dilated cardiomyopathy, and discoloration of the skin. The skin classically turns a 'slate grey' colour, lending to the alternative name of 'bronzed diabetes'.

> ## Key points: Inherited causes of chronic liver disease
>
> ◆ Wilson's disease is an inherited disorder of copper metabolism, leading to accumulation of copper in the liver, brain, and iris. Accumulation in the liver leads to chronic liver disease. Wilson's disease is treatable if diagnosed early, and should be considered in any patient presenting with liver disease.
>
> ◆ α_1-Antitrypsin deficiency leads to chronic liver disease and emphysema.
>
> ◆ Hereditary haemochromatosis is an inherited disorder of iron handling leading to absorption of excess iron from the gut and deposition in a number of organs including the liver. Chronic liver disease and hepatocellular carcinoma are the main problems in patients with hereditary haemochromatosis.

Cirrhosis

Cirrhosis represents the final result of progressive liver fibrosis

Cirrhosis is the end result of a chronic liver disease causing progressive fibrosis in the liver. It is an *irreversible* process whereby the normal architecture of the liver is *completely* replaced by nodules of regenerating hepatocytes separated by bands of fibrosis (Fig. 9.9).

The hepatic stellate cell is key to the development of liver fibrosis

The key cell implicated in the development of fibrosis and cirrhosis in the setting of chronic liver injury is the

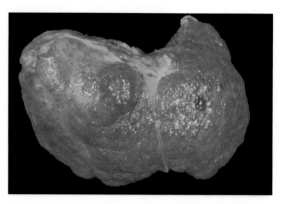

Fig. 9.9 Cirrhotic liver. This liver was removed at post-mortem from a patient known to abuse alcohol. The whole of the liver is studded with nodules. Microscopically, the liver showed nodules of regenerating hepatocytes separated by dense bands of fibrosis, confirming established cirrhosis.

hepatic stellate cell. Normally this is a relatively quiescent cell which lives just underneath the endothelial lining of the liver sinusoids next to the liver cell plates in the space of Disse. In the setting of persistent liver injury, however, cytokines released from Kupffer cells and hepatocytes activate hepatic stellate cells. Activated hepatic stellate cells then start secreting large quantities of collagen, leading to fibrosis and eventually cirrhosis (Fig. 9.10).

Cirrhosis is classified according to its cause

Early classifications of cirrhosis described two types based on the size of the regenerative nodules. Micronodular cirrhotic nodules were up to 3 mm, while macronodular cirrhotic nodules were larger than 3 mm. This distinction has no clinical relevance at all, so it has been replaced by a classification according to the underlying cause.

Cirrhosis may occur as a result of a number of diseases causing chronic liver injury (Table 9.4). It should be emphasized that of all patients with chronic liver injury, only a minority develop fibrosis and progress to cirrhosis. By far the most common causes are alcohol and chronic viral hepatitis due to the HBV and HCV. Very often no definite cause can be found and the cirrhosis is called cryptogenic. As we mentioned earlier, it is now thought that many of these may represent end-stage cases of the entity NASH.

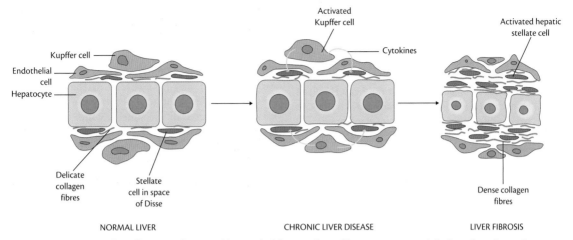

Fig. 9.10 Pathogenesis of liver fibrosis. In the normal liver, only delicate collagen fibres are present and the hepatic stellate cells are quiescent cells in the space of Disse. In the setting of chronic liver disease, Kupffer cells lining the vascular sinusoids release cytokines which activate the hepatic stellate cells. Activated hepatic stellate cells proliferate and secrete large quantities of dense collagen, leading to irreversible liver fibrosis.

Patients with cirrhosis may come to medical attention in two settings

The patient with cirrhosis may be picked up in one of two ways. It may develop in patients who are already known to have a chronic liver disease and are being followed-up with intermittent liver biopsies to assess fibrosis. Alternatively, cirrhosis may be the presenting feature of a pre-existing chronic liver disease which was entirely asymptomatic during its evolution and was not picked up serendipitously on a blood test.

The development of cirrhosis has important consequences

Cirrhosis has a number of important consequences which justify its distinction from chronic liver disease with milder degrees of fibrosis. Nodules of regenerating hepatocytes lack the structural organization of normal liver lobules and so surviving hepatocytes do not function optimally. Diffuse scarring disrupts hepatic sinusoids and increases resistance to flow of blood into the liver from the portal venous system, leading to **portal hypertension**. The repeated cycles of liver cell loss and regeneration predispose hepatocytes to developing genetic mutations, which can lead to **hepatocellular carcinoma**.

Portal hypertension has some potentially very dangerous consequences

The development of portal hypertension has a number of knock-on effects, most notably **splenomegaly** and the development of **portosystemic anastomoses**. Portosystemic anastomoses are new vascular channels that open up between the portal venous system and the systemic venous system in an attempt to bypass the

TABLE 9.4	Causes of cirrhosis
Common	
Alcohol	
Chronic viral hepatitis	
NASH	
Cryptogenic	
Less common	
Primary biliary cirrhosis	
Primary sclerosing cholangitis	
Autoimmune hepatitis	
Haemochromatosis	
α_1-Antitrypsin deficiency	
Wilson's disease	

high pressure created in the liver. There are two important sites in which they develop:

- The lower oesophagus, where dilated vessels called **oesophageal varices** develop. One of the most feared complications of portal hypertension is rupture of an oesophageal varix. Not only can this lead to a massive upper gastrointestinal bleed, but it can also precipitate the development of decompensated hepatic failure, both of which are life-threatening conditions.

- The periumbilical veins where the dilated channels may be visible on the anterior abdominal wall as **caput medusae**.

Cirrhotic patients have many clinical signs but relatively few symptoms

Patients with cirrhosis may manifest a number of clinical signs on physical examination. As well as all the features of chronic liver disease, they may also have palpable splenomegaly and visible caput medusae (Fig. 9.11). Note that in stable compensated cirrhosis, *jaundice is usually absent*. This is because the liver still manages to maintain adequate bilirubin metabolism despite loss

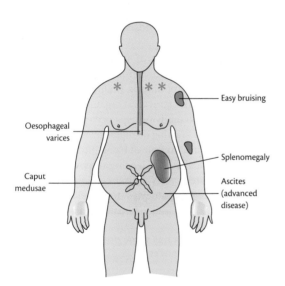

Fig. 9.11 Clinical features of cirrhosis. Patients with cirrhosis may show any of the features of chronic liver disease, together with features of portal hypertension, i.e. splenomegaly, caput medusae, and ascites. Note that some patients with cirrhosis may show none of these features at all.

Oesophageal varices

Caput medusae

Easy bruising

Splenomegaly

Ascites (advanced disease)

of a large proportion of the functional hepatic mass. The development of jaundice usually implies the onset of hepatic failure.

Remarkably, most patients with stable compensated cirrhosis are relatively free of symptoms and *may even have normal liver function tests*. As the disease progresses, however, symptoms become more prominent. Patients feel tired all the time, become anorexic and lose weight, particularly muscle bulk. With advancing disease, impaired synthesis of clotting factors leads to easy bruising, and ascites may develop.

Ascites is commonly seen in patients with advanced cirrhosis

Cirrhosis is one of the common causes of ascites, though the precise mechanism is still not clearly understood. Current thinking is that a reduction in effective renal blood flow in advanced cirrhosis causes secondary hyperaldosteronism; stimulation of sodium and water retention by the kidneys in the presence of portal hypertension then leads to ascites.

Whatever the mechanism, the development of ascites in a patient with cirrhosis is an ominous sign as it usually implies severe end-stage liver disease. Only half of cirrhotic patients with ascites survive beyond 2 years.

The natural history of cirrhosis is an inexorable progression to hepatic failure and death

The development of hepatic failure in a patient with cirrhosis is known as **decompensated hepatic failure**. The transition from compensated cirrhosis to decompensated hepatic failure is an extremely important cause of an abrupt deterioration in patients with cirrhosis and often leads to death. Common precipitants of decompensation include:

- Alcohol binge

- Intercurrent infection

- Variceal bleed

- Development of hepatocellular carcinoma.

Decompensated hepatic failure is difficult to manage and carries a poor prognosis

Decompensated hepatic failure has a large number of possible clinical features (Fig. 9.12). It is important to realize that an individual patient will not necessarily display all of these features; however, the more severe

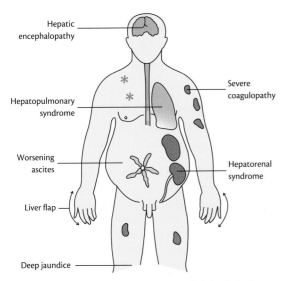

Fig. 9.12 Clinical features of decompensated cirrhosis. Patients with decompensated hepatic failure show the features of advanced cirrhosis together with the features of hepatic failure such as deep jaundice, hepatic encephalopathy, and a severe coagulopathy.

the disease, the more problems a patient is likely to develop. Furthermore, there is often a snowballing effect whereby the development of one complication increases the likelihood of more occurring.

The combination of all these problems makes decompensated hepatic failure extremely difficult to manage. The outlook is grave, and the patient and their relatives should be informed of the poor prognosis.

Key points: Cirrhosis

- Cirrhosis is an irreversible state in which the liver is diffusely replaced by bands of fibrosis separating nodules of regenerating hepatocytes.

- Cirrhosis represents the end stage of a chronic liver disease causing progressive fibrosis in the liver. The most common causes are alcoholic liver disease, chronic viral hepatitis, and non-alcoholic steatohepatitis.

- The development of cirrhosis leads to a loss of synthetic capacity of the liver, portal hypertension, and a risk of developing hepatocellular carcinoma.

- Many patients with stable cirrhosis have minimal symptoms, though physical examination may reveal a number of stigmata.

- Eventually patients with cirrhosis develop decompensated hepatic failure which often leads to death.

Liver tumours

Tumours of the liver may be benign or malignant.

Haemangioma is the most common benign neoplasm of the liver

A **haemangioma** is a benign tumour composed of neoplastic endothelial cells forming vascular channels of varying sizes. Haemangiomas commonly arise within the liver, affecting about 3 per cent of the population. The aetiology is unknown. Most liver haemangiomas are small and asymptomatic, being detected when the liver is imaged during an ultrasound or CT scan. Occasionally a large haemangioma may cause symptoms of discomfort, in which case surgical excision may be performed.

Liver cell adenoma is a benign neoplasm of hepatocytes seen mostly in young women

Liver cell adenoma is a benign neoplasm composed of hepatocytes. The hepatocytes are arranged in sheets and cords but the normal lobular architecture of the liver is not present as there are no portal tracts or central veins within a liver cell adenoma.

Liver cell adenoma is seen mostly in young women and is said to be related to use of the oral contraceptive pill. Liver cell adenomas may occur anywhere in the liver, but are often found near the surface of the liver right underneath the capsule. The subcapsular location is relevant as liver cell adenomas can occasionally rupture through the liver capsule, causing massive bleeding into the peritoneal cavity.

The most common malignancy in the liver is metastatic tumour

The liver is a very common site for metastases. Lung, breast, and colonic carcinomas are the most common primary tumours that spread to the liver. Small tumour deposits in the liver usually remain asymptomatic and may only be picked up when the liver is imaged as part of the staging of a patient with cancer.

Sometimes the presence of hepatic metastases is suggested when liver function tests reveal an isolated rise in ALP and GGT, a pattern suggestive of hepatic infiltration which should always be investigated. Extensive liver metastases may manifest clinically with jaundice and an enlarged craggy palpable liver.

The most common primary tumour of the liver is hepatocellular carcinoma

Hepatocellular carcinoma (HCC) is a malignant tumour derived from hepatocytes. HCC usually develops in a liver already affected by cirrhosis, presumably because repeated cycles of cell death and regeneration predispose hepatocytes to developing genetic mutations. Different causes of cirrhosis carry quite varying risks of hepatocellular carcinoma, those with the highest being:

◆ Chronic hepatitis B and C

◆ Alcohol

◆ Haemochromatosis.

Worldwide, HCC is a very common cancer and this is largely due to the very high rates seen in areas of South East Asia with high rates of chronic HBV infection. In the Western world where HBV is not so prevalent, chronic hepatitis C and alcohol are the most common causes of HCC.

In patients with cirrhosis, HCC often presents with decompensated liver failure as the growing tumour obliterates residual hepatocyte function. Some patients may be diagnosed at an earlier stage if they are found to have a rising level of **α-fetoprotein** and imaging of the liver reveals a tumour. α-Fetoprotein is a glycoprotein which is synthesized by the yolk sac and fetal liver and gut. In adult life, only minimal amounts of α-fetoprotein are present in plasma. Most hepatocellular carcinomas secrete α-fetoprotein, making it a valuable marker for the tumour. Regular measurement of α-fetoprotein should be a routine part of the management of patients known to have cirrhosis.

The outlook for patients with HCC is extremely poor. The only curative treatment is surgical resection, but only a small minority of patients are suitable for attempted resection.

Intrahepatic bile duct carcinoma presents late and has a poor prognosis

Carcinomas developing from intrahepatic bile ducts are best considered as liver tumours since they present with symptoms related to a liver mass rather than signs localizing to the biliary tree (they do not cause jaundice unlike carcinomas of extrahepatic bile ducts). Intrahepatic bile duct carcinomas cause very non-specific symptoms of abdominal discomfort and weight loss. Because it presents late, the prognosis is very poor, with many patients having metastases at presentation.

Key points: Liver tumours

◆ Liver tumours may be benign or malignant.

◆ Benign liver tumours include haemangioma and liver cell adenoma.

◆ Most malignant tumours of the liver are metastases, particularly from the gastrointestinal tract.

◆ The most common primary liver malignancy is hepatocellular carcinoma which usually develops on the background of cirrhosis. A rising α-fetoprotein in a patient with cirrhosis is highly suggestive of the development of hepatocellular carcinoma.

◆ Intrahepatic bile duct carcinoma is a primary liver malignancy derived from small intrahepatic bile ducts. It presents late and has a poor prognosis.

Gallbladder

Gallstones

The two most important points to appreciate about gallstones is first that they are extremely common, and secondly the vast majority of patients with gall-stones never experience any symptoms from them. Nevertheless, the small proportion of patients with symptomatic gallstones represent a significant work-load to the health service.

Gallstones are often classified according to their pre-dominant constituents as either **cholesterol** or **pigmented** (containing mostly calcium bilirubinate). There does not appear to be any correlation between the type of stone and the clinical consequences.

Eighty per cent of all gallstones in the Western world contain mostly cholesterol. Cholesterol stones form when bile becomes supersaturated with cholesterol and crystallizes out. Cholesterol secretion is highest in overweight women, and this group of people are at par-ticular risk of gallstone disease.

LINK BOX

Gallstones and Crohn's disease

Gallstones are very common in patients with Crohn's disease due to malabsorption of bile salts from the terminal ileum (p. 156).

Gallstones can cause a number of diseases according to their location

Gallstones may cause several diseases (Fig. 9.13). Stones impacting in the cystic duct cause a severe pain known as **biliary colic** as the gallbladder contracts firmly against the acutely obstructed duct. If an impacted stone incites an acute inflammatory response, a more marked systemic illness occurs known as **acute chole-cystitis**. The inflammation is initially *sterile*, due to

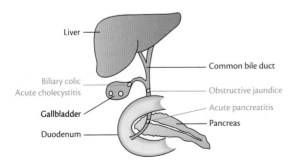

Fig. 9.13 Diseases caused by gallstones.

irritant effects of retained bile. It has been suggested that external compression of the nearby cystic artery by the impacted stone may contribute by causing mucosal ischaemia.

Smaller stones passing out of the cystic duct may lodge in the common bile duct, causing intermittent or persistent **obstructive jaundice**. This may be compli-cated by the development of infection and **ascending cholangitis**. Finally, stones impacting more distally may affect drainage of pancreatic secretions. As we shall see, gallstones are a very common cause of **acute pancreatitis**.

Biliary colic is characterized by severe pain which spontaneously resolves

Intermittent obstruction of the cystic duct giving rise to episodes of biliary colic is probably the most common type of symptom attributed to gallstones. The pain is severe, typically rising to a plateau over a few minutes and then continuing unrelentingly. *True 'colicky' intermit-tent pain is actually quite rare.* The pain usually resolves spontaneously after several hours. A bout of vomiting usually ends the attack and the patient feels washed out and sore for the next day or so. Commonly a history of previous episodes exists. An ultrasound scan will confirm the presence of gallstones, and cholecystec-tomy is the definitive treatment.

Acute cholecystitis is a more severe prolonged illness than biliary colic

In contrast to straightforward biliary colic, the patient with acute cholecystitis is systemically unwell with fever and tachycardia. The course is much more pro-longed than simple biliary colic, often lasting several days before settling or precipitating urgent surgery.

Treatment is supportive, with antibiotics and analge-sia. Oral intake is limited to fluids only. Usually once the episode is over, the patient is listed for cholecystec-tomy after about 3 months. This is to allow time for the inflammatory episode to settle down completely for easier removal of the organ. Some surgeons advise early surgical intervention within 48 h of an attack of acute cholecystitis as the dissection is actually facili-tated by oedema of the adjacent tissues.

Chronic cholecystitis should be a histopathological diagnosis only

The term **chronic cholecystitis** is another one of those entities with little agreement as to its actual definition.

We think it is best restricted to being a pathological diagnosis, i.e. *it should only be made by histological examination of a resected gallbladder specimen.* Chronic cholecystitis is a common finding in the gallbladder following episodes of biliary colic or acute cholecystitis. The pertinent features are fibrosis in the gallbladder wall and formation of outpouchings of mucosa through the muscular layer (Fig. 9.14).

Unfortunately the term chronic cholecystitis is sometimes still used inappropriately as a *clinical* diagnosis in patients presenting with non-specific dyspeptic symptoms (such as discomfort in the upper abdomen) who are found to have gallstones. It is tempting to assume cause and effect, but gallstones are rarely responsible for such symptoms, and cholecystectomy does not improve these symptoms. Such patients are best labelled as having **non-ulcer dyspepsia** (p. 174) and managed conservatively.

Key points: Gallstones

♦ Gallstones are very common and may be predominantly cholesterol or pigmented.

♦ Many people with gallstones remain completely asymptomatic throughout life.

♦ Symptomatic gallstone disease includes biliary colic, acute cholecystitis, obstructive jaundice, and acute pancreatitis.

♦ Biliary colic is a severe pain which lasts for several hours due to impaction of a gallstone in the cystic duct.

♦ Acute cholecystitis is a systemic disease due to inflammation in the gallbladder wall set up by an impacted gallstone.

♦ Chronic cholecystitis is a *histological* term for the changes seen in a gallbladder affected by previous episodes of biliary colic or acute cholecystitis.

Extrahepatic bile ducts

A variety of diseases can involve the extrahepatic bile ducts, all of which tend to present with obstructive jaundice due to mechanical obstruction of the bile duct. In most instances, the obstruction is not due to

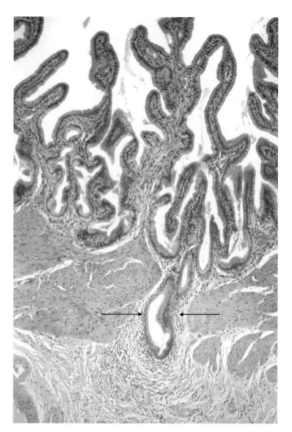

Fig. 9.14 Chronic cholecystitis. This is a microscopic image from a gallbladder specimen removed from a patient several weeks after an attack of acute cholecystitis. The gallbladder wall shows the features of chronic cholecystitis, with hypertrophy of the muscular layer of the wall, chronic inflammation, and formation of Rokitansky–Aschoff sinuses (pouches of epithelium which have herniated through the muscular layer of the gallbladder wall—arrows).

disease of the bile duct itself but rather something lodging in the bile duct (e.g. a gallstone) or something squashing it from outside (e.g. a carcinoma of the head of the pancreas). Primary diseases of the extrahepatic bile ducts do also occur, and include primary sclerosing cholangitis (discussed earlier) and carcinoma of an extrahepatic bile duct.

Extrahepatic bile duct carcinomas carry a poor prognosis

Carcinomas of extrahepatic bile ducts are usually well differentiated adenocarcinomas derived from the glandular epithelium lining the bile ducts. Primary sclerosing cholangitis is a well established risk factor for the development of carcinoma of an extrahepatic bile duct. Gallstones in bile ducts do not seem to play a role.

The tumour usually presents early, as obstructive jaundice occurs when the tumour is still relatively small and before widespread dissemination has occurred. If cholangitis develops, there may be fever and chills. An ultrasound usually shows dilated bile ducts, and ERCP allows precise localization of the carcinoma. Although the tumours are often small when diagnosed, surgical resection is rarely achievable and most patients are treated symptomatically. Progressive deterioration is the rule and survival is not good.

Exocrine pancreas

The pancreas has two components: exocrine and endocrine. Disorders of the endocrine function of the pancreas, such as diabetes mellitus, are discussed in Chapter 14. For now, we are concerned with the exocrine part of the pancreas, whose function is the secretion of an alkaline fluid containing various digestive enzymes including proteases (trypsin, chymotrypsin), lipase, and amylase. The major disorders of the exocrine pancreas are acute pancreatitis, chronic pancreatitis, and carcinoma of the pancreas.

Acute pancreatitis

Acute pancreatitis is a condition in which acute inflammation of the pancreas leads to the activation and release of enzymes which autodigest the pancreas and peripancreatic tissues. It is a common and important cause of acute abdominal pain and emergency admission to hospital. Acute pancreatitis has many causes (Table 9.5), with the final common pathway being injury to the pancreas with escape of activated digestive enzymes.

Alcohol and gallstones account for most cases of acute pancreatitis

Acute pancreatitis due to alcohol usually follows a bout of heavy drinking. Alcohol and its metabolites have a direct toxic effect on pancreatic exocrine cells, leading to the release and activation of digestive enzymes.

In patients who do not drink alcohol, most cases of acute pancreatitis are due to gallstones. The hypothesized

TABLE 9.5	Causes of acute pancreatitis
Common	
Gallstones	
Alcohol	
Post-ERCP	
Idiopathic	
Less common	
Blunt trauma to the pancreas	
Post-surgical	
Drugs, e.g. azathioprine	
Metabolic, e.g. hypercalcaemia	

mechanism is obstruction of the common bile duct and the main pancreatic duct when a gallstone becomes lodged at the ampulla of Vater. Reflux of bile and duodenal contents into the pancreas leads to parenchymal injury.

Despite the many possible causes of acute pancreatitis, in as many as 25 per cent of cases no cause can be identified. It is thought that many of these cases are caused by occult small gallstones. It is important to attempt to identify the underlying cause, as treatment (e.g. removal of common bile duct stones) may prevent the pancreatitis from worsening and stop recurrent attacks in the future.

Acute pancreatitis presents with acute upper abdominal pain and vomiting

The typical clinical history of acute pancreatitis is the sudden onset of severe upper abdominal pain, often radiating to the back. Note that features of peritonitis such as guarding and rebound tenderness are absent because the inflammation is retroperitoneal, a helpful distinguishing feature from a perforated duodenal ulcer. Nausea and vomiting, and a low grade fever are common.

Biochemical results are extremely important in acute pancreatitis

Biochemical investigations are essential in the diagnosis and management of acute pancreatitis. In a patient with a compatible history, the finding of a significantly raised plasma **amylase** is virtually diagnostic of acute pancreatitis. However, it is important to realize that there are other causes of an increased plasma amylase, including other acute abdominal conditions such as a perforated duodenal ulcer and intestinal obstruction.

Biochemical parameters also form part of prognostic scoring systems designed to establish the severity of an episode of acute pancreatitis. Poor prognostic factors include raised levels of blood glucose, lactate dehydrogenase, AST, urea, and C-reactive protein (CRP), and a reduced level of calcium.

Patients with acute pancreatitis can deteriorate very rapidly

The severity of acute pancreatitis varies considerably, ranging from a mild self-limiting illness lasting 1–2 days, to death from fulminant haemorrhagic pancreatic necrosis, shock, and multiorgan failure. One of the important, and worrying, features of acute pancreatitis is that patients can very rapidly deteriorate from an initially mild picture to a severe, life-threatening illness. Regular reassessment of patients with acute pancreatitis is therefore extremely important. Deterioration is suggested by the development of the following:

- Hypovolaemia. This is due to massive exudation of plasma into the retroperitoneal space. Early signs are a postural drop in blood pressure and a declining urine output.

- Paralytic ileus. This is a reaction to extensive inflammation occurring in the vicinity of the bowel together with an electrolyte imbalance. The development of ileus also worsens hypovolaemia as an immotile gut accumulates large amounts of fluid within it.

- Hypoxia. Hypoxia is common in severe pancreatitis and is a useful marker of severity. The underlying mechanism remains unclear, but suffice it to say that a raised respiratory rate should alert the astute doctor to measure arterial blood gases and reassess the patient for other markers of severity.

Infection of a necrotic pancreas is an ominous complication of acute pancreatitis

Superadded infection of an extensively necrotic pancreas is a major problem in severe cases of acute pancreatitis. It is believed that the organisms spread from the transverse colon into the necrotic peripancreatic tissue. Infection can spread rapidly through the devitalized tissue leading to severe hypovolaemic shock, acute disseminated intravascular coagulation, and multiorgan failure (acute respiratory distress syndrome and acute

renal failure being particular risks). These are ominous developments which carry a high mortality.

INTERESTING TO KNOW

Feeding in severe acute pancreatitis

There was a long-held belief that patients with severe acute pancreatitis should not be allowed to eat or drink. The reasoning behind this was to 'rest' the gut and reduce the stimulation to pancreatic exocrine secretion. This concept has now been shown to be erroneous. Once symptoms develop, pancreatic enzyme synthesis stops and it is not possible to stimulate the pancreas. Furthermore, starving the patient may be harmful because it deprives the gut mucosa of nutrients and increases the chance of penetration of the mucosal barrier by bacteria and toxins. It is now accepted that early nasojejunal nutrition, if tolerated by the patient, is safe in acute pancreatitis.

Pancreatic pseudocyst is a common late complication of acute pancreatitis

Collections of fluid in the region of the pancreas are common in acute pancreatitis, and these frequently resolve spontaneously. A diagnosis of a **pancreatic pseudocyst** should be reserved for a fluid collection that is present beyond 4 weeks from the onset of the episode of acute pancreatitis. The term pseudocyst is used as the collection is not lined by epithelium.

Pancreatic pseudocysts usually form in the lesser sac, and one of the most reliable ways of treating them is **cystogastrostomy**. A cystogastrostomy is a surgical technique which creates a communication between the cyst and the stomach, allowing drainage of the fluid into the stomach.

Key points: Acute pancreatitis

- Acute pancreatitis is caused by acute inflammation in the pancreas leading to destructive autodigestion of the pancreas and surrounding tissues.

- The most common causes of acute pancreatitis are alcohol and gallstones. In up to a quarter of cases, no cause can be found.

Key points: Acute pancreatitis—cont'd

- Acute pancreatitis presents with severe upper abdominal pain and vomiting. The diagnosis is usually established upon finding a markedly raised plasma amylase.

- The severity of acute pancreatitis varies markedly, from a mild illness which resolves over a few days to a very severe life-threatening disorder with hypovolaemic shock and multiorgan failure.

- Infection of an extensively necrotic pancreas is an ominous development associated with rapid deterioration.

Chronic pancreatitis

We have seen how acute pancreatitis is a process which occurs in a previously normal pancreas which usually returns to normal after the episode. **Chronic pancreatitis**, however, is associated with persistent inflammation in the pancreas which leads to scarring and the irreversible destruction of the gland.

The most common cause of chronic pancreatitis is alcohol

By far the most common cause of chronic pancreatitis is alcohol. Unlike their role in acute pancreatitis, gallstones do not appear to be important in the development of chronic pancreatitis; however, this may merely be a reflection of the fact that symptomatic gallstones are usually treated with cholecystectomy before chronic pancreatitis develops. Almost all patients with cystic fibrosis develop established chronic pancreatitis due to blockage of the duct system with thick secretions.

Chronic pancreatitis presents with persistent abdominal pain and weight loss

Patients usually come to medical attention because of persistent abdominal pain and weight loss. Eventually development of malabsorption occurs due to lack of digestive enzymes. Steatorrhoea is typical of malabsorption due to pancreatic insufficiency. The onset of diabetes mellitus due to lack of insulin occurs late in the disease history as islet cells seem to be lost more slowly than the exocrine glands.

Chronic pancreatitis may closely mimic a pancreatic carcinoma

One of the main problems of chronic pancreatitis is distinguishing it from carcinoma of the pancreas. Both can present with very similar symptoms, and sometimes the features on imaging can be very similar. Even at laparotomy, a pancreas affected by chronic pancreatitis may feel like a carcinoma because the dense scarring makes it very hard and firm. In equivocal cases, biopsy may be required.

Avoiding alcohol is the most beneficial course of action in chronic pancreatitis

Management of chronic pancreatitis is supportive, with appropriate pain relief. The most important action is avoidance of alcohol, which halts progression of the disease and alleviates the pain. Despite these clear benefits, many patients are unable to stop drinking alcohol.

Key points: Chronic pancreatitis

- Chronic pancreatitis is characterized by ongoing inflammation in the pancreas, leading to scarring and destruction of the gland.

- The most common cause of chronic pancreatitis is alcohol.

- Patients present with persistent abdominal pain and weight loss. Features of malabsorption do not occur until large areas of the pancreas have been lost.

- The diagnosis can usually be made on imaging of the pancreas, but sometimes chronic pancreatitis can closely mimic carcinoma of the pancreas, necessitating biopsy to distinguish the two diseases.

- Chronic pancreatitis is managed with pain relief and avoidance of alcohol.

Carcinoma of the pancreas

Almost all pancreatic carcinomas are adenocarcinomas

Almost all carcinomas of the pancreas are adenocarcinomas derived from the glandular epithelial cells

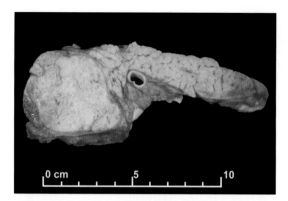

Fig. 9.15 Carcinoma of the head of the pancreas. The head of this pancreas is replaced by a large white tumour. Microscopically this was shown to be an adenocarcinoma.

lining the pancreatic ducts. Most cases are seen in elderly males. Very little is known about the cause of pancreatic cancer, with smoking being the only well recognized risk factor.

Most pancreatic carcinomas arise in the head of the pancreas

Most adenocarcinomas involve the head of the pancreas (Fig. 9.15). In this location, they tend to present early because the mass compresses the common bile duct as it passes through the head of the pancreas, leading to obstructive jaundice.

Adenocarcinomas of the body and tail present later, usually with persistent upper abdominal pain due to extensive local infiltration by tumour. Weight loss is very common in carcinoma of the pancreas and can be very severe and rapid.

Virtually all patients diagnosed with pancreatic carcinoma die within a few years

The majority of patients with pancreatic carcinoma have advanced disease at the time of diagnosis, and treatment is palliative. If there is obstructive jaundice, this should be relieved by placing a metal stent in the common bile duct. The prognosis is very poor.

The only possible cure for carcinoma of the pancreas is surgical resection of the tumour, but this can only be attempted if the tumour appears to be confined to the pancreas. Only a very small minority of patients have an operable tumour, and even those that appear to have organ confined disease at the time of surgery often suffer recurrence at some point after surgery.

> ## Key points: Carcinoma of the pancreas
>
> ◆ Most carcinomas of the pancreas are adenocarcinomas derived from the glandular epithelium lining the pancreatic ducts.
>
> ◆ The head of the pancreas is the most common location for carcinomas, but they may also arise in the body and tail.
>
> ◆ Carcinomas of the head of the pancreas present early with obstructive jaundice.
>
> ◆ Carcinomas in the body and tail present later with persistent pain.
>
> ◆ Severe weight loss is common in patients with carcinoma of the pancreas.
>
> ◆ The only hope for cure is surgical resection of the tumour, but this can only be attempted in the small number of patients who have disease limited to the pancreas at presentation.
>
> ◆ Most patients have advanced disease at diagnosis and die within a few years.

Renal disease

Introduction

The main function of the kidneys is the production of urine, allowing the excretion of waste products, maintenance of extracellular fluid volume, and control of acid balance. In addition, the kidneys have an endocrine function, producing the hormones **renin**, **erythropoietin**, and **calcitriol** (the hormonally active form of vitamin D). With so many diverse roles, it is not surprising that diseases of the kidneys can give rise to many different problems.

The basic functional unit of the kidney is the **nephron**, of which there are approximately 1 million per kidney. Each nephron consists of a **glomerulus** connected to a complex **tubule system**. The glomeruli filter plasma under pressure (ultrafiltration), and the tubules process the filtrate as it flows along the tubular system to form urine. Urine formed by nephrons then drains into **collecting ducts** which open onto the surface of the **renal papillae** projecting into the **calyces** (Fig. 10.1).

The best way to consider kidney disease is to divide the organ into its main structural components, each of which is affected by different types of disease processes:

- **Blood vessels**. The renal blood vessels are affected by the common diseases of arteries, particularly atherosclerosis and hypertension.
- **Glomeruli**. Glomeruli are prone to *structural* conditions that disrupt the delicate filtration system.
- **Tubules**. Processing of the filtrate requires large amounts of energy, making the tubules the most metabolically active part of the nephron. The tubules are therefore particularly sensitive to the effects of *ischaemia*, *toxins*, and *metabolic disorders*.

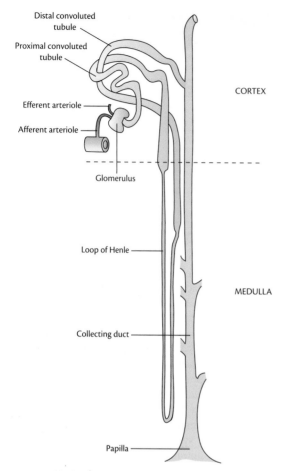

Distal convoluted
tubule

Proximal convoluted
tubule

CORTEX

Efferent arteriole

Afferent arteriole

Glomerulus

Loop of Henle

MEDULLA

Collecting duct

Papilla

Fig. 10.1 Nephron structure.

- **Interstitium**. The interstitium is the tissue that surrounds the nephrons in which the blood vessels of the kidney are embedded. Any molecule transiting between the tubules and the blood must therefore pass through the interstitium. Diseases affecting the interstitium, which are most often due to *drug toxicity*, can therefore have a profound effect on the function of the nephrons.

- **The outflow tract**. This includes the renal papillae, the calyces, and the renal pelvis. *Infections* ascending from the lower urinary tract are important, as are the effects of *obstruction* in the urinary tract.

Although this approach is a convenient way of dividing up renal diseases, it is important to appreciate

that each of these components is functionally linked together, such that a disease affecting one component will eventually damage other areas too. For example, scarring of a glomerulus due to a glomerular disease leads to loss of the associated tubular system of that nephron.

Measuring renal function

Measuring renal function is important in the diagnosis and monitoring of renal disease. The most commonly used tests of renal function are those that assess glomerular function.

Plasma creatinine concentration is a simple reliable test of glomerular function

Creatinine is a substance derived largely from turnover of creatine phosphate in muscle. Creatine phosphate is used as a storage form of high energy phosphate, such that when energy demand is high (e.g. during exercise) creatine phosphate donates its phosphate to ADP to yield ATP, generating creatinine. The amount of creatinine produced is related to muscle mass and remains remarkably constant from day to day.

Creatinine is a useful estimate of glomerular function because it is freely filtered by the glomerulus but not significantly reabsorbed by the tubules back into the blood. The main drawback with the use of plasma creatinine as an assessment of glomerular function is that the glomerular filtration rate (GFR) needs to decrease by as much as 50 per cent before the plasma creatinine level begins to rise above the normal range. Plasma creatinine is therefore not a sensitive indicator of mild to moderate renal impairment. *A normal plasma creatinine therefore does not necessarily imply normal renal function, but a raised creatinine concentration is usually indicative of impaired renal function.*

Urea is not as accurate as creatinine for assessing glomerular function

Plasma urea concentration is also often measured along with creatinine as an indicator of renal function, but it is not as accurate as creatinine. The main problem is that urea is filtered at the glomerulus but significant tubular reabsorption occurs through passive diffusion. When urinary flow rate is low, for instance in fluid-depleted patients, tubular reabsorption of urea increases, which raises the plasma urea concentration. *Plasma urea concentration may therefore be raised in the presence of normal renal function, particularly in fluid-depleted patients.*

Renal failure

Renal failure is a clinical syndrome which develops when there is widespread loss of kidney function. Renal failure may complicate virtually any renal disease if the disease is severe enough. Very often the onset of renal failure is the presenting feature of a patient with an underlying renal disease. Renal failure may be acute or chronic depending on whether the loss of renal function occurs suddenly (hours to days) or over a longer period of time (months to years).

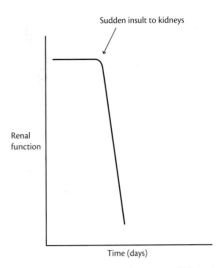

Fig. 10.2 Graphical representation of acute renal failure. In acute renal failure, a massive insult to previous healthy kidneys causes them suddenly to fail. If acute renal failure is due to hypoperfusion alone and circulating volume is restored before intrinsic kidney damage occurs, then renal function may rapidly return to normal. If, however, intrinsic renal damage occurs (e.g. acute tubular necrosis), then renal failure will be prolonged and the patient will need support until regeneration occurs.

JARGON BUSTER

Uraemia and azotaemia

The term **uraemia**, which literally means 'urine in the blood', is often used synonymously for renal failure. The term **azotaemia**, which refers to an increase in nitrogenous compounds in the blood, is also sometimes used in a similar context.

Acute renal failure

Acute renal failure occurs when the kidneys suddenly stop working

Acute renal failure occurs when both kidneys suddenly stop working (Fig. 10.2). Often acute renal failure develops as a complication in a patient who is already very unwell in hospital, or the patient may present in acute renal failure.

The onset of acute renal failure is usually heralded by **oliguria** (passing small volumes of urine), and the diagnosis is confirmed when blood tests reveal high concentrations of urea and creatinine. Biochemical testing also reveals a metabolic acidosis due to an inability to excrete hydrogen ions, and hyperkalaemia due to impaired excretion of potassium ions.

Hyperkalaemia is a potentially lethal feature of acute renal failure

Hyperkalaemia (a plasma potassium ion concentration >6 mmol/l) is the most pressing problem in acute renal failure. Hyperkalaemia reduces the threshold for initiation of action potentials and disturbs the normal electrical conducting system of the heart. Cardiac arrest due to a lethal arrhythmia may be the first and only sign of hyperkalaemia.

The causes of acute renal failure are best divided into pre-renal, renal, and post-renal

There are many causes of acute renal failure. To help make the list more manageable, the causes are often broken down into *pre-renal*, *renal*, and *post-renal* causes depending on the site of the problem (Table 10.1). By far the most common causes of acute renal failure are **hypoperfusion** and **acute tubular necrosis**.

Pre-renal failure refers to acute renal failure due to hypoperfusion alone

The term pre-renal failure is used when acute renal failure is *entirely attributable to hypoperfusion of the kidneys*. Acute renal failure is therefore a risk in any patient with shock (p. 68). In pre-renal failure, renal failure occurs simply because there is insufficient blood supply to the kidneys to produce enough urine to clear waste products. The kidneys themselves are not intrinsically

TABLE 10.1 Common causes of acute renal failure
Pre-renal
Hypoperfusion
Renal
Acute glomerular injury
Acute tubular necrosis
Acute interstitial nephritis
Hypertensive emergency
Post-renal
Bilateral obstruction

damaged, so prompt restoration of renal perfusion leads to rapid normalization of plasma urea and creatinine levels.

Acute tubular necrosis is the most common cause of 'renal' acute renal failure

'Renal' acute renal failure is the result of massive damage to one of the intrinsic component of the kidneys. The most common cause is acute tubular necrosis, i.e. widespread destruction of tubular epithelial cells. We discuss this in more detail later in the chapter. Briefly, the most common cause of acute tubular necrosis is ischaemia due to prolonged renal hypoperfusion. Thus 'pre-renal' renal failure and 'renal' renal failure due to ischaemic acute tubular necrosis are in reality part of the same spectrum of disease: prolonged hypoperfusion, initially causing pre-renal failure, will eventually lead to ischaemic acute tubular necrosis and full-blown 'renal' renal failure. Once acute tubular necrosis has occurred, restoration of renal perfusion will not normalize urea and creatinine levels, and the patient will need to be supported until the tubules regenerate.

Excluding a post-renal cause of acute renal failure is important

One of the benefits of using the pre-renal, renal, post-renal classification for acute renal failure is that it serves as a useful reminder to consider the possibility of a post-renal cause. Ruling out obstruction in the renal tract is a vital part of the early investigations in a patient with acute renal failure. Relief of an obstruction is usually a simple intervention, and if done early can have a considerable impact on survival.

Key points: Acute renal failure

♦ Acute renal failure occurs when kidney function abruptly ceases.

♦ The diagnosis is usually made when a patient develops oliguria and blood tests reveal a high plasma urea and creatinine.

♦ Hyperkalaemia is a potentially life-threatening feature of acute renal failure which must be treated as an immediate priority.

♦ The causes of acute renal failure can be divided into pre-renal, renal, and post-renal. The most common causes are hypoperfusion and acute tubular necrosis.

♦ Pre-renal acute renal failure can be rapidly reversed if circulating volume is restored.

♦ Patients with established acute renal failure require supportive treatment while the underlying cause is being treated.

♦ The possibility of post-renal failure should always be ruled out in a patient with acute renal failure as relieving an obstruction may promptly reverse the renal impairment.

Chronic renal failure

Chronic renal failure is a gradual and progressive loss of kidney function

Chronic renal failure is characterized by a slowly progressive irreversible decline in renal function as nephrons are insidiously 'picked off' over many years and replaced by scar tissue (Fig. 10.3). An unfortunate problem with chronic renal failure is its inevitable progressive nature. This appears to be because a greater functional burden is borne by fewer nephrons, and compensatory hyperfiltration by remaining healthy nephrons predisposes them to scarring and destruction as well. As a result, the rate of nephron destruction increases, speeding the progression of chronic renal failure. *Chronic renal failure is therefore an ever-increasing burden that patients carry for the rest of their lives.* Although the rate of deterioration can be slowed with treatment, it cannot be stopped nor reversed.

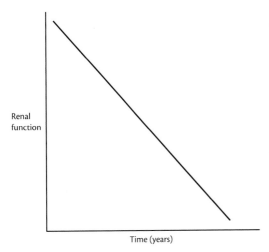

Fig. 10.3 Graphical representation of chronic renal failure. Chronic renal failure is the result of a gradual insidious decline in renal function. No symptoms occur until chronic renal failure is relatively advanced, so the diagnosis will only be picked up if renal function is measured for another reason. Lost nephrons in chronic renal failure can never be recovered.

TABLE 10.3	Severity of chronic renal failure		
Severity	**GFR (ml/min)**	**Creatinine (µmol/l)**	**Clinical manifestations**
Mild	30–50	170	Hypertension
Moderate	10–30	350	Anaemia
Severe	<10	700	Anorexia
End stage	<5	1500	Acidosis, hyperkalaemia, coma, death

Chronic renal failure is caused by slowly progressive kidney diseases

A number of kidney diseases may terminate in chronic renal failure (Table 10.2). All of these entities are explained in further detail throughout the rest of this chapter. For now, two important points should be stressed. First, note that the diseases leading to chronic renal failure are chronic and slowly progressive in nature (contrast this with the causes of acute renal failure which are sudden and catastrophic). Secondly, in a significant proportion of patients with chronic renal failure, no definite underlying cause can be found; there are no clues in the history, and imaging reveals two small shrunken kidneys which, although unsafe to biopsy, would only show non-specific scarring throughout the kidneys.

The severity of chronic renal failure is graded according to the amount of kidney function remaining

The severity of chronic renal failure can be graded according to the GFR and creatinine concentration (Table 10.3). This categorization is useful because it gives an indication of the likely problems to be expected and allows decisions to be made about current and future treatments. **End-stage renal failure** (ESRF) occurs when renal function becomes so poor that death will occur unless renal replacement therapy (e.g. dialysis) is given.

Chronic renal failure is often asymptomatic during its evolution

In the early stages of chronic renal failure, patients may be completely asymptomatic because the remaining healthy nephrons compensate for those that have been lost. Mild to moderate chronic renal failure is therefore often diagnosed incidentally when a routine blood test reveals a raised urea and creatinine, or renal function is measured as part of the work-up of a patient with hypertension. Explaining to these patients, who otherwise feel completely well, that they have a serious disease which will eventually terminate in ESRF can be a very difficult task indeed.

TABLE 10.2	Common causes of chronic renal failure
Chronic glomerulonephritis	
Diabetic nephropathy	
Hypertensive nephropathy	
Ischaemic nephropathy	
Reflux nephropathy	
Obstructive nephropathy	
Autosomal dominant polycystic kidney disease	

Chronic renal disease and hypertension

The development of hypertension occurs early in chronic renal failure and is extremely important for two reasons. First, it accelerates the rate of progression of the chronic renal failure (hypertension itself is a cause of chronic renal failure) and, secondly, it increases the risk of cardiovascular disease which is a big problem in patients with chronic renal failure. Renal function should always be checked as part of the routine investigation of any patient with hypertension. Remember that chronic renal disease is the most common cause of secondary hypertension (p. 73).

By the time symptoms of chronic renal failure occur, most of the renal mass has been destroyed

Because of the lack of symptoms, many patients with mild to moderate chronic renal failure go undiagnosed and do not present until symptoms of chronic renal failure occur. By this time, a considerable amount of renal mass has been irreversibly lost. In fact, over a quarter of all patients with chronic renal failure require dialysis for ESRF within 3 months of first being diagnosed.

Often the first symptom to be noticed is **nocturia** as renal concentrating ability becomes impaired. Nocturia in old men is very often due to benign prostatic enlargement, but nocturia in a young man or a woman should be taken very seriously and fully investigated. Non-specific feelings of malaise and tiredness are also very common. With progression, patients become more unwell as uraemia worsens, leading eventually to death if renal replacement therapy is not begun.

There are a number of biochemical consequences of chronic renal failure

As chronic renal failure progresses and renal function gets worse, a number of biochemical changes occur. The typical biochemical features of chronic renal failure are as follows:

* **Raised urea and creatinine**, due to impaired excretion of waste products

* **Hypocalcaemia** and **hyperphosphataemia**. Hypocalcaemia occurs because of the lack of active

calcitriol stimulating calcium absorption from the gut. Hyperphosphataemia occurs due to impaired excretion of phosphate via the kidneys.

* **Anaemia,** due to reduced erythropoietin synthesis.

* **Metabolic acidosis,** due to impaired acid–base balance. Acidosis is usually a late feature of chronic renal failure when the capacity of the kidneys to excrete hydrogen ions becomes inadequate.

Of note, sodium and potassium balance is usually maintained in chronic renal failure until the GFR falls to a very low level. Hyperkalaemia is therefore a late feature of chronic renal failure.

Virtually every organ system is affected by the effects of reduced renal function (Fig. 10.4); the most important

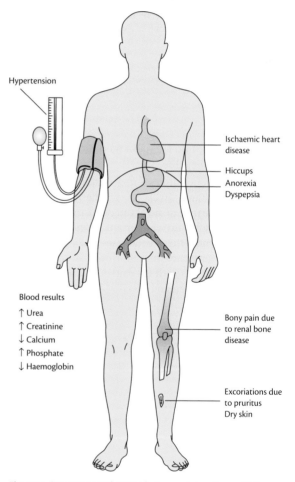

Fig. 10.4 Symptoms and signs of advanced chronic renal failure.

are the cardiovascular, skeletal, and dermatological complications.

Cardiovascular disease is the leading cause of death in patients with chronic renal failure

Cardiovascular disease in chronic renal failure is very common and the leading cause of death in patients with ESRF. Patients with chronic renal failure suffer from markedly accelerated atherosclerosis due to the combined effects of chronic hypertension, hyperlipidaemia, and vascular calcification. Patients are at a much greater risk of heart failure, myocardial infarction, arrhythmias, and sudden death.

Skeletal disorders in patients with chronic renal failure are called renal osteodystrophy

A variety of bone disorders may be seen in chronic renal failure. These are often grouped together under the general heading **renal osteodystrophy**. The most common bony problem is **hyperparathyroid bone disease** caused by secondary hyperparathyroidism as a result of loss of the normal negative feedback exerted on parathyroid hormone secretion by calcitriol. The parathyroid glands undergo hyperplasia and secrete large quantities of parathyroid hormone, leading to hyperparathyroidism.

Hyperparathyroid bone disease reflects a combination of osteoclastic bone resorption and fibrosis of the bone marrow and can be easily identified radiologically long before symptoms develop. A characteristic feature is subperiosteal bone resorption on the radial side of the middle phalanges of the index and middle fingers seen on hand radiographs. The main symptom of hyperparathyroid bony disease is bone pain, though this does not usually occur until ESRF is reached and the patient has started dialysis.

The mainstay of treatment of secondary hyperparathyroidism is dietary restriction of phosphate, oral calcium supplements, and oral calcitriol. There is now an increasing vogue to start treatment as soon as parathyroid hormone levels persistently rise above twice the upper limit of normal, even in the absence of radiological evidence of hyperparathyroid bone disease. Early treatment appears to be better at controlling parathyroid hyperplasia and keeping parathyroid hormone levels down. Patients with markedly raised parathyroid hormone levels with marked enlargement of the parathyroid glands despite medical treatment often require surgical reduction of the parathyroid glands.

Osteomalacia may also develop as part of renal osteodystrophy. Osteomalacia is characterized by poor mineralization of bone (p. 405) and in chronic renal failure is due to a combination of low calcitriol, low calcium, and a metabolic acidosis which promotes demineralization of bone. The main manifestation of osteomalacia is pain and deformity of long bones.

LINK BOX

Hyperparathyroidism

The hyperparathyroidism in chronic renal failure is known as secondary hyperparathyroidism because the parathyroid glands are responding appropriately to the low calcium and high phosphate. Contrast this with **primary hyperparathyroidism**, where the problem lies within the parathyroid glands which *inappropriately* secrete large quantities of parathyroid hormone (p. 321).

Dryness of the skin and pruritus are common problems in chronic renal failure

Dryness of the skin is the most common cutaneous abnormality in chronic renal failure. The pathogenesis is not known, but may be related to an impairment of sweat gland function. Chronic renal failure is also a common cause of persistent pruritus. The pruritus tends to get worse with increasing severity of chronic renal failure and in many instances persists even after dialysis is started. Again, the cause is not clear but does seem to be independent of the effects of dry skin.

Management of chronic renal failure is supportive

Unfortunately there is no cure for chronic renal failure. Management therefore aims to slow the progression of the disease, treat any symptoms related to the effects of chronic renal failure, and prepare in advance for eventual renal replacement therapy.

One of the most important management strategies in chronic renal failure is controlling hypertension. Hypertension is a big problem in patients with chronic renal failure for two reasons: first, the hypertension itself increases the rate of progression of the disease (remember hypertension itself is a cause of chronic renal failure) and, secondly, hypertension is a risk factor for cardiovascular disease which as we have seen is a major killer in patients with chronic renal failure. Hypertension should therefore be aggressively treated in patients with chronic renal failure.

Key points: Chronic renal failure

- Chronic renal failure is characterized by a gradual and irreversible loss of kidney function.

- The most common causes of chronic renal failure are a chronic glomerulonephritis, diabetic nephropathy, hypertension, and ischaemic nephropathy.

- Chronic renal failure is usually asymptomatic in its early stages and is therefore only diagnosed if a blood test is performed for another reason, or if hypertension is investigated.

- By the time symptoms of chronic renal failure occur, most of the renal mass has been irreversibly lost.

- Chronic renal failure has a number of consequences on most of the organ systems of the body.

- The most important effects are related to the cardiovascular system. Patients with chronic renal failure are at much greater risk of ischaemic heart disease, and this is a common cause of death.

- The most common skeletal disorder in chronic renal failure is hyperparathyroid bone disease due to secondary hyperparathyroidism. Even though symptoms of bone pain do not occur until end-stage renal failure is reached, early treatment is advised as it is much easier to control hyperparathyroidism if parathyroid hyperplasia is controlled from early on.

- There is no cure for chronic renal failure. Management aims to slow the progression of the disease and control any symptoms. Aggressively treating hypertension is particularly important.

Vascular disease of the kidney

We have already seen how a global reduction in blood supply to the kidneys is a common cause of acute renal failure. Here we turn our attention to specific diseases of blood vessels that can affect the kidneys, of which the most important are the two familiar enemies of blood vessels: hypertension and atherosclerosis.

Hypertension

Hypertension is a common cause of chronic renal failure

Long-standing hypertension, of any cause, has important structural effects on blood vessels. The walls of small muscular arteries and arterioles become thickened, narrowing the lumen of the vessels and reducing the flow of blood through them. Chronic and progressive reduction in blood flow to the kidneys causes chronic ischaemia, leading to the irreversible loss of nephrons slowly over many years. When sufficient numbers of nephrons have been lost in both kidneys, the patient develops chronic renal failure, an important complication of hypertension.

Atherosclerotic renovascular disease

Atherosclerosis affecting the main renal arteries is known as atherosclerotic renovascular disease

Atherosclerosis commonly affects the abdominal portion of the aorta and may co-involve the origins of the renal arteries. Narrowing of one or both renal arteries by atherosclerosis is known as **atherosclerotic renovascular disease** (ARVD). Patients with evidence of other atherosclerotic diseases such as peripheral vascular disease, coronary artery disease, or aortic aneurysm are also at high risk of atherosclerotic renovascular disease. Many patients have asymptomatic disease that may be detected incidentally during investigation for other atherosclerotic diseases. ARVD is associated with two common clinical problems: hypertension and chronic renal failure.

ARVD is a common cause of secondary hypertension

Hypertension may occur with unilateral or bilateral ARVD, although the mechanisms causing hypertension are slightly different. In patients with unilateral renal artery stenosis, the mechanism of the hypertension is renin mediated, i.e. underperfusion of one kidney stimulates release of renin and the production of angiotensin II which increases blood pressure by causing vasoconstriction. Secondary hypertension in patients with bilateral renal artery stenosis is largely due to volume overload as a result of high levels of aldosterone stimulating sodium and water retention by both kidneys.

ARVD is increasingly recognized as a common cause of chronic renal failure

Extensive ARVD is a common cause of chronic renal failure. The cause of the renal impairment is mostly due to ischaemic injury related to the narrowed renal arteries (**ischaemic nephropathy**), though damage from secondary hypertension is also contributory.

Ischaemic nephropathy is being increasingly recognized as a common cause of chronic renal failure in older individuals; it is now thought to be the cause of chronic renal failure in up to a quarter of patients aged over 60 requiring dialysis. In fact, it seems likely that many patients diagnosed with hypertensive chronic renal failure actually have ischaemic nephropathy, a theory supported by the increase in ESRF attributed to renal vascular disease despite improved control of blood pressure in the population.

INTERESTING TO KNOW

Fibromuscular dysplasia

A small proportion of patients with renal artery stenosis do not have atherosclerosis. Instead they have a condition called **fibromuscular dysplasia**, a disease characterized by structural abnormalities in medium sized arteries leading to areas of narrowing. The condition usually affects the renal arteries, causing renal artery stenosis, and comes to light when a young person is found to be hypertensive.

Although uncommon, fibromuscular dysplasia is important to be aware of as it is one of the rare situations where treatment (stenting the artery) can completely cure hypertension and avoid lifelong antihypertensive drugs. Fibromuscular dysplasia can involve other similar sized arteries, such as the internal carotid artery, where it can cause stroke in a young person.

There are many controversial areas in ARVD

There remains a lot of controversy surrounding the management of ARVD. If a hypertensive patient is found to have anatomical renal artery stenosis, this does not necessarily prove that the hypertension is due to the renal artery stenosis, as the patient may have primary hypertension leading to accelerated atherosclerosis involving the renal arteries coincidentally. Furthermore, treating the stenosis by angioplasty or stenting may improve blood pressure control, but rarely cures the hypertension. There are currently ongoing trials to assess the benefits of revascularization in patients with ARVD.

Glomerular disease

The glomerular diseases commonly top polls of diseases most difficult to understand in medicine! Much of this is related to the terminology, which is complicated and often confusing. Many books fall into the trap of launching into detailed explanations of individual entities with little in the way of a general introduction first. This is unfortunate, as certain conceptual hurdles must first be overcome before one really has a hope of understanding the individual glomerular diseases.

Glomerular diseases are those where the glomeruli are the predominant site of injury

Glomerular diseases are a diverse group of conditions characterized by injury to glomeruli. Each glomerulus consists of a complex knot of capillaries (the '**capillary tuft**') which projects into the urinary space of the Bowman's capsule. The capillary tuft is supported by a scaffold known as the **mesangium** which comprises mesangial cells embedded in loose connective tissue known as the mesangial matrix (Fig. 10.5).

The glomeruli are the site of ultrafiltration

The role of the glomeruli is to filter the plasma under pressure, a process known as ultrafiltration. Ultrafiltration occurs across the **filtration barrier** which is composed of three layers (Fig. 10.6):

◆ The endothelial cell lining of the glomerular tuft capillaries

◆ The basement membrane of the capillaries

◆ The foot processes of podocytes (the epithelial cells lining the urinary space).

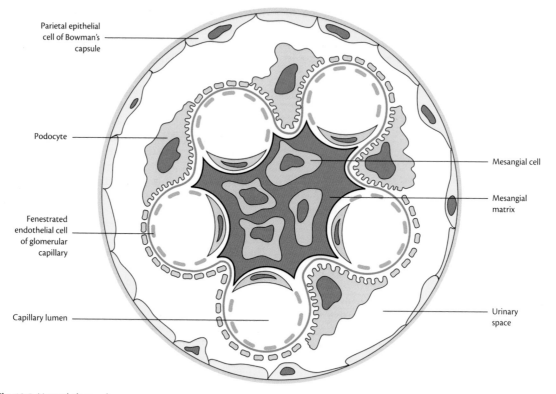

Fig. 10.5 Normal glomerulus.

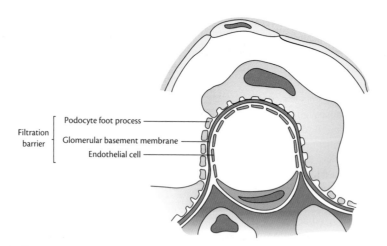

Fig. 10.6 The glomerular filtration barrier. There are three elements to the glomerular filter: the fenestrated endothelium of the capillary loops, the thin glomerular basement membrane, and the foot processes of the podocytes which line the urinary space.

Correct functioning of the glomerulus is reliant on the integrity of this complex filtration system. Glomerular diseases are therefore often the result of conditions which lead to structural damage to the filtration barrier.

Glomerular damage is usually caused by the deposition of material in the glomerulus

Most glomerular diseases are caused by the deposition of material within the filtration barrier, disrupting the function of the filtration system. In most cases, the material is derived from constituents of the immune system, particularly immune complexes (antibodies which have bound to their corresponding antigen). The immune complexes usually form at a site distant from the kidneys but circulate in the blood to the kidneys where they become lodged in the glomeruli. The glomeruli are therefore innocent bystanders damaged by circulating immune complexes formed at a distant site.

Very often the source of these immune complexes cannot be determined, in which case the glomerulopathy is termed 'primary'. It is essential to consider and exclude a systemic disorder as the underlying cause in all cases of glomerulopathy. Common disorders associated with glomerular disease include underlying malignancy, systemic lupus erythematosus, and persistent infections such as endocarditis, hepatitis B, or hepatitis C.

There are also some important glomerular diseases which are caused by deposition of non-immune material in the glomerulus. Two important such examples are **diabetes mellitus** and **amyloidosis**.

JARGON BUSTER

Glomerulonephritis

The term **glomerulonephritis** is often used to refer to a glomerular disease which is immune mediated. Strictly the term means 'inflammation in the glomerulus' and in fact many glomerulonephritides do not actually have an associated inflammatory cell infiltrate, but nevertheless are immune mediated.

Direct immune attack of components of the glomerulus may also lead to glomerular damage

The other main cause of glomerular damage is a specific immune attack targeted directly against the glomerulus.

Two well recognized examples of this are a **small vessel vasculitis** attacking the endothelial cells of the capillary tuft, and the condition **antiglomerular basement membrane disease** in which there is antibody-mediated attack of the glomerular basement membrane. Both of these problems lead to very severe glomerular injury.

A damaged glomerulus leaks protein and blood

The intact glomerulus is a selective filter which does not allow large protein molecules or red blood cells to pass into the tubular system. A damaged glomerulus, however, leaks protein and erythrocytes into the tubular system. Glomerulopathies are therefore characterized by the presence of haematuria and proteinuria. Although both red blood cells and protein are usually present in the urine, usually one is more florid and will dominate the clinical picture.

The glomerulus responds to damage in three main ways

When glomeruli become injured, there are certain patterns of response that can occur. In a broad sense, these can divided into three main patterns (Fig. 10.7):

◆ A *proliferative response*, characterized by proliferation of the cellular elements of the glomerular tuft, i.e. endothelial and mesangial cells.

◆ A *structural response*, characterized either by thickening of the glomerular basement membrane or by scarring of an area of the glomerulus (glomerulosclerosis).

◆ A *necrotizing response*, characterized by necrosis of the capillary walls of the glomerular tuft. Necrosis tends to signify severe glomerular injury and is often associated with thrombosis within the glomerular capillaries. If the soft necrotic capillary loops rupture, allowing intravascular contents to escape into the Bowman's space, an intense proliferative response occurs within Bowman's space leading to the formation of a cellular structure called a **crescent** which surrounds and destroys the glomerular tuft. Diseases which lead to widespread crescent formation ('diffuse crescentic glomerulonephritis') can disrupt renal function sufficiently to cause acute renal failure. More about these later.

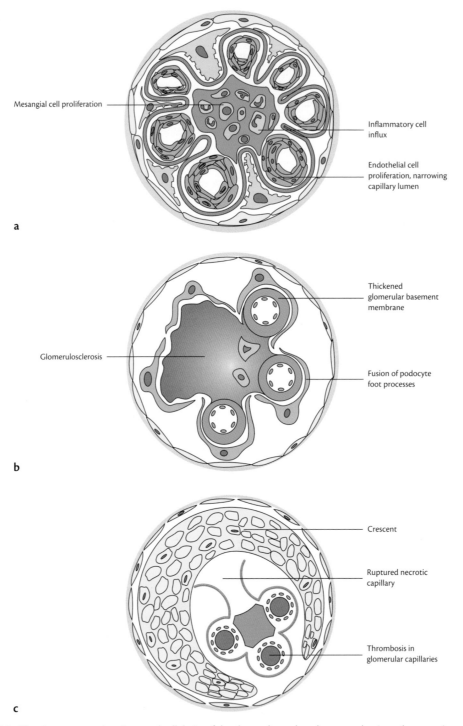

Mesangial cell proliferation

Inflammatory cell influx

Endothelial cell proliferation, narrowing capillary lumen

a

Thickened glomerular basement membrane

Glomerulosclerosis

Fusion of podocyte foot processes

b

Crescent

Ruptured necrotic capillary

Thrombosis in glomerular capillaries

c

Fig. 10.7 (a) Proliferative responses show increased cellularity of the glomerulus and tend to cause dominant haematuria. (b) Structural responses may include thickening of the glomerular basement membrane or glomerular sclerosis. These are associated with podocyte foot process fusion which causes proteinuria. (c) A necrotizing response is associated with glomerular capillary thrombosis and rupture, stimulating the formation of crescents which compress and obliterate the capillary tuft. Widespread crescent formation is associated with the development of acute renal failure.

It is vital at this point to stress some important points

First, one must understand that these three responses are descriptive terms for what is seen when glomeruli are scrutinized under the microscope. Terms such as 'proliferative glomerulonephritis' merely mean that, down the microscope, the glomeruli show proliferative changes. *The term has no clinical meaning and does not imply a specific disease, but may come about as a result of numerous causes.*

Secondly, these patterns are not mutually exclusive. Whilst they may occur individually, they may also occur in various combinations either within the same glomerulus or in different glomeruli. For instance, a severe proliferative glomerulonephritis may result in glomerular necrosis in some glomeruli and the formation of crescents in other glomeruli.

Thirdly, the clinical presentation provides clues to the nature of the response in the glomeruli. Proliferative changes tend to cause a clinical picture dominated by **haematuria** or the **nephritic syndrome**, whereas structural changes give rise to dominant **proteinuria** or the **nephrotic syndrome**. These will all be discussed shortly.

Finally, it should be appreciated that the clinical picture or renal biopsy is diagnostic in only a few select conditions. Making a final diagnosis in a patient with a glomerular disease is therefore an integrated process in which one must analyse all the clinical and biopsy features to arrive at the best overall diagnosis.

Proliferative changes

Proliferative changes cause haematuria or the nephritic syndrome

Depending on how many glomeruli are affected, proliferative glomerulopathies can be described as **diffuse**, where all glomeruli are affected, or **focal**, where only some glomeruli are involved. Focal proliferative glomerulonephritis usually causes varying degrees of haematuria with minor proteinuria and no other symptoms. More florid proliferative changes involving many glomeruli may cause the nephritic syndrome.

The **nephritic syndrome** occurs when there is marked haematuria and proteinuria. The macroscopically visible haematuria may be bright red, but more often (after stagnating in the bladder) it has a brown hue, likened to tea or Coca-Cola. Usually there is associated oliguria, with circulatory overload and hypertension.

IgA nephropathy is a common cause of haematuria

IgA nephropathy is the most common glomerular disease. It is defined by the presence of deposits of IgA in the mesangium, which is usually accompanied by proliferation of mesangial cells ('mesangioproliferative glomerulopathy'). The mechanisms which lead to the deposition of IgA immune complexes in the mesangium remain poorly understood.

The typical presentation is a young male with recurring episodes of macroscopic haematuria, usually occurring within 12–24 h of an otherwise simple bout of pharyngitis. The urine is usually frankly bloody for between 1 and 5 days. Blood pressure remains normal, there is no oedema, and recovery is rapid. In some patients, the diagnosis is made following discovery of microscopic haematuria. In some adults, the disease becomes progressive, leading to nephron destruction and the slow development of chronic renal failure over a period of 15–20 years.

Systemic disorders can also lead to focal proliferative glomerulopathy

A focal proliferative pattern causing haematuria or nephritic syndrome can occur in association with systemic diseases which lead to the production of circulating immune complexes. Common examples include systemic lupus erythematosus and infectious endocarditis.

Diffuse proliferative glomerulonephritis is usually a reaction to a streptococcal pharyngitis

The most common cause of a diffuse proliferative glomerulonephritis is a reaction to a pharyngeal infection with particular 'nephritogenic' strains of streptococci. Not all strains cause this disease. This is often called 'post-streptococcal glomerulonephritis' to indicate its link to the bacterial infection. Immune complexes generated in response to the infection become lodged in the glomeruli and activate complement.

Fixation of complement leads to the recruitment of neutrophils into the glomerulus (i.e. a genuine 'glomerulonephritis'), which degranulate and damage the glomerulus. In response, the endothelial and mesangial cells proliferate. Glomerular capillaries become obliterated by the proliferating endothelial cells, leading to oliguria and circulatory overload.

Treatment is aimed at eradicating the infection and providing symptomatic relief of the consequences of the nephritic syndrome until the episode resolves. It is unusual for dialysis to be required. It usually takes a few weeks for the immune complexes to be cleared from the glomerular basement membrane. With resolution of disease, the proliferating cells are shed and the capillaries become patent again, restoring renal function to normal.

Structural changes

Structural changes cause proteinuria and the nephrotic syndrome

Persistent proteinuria is always considered to be abnormal and indicates some form of intrinsic renal disease. Glomerular disease is by far the most common cause of proteinuria.

The patient with mild to moderate proteinuria will be asymptomatic. The urine looks normal. If there is very heavy protein loss in the urine, a clinical state called the **nephrotic syndrome** arises, characterized by the onset of hypoproteinaemic oedema. The patient develops pitting oedema with facial swelling in the morning and ankle oedema at night. Scrotal oedema in boys and men can be very prominent. *Only a glomerular disorder can cause proteinuria heavy enough to result in the nephrotic syndrome.*

The nephrotic syndrome is usually suspected when a patient presents with peripheral oedema and urine stick testing reveals large amounts of protein in the urine. Confirmation of the diagnosis of nephrotic syndrome requires measurement of albumin to prove hypoproteinaemia, and quantitation of the degree of proteinuria by performing a 24 h urine collection.

Nephrotic patients are at increased risk of infection and thrombosis

A number of complications are recognized in patients with the nephrotic syndrome which result from persistent loss of proteins into the urine. Loss of immunoglobulin and complement components in the urine leads to an increased susceptibility to bacterial infections. A streptococcal cellulitis is common and can spread very quickly. Children are particularly vulnerable to the development of peritonitis due to *Streptococcus pneumoniae*.

Nephrotic patients are also at increased risk of thrombosis, both arterial and venous. Part of this is mediated by loss of natural anticoagulants such as antithrombin III into the urine. Fortunately, mortality from thromboembolism is low in patients with the nephrotic syndrome and it is not standard practice to anticoagulate patients routinely unless an individual is at particular risk.

Almost all cases of heavy proteinuria and nephrotic syndrome are due to one of five possibilities

A large percentage of cases of heavy proteinuria and the nephrotic syndrome are caused by five main types of glomerulopathies:

- Minimal change disease
- Membranous glomerulopathy
- Focal segmental glomerulosclerosis
- Diabetic glomerulosclerosis
- Amyloidosis.

Minimal change disease is a common cause of nephrotic syndrome in childhood

Minimal change disease is a glomerulopathy which causes proteinuria heavy enough to cause the nephrotic syndrome. The glomerulopathy is called minimal change disease because if a renal biopsy is taken, the glomeruli appear normal down the light microscope. Electron microscopy is required to visualize the typical abnormality, which is *fusion of the foot processes of the podocytes*. Although podocyte foot fusion can occur in many glomerular diseases, in the absence of any changes seen with the light microscope, it is highly suggestive of minimal change disease.

Over three-quarters of all children with the nephrotic syndrome have minimal change disease. Minimal change disease has a good prognosis. Although relapses may occur, their frequency diminishes over time and most children with minimal change disease go into complete remission by the time they are 30 years old. The development of chronic renal failure is extremely rare.

Membranous glomerulopathy is characterized by thickening of the glomerular basement membrane in all glomeruli

Membranous glomerulopathy is a common cause of heavy proteinuria and the nephrotic syndrome in adults.

It is associated with a diffuse thickening of the basement membrane caused by widespread deposition of immune complexes within it. The abnormality of the basement membrane renders it unable to filter proteins selectively, leading to heavy proteinuria and the nephrotic syndrome. There are no associated proliferative changes, nor any inflammation.

Most cases of membranous nephropathy have no apparent underlying cause for the deposition of immune complexes (**primary** or **idiopathic membranous glomerulopathy**). In about 10 per cent of cases, a reason for the circulating immune complexes can be found. These are usually as a result of persistent diseases that form immune complexes, such as chronic infections (e.g. hepatitis B) and malignancy.

The routine investigation of all nephrotic patients should include antinuclear antibodies, hepatitis B surface antigen, and antihepatitis C antibodies. Malignancy should always be considered in older patients and common sites investigated, e.g. chest radiography and investigation of the gastrointestinal tract.

Focal segmental glomerulosclerosis has a poor prognosis

As its name suggests, **focal segmental glomerulosclerosis** (FSGS) is characterized by the obliteration of segments of glomerular capillary loops by sclerosis (scarring). FSGS can be an idiopathic primary disease, but may also be seen as a secondary response to other conditions. The aetiology of the primary form is unknown, but it is known to recur in transplanted kidneys, sometimes within days of transplantation. This has led to the hypothesis that a circulating factor may be involved. FSGS has a poor prognosis. Over time, the focal segmental sclerosis becomes global, leading to progressive loss of nephrons and the development of chronic renal failure in about half of all patients.

Diabetes mellitus and amyloidosis can also cause proteinuria and nephrotic syndrome

Diabetes mellitus is a very common cause of proteinuria. The hallmark of diabetic nephropathy is glomerulosclerosis due to deposition of extracellular material in the glomerular basement membrane and mesangium. Diabetic nephropathy is almost always diagnosed when a patient known to have diabetes is found to have proteinuria as part of their regular monitoring.

Amyloidosis is another cause to consider in the differential diagnosis of a patient with proteinuria or the nephrotic syndrome. In this instance, it is deposition of amyloid fibrils in the glomerulus that causes protein leakage. The kidney is the most common and important organ to be affected by amyloidosis.

Necrotizing changes

Necrosis and crescent formation are associated with the development of acute renal failure

The most severe forms of glomerular damage lead to necrosis of the capillary tufts and thrombosis within the vessels. Crescents are structures that form when there is severe necrotizing damage to glomerular capillaries allowing intravascular contents to leak into Bowman's space.

A necrotizing pattern is typically seen in patients with a small vessel vasculitis affecting the glomeruli, e.g. **microscopic polyarteritis** and **Wegener's granulomatosis**, and in the condition antiglomerular basement membrane disease. The severe glomerular injury leads to the rapid onset of renal failure. The clinical picture of acute renal failure plus evidence of severe acute glomerular injury is often called 'rapidly progressive glomerulonephritis'. This is a non-specific clinical term and not a histological pattern or actual disease entity.

Chronic glomerulonephritis

A chronic glomerulonephritis is a common cause of chronic renal failure

Many episodes of glomerulopathy are temporary and reversible conditions, from which the patient fully recovers without lasting renal damage. In some patients, the disease is more persistent and the damage leads to permanent scarring of the glomerulus. Loss of the glomerulus leads to atrophy of the associated tubular system and irreversible loss of whole nephrons.

The term **chronic glomerulonephritis** is used to describe a glomerular disease that becomes persistent and leads to chronic renal failure. *A chronic glomerulonephritis is one of the most common causes of chronic renal failure.* Chronic glomerular disease is typically recognized by the presence of renal insufficiency (raised urea and creatinine) and the presence of chronic proteinuria and/or haematuria on urinalysis.

Key points: Glomerular disease

♦ Glomerular diseases are renal diseases in which the glomeruli are the primary site of injury.

♦ Glomeruli may be damaged by the deposition of material in the delicate filtration system (usually immune material) or by direct immune attack targeted against a component of the glomerulus.

♦ Damaged glomeruli are unable to act as selective filters and leak blood and/or protein into the urine. Haematuria and proteinuria are therefore common manifestations of glomerular disease.

♦ Glomeruli respond to damage in three main ways: a proliferative response, a structural response, and a necrotizing response.

♦ Proliferative changes tend to be associated with dominant haematuria, whereas structural changes tend to cause dominant proteinuria. A necrotizing response is a marker of severe glomerular injury which may cause acute renal failure.

♦ Making a diagnosis in a patient with a glomerular disease involves analysing all the available clinical and biopsy features to arrive at the best diagnosis.

♦ A chronic glomerulonephritis is a common cause of chronic renal failure.

Tubular disease

Acute tubular necrosis

Acute tubular necrosis is the most common cause of acute renal failure

Necrosis of large numbers of tubular epithelial cells leading to acute renal failure is known as **acute tubular necrosis** (ATN). The tubular epithelial cells are very metabolically active, as they are constantly reabsorbing and secreting substances to and from the urine passing through the tubular lumen. The tubules are therefore exquisitely sensitive to metabolic disruption, either through deprivation of blood supply or by toxic molecules. There are two main types of acute tubular necrosis: **ischaemic ATN** and **toxic ATN**.

We have already briefly mentioned ischaemic ATN in the section on acute renal failure. Ischaemic ATN is by far the more common type and is caused by a prolonged reduction in renal perfusion. Acute tubular necrosis may also occur with normal renal perfusion if a substance toxic to tubular epithelial cells passes through the tubules. Such toxins may be certain drugs, poisons such as paraquat, or large quantities of endogenous toxins such as myoglobin or haemoglobin. The development of acute renal failure in patients with massive trauma who appear to have an adequate circulating volume is usually due to the release of large volumes of myoglobin from crushed muscles which is toxic to tubular epithelial cells.

The initial problem in ATN is the direct destruction and loss of tubular epithelial cells, leading to a sudden cessation of renal function. Once this damage has been sustained, persistence of excretory failure is thought to be exacerbated by blockage of distal tubules by the cellular debris. Renal function can be recovered through regeneration of tubular cells, but only if the insult is reversed and the patient is supported during the reparative stages.

LINK BOX

Acute renal failure in malaria

Patients with severe *Plasmodium falciparum* infection may develop acute renal failure because large quantities of haemoglobin released from destroyed erythrocytes enter the tubules and cause toxic acute tubular necrosis (p. 27).

Renal tubular disorders

Renal tubular disorders present with defects of tubular function

Less dramatic conditions affecting tubular function alone are generally uncommon. Single or multiple tubular functions may be affected, with either excessive loss of substances normally reabsorbed by the tubules (e.g. phosphate, glucose, and amino acids), or inadequate excretion of substances normally secreted by the tubules (e.g. hydrogen ions). As a group, they are collectively known as **renal tubular disorders** and may be congenital or acquired.

One of the most common acquired diseases presenting with tubular dysfunction is **nephrocalcinosis**. Nephrocalcinosis refers to the deposition of calcium within the renal tubules and interstitium, and is usually associated with hypercalcaemia. The calcium damages mitochondria and other organelles in the tubular epithelial cells, leading to impaired tubular function.

The earliest functional defect is insensitivity to the actions of antidiuretic hormone (ADH), leading to polyuria. With further damage, a slowly progressive chronic renal failure develops. Often this is contributed to by other complications of hypercalcaemia in the kidneys, e.g. formation of calcium-containing renal stones.

Interstitial disease

Interstitial diseases are characterized by an inflammatory reaction that affects predominantly the interstitial space. It is important to appreciate that the interstitial compartment is commonly secondarily involved by diseases of the kidney which started elsewhere (e.g. glomeruli), but such secondary interstitial inflammation is different from a primary interstitial disease.

Disorders affecting primarily the interstitial compartment of the kidneys are usually caused by reactions to drugs. Unlike glomerular diseases, where the microscopic pattern of change within the glomeruli can provide useful information about the underlying cause, interstitial disease usually presents with a fairly non-specific inflammatory infiltrate within the interstitium, known as interstitial nephritis. The term interstitial nephritis, when used in practice, has a *clinicopathological* definition, meaning that the diagnosis should only be made when a patient fits both clinical and histological criteria.

Acute interstitial nephritis

Acute interstitial nephritis presents with acute renal failure

Acute interstitial nephritis refers to the development of acute renal failure due to a dramatic inflammatory infiltration of the interstitial compartment of the kidneys. Current evidence points towards an immediate (type I) hypersensitivity reaction, and in many cases an offending drug can be identified.

Almost any drug can cause acute interstitial nephritis, but the most common offenders are antibiotics and non-steroidal anti-inflammatory drugs (NSAIDs). Extensive oedema formation in the interstitium leads to stretching of the renal capsule, which often results in tenderness in the flanks. It is important to remember drug-induced acute interstitial nephritis as a possible cause of acute renal failure because withdrawal of the offending drug is usually followed by complete renal recovery.

Chronic interstitial nephritis

Chronic interstitial nephritis is a slower disease which leads to chronic renal failure

The defining feature of **chronic interstitial nephritis** is the presence of *interstitial fibrosis*, which indicates some degree of irreversible renal injury. Chronic interstitial nephritis also appears to be due to an inflammatory response to drugs, but the natural progression of the disease is much slower than acute interstitial nephritis.

The clinical presentation is therefore relatively late in the disease with features of chronic renal failure, picked up either through a routine blood test, or the investigation of hypertension, or with symptoms of chronic renal failure. Although a variety of drugs have been implicated in causing chronic interstitial nephritis, the most important are analgesics and NSAIDs.

Analgesic nephropathy is an example of chronic interstitial nephritis

Analgesic nephropathy is a condition in which chronic interstitial nephritis is caused by prolonged and excessive consumption of analgesics, particularly compound analgesics containing combinations of different agents. After many years of exposure to damaging analgesics, the renal papillae undergo necrosis. In response to the gradual development of papillary necrosis, a chronic interstitial nephritis develops leading to progressive chronic renal failure.

Fortunately, the incidence of analgesic nephropathy has declined following the restriction of over the counter sales of analgesic mixtures.

Key points: Interstitial diseases

◆ Interstitial diseases are those in which damage to the interstitium is the primary site of renal damage.

Continued

Outflow tract disease

The outflow tracts of the kidney are affected predominantly by bacterial infection and by obstruction in the urinary tract. The term **pyelonephritis** is defined as a bacterial infection of the kidney involving the renal parenchyma, calyces, and pelvis.

Pyelonephritis was traditionally divided into acute and chronic forms. Whilst the term acute pyelonephritis remains in common clinical use, the term chronic pyelonephritis has been replaced by the term **reflux nephropathy**.

Acute pyelonephritis

Acute pyelonephritis is usually the result of ascending infection from the lower urinary tract

Lower urinary tract infections are common and are usually caused by Gram negative bacilli from the patient's own endogenous faecal flora, particularly *Escherichia coli*. In most cases, infection remains confined to the bladder. Spread of infection into the upper urinary tract is a rare complication, but can occur in susceptible individuals. Common risk factors for ascending infection into the kidney include obstruction and pregnancy.

The classic clinical presentation of acute pyelonephritis is an abrupt onset of high fever and flank pain, often accompanied by vomiting. These so-called 'upper tract signs' are often accompanied by dysuria, increased urinary frequency, and urgency. The diagnosis of acute pyelonephritis is usually made on the basis of such a clinical picture, and the presence of upper tract infection is presumed.

Most cases of acute pyelonephritis follow an uncomplicated course if treated promptly with suitable antibiotics. The development of severe infection carries a high risk of bacteraemia, sepsis, and death, and is mostly a problem in people with obstruction in the urinary tract and diabetics.

Acute papillary necrosis is a complication of acute pyelonephritis seen mostly in diabetics

Ischaemic necrosis of the renal papillae can occur as a complication of acute pyelonephritis, usually in people with an already tenuous blood supply to their renal papillae. It occurs particularly in diabetic patients with acute pyelonephritis. The development of papillary necrosis is usually suggested by the onset of haematuria, flank pain, and renal colic as the necrotic papillae crumble and pass through the urinary tract.

Treatment usually involves intense fluid hydration and antibiotic treatment. If papillary necrosis is extensive and bilateral, it can present as a devastating fulminant condition leading to acute renal failure. Thankfully this is rare.

Reflux nephropathy

Reflux nephropathy has replaced the term chronic pyelonephritis

Historically the term chronic pyelonephritis was used to refer to a scarred kidney with chronic inflammation involving the renal parenchyma, calyces, and pelvis. This distinguished the condition from cases of chronic glomerulonephritis where the glomeruli were the primary site of damage. The underlying problem of chronic pyelonephritis was presumed to be bacterial infections, but very often it was impossible to prove recent or remote episodes of infection.

It soon became recognized that almost all cases of chronic pyelonephritis were associated with evidence of retrograde reflux of urine from the bladder into the ureters (**vesicoureteric reflux**) and that the renal damage was due to reflux of urine into the kidneys causing scarring. The term reflux nephropathy was therefore introduced to reflect the underlying cause of the renal scarring.

Reflux nephropathy is renal scarring that occurs in association with severe vesicoureteric reflux

The normal vesicoureteric junction acts as a one-way valve, such that the ureter is shut off when the bladder contracts, preventing reflux of urine back up the ureter. In some infants and children, this valve mechanism does not work properly, such that contraction of the bladder causes a jet of urine to reflux back up into the ureter. Vesicoureteric reflux is almost always a problem one is born with, and there is a strong tendency for it to run in families. In most cases, it causes no problems or minimal problems. The main concern with vesicoureteric reflux is that in a small number of cases it can lead to progressive damage to the kidneys (reflux nephropathy).

If reflux is sufficiently severe, retrograde flow of urine into the kidneys incites an inflammatory response which heals with scarring. Whether or not scarring is induced by sterile urine, or whether infection is mandatory remains disputed and uncertain. Certainly the presence of infection is likely to worsen any inflammation or scarring.

Reflux nephropathy may be picked up due to hypertension or chronic renal failure

Reflux nephropathy is usually a unilateral condition which may only come to attention if the scarring is sufficient to cause secondary hypertension and the diagnosis is picked up on investigation of the kidneys for hypertension. The serum urea and creatinine are usually within the normal range as the reduced function of the affected kidney is masked by compensation by the opposite kidney.

Bilateral reflux nephropathy may also come to clinical attention because of hypertension, but may also present due to chronic renal failure (Fig. 10.8). Reflux nephropathy is an important cause of chronic renal

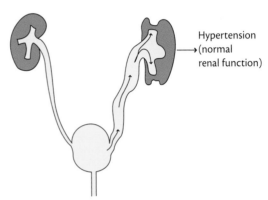

UNILATERAL REFLUX NEPHROPATHY

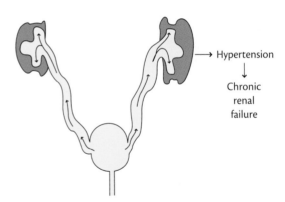

BILATERAL REFLUX NEPHROPATHY

Fig. 10.8 Reflux nephropathy. Unilateral reflux nephropathy typically presents with hypertension. Provided the other kidney is normal and compensates, renal function remains normal. Bilateral reflux nephropathy initially causes hypertension but eventually leads to chronic renal failure. This is one of the most common causes of chronic renal failure in children and young adults.

failure, especially in children and young adults. Overall it accounts for about 15 per cent of people reaching ESRF.

Reflux nephropathy does not appear ever to begin during adult life

Reflux of urine into the kidneys only causes permanent scarring during early childhood. The kidney appears to become much less vulnerable to permanent damage with increasing age. After about age 4, the development of new scars is uncommon and it is unlikely that reflux nephropathy ever starts in adult life. Reports of reflux nephropathy developing in adults almost certainly reflect misinterpretation of the radiological features of an alternative cause of renal impairment such as papillary necrosis or obstructive nephropathy for reflux nephropathy.

Key points: Reflux nephropathy

+ Reflux nephropathy is now the preferred term for what was once called chronic pyelonephritis.

+ Reflux nephropathy refers to the presence of renal scarring as a result of persistent vesicoureteric reflux.

+ Only a minority of children with vesicoureteric reflux develop renal scarring, which occurs because the presence of refluxed urine in the kidney incites an inflammatory response which heals with scarring, leading to permanent damage.

+ It remains unclear whether sterile urine can initiate renal inflammation and scarring, or if infection must be present as well.

+ Reflux nephropathy is a common cause of hypertension in children and a leading cause of chronic renal failure in children and young adults.

Obstructive nephropathy

Obstruction in the urinary tract may also lead to renal damage

Obstruction in the urinary tract is dealt with in more detail in Chapter 11. The main concern with urinary tract obstruction is the development of renal damage.

Renal damage due to the effects of obstruction is known as **obstructive nephropathy**. If obstruction affects both kidneys, or a solitary kidney, then renal impairment will occur.

The importance of obstructive nephropathy is that the decline in renal function can be halted or even reversed if obstruction is relieved, so obstruction must be excluded early in the course of investigation of all patients with unexplained renal failure, whether acute or chronic.

Obstructive nephropathy is a major cause of chronic renal failure in children, as a result of congenital anomalies of the urinary tract. The condition declines in adults until the age of 60, when the incidence rises, particularly in men because of benign nodular hyperplasia of the prostate.

Autosomal dominant polycystic kidney disease

Autosomal dominant polycystic kidney disease is an inherited cause of chronic renal failure

Autosomal dominant polycystic kidney disease (ADPKD) is an inherited disease which results in replacement of both kidneys with multiple fluid-filled cysts (Fig. 10.9). Progressive enlargement of the renal cysts destroys the renal parenchyma, leading to renal failure. Half of all patients with the disease eventually develop ESRF.

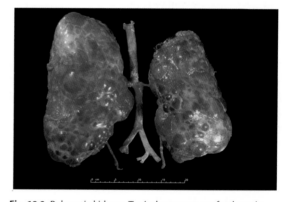

Fig. 10.9 Polycystic kidneys. Typical appearance of polycystic kidney disease with bilateral replacement of the kidneys with numerous fluid-filled cysts.

Most cases of ADPKD are caused by mutations in the PKD1 gene

The PKD1 (polycystic kidney disease 1) gene is very large and codes for a membrane protein called polycystin-1 which appears to be involved in cell–cell and cell–matrix interactions. Defects in the function of the protein lead to cystic change in the renal tubules and loss of normal renal tissue. Although the mutation is carried by all nephrons, only a small percentage become cystic. This is probably because two 'hits' are needed to produce cysts, the first hit is the inherited PKD1 mutation, and then some nephrons acquire a second somatic hit during life which inactivates the remaining normal allele, leading to cyst formation.

Most patients with ADPKD do not develop manifestations of the disease until middle age

Hypertension is a common manifestation of ADPKD which occurs early, usually before there is any biochemical evidence of renal impairment. Very often the diagnosis is made following investigation for hypertension. Current opinion is that the hypertension is due to release of renin in response to ischaemia brought about by compression and distortion of renal blood vessels by the growing cysts.

Flank pain is also a common presenting symptom of ADPKD. Persistent chronic pain is probably related to compression of surrounding tissues and stretching of the renal capsule by the cysts. Generally speaking, the severity of the pain correlates with the size of the kidneys. Sudden acute pain may occur and is usually due to bleeding into a cyst from the richly vascularized cyst wall.

Some patients do not present until they have symptoms of severe chronic renal failure.

Care must be taken when diagnosing ADPKD

The sensitivity of diagnosing ADPKD using ultrasound scanning is poor in those aged under 20 as the cysts may be too small to be detected. The specificity, however, is good because solitary cysts in the kidneys are extremely rare in those under 20, especially if bilateral. In contrast, renal cysts (even if bilateral) are relatively common in patients aged over 50, so strict criteria are needed before making the diagnosis in older patients.

ADPKD patients often have abnormalities in other organs too

Although the major consequences of PKD1 mutations are seen in the kidneys, ADPKD is a systemic disorder, and anomalies in other organs are well recognized. Over half of all patients also have liver cysts which develop from biliary epithelium. Liver cysts are usually asymptomatic and do not cause an impairment of liver function. Berry aneurysms can arise in intracranial arteries. Subarachnoid haemorrhage resulting from rupture of a berry aneurysm is a serious complication of ADPKD and is a common cause of sudden death.

Key points: Autosomal dominant polycystic kidney disease

- ADPKD is by far the most frequent inherited kidney disease, with a prevalence of up to 1 in 400.

- ADPKD is characterized by the development of multiple cysts in both kidneys which terminates in end-stage renal failure by the age of 60.

- ADPKD accounts for up to 10 per cent of patients requiring dialysis for end-stage renal failure.

- Most cases of ADPKD are due to mutations in the gene PKD1 which codes for a large protein called polycystin-1.

- Common manifestations of ADPKD are hypertension, flank pain, and gross haematuria.

- ADPKD is also associated with extrarenal manifestations including cysts in the liver and berry aneurysms in the brain.

Urological disease

Introduction

Urology deals with diseases of the urinary tract and male genital system. The urinary tract is often divided into the **upper urinary tract** comprising the kidneys and ureters, and the **lower urinary tract** which includes the bladder and urethra. The male genital tract includes the penis, scrotum, testes, and prostate (Fig. 11.1).

Three broad problems account for the majority of a urologist's workload: obstruction in the urinary tract, tumours of the genitourinary tract, and infections of the urinary tract. As we shall see, these three problems are often inter-related. For instance, a tumour may obstruct the urinary tract, and obstruction in the urinary tract increases the risk of developing infection.

Urinary tract obstruction

Urinary tract obstruction (**obstructive uropathy**) is a blockage in the flow of urine at some point in the urinary tract, and has many possible causes (Fig. 11.2). Obstruction in the urinary tract has a number of consequences, including an increased susceptibility to infection, stone formation, and most importantly renal damage. *Renal damage due to obstruction is called obstructive nephropathy and is the most important consequence of obstructive uropathy.*

Unrelieved obstruction leads to dilation of the urinary tract and destruction of the kidney

Obstruction in the urinary tract leads to dilation of the urinary tract above the point of obstruction. Dilation of a ureter is known as **hydroureter** and dilation of the

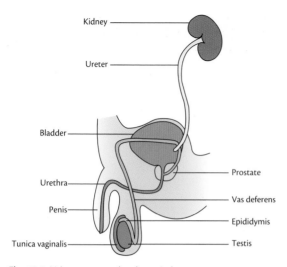

Fig. 11.1 Urinary tract and male genital tract.

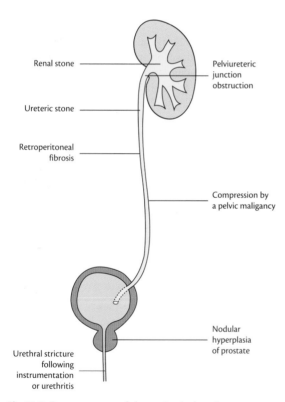

Fig. 11.2 Common causes of obstruction in the urinary tract.

renal pelvis and calyces is known as **hydronephrosis**. Prolonged hydronephrosis leads to atrophy of the renal parenchyma with gradual loss of function of the involved kidney.

The changes in the renal parenchyma are due to a combination of *pressure atrophy* from an increase in pelvic pressure and *ischaemic atrophy* due to compression of vessels within the kidney. Eventually the kidney is completely destroyed, converted into a thin-walled, fluid-filled sac which is liable to secondary infection. Such an end-stage hydronephrotic kidney is only seen in patients with unilateral obstruction, as patients with bilateral obstruction develop renal failure before both kidneys have been able to develop such terminal changes.

Urinary tract obstruction may come to clinical attention in a variety of ways

The presence of obstruction in the urinary tract should be considered in any patient presenting with:

- Symptoms directly suggestive of obstruction.
- Impaired renal function found on biochemical testing.
- Recurrent urinary tract infections.

The manner in which an individual patient with obstruction presents depends on the precise nature of the obstruction: whether it is *acute or chronic*, whether it involves the *upper or lower tract*, and whether it is *unilateral or bilateral*.

LINK BOX

Post-renal renal failure

Remember that *all* patients presenting in renal failure, whether acute or chronic, should have the possibility of obstruction ruled out as a priority.

Acute upper tract obstruction causes severe flank pain

Patients with acute urinary tract obstruction usually present immediately, due to the sudden onset of severe pain. Acute upper urinary tract obstruction causes pain in the flank which may radiate down towards the groin.

The pain can be extremely severe, usually waxing and waning in intensity. The most common cause of acute upper tract obstruction is a ureteric stone.

Acute lower tract obstruction causes severe suprapubic pain

Acute lower urinary tract obstruction causes **acute urinary retention**. Acute urinary retention causes severe suprapubic pain and inability to pass urine. The combination of these symptoms with the presence of a palpably enlarged bladder in the lower abdomen is usually sufficient to establish the diagnosis. By far the most common cause of acute urinary retention is prostatic nodular hyperplasia.

Chronic lower tract obstruction causes lower urinary tract symptoms

Chronic lower urinary tract obstruction usually presents with symptoms such as poor stream and terminal dribbling. By far the most common cause is nodular hyperplasia of the prostate, although prostatic carcinoma and urethral strictures may also be responsible.

Chronic upper tract obstruction presents late

Chronic upper urinary tract obstruction is potentially more dangerous because there may be no symptoms alerting the patient or doctor to the problem. The obstruction goes unrelieved leading to dilation of the involved upper urinary tract and gradual destruction of the kidney. The final outcome depends on whether the obstruction is unilateral or bilateral.

Chronic *unilateral* upper tract obstruction usually leads to complete destruction of the kidney. As the other kidney can provide adequate renal function, patients usually present with symptoms related to the presence of a large hydronephrotic kidney.

In chronic *bilateral* upper urinary tract obstruction, the earliest manifestation is an inability to concentrate the urine, causing nocturia and polyuria. Hypertension is also commonly found, and with progression there is biochemical evidence of chronic renal failure.

Having considered some general points about obstructive uropathy, we now move on to consider the important causes in more detail.

> ## Key points: Urinary tract obstruction
>
> - Obstruction may occur at any point in the urinary tract and may affect one or both tracts.
>
> - Obstruction predisposes to infection, stone formation, and, most importantly, renal damage (obstructive nephropathy).
>
> - Acute upper tract obstruction presents with severe loin pain. The most common cause is a ureteric calculus.
>
> - Acute lower tract obstruction presents with inability to pass urine and painful enlargement of the bladder. The most common cause is nodular hyperplasia of the prostate.
>
> - Chronic lower tract obstruction causes symptoms of poor stream and terminal dribbling. Nodular hyperplasia of the prostate is the most common cause.
>
> - Chronic upper tract obstruction often presents late. A single end-stage hydronephrotic kidney may be picked up on imaging or abdominal examination. Bilateral upper tract obstruction is often not discovered until hypertension or renal failure is investigated.

Renal stones

Renal stone disease continues to be a common problem across the world. The lifetime risk of stone formation has been reported to be up to 10 per cent of the population. The risk is generally higher in men, although stone disease appears to be becoming more common in women.

Stones may form anywhere in the urinary tract, but most commonly arise in the renal calyces and pelves. Most stones tend to remain small (2–3 mm). On occasion, progressive enlargement of a renal stone creates a large branching mass known as a **staghorn calculus** which fills the entire renal pelvis and calyces.

The most common types of renal calculi are:

- Calcium oxalate or a mixture of calcium oxalate and calcium phosphate (70 per cent)

- Magnesium ammonium phosphate, 'triple', or 'struvite' stones (15 per cent)

- Uric acid stones (5 per cent).

Most people with calcium stones have hypercalciuria without hypercalcaemia

Most calcium stone formers have **hypercalciuria** (high levels of calcium in their urine) but do not have high serum calcium levels. Many of these people appear to absorb calcium from their gut too well ('absorptive hypercalciuria'), a tendency which can run in families. Others have something wrong with their renal tubules which impairs renal tubular absorption of calcium in the proximal tubule ('renal hypercalciuria'). Only a minority of patients have hypercalciuria due to hypercalcaemia, which is usually due to primary hyperparathyroidism.

Magnesium ammonium phosphate stones are associated with infections

Triple stones are formed largely as a result of infections with particular types of organisms (e.g. *Proteus*) that produce the enzyme urease which splits urea in the urine to ammonia. The ammonia alkalinizes the urine and promotes the precipitation of magnesium ammonium phosphate salts. Triple stones can become very large indeed, and most staghorn calculi are of this type.

Most patients with uric acid stones have no detectable abnormality in uric acid metabolism

Uric acid stones are known to form in patients with hyperuricaemia, for instance patients with gout and conditions associated with rapid cell turnover, e.g. leukaemias. However, most patients with uric acid stones do not have hyperuricaemia nor increased urinary excretion of uric acid. It has been speculated that these patients have a tendency to make slightly acidic urine which is prone to forming uric acid stones.

Stones cause a variety of symptoms depending on their size and location

Large renal stones tend to remain confined to kidney and may cause no symptoms for long periods of time. Their presence may be picked up following investigation of haematuria or recurrent urinary tract infections.

Smaller stones tend to be more of a problem because they can pass into the ureter and cause **ureteric colic**. Ureteric colic is an agonizing pain which starts suddenly and comes in waves lasting several minutes, originating in the loin and radiating towards the groin. If a stone becomes lodged in the ureter, then the pain becomes even more severe and constant.

There are three common places that ureteric stones become impacted:

- The pelviureteric junction where the large diameter of the renal pelvis decreases to that of the ureter.
- The pelvic brim as the ureters arch over the iliac vessels.
- The vesicoureteric junction. This is the most common area for stones to impact.

These areas should be particularly scrutinized when examining a plain radiograph for stones.

Immediate intervention is necessary if there is superadded infection

Obstruction in the urinary tract increases the risk of developing infection. Infection in a blocked urinary tract is bad news, as it can lead to rapid destruction of the kidney and the development of life-threatening sepsis. Patients with evidence of severe infection require immediate treatment to bypass the obstruction without delay. This is usually achieved by inserting a tube through the abdominal wall into the renal pelvis through which urine can drain freely, a procedure known as a **nephrostomy** which is performed by radiologists under imaging guidance.

Urgent intervention is needed if there is complete obstruction

If there is evidence of progressive obstruction of the kidney, urgent removal of the stone is necessary even if the stone is small. Non-resolving or increasing pain is the usual indication of worsening obstruction, and this should be taken seriously. Usually stones can be removed by passing instruments up into the ureter via the urethra and bladder, a technique known as ureteroscopy.

A watch and wait policy is appropriate for stones less than 5 mm

Small ureteric stones measuring less than 5 mm are likely to pass naturally. This may take several months, but it is safe simply to follow the patient up with repeat radiographs every 6–8 weeks provided there is no obstruction. Renal stones that fail to pass spontaneously or larger stones require active intervention. Options include extracorporeal shock wave lithotripsy (ESWL) and endoscopic stone removal. Open surgical stone removal, once the only available method for removing renal calculi, is now rarely performed.

Patients with renal stones have a high chance of recurrence

Because of the high chance of recurrence, it is important for patients with renal stone disease to be counselled about stone prevention. Patients should be strongly encouraged to drink at least 3 l of fluid every day and maintain a daily urine volume of at least 2 l. Fluid intake should occur regularly during the day, and just before bedtime. Patients should drink enough to need to get up in the night, and should drink again when they are up. Despite the fact that most stones are calcium oxalate, current evidence suggests that reducing calcium intake in the diet is not effective at preventing stone formation.

> # Key points: Renal stones
>
> - Renal stones are very common and often recurrent.
>
> - Most are composed of calcium and are visible on plain radiographs.
>
> - Large stones tend to remain confined to the kidneys and may remain clinically silent or come to light when haematuria or recurrent urinary tract infections are investigated.
>
> - Small stones are more hazardous because they can enter the ureter and cause ureteric colic.
>
> - Most small stones pass spontaneously and can be treated conservatively.
>
> - The presence of infection in a tract obstructed by a stone is dangerous and requires urgent surgical intervention even if the stone is small.
>
> - Drinking at least 3 l of water a day can halve the risk of developing further stones.

Prostatic nodular hyperplasia

The prostate is a small organ situated beneath the bladder in men. Its role is to produce an alkaline secretion which acts to neutralize the acidic environment of the vagina and nourish the spermatozoa. The prostate is made up of numerous acini and ducts which are embedded in a fibromuscular stroma composed of smooth muscle cells and fibroblasts (Fig. 11.3).

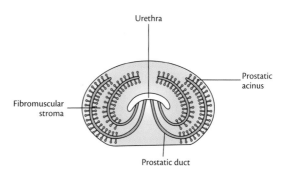

Fig. 11.3 Diagram of a prostate gland showing the arrangement of acini and ducts with intervening fibromuscular stroma.

The prostatic acini secrete prostatic juice which drains into the prostatic urethra via the duct system. The stromal cells have a crucial role in maintaining suitable levels of androgens in the prostate by converting testosterone into its more potent derivative **dihydrotestosterone**. This is achieved by the action of the enzyme **5α-reductase**, located principally in stromal cells.

Prostatic nodular hyperplasia results from overgrowth of the cellular elements of the prostate

Prostatic nodular hyperplasia, also often known as **benign prostatic hyperplasia**, is an extremely common cause of urinary tract obstruction in men. The obstruction arises due to the formation of large nodular overgrowths of prostatic tissue in the transition zone of the prostate, leading to compression of the prostatic urethra.

The nodules form due to hyperplasia of all the cellular elements of the prostate, i.e. epithelial, muscular, and fibrous. The contribution of each of these three components varies markedly, and this may account for the poor reliability of the prediction of responsiveness to a specific medical therapy.

Nodular hyperplasia is thought to arise due to subtle hormonal imbalances occurring with age

The pathogenesis of nodular hyperplasia is almost certainly related to the action of androgens, in particular increased levels of dihydrotestosterone locally in the prostate. Although androgen levels do not appear to rise in peripheral blood with age, oestrogen levels do, and oestrogens are known to induce androgen receptors in prostate tissue. This leads to an increased level of androgens locally within the prostate, causing growth of stromal and epithelial cells. This creates a vicious circle as more stromal cells produce more potent androgens which induce more growth, and so on.

Enlarging prostatic tissue causes symptoms of bladder outflow obstruction

There are two components underlying the development of obstruction in nodular hyperplasia:

- Increased tone of smooth muscle in the prostate, making the organ more contracted around the urethra.

- A mechanical effect due to the physical bulk of the prostate.

The relative effects of each will vary between individuals, and may explain why there seems to be a very poor correlation between the size of the prostate and the degree of obstruction.

Bladder outflow obstruction may present with acute retention or LUTS

There are two ways in which patients with bladder outflow obstruction may present: with **acute retention** or with **lower urinary tract symptoms** ('LUTS'). LUTS covers a number of symptoms suggestive of a problem in the bladder or prostate. They are by no means specific for any particular pathology. LUTS include frequency, urgency, nocturia, hesitancy, poor flow, and terminal dribbling. Acute urinary retention causes a sudden inability to pass urine associated with a painful distension of the bladder.

Unrelieved bladder outflow obstruction may lead to chronic urinary retention and renal damage

As the condition progresses, pressure rises within the bladder and the muscle wall of the bladder undergoes hypertrophy leading to visible trabeculations of the wall (Fig. 11.4). If obstruction continues unrelieved, eventually the bladder 'decompensates' and begins to dilate until it is converted into a big flabby sac with little power of contraction. Patients with chronic lower urinary retention have a palpably enlarged massively distended bladder which may contain litres of urine, and suffer from overflow incontinence.

Chronic retention differs from acute retention in that the distension of the bladder is almost painless. These patients are at particular risk of developing bilateral

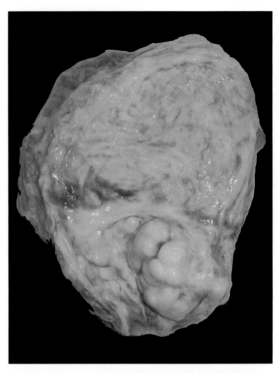

Fig. 11.4 A huge benign nodular hyperplastic prostate gland bulging up into the base of the bladder. The bladder wall is trabeculated due to hypertrophy of the smooth muscle layer developing in response to the bladder outflow obstruction.

upper tract dilation and obstructive nephropathy. Nodular hyperplasia is one of the most common causes of obstructive nephropathy in adults. Fortunately most patients will seek medical attention with symptoms of bladder outflow obstruction before renal impairment develops.

Treatment of nodular hyperplasia may be medical or surgical

The mainstay of medical therapy of nodular hyperplasia is with **α-blockers** (e.g. tamsulosin) and **5α-reductase inhibitors** (e.g. finasteride). α-Blockers work by causing relaxation of smooth muscle cells in the prostate, and it is thought that they give a better response in patients whose nodules have a significant smooth muscle component. Those with predominant epithelium probably respond better to a 5α-reductase inhibitor as it reduces the amount of active dihydrotestosterone which is a strong stimulator of prostate epithelial growth. Patients with large amounts of fibrous tissue may not respond to either form.

Surgical treatment is indicated in patients who respond poorly to medical treatment or in patients with advanced disease, e.g. those with chronic retention. The most common procedure performed is a **transurethral resection of prostate** (TURP). In this procedure, a resectoscope is passed up into the prostatic urethra and the enlarged prostate is cored away using a wire loop that carries an electric current (Fig. 11.5).

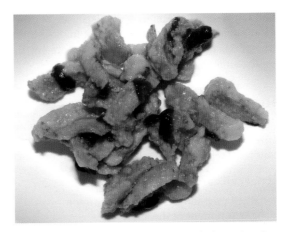

Fig. 11.5 Prostate chippings from a transurethral resection of the prostate in a patient with benign nodular hyperplasia.

Key points: Benign nodular hyperplasia

- Benign nodular hyperplasia of the prostate is an extremely common condition in men.

- The prostate enlarges due to the formation of hyperplastic nodules in the transition zone of the organ.

- The nodules contain varying amounts of epithelial, muscular, and fibrous elements.

- Most men present with LUTS or the sudden onset of acute urinary retention.

- There is a poor correlation between the size of the prostate and the severity of symptoms.

- In some cases, long-standing unrelieved obstruction leads to bilateral obstructive nephropathy and chronic renal failure.

- Treatment of nodular hyperplasia includes medical and surgical options.

Pelviureteric junction obstruction

Pelviureteric junction obstruction is a functional obstruction due to failure of peristalsis at the junction of the renal pelvis and ureter. Pelviureteric junction obstruction is the most common cause of urinary tract obstruction in childhood, where it is often bilateral, but about a quarter of cases occur in adults, where it is usually unilateral.

The condition may be asymptomatic, but patients may notice the insidious onset of a dull ache in the loin. Patients often describe a sensation of a dragging heaviness that is made worse by drinking large volume of fluid. Ultrasound scanning is an easy means of detecting the hydronephrotic kidney.

Patients with evidence of increasing hydronephrosis and renal parenchymal damage should undergo surgical treatment to conserve the remaining functional renal mass. The surgical operation is known as a **pyeloplasty**; the area of obstruction is removed followed by reconstruction of the pelviureteric junction. Removal of the entire kidney should only be performed if most of the functional renal parenchyma has been destroyed.

Idiopathic retroperitoneal fibrosis

Idiopathic retroperitoneal fibrosis or periaortitis is a condition in which one or both ureters become embedded in dense fibrous tissue with resultant obstruction. It is thought that the fibrosis may be the end result of an immune response to leakage of atherosclerotic material from an aorta diseased by atherosclerosis.

The disease usually manifests with nonspecific persistent pain in the abdomen, flank, and back. The diagnosis is often overlooked in its early stages until patients present in chronic renal failure and are found to have bilateral hydronephrosis. *It is very important to rule out a retroperitoneal malignancy masquerading as idiopathic retroperitoneal fibrosis by taking multiple biopsies of the area.*

Once the diagnosis has been confirmed, treatment aims to conserve as much renal function as possible. In the early stages of the disease, treatment with steroids has been reported to achieve good responses, but they are of minimal value in advanced cases. In these cases, prompt relief of obstruction is required by freeing the ureters surgically ('ureterolysis').

Tumours of the kidney

Tumours of the kidney are common and important. Only two are worth knowing about in detail: the malignant renal cell carcinoma and the benign oncocytoma.

Renal cell carcinoma

Renal cell carcinoma is the most common malignant tumour of the kidney

Renal cell carcinomas are adenocarcinomas derived from the epithelium lining the renal tubules. They account for over 90 per cent of all malignant renal tumours. Smoking appears to be the only factor that can be consistently linked to the development of renal cell carcinoma. Gender is also important as the incidence is about four times greater in men than in women. Most cases occur in people aged over 50.

Many renal cell carcinomas are picked up incidentally on imaging

Most renal cell carcinomas remain confined to the kidney for a substantial period of time and cause no change in renal structure or function, thus remaining asymptomatic. In fact, about half of all renal cell carcinomas are now found incidentally on a scan performed for an unrelated reason.

Haematuria is the most common presenting symptom of a renal cell carcinoma

Of patients presenting with symptoms due to a renal cell carcinoma, haematuria is the most common symptom. The haematuria is usually visible, painless, and intermittent. Any patient with otherwise unexplained haematuria should have imaging of the kidneys to exclude a renal cell carcinoma. Many non-specific symptoms, such as fever, weight loss, fatigue, and nausea are also commonly observed.

Renal cell carcinomas have been associated with paraneoplastic syndromes

Renal cell carcinomas may also produce a number of paraneoplastic syndromes due to abnormal hormone production, including polycythaemia due to erythropoietin production and hypercalcaemia due to parathyroid hormone-related protein production.

Hypertension is often stated as a common feature in patients with renal cell carcinoma and is postulated to be related to the secretion of renin or a renin-like substance by the tumour. This theory is attractive, but it should be remembered that primary hypertension is common and the frequency of hypertension in patients with renal cell carcinomas is in fact no greater than in age-matched patients without the malignancy.

Some patients may present with signs or symptoms of metastatic disease

Renal cell carcinomas have a great tendency to metastasize before giving rise to any local symptoms. Up to a quarter of all patients are found to have distant metastases when they are diagnosed with a renal cell carcinoma. The most common location of metastases are the lungs and bones, and these may cause breathlessness or persistent bony pain.

Any patient with a solid renal mass should have a radical nephrectomy

The first line investigation for a patient suspected of having a renal tumour is an abdominal ultrasound. If a renal mass is found, then CT scanning of the chest and abdomen should be performed to detail further the nature of the mass and to look for evidence of metastatic disease.

If the renal mass appears to be confined to the kidney, then a radical nephrectomy is the recommended treatment. Radical nephrectomy involves surgical removal of the kidney, adrenal gland, and perinephric fat. The specimen should be placed in a large volume of formalin for fixation and sent to histopathology for examination (Fig. 11.6).

The pathologist will report the tumour type, the grade, and the stage

The pathologist will examine the specimen and sample suitable areas for microscopic examination. Three important pieces of information will be reported by the pathologist. The first is the precise histological type of tumour. There are three main types of renal cell carcinoma, which are distinguished by their appearance down the light microscope:

◆ **Clear cell carcinoma** (80 per cent). These tumours are made up of cells with clear cytoplasm and are not papillary (Fig. 11.7).

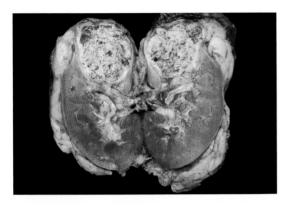

Fig. 11.6 This patient presented with macroscopic haematuria and was found to have a solid renal mass on CT imaging. A nephrectomy was performed and sent to pathology. The kidney has been sliced open by the pathologist to reveal a large tumour in the upper pole of the kidney. Subsequent microscopic examination of samples of the tumour revealed this to be a clear cell renal cell carcinoma.

- ◆ **Papillary carcinoma** (15 per cent). These tumours are defined by a papillary growth pattern.

- ◆ **Chromophobe carcinoma** (5 per cent). These uncommon tumours are made up of large pale cells with prominent cell borders.

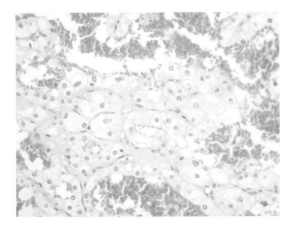

Fig. 11.7 Typical appearance of a clear cell renal carcinoma. Note the strikingly clear cytoplasm of the malignant cells. These tumours are typically highly vascular, and this can also be appreciated here; look at all the red blood cells in the background.

As well as typing the tumour, the pathologist will provide a histological **grade** of the tumour and assess the **stage** of the malignancy, i.e. the amount of spread. The stage of the tumour and the histological grade have an important impact on long-term survival. The most widely used grading system is that described by **Fuhrman**. Based on the features of the nuclei of the malignant cells, a Fuhrman grade between 1 and 4 is assigned, with grade 4 being the most abnormal.

Clear cell renal carcinomas have a deleted VHL gene

There has been a significant increase in our understanding of the genetics of renal cell carcinomas in recent years. *Almost all clear cell renal cell carcinomas are consistently associated with a deletion of the short arm of chromosome 3* (3p). This region harbours a gene called the VHL gene, which is the gene deleted in the inherited condition von Hippel–Lindau syndrome.

The VHL gene is a tumour suppressor gene which when inactivated promotes cell growth and angiogenesis. The angiogenesis probably accounts for the fact that clear cell carcinomas are highly vascular tumours and why haematogenous spread to distant sites is so common.

INTERESTING TO KNOW

von Hippel–Lindau syndrome

In this genetic syndrome, patients are born with an inherited loss of one of their two VHL gene alleles. As well as being predisposed to the development of clear cell renal cell carcinoma, patients with VHL syndrome are also prone to tumours called **haemangioblastomas**. These are probably not true neoplasms but rather abnormal overgrowths of blood vessels which are thought to develop in response to a pseudohypoxic state.

A pseudohypoxic state is seen in VHL syndrome because the VHL protein targets a protein called hypoxia-inducible factor 1 (HIF-1), which is normally upregulated in states of hypoxia, for degradation. If a cell in a patient with von Hippel–Lindau syndrome spontaneously loses its remaining functional VHL gene, the cell will have persistently high HIF-1 levels. This mimics a hypoxic state and stimulates blood vessel overgrowth.

Papillary renal cell carcinomas have MET mutations

Papillary renal cell carcinomas tumours arise through a different genetic pathway which may involve gain of chromosomes 7 and 17. The most common genetic abnormality in papillary renal cell carcinomas are activating mutations of the oncogene MET which encodes a growth-stimulating tyrosine kinase receptor.

Key points: Renal cell carcinoma

- Renal cell carcinomas are adenocarcinomas derived from the epithelium of the renal tubules.

- Renal cell carcinomas account for over 90 per cent of all malignant renal tumours.

- Most renal cell carcinomas are found incidentally on imaging of the kidneys. The remainder present with haematuria or symptoms of metastatic disease.

- Patients with a renal mass and no evidence of metastatic disease should undergo radical nephrectomy.

- Clear cell carcinoma is the most common type of renal cell carcinoma, composed of cells with clear cytoplasm. Almost all clear cell renal cell carcinomas demonstrate loss of a region of chromosome 3p carrying the VHL gene.

- Papillary carcinoma is the second most common type of renal cell carcinoma, composed of a tumour with a papillary architecture. Activating mutations of the oncogene MET are often present in these tumours.

- The type of tumour, the histological grade, and the stage of the tumour are all important prognostic factors.

Oncocytoma

Oncocytoma is the most common benign tumour of the kidney

Oncocytoma is a benign renal epithelial neoplasm which is thought to arise from cells of the collecting duct of the nephron. The majority of oncocytomas are asymptomatic, most being picked up when the kidneys are imaged for an unrelated reason. Only a few patients present with symptoms such as haematuria.

Oncocytomas are mainly of clinical significance because they are solid renal masses which mimic renal cell carcinomas on imaging and therefore are often removed by nephrectomy despite being benign tumours.

Tumours of the urothelial tract

The entirety of the renal pelvis, ureter, bladder, and urethra is lined by **transitional cell epithelium** or **urothelium**. Urothelium is a specialized epithelium which is several cell layers thick, allowing it to stretch and distend as needed.

The most common cancer of the urothelial tract is the **transitional cell carcinoma** or **urothelial carcinoma**. Squamous cell carcinomas and adenocarcinomas can develop, but these are much rarer. Cigarette smoking is the major established risk factor for urothelial carcinomas. Exposure to certain industrial dyes and solvents has also been associated with urothelial carcinomas.

Because the renal pelvis, ureter, and bladder are all exposed to a similar environment, very often there is a 'field change' effect whereby the whole urothelial tract becomes unstable and prone to developing tumours. Patients with bladder tumours are also at risk of tumours in the renal pelvis and ureter.

The ratio of bladder to renal pelvis to ureteric carcinomas is in the region of 50:3:1. Bladder carcinomas are probably so much more common because carcinogens passing through the urinary tract dwell in the bladder and come into contact with the transitional cell epithelium of the bladder for longer periods of time. We will therefore concentrate on bladder carcinomas and only briefly mention tumours of the renal pelvis and ureter.

Bladder tumours classically present with painless macroscopic haematuria

Almost all bladder tumours present when the patient notices blood in their urine. Even a single episode of macroscopic haematuria should be investigated, even if it appears to resolve. Some hospitals offer haematuria clinics which combine clinical examination, urine cytology, imaging of the upper tracts, and cystoscopy

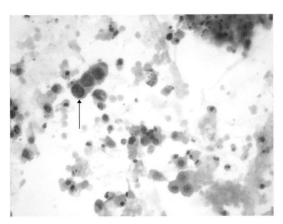

Fig. 11.8 Urine cytology from a patient with a high grade transitional cell carcinoma of the bladder. Clusters of malignant transitional epithelial cells are seen with large irregular nuclei filling the cells (arrow).

all in one visit. Urinary cytology is particularly good at detecting high grade cancers and carcinoma in situ but is less reliable at picking up low grade carcinomas (Fig. 11.8).

Transitional cell carcinomas show a wide range of behaviour

Transitional cell carcinomas of the bladder have a wide spectrum of biological behaviour, ranging from very well differentiated papillary lesions to poorly differentiated infiltrating urothelial carcinomas which can widely metastasize. In clinical practice, three types of transitional cell carcinoma are recognized: superficial transitional cell carcinoma, muscle invasive transitional cell carcinoma, and carcinoma in situ (Fig. 11.9).

Superficial bladder tumours are prone to recurrence

Superficial bladder tumours are frond-like papillary growths which project in an exophytic fashion into the bladder lumen. Such tumours can be removed at cystoscopy, a technique known as transurethral resection of a bladder tumour (TURBT). The fragments of the tumour are then sent for histopathology. The pathologist gives the urologist two crucial pieces of information: the **grade** and **stage** of the tumour. A grade between 1 and 3 is assigned depending on how abnormal the cells

appear, with 3 being the worst. The stage is a reflection of how far (if at all) the tumour has spread into the bladder wall (Fig. 11.10).

Superficial bladder tumours have a high propensity to recur. Although only a minority of patients with superficial tumours will develop a subsequent muscle invasive tumour, if this occurs the patient's prognosis worsens considerably. All patients diagnosed with superficial bladder transitional cell carcinoma therefore require check cystoscopies at regular intervals for at least 10 years from diagnosis, and possibly for life.

Given the high frequency of superficial bladder tumours, this represents a large burden to the health service and to patients. The main problem is that, at the present time, histopathological evaluation of tumour grade and stage is inadequate to accurately predict the behaviour of most superficial bladder tumours. There is, therefore, great interest in identifying markers which will reliably predict the expected clinical course of an individual bladder tumour.

Muscle invasive transitional cell carcinomas carry a much worse prognosis

Muscle invasive bladder carcinomas are invasive tumours which have infiltrated into the muscle coat of the bladder or beyond. These tend to be solid tumours, which are often large and broad based with an irregular ulcerated appearance. Muscle invasive disease carries a much worse prognosis as they are more likely to spread to regional lymph nodes and metastasize to distant organs. Treatment requires removal of the entire bladder (cystectomy).

Carcinoma in situ is a flat lesion containing urothelial cells which appear frankly malignant

Carcinoma in situ is defined as a non-papillary (i.e. flat) lesion in which the urothelium contains cells that appear obviously malignant, *but showing no invasion through the basement membrane*. The abnormal urothelium loses its normal cohesiveness and begins to fall apart. The loss of the urothelium often leads to intense lower urinary tract symptoms such as dysuria and increased frequency of urination.

At cystoscopy, areas of carcinoma in situ may be visible as red patches, but they may be indistinguishable from the surrounding normal urothelium and thus not apparent. Urine cytology is very good at picking up carcinoma in situ because the highly atypical cells are shed into

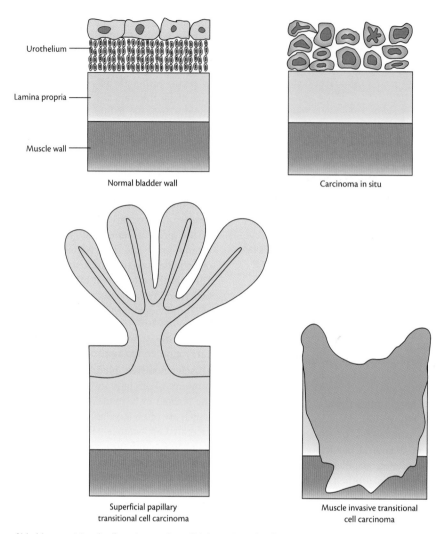

Urothelium

Lamina propria

Muscle wall

Normal bladder wall

Carcinoma in situ

Superficial papillary
transitional cell carcinoma

Muscle invasive transitional
cell carcinoma

Fig. 11.9 Types of bladder transitional cell carcinoma. Superficial transitional cell carcinomas are usually frond-like lesions made up of bland looking cells with no invasion or minimal invasion. Muscle invasive transitional cell carcinomas are usually solid lesions which infiltrate into the muscle coat of the bladder wall. Carcinoma in situ is a flat lesion in which the full thickness of the urothelium is replaced by malignant appearing cells but with no invasion.

the urine. Cytology therefore complements cystoscopic examination of the bladder very well in that it will tend to detect the lesions which may be missed at cystoscopy.

Carcinoma in situ is notoriously unpredictable, and is a much more ominous diagnosis than a superficial papillary transitional cell carcinoma showing no invasion. Around 20–50 per cent of cases of carcinoma in situ turn into muscle invasive cancer within 5 years. A diagnosis of carcinoma in situ of the bladder is therefore very serious, as there is a very high chance of progression to muscle invasive disease. In fact, it is very likely that most muscle invasive bladder cancers develop from areas of carcinoma in situ, rather than from superficial papillary lesions.

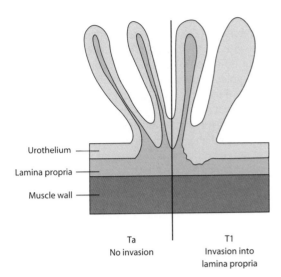

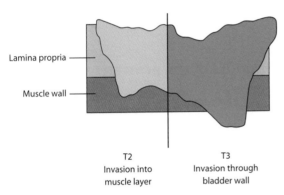

Fig. 11.10 Bladder cancer staging.

Biologically, there is a significant difference between non-invasive low grade tumours (i.e. grade 1 and 2 Ta tumours) when compared with grade 3 and muscle invasive tumours. The low grade non-invasive neoplasms have only a few genetic changes, suggesting that these are genetically stable lesions. Grade 3 non-invasive tumours, however, genetically resemble the muscle invasive tumours, being genetically highly unstable with many different chromosomal abnormalities.

The take home message is that although in practice we group all Ta and T1 tumours together as 'superficial tumours', at the genetic level all grade 3 tumours and T1 tumours have more in common with the muscle invasive tumours than with the other low grade non-invasive tumours.

Squamous cell carcinomas and adenocarcinomas of the bladder are rare

Squamous cell carcinomas, as elsewhere in the body, are malignant epithelial tumours defined by the presence of squamous differentiation, i.e. intercellular bridges and/or formation of keratin. Squamous cell carcinomas of the bladder are rare in Western countries but are more common in sub-Saharan Africa where there is a higher incidence of bladder schistosomiasis due to *Schistosoma haematobium*. Presumably the squamous cell carcinomas arise in areas of squamous metaplasia which develop in response to chronic infection of the bladder.

Adenocarcinomas are epithelial malignancies that show evidence of gland formation and/or mucin production. Adenocarcinomas of the bladder have been described but are extremely rare.

Squamous cell carcinomas and adenocarcinomas of the bladder—cont'd

True squamous cell carcinomas and adenocarcinomas should only be diagnosed by a pathologist when the *entire* tumour appears squamous or glandular, respectively.

In comparison with the bladder, carcinomas of the renal pelvis and ureter are not common

The majority of tumours of the renal pelvis and ureter are also transitional cell carcinomas and, as with bladder transitional cell carcinomas, the main risk factor is smoking. Because the tumours fragment easily, they often become clinically apparent early due to macroscopic haematuria. Patients may experience episodes of ureteric colic due to transient obstruction by tumour fragments or blood clots. Persistent obstruction may lead to unilateral hydronephrosis with the development of flank pain and a mass.

Key points: Tumours of the urothelial tract

+ Tumours of the urothelial tract are almost all transitional cell carcinomas (TCCs) arising from the transitional epithelium (urothelium) lining the urothelial tract.

+ Smoking is the major aetiological factor in TCCs of the urothelial tract.

+ The vast majority of TCCs occur in the bladder. TCCs of the renal pelvis and ureter are much less common.

+ Managing bladder TCC represents a significant proportion of the urologist's workload.

+ Bladder TCC almost always presents with painless haematuria.

+ Urologists tend to divide bladder TCCs into superficial, muscle invasive, and carcinoma in situ.

+ Superficial TCCs tend to be frond-like papillary growths which can be resected at cystoscopy and sent off for histological examination to determine the grade and stage of the tumour. Superficial TCCs are often recurrent, and some patients will develop a muscle invasive tumour at some point in the future. At the moment, it is difficult to predict reliably which patients are at greatest risk of developing muscle invasive tumours.

+ Muscle invasive TCCs are much more likely to metastasize and so carry a much worse prognosis. Radical treatment is required for cure, usually cystectomy.

+ Carcinoma in situ is a flat lesion composed of malignant urothelial cells but with no invasion. It is a serious condition which has a high chance of progressing to muscle invasive carcinoma.

Tumours of the prostate

Although a variety of tumours can arise in the prostate, only one is important: **prostate carcinoma**. Prostate carcinoma is one of the most common malignancies in men, but has a low mortality rate. Many men remain alive and well following a diagnosis of prostate carcinoma. In fact, over 50 per cent of all men aged over 50 have microscopic evidence of prostate carcinoma, but only 3 per cent of them will die of it. Most of these neoplasms are tiny and remain latent for many years.

Prostate carcinomas arise from areas of prostatic intraepithelial neoplasia

Prostate carcinomas are adenocarcinomas derived from the glandular epithelial cells lining the glands and ducts of the prostate. Most carcinomas arise in the peripheral zone of the prostate. Prostatic adenocarcinoma is thought to arise from a precursor lesion called **prostatic intraepithelial neoplasia** (PIN) which refers to glands containing abnormal cells with atypical features, but where no invasion into surrounding tissue has occurred (Fig. 11.11).

A number of observations support the theory that PIN progresses into carcinoma: PIN is often seen close to a focus of invasive cancer; similar molecular changes are found in PIN and in carcinoma; and if patients with

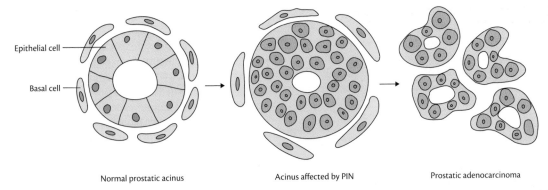

Epithelial cell

Basal cell

Normal prostatic acinus   Acinus affected by PIN   Prostatic adenocarcinoma

Fig. 11.11 Evolution of prostate cancer. Prostatic adenocarcinoma develops from a precursor stage known as prostatic intraepithelial neoplasia (PIN) which microscopically shows neoplastic cells confined to the duct system.

PIN alone are followed up regularly with repeat biopsies, carcinoma invariably develops within a 10 year period.

Prostate carcinoma may be symptomatic or latent

There are two distinct ways in which prostate carcinoma may present. Patients either present with symptoms related to the cancer, or the carcinoma is picked up when the patient is asymptomatic.

The first group either present with symptoms of bladder outflow obstruction, or with symptoms related to metastatic disease. Bony metastases are very common, with persistent back pain from vertebral metastases being a particularly common symptom of metastatic prostate carcinoma (Fig. 11.12). Patients presenting with symptoms due to prostate carcinoma will almost always have advanced disease which, although controllable, is not curable. Historically, virtually all cases of prostate carcinoma presented in this fashion.

Nowadays, however, many patients with prostate carcinoma are diagnosed at a much earlier stage when they have no symptoms from the carcinoma. Sometimes carcinoma is picked up as an incidental finding when chippings from a TURP resection are found to contain carcinoma, but increasingly patients with latent disease are being picked up as a result of PSA testing followed by transrectal ultrasound guided prostate biopsies.

Prostate specific antigen (PSA) is produced by the prostatic glands and is secreted into the ductal system. It is a protease enzyme which acts to break down

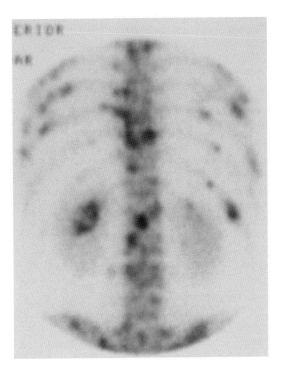

Fig. 11.12 A bone scan from a patient with a very high prostate specific antigen level shows multiple metastatic bony deposits in the vertebral bodies and ribs.

proteins in seminal fluid, thinning the ejaculate and increasing sperm mobility. Large amounts of PSA are secreted into the semen, but small amounts diffuse into the plasma where it can be measured. PSA levels tend to increase in prostatic cancer but the sensitivity and specificity of PSA as a marker are limited by the fact that PSA is detectable in the plasma of normal men and because its concentration rises with age and in benign nodular hyperplasia (which is very common in elderly men). The finding of an elevated PSA is therefore not diagnostic of prostate cancer, but should prompt biopsy of the prostate.

The management of latent prostate carcinoma is extremely challenging for urologists

The main problem with latent prostate carcinoma is that many of the cancers that are picked up are tiny and if left would remain small and never cause the patient any problems. A minority would be aggressive malignancies which would result in the death of the patient. Our current problem is that we have no completely reliable means of predicting how each carcinoma will behave. Discovering a test which will reliably achieve this is the Holy Grail of prostate pathology!

Patients diagnosed with latent prostate cancer may be managed in a number of ways

There are three main options for patients found to have prostate carcinoma confined to the prostate: active surveillance, radical prostatectomy, or radical radiotherapy. The choice depends on a number of factors including the age and general health of the patient, and the **grade** of the prostate cancer. The grade of the cancer is assessed by the pathologist examining a biopsy of the prostate.

The most widely used grading system is known as the **Gleason** system. On the basis of the architectural features of the malignant glands, prostate cancers are assigned a grade on a scale from 1 to 5, where 1 is well differentiated and 5 is poorly differentiated. Most tumours contain more than one pattern, so a sum score from 2 to 10 is generated by adding together the most dominant grade and the second most dominant grade seen. The lower the score, the better the prognosis for the patient.

The Gleason grading is therefore one important factor that is considered when deciding on the best management option for the patient. The majority of potentially treatable cancers detected on needle biopsy have Gleason scores of 5–7. Tumours with Gleason scores of 8–10 tend to be advanced cancers that spread widely and are unlikely to be curable.

PSA testing is a useful way of monitoring a patient's disease

After a diagnosis of prostate carcinoma has been made, serial PSA measurements are extremely useful in monitoring disease activity. In patients who are being actively watched, the PSA levels provide a useful indicator of when and if to intercede. In patients who have been treated radically with prostatectomy or radiotherapy, PSA levels should fall to virtually zero and stay there. A rising PSA is a quick and easy test which can be used to screen for possible recurrence.

Currently there are no plans for a national screening programme for prostate cancer in the UK

It has been suggested that PSA testing could be used as a screening test for prostate cancer. Although this would be a cheap and acceptable test, the low specificity of the test means that many men without prostate cancer would undergo biopsy unnecessarily. A raised PSA would condemn many men to a prolonged period of follow-up and rebiopsying in the hunt for a tumour that may not even exist.

Even in those men who are diagnosed with prostate cancer, we still have no way of knowing which cancers would progress. Many of them would remain latent and the patient would die of other causes. These men would be overtreated for a disease which would never have caused them any problems.

Until we have a better understanding of the natural history of prostate cancer, a screening programme is unlikely to be successful. Routine measurement of PSA is not indicated under any circumstances in an asymptomatic man. PSA should only be measured in patients with symptoms of bladder outflow obstruction or in men with metastatic malignancy to rule out a prostatic primary.

> ## Key points: Prostate cancer
>
> - Prostate cancer is an extremely common malignancy but has a low fatality rate compared with other carcinomas.
>
> - Almost all prostate cancers are adenocarcinomas which develop from a precursor lesion known as prostatic intraepithelial neoplasia (PIN).

Key points: Prostate
cancer—cont'd

- The spectrum of biological behaviour is extremely wide. The majority of prostate cancers are of no clinical significance, and many patients die of unrelated causes.

- Finding a way of reliably separating those patients with indolent cancers from those whose cancer will progress is the Holy Grail of prostate pathology.

- Screening for prostate cancer is unlikely to be successful until we have a better understanding of the natural history of all prostate cancers.

Tumours of the testis

Testicular tumours are not as common numerically as the other urological tumours but they are important as most of them occur in young men and, unlike most solid tumours, are curable in the majority of cases. There are three main groups of testicular tumours to know about: germ cell tumours, sex cord stromal tumours, and testicular lymphomas (Table 11.1).

Germ cell tumours are the most common type of testicular tumour, accounting for over 90 per cent of all tumours. Germ cell tumours are so called because they are derived from the germ cells of the testis which develop into mature spermatozoa. Embryologically, they originate in the fetal yolk sac and then migrate into the developing testes where they become enclosed within the seminiferous tubules (Fig. 11.13).

TABLE 11.1 Testicular tumours

Germ cell tumours
Seminoma
Non-seminomatous germ cell tumour
Sex cord stromal tumours
Leydig cell tumour
Sertoli cell tumour
Lymphomas
Diffuse large B cell lymphoma

Sex cord stromal tumours are much less common than germ cell tumours, accounting for about 5 per cent of all testicular tumours. They are called sex cord stromal tumours because they originate from cells derived from the sex cords of the primitive gonad. The sex cords are groups of cells which grow into the developing testis and engulf the migrating germ cells. Most of them develop into Sertoli cells in seminiferous tubules which support the developing germ cells. Those that do not become incorporated into seminiferous tubules are left behind in the interstitium and instead develop into Leydig cells which synthesize testosterone. The two main sex cord stromal tumours are therefore known as **Leydig cell tumours** and **Sertoli cell tumours**.

Lymphomas account for some 5 per cent of all testicular tumours. Strictly speaking lymphomas are not primary testicular tumours (they are haematological malignancies derived from mature B lymphocytes which happen to involve the testis), but they are best considered here because they present as a testicular mass.

Germ cell tumours

Testicular germ cell tumours are the most common solid cancers in men aged between 20 and 45. Despite being malignant tumours capable of wide dissemination, they are one of the most curable forms of cancer with less than 100 deaths each year in the UK.

Testicular germ cell tumours arise from intratubular germ cell neoplasia

Intratubular germ cell neoplasia (ITGCN) refers to the presence of abnormal neoplastic germ cells located within the seminiferous tubules. In essence, it is a form of testicular carcinoma in situ analogous to that described in other organs. There is a very strong and very specific association between ITGCN and testicular germ cell tumours. ITGCN is almost always present in the testis adjacent to a testicular germ cell tumour, and the condition has never been known to resolve spontaneously.

Our current thinking is that the disease process leading to testicular germ cell tumours begins early in life, causing the abnormal differentiation of the primordial germ cells in the fetus, which leads to persistent ITGCN which then inevitably progresses into an invasive germ cell tumour in early adult life. This line of thinking is supported by several pieces of evidence:

- Abnormalities of the developing testis are associated with a higher incidence of testicular germ cell tumours.

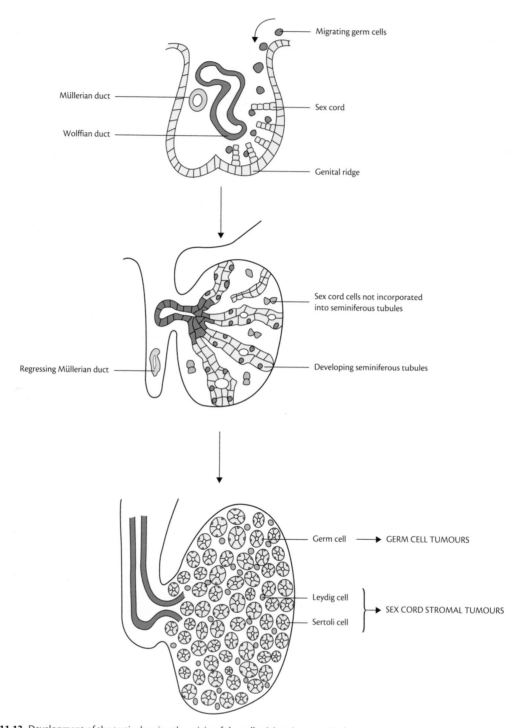

Fig. 11.13 Development of the testis showing the origin of the cells giving rise to testicular tumours.

For instance, undescended testis (cryptorchidism) has a high risk of testicular germ cell tumour.

- The decline in incidence of testicular germ cell tumours after 40 years of age may be due to the loss of susceptible individuals with ITGCN as these will have all progressed to invasive germ cell tumours by age 40.

There are many types of germ cell tumours depending on how the neoplastic cells differentiate

Malignant germ cells have the capacity to differentiate along various cell lineages, giving rise to a host of different tumour subtypes. If the neoplastic germ cells do not differentiate, the tumour is called a **seminoma** and is composed of cells resembling immature spermatogonia. If some differentiation does occur, it may happen down various possible pathways giving rise to the following tumours:

- **Embryonal carcinoma**, consisting of cells which appear malignant and highly primitive, somewhat resembling the cells of the inner cell mass of the blastocyst.

- **Teratomas**, composed of tissues from all the different germinal layers (endoderm, mesoderm, and ectoderm). They may be composed of exclusively well differentiated mature tissues or have immature fetal-like tissues.

- **Yolk sac tumours**, made up of cells with features reminiscent of the fetal yolk sac.

- **Choriocarcinomas**, containing cells resembling trophoblast.

Germ cell tumours may contain a single element or combinations of more than one element

Some germ cell tumours are composed entirely of one of the above five elements, for instance a pure seminoma. Often, however, there is differentiation down several of these pathways leading to a mixture of various different elements within the same tumour. Any combination is possible, though certain mixtures are seen more often, e.g. embryonal carcinoma with teratoma.

For treatment purposes, germ cell tumours are divided into seminomas and non-seminomatous germ cell tumours

In everyday practice, the classification of germ cell tumours is actually quite simple because treatment is the same for all types of germ cell tumour except the pure seminoma. Clinicians therefore simply divide all germ cell tumours into seminomas and non-seminomatous germ cell tumours (NSGCTs). *Any germ cell tumour other than a pure seminoma is considered to be a NSGCT for the purposes of treatment.*

The NSGCTs (60 per cent) are slightly more common than pure seminomas (40 per cent). NSGCTs have a peak incidence in men between 20 and 30 years. NSGCTs tend to be more aggressive than pure seminomas, spreading earlier via the blood stream, with most patients having disease outside the testis at presentation.

Pure seminoma is seen in slightly older men than NSGCTs, with a peak incidence between 30 and 40 years of age. These tumours usually spread late via lymphatics to the para-aortic lymph nodes.

INTERESTING TO KNOW

Extratesticular germ cell tumours

Germ cell tumours can arise in other midline structures in the body including the thymus (causing an anterior mediastinal mass) and the pineal gland. Presumably they originate from viable germ cells which never made it to the testes during development.

Most testicular germ cell tumours present with a painless lump in the testis

The majority of patients present with a painless lump in the testis. Occasionally sudden severe scrotal pain may occur due to bleeding into the tumour. Examination of the testis reveals a hard irregular mass in the testis. An ultrasound scan is a simple investigation which can confirm that the mass is within the testis and the echo pattern is usually suggestive of a tumour (most tumours are hypoechoic compared with the surrounding testis).

Tumour markers are useful to measure in patients with testicular germ cell tumours

There are three tumour markers which are widely used in the assessment and management of testicular germ cell tumours:

- **α-Fetoprotein** (AFP). Serum AFP levels are normally only found in trace amounts beyond the age of 1 year.

AFP may be produced by any NSGCT but is not expressed by pure seminomas. Marked elevation of serum AFP is typical of yolk sac tumours.

◆ **Human chorionic gonadotrophin** (HCG). HCG is normally synthesized by syncytiotrophoblast cells of the placenta. Choriocarcinomas often produce high serum levels of HCG.

◆ **Lactate dehydrogenase** (LDH). LDH is produced in many tissues and is not a specific marker for testicular tumours. However, the degree of LDH elevation corresponds well with the bulk of the tumour and is therefore useful in assessing tumour burden.

These tumour markers are therefore useful in the initial assessment of testicular masses, monitoring response to therapy, and in long-term follow-up for recurrence.

Patients with testicular cancer should have orchidectomy

The primary treatment for all testicular tumours is radical orchidectomy ('orchiectomy' in the USA). This involves removal of the testis together with the epididymis and spermatic cord through a groin incision. The specimen should be sent to histopathology (Fig. 11.14). The results of the histopathology are essential to guide further treatment. The pathologist provides several important pieces of information:

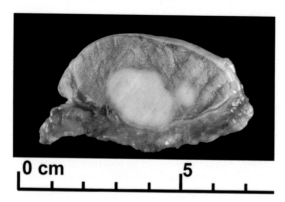

Fig. 11.14 This is a testis from a young man who presented with an enlarging testicular lump. Following an ultrasound scan which was suspicious for a neoplasm, he underwent orchidectomy. The testis has been sliced in the pathology department revealing this white solid mass in the testis. This appearance is typical of a seminoma, and microscopic examination confirmed this.

◆ The tumour type. Microscopic examination of sections of the tumour is required to type the tumour, e.g. pure seminoma or NSGCT.

◆ The local spread of the tumour.

◆ If there is vascular or lymphatic invasion. This is important, particularly in NSGCTs as these patients may be considered for adjuvant chemotherapy.

Sex cord stromal tumours

Leydig cell tumours and Sertoli cell tumours are much less common than germ cell tumours

Of the two main sex cord stromal tumours, Leydig cell tumours are more common. Sertoli cell tumours are very rare and most are benign.

Leydig cell tumours are seen in two groups of people: children aged 5–10 years and young men aged 25–35 years. Because Leydig cells produce testosterone, prepubertal boys with Leydig cell tumours often present with virilization, whereas adult men present with a testicular mass. Most Leydig cell tumours are benign and prognosis is excellent.

Testicular lymphomas

Testicular lymphomas usually occur in elderly men

Testicular lymphomas are usually seen in elderly men. In men aged 60–80 years, a testicular lymphoma is the single most frequent testicular tumour. They usually present with unilateral enlargement of a testis. Most are high grade lymphomas, the most common being the **diffuse large B cell lymphoma**. Patients usually have disseminated disease with involvement of other sites as well as the testis. Prognosis is very poor.

Key points: Testicular tumours

◆ Testicular tumours may be divided into germ cell tumours, sex cord stromal tumours, and lymphomas.

◆ Testicular germ cell tumours are common in young men and have an excellent cure rate.

◆ Germ cells tumours are easily divided into seminomas and non-seminomatous germ cell tumours (NSGCTs).

Key points: Testicular tumours—cont'd

◆ Seminomas occur in men aged 30–40 years and are usually confined to the testis at presentation. Spread occurs late, usually to retroperitoneal lymph nodes.

◆ Non-seminomatous germ cell tumours occur in younger men aged 20–30 years. They are more aggressive tumours which spread early via the blood, and are often advanced when the patient presents.

◆ Orchidectomy is the primary treatment for a testicular germ cell tumour which may be followed by further adjuvant treatment if required. For seminomas, this is radiotherapy to the retroperitoneal nodes. For NSGCTs, systemic chemotherapy is administered.

◆ The tumour markers AFP, HCG, and LDH are useful in the management of patients with testicular germ cell tumours.

◆ Sex cord stromal tumours are much less common than germ cell tumours and comprise two tumours: Leydig cell tumour and Sertoli cell tumour.

◆ Testicular lymphomas typically occur in elderly men. Most are high grade lymphomas and the prognosis is poor.

Tumors of the penis

Penile cancer is uncommon, mostly occurring in elderly men. Almost all penile cancers are squamous cell carcinomas. The main risk factors are being uncircumcized and human papillomavirus infection. The most common presentation is a hard painless lump on the glans penis. Often the tumour is surprisingly large at presentation, because it either has gone unnoticed under the foreskin or has been ignored.

Urinary tract infection

Lower urinary tract infection

With the exception of the terminal portion of the urethra, the urinary tract is normally sterile. The most essential natural defence is the flushing effect of urine preventing bacterial colonization. The urine also has properties that inhibit bacterial colonization and growth, for instance the Tamm–Horsfall glycoprotein inhibits bacterial adherence.

Consequently any structural abnormality that impedes urinary flow increases the risk of urinary tract infection (UTI), particularly obstruction at any level of the urinary tract. Similarly, foreign bodies, e.g. stones and catheters, allows bacteria to hide away from the natural defences.

Urinary tract infections result from ascending spread of bacteria up the urethra

Virtually all UTIs are caused by ascending spread of gastrointestinal bacteria up the urethra. The shorter urethra of women and its closer proximity to the rectum is thought to be the main reason why females are more susceptible than males to UTI throughout life. It is also likely that sexual intercourse assists the access of bacteria into the bladder in women.

The most common microbe causing urinary tract infection is E. coli

Escherichia coli is a common cause of UTI. Of the many strains of *E. coli*, only some are common causes of urinary tract infection due to increased ability to adhere to urothelial cells. They possess pili with protein components that preferentially bind to galactose-containing receptors on the cell surface of urothelial cells.

Once attachment to urothelial epithelial cells has occurred, other virulence factors become important, such as the production of haemolysin which allows tissue invasion, and the presence of the K antigen on the invading bacteria protects them from phagocytosis by neutrophils. These factors allow the bacteria to escape the host defences.

INTERESTING TO KNOW

Cranberry juice and urinary tract infection

The folk wisdom that cranberry juice prevents and helps cure bladder infections has been shown to be true; it prevents *E. coli* from forming fimbriae and so they cannot bind to urothelial cells.

Frequency and dysuria are the main symptoms of lower urinary tract infection

The most common symptoms of UTI are frequent urination (**frequency**), an urgent desire to urinate (**urgency**), and painful urination (**dysuria**). There may also be suprapubic pain. Confirming the diagnosis relies on urinalysis and urine culture. Urinalysis provides a rapid screen for UTI, but the gold standard for identification of UTI is culturing of the urine for bacteria.

A correctly collected midstream urine specimen is the ideal specimen to confirm UTI

The ideal specimen is a correctly collected midstream urine specimen (MSU) which should be sent to the microbiology laboratory as soon as possible after voiding (urine specimens deteriorate very quickly at room temperature).

In the laboratory, the specimen is examined under the microscope and the numbers of neutrophils and erythrocytes are counted. Significant pyuria suggestive of UTI is present when there are greater than 10^8 cells/ml urine. The urine is then diluted and spread onto culture plates. The number of bacterial colonies which grow are counted and adjusted per millilitre of urine (colony-forming unit (c.f.u)/ml).

The significance of bacteria isolated from a urine culture depends on the number of c.f.u/ml and the number of bacterial species present. A threshold of 10^5 c.f.u/ml is generally used. Contamination of the specimen is usually indicated by very low counts of organisms or mixed species.

Pyuria in the absence of significant bacterial growth is known as 'sterile pyuria'. Possible reasons for sterile pyuria include antibiotic treatment prior to urine collection, or infection with organisms that do not grow on the routine media for urine culture, such as mycobacteria and anaerobic bacteria.

Renal tuberculosis

Only a small percentage of patients with pulmonary tuberculosis develop genitourinary disease, although urinary disease is one of the more common forms of extrapulmonary tuberculosis. The organisms reach the kidneys by haematogenous spread from the lungs during the initial infection. In most cases, the immune response contains the infection. If, however, the organisms are of high virulence or there is a poor immune response, infection may become established.

Tuberculosis of the kidney develops slowly over a period of 15–20 years. During this period, there are usually no symptoms, so much so that renal tuberculosis is probably underdiagnosed. Many cases are diagnosed as a result of the chance finding of sterile pyuria on urine stick testing. Patients with symptoms due to renal tuberculosis have more advanced disease, with considerable destruction of renal tissue. Infected material passing through the urinary tract can lead to spread to other organs including the bladder, prostate, epididymis, and testes.

The diagnosis of genitourinary tuberculosis requires isolation of *Mycobacterium tuberculosis* in the urine following suitable culture. The urine is processed to suppress faster growing commensal bacteria and then cultured for mycobacteria on a specialized medium (e.g. Lowenstein–Jensen). Early morning urine is more likely to grow the organism than samples obtained at other times.

Urethritis

Urethral discharge in males is usually caused by sexually transmitted infection

Urethritis is often caused by sexually transmitted infection. Clinically, urethritis is divided into gonococcal urethritis and non-gonococcal urethritis.

Non-gonococcal urethritis is much more common in the UK. Most of these are due to *Chlamydia trachomatis*, and patients typically describe a sensation of urethral 'itching'. Gonococcal urethritis is due to sexually transmitted infection with *Neisseria gonorrhoeae*. Patients with gonococcal urethritis tend to present with a more purulent discharge and dysuria, i.e. pain on urination.

A Gram stain performed on a smear of purulent urethral discharge is a good means of detecting *N. gonorrhoeae*, which appear as intracellular Gram negative diplococci. If these organisms cannot be detected but the presence of numerous neutrophils confirms a urethritis, then a non-gonococcal urethritis is diagnosed. Detection of *C. trachomatis* traditionally required culturing the organism from a distal urethral swab. However, culturing *Chlamydia* is slow and unreliable and so is being replaced by molecular methods such as polymerase chain reaction (PCR) on a first void urine specimen.

Treatment for gonococcal urethritis is usually a single dose of ciprofloxacin. Chlamydial urethritis requires a 7 day course of doxycycline. A single dose of azithromycin is also effective for chlamydial urethritis but costs more; however, this may be preferred if compliance is likely to be a problem.

Prostatitis

Acute bacterial prostatitis is inflammation of the prostate associated with a UTI. The infection is thought to occur from ascending urethral infection and reflux of infected urine from the bladder into prostatic ducts. Patients present feeling unwell with fever and urinary symptoms. Digital rectal examination reveals a swollen tender prostate. It frequently affects adult men. *Escherichia coli* is the most common organism.

Epididymitis

Infection of the epididymis most often results from ascending infection from the lower urinary tract. In men under 35, it is usually due to a sexually transmitted organism such as *C. trachomatis* or *N. gonorrhoeae*. In men over 35, it is usually due to ascending infection with *E. coli*.

Epididymitis tends to present with severe, unilateral testicular pain developing over a number of hours or days. The main problem in young men is that it may be impossible to differentiate from testicular torsion, in which case immediate hospital referral is mandatory. Once correctly diagnosed, antibiotic treatment is usually successful, though it is important to remember that in cases due to a sexually transmitted organism, taking a sexual history and screening sexual partners is mandatory.

Common miscellaneous urological conditions

Hydrocele

A hydrocele is a collection of fluid in the tunica vaginalis

A **hydrocele** occurs when fluid accumulates in the space between the two layers of the tunica vaginalis. The tunica vaginalis is a mesothelial-lined sac which surrounds the testis and epididymis. Hydroceles are one of the most common causes of a scrotal swelling

and are usually a reaction to underlying pathology such as epididymitis, orchitis, or a tumour. One should therefore always be suspicious of an acute hydrocele developing in a young man and always be sure to rule out the possibility of an underlying neoplasm.

Varicocele

A varicocele is a persistent dilation of the testicular veins

A **varicocele** is a persistent abnormal dilation of the pampiniform plexus of veins in the spermatic cord. Varicoceles are more common on the left side where the testicular vein drains vertically into the renal vein. They are usually apparent as a nodularity on the lateral side of the scrotum. Most varicoceles are asymptomatic, but they can ache, especially after prolonged standing or towards the end of the day. More importantly, it is thought that varicoceles may be a cause of male subfertility because the increased blood flow raises scrotal temperature and impairs spermatogenesis.

Epididymal cysts

Epididymal cysts are common and benign

Epididymal cysts are common and are found in a high percentage of men who have ultrasonography. They may contain serous fluid or spermatozoa. Most epididymal cysts do not cause pain, but men can be alarmed on finding them. Epididymal cysts are entirely benign, and treatment is generally not required unless they are very large and bothersome.

Torsion of the testis

Torsion of the testis is a surgical emergency

In some men, the testis is particularly mobile due to an inappropriately high attachment of the tunica vaginalis. This so-called 'bell clapper' deformity allows the testis to swing freely on the spermatic cord. If the testis spontaneously twists completely around the spermatic cord, then the venous drainage is cut off leading to venous infarction of the testis.

Testicular torsion is most often seen in men younger than 30 years, with most presenting between 12 and 18 years of age. The typical presentation is the sudden onset of severe scrotal pain with swelling. Timing is critical in suspected testicular torsion. Nearly all testicles untwisted and fixed within 6 h will survive; the majority treated after 12 h will suffer at least some atrophy.

Balanitis xerotica obliterans

Balanitis xerotica obliterans is a common cause of phimosis in adult men

Balanitis is inflammation of the glans penis. Balanitis xerotica obliterans is an idiopathic chronic inflammatory condition of the glans and prepuce characterized by formation of hard white plaques and fissures. It is most commonly seen in the 30–50 year age group. The tissue underneath the squamous epithelium becomes scarred and thickened such that the foreskin cannot be retracted (**phimosis**). Balanitis xerotica obliterans is therefore a common indication for circumcision.

LINK BOX

Balanitis xerotica obliterans and lichen sclerosus

Balanitis xerotica obliterans has precisely the same microscopic appearances as the vulval lesion lichen sclerosus seen in women (p. 252), and the two conditions are considered to be the same.

Gynaecological disease

Introduction

The female genital tract comprises the vulva, vagina, uterus, fallopian tubes, and ovaries. Note that the cervix is part of the uterus, but it is useful to consider it separately from the rest of the uterus as the diseases which affect the cervix are quite distinct from those of the main body of the uterus. Often the vulva, vagina, and cervix are collectively referred to as the 'lower genital tract' and the rest of the uterus, fallopian tubes, and ovaries are known as the 'upper genital tract'.

Diseases of the female genital tract are extremely common. Infections and malignant tumours are the most important types of diseases affecting the female genital tract. Infections predominantly arise in the lower genital tract but can spread by ascending infection into the upper genital tract with potentially serious consequences such as infertility.

Malignant tumours of the lower genital tract are usually squamous cell carcinomas, most of which are driven by persistent infection with human papillomavirus (HPV). Malignant tumours of the upper genital tract are usually adenocarcinomas and are not associated with HPV infection.

As it is a major cause of female genital tract disease, it is worthwhile at this point briefly to discuss HPV infection.

Human papillomavirus infection of the female genital tract

Human papillomavirus is a DNA virus that infects the surface epithelium of skin and mucosa (e.g. genital tract and oral cavity). Infection is initiated when minor trauma (e.g. sexual intercourse or skin abrasion) exposes the basal cells of the epithelium to infectious virus particles. The virus infects the basal cells and stimulates their proliferation.

There are over 100 different types of HPV, and each is specific to a site of infection, i.e. cutaneous HPV types do not readily infect mucosal epithelium, and vice versa. The HPV types most relevant to the genital tract are types 6, 11, 16, and 18.

Almost all young women are exposed to HPV once they become sexually active. The infection may involve the epithelium of the vulva, vagina, and cervix. Co-involvement of the perineum and anus may also occur. Most HPV infections are of relatively short duration as most women will clear the virus. Only a small proportion of women (<10 per cent) exposed to HPV become persistently infected and continue to have detectable levels of HPV DNA in the genital epithelium. It is these persistently infected women who are at risk of developing neoplasms.

Anogenital warts are benign proliferations caused by infection with so-called 'low risk' types of HPV (types 6 and 11). Whilst these may be troublesome and recurrent, they are not associated with malignant transformation. Persistent infection with 'high risk' types of HPV (types 16 and 18) are more worrying as these can lead to the development of dysplasia and eventually carcinoma in a small proportion of women.

> ## Key points: Human papillomavirus infection of the female genital tract
>
> - HPV infects the basal epithelial cells of skin and mucosal surfaces following minor trauma.
> - HPV infection of the genital tract is almost universal in sexually active young women.
> - Most women develop transient infection and clear the virus.
> - Persistent infection leads to sustained proliferation of the infected epithelium.
> - Low risk HPV types cause benign warts of the vulva, vagina, and cervix.
> - High risk HPV types can lead to malignant transformation of the epithelium and eventually give rise to carcinomas of the vulva, vagina, or cervix in a small proportion of women.

Vulva

The **vulva** encompasses the entirety of the female external genitalia which includes the mons pubis, labia majora, labia minora, clitoris, and vestibule. The vulva is covered mostly by skin, and so most vulval disorders are skin diseases. Neoplasms of the vulva are less common but are important to be aware of.

TABLE 12.1	Common vulval skin disorders
Atopic dermatitis	
Contact dermatitis	
Psoriasis	
Lichen sclerosus	
Lichen planus	

Vulval skin disorders

A number of common dermatological conditions commonly affect the vulva (Table 12.1). Distinguishing between them can be challenging as women often present late due to embarrassment, by which time the typical features of the skin disorder may have been masked by the effects of scratching and attempts at self-treatment.

Seborrhoeic dermatitis is the most common vulval dermatitis

Seborrhoeic dermatitis is an inflammatory skin disorder which affects the sebum-rich areas of skin such as the scalp, eyebrows, face, and genitalia. Vulval seborrhoeic dermatitis presents with vulval itching and erythema. Thickening and excoriations may develop secondary to scratching. The main difficulty with seborrhoeic dermatitis is distinguishing it from psoriasis, which can look identical both clinically and microscopically.

Psoriasis of the vulva may not show the typical appearances seen elsewhere in the body

Psoriasis is a common chronic relapsing and remitting inflammatory skin disorder characterized by scaling pink plaques. The vulva may be affected in isolation or as a part of a more generalized complaint. Women with widespread psoriasis elsewhere may have co-involvement of the perineum and labia, in which case the diagnosis is not difficult. Occasionally, however, the disease can be confined to the vulva which may make diagnosis more problematic, especially if the patient has the flexural variant of psoriasis. This variant lacks the typical scales of classical psoriatic plaques, making it look very similar to seborrhoeic dermatitis (Fig. 12.1).

Irritant contact dermatitis commonly affects the vulva

The delicate vulval skin is particularly susceptible to irritant contact dermatitis as it is exposed to a number

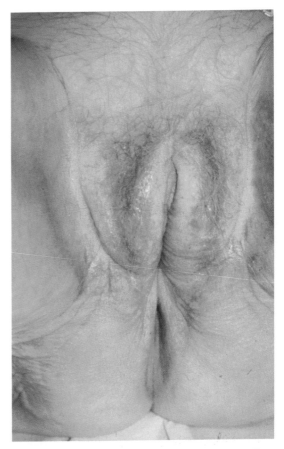

Fig. 12.1 Psoriasis of the vulva, flexural variant. Note the well demarcated, intensely erythematous eruption involving the vulva and groins. Scaling is typically absent in flexural disease.

of potential irritants such as soaps, bubble baths, washing powders, and fabric conditioners. Sweating may exacerbate any irritation, as will mechanical trauma from towels or from scratching.

Avoidance of fragranced toiletries, wearing loose fitting clothing, and applying simple barrier ointments is the first-line strategy in managing irritant dermatitis. Only if these simple measures fail should topical steroids be considered.

Lichen planus is an intensely itchy inflammatory skin disease

Lichen planus is an inflammatory disease of skin and mucosa of unknown cause which often involves the vulva. Patients with vulval lichen planus have a wide age range, but it presents most commonly in women below 40 years of age. The appearances may be highly variable, ranging from small purple papules to an erosive process with ulceration. White lace-like plaques involving the vaginal mucosa may also be present.

Because of the variable appearances, lichen planus is probably the most underdiagnosed vulval inflammatory skin disorder. Most cases of lichen planus resolve over a period of weeks to months with topical steroid treatment, though the erosive form may heal with permanent scarring.

Lichen sclerosus predisposes to the development of squamous cell carcinoma of the vulva

Lichen sclerosus is an inflammatory vulval skin disorder of unknown cause that affects about 1 in 1000 women. Severe persistent vulval itching, particularly at night, is the typical presentation of lichen sclerosus.

The appearance can vary considerably, but classically the affected skin becomes white, thin, and parchment like with fine wrinkling. Scattered purpuric areas are common (Fig. 12.2). Long-standing disease results in the development of vulval deformities with shrinkage of the labia minora.

Biopsy of the area is usually performed to confirm the diagnosis and rule out any co-existing neoplasia. Correct recognition and treatment with topical steroids can stop the distressing symptoms and prevent vulval deformities.

Patients with lichen sclerosus require long-term follow-up because it is associated with a small but significant risk of differentiated vulval intraepithelial neoplasia (VIN) and subsequent invasive squamous cell carcinoma in later life (see below).

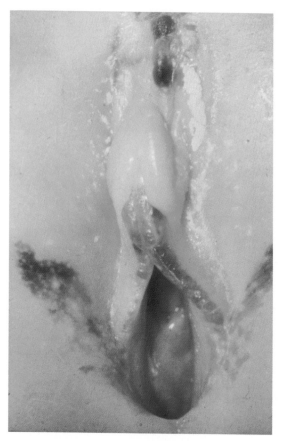

Fig. 12.2 Lichen sclerosus of the vulva. Note symmetrical white lesions with marked atrophy and spots of haemorrhage.

LINK BOX

Balanitis xerotica obliterans and lichen sclerosus

Lichen sclerosus of the vulva is identical to the disease **balanitis xerotica obliterans** which affects the foreskin of the penis in men and can lead to phimosis (p. 248).

Key points: Vulval skin disorders

- The vulva is covered with skin so dermatological complaints are common vulval problems.

- Many women present late due to embarrassment, by which time the typical appearances of the skin disease may have been altered by the effects of rubbing, scratching, and attempts at self-treatment.

- Seborrhoeic dermatitis is the most common vulval skin disorder and may appear very similar to psoriasis.

Key points: Vulval skin disorders—cont'd

- ◆ Psoriasis can affect the vulva as part of a generalized disease or in isolation. Isolated vulval psoriasis may be difficult to diagnose especially if the appearance is not typical.

- ◆ Irritant contact dermatitis is common due to contents of soaps, bubble baths, and washing powders, together with the effects of sweating and mechanical trauma.

- ◆ Lichen planus is an intensely itchy inflammatory skin disease with a variety of possible appearances which usually resolves over a period of weeks to months with steroid treatment.

- ◆ Lichen sclerosus is an inflammatory skin disorder of unknown cause which leads to thinning of the epidermis. It is associated with a small risk of developing differentiated vulval intraepithelial neoplasia and vulval squamous cell carcinoma.

Vulval neoplasms

The role of HPV in the vulva is similar to that in the vagina and cervix. By infecting the squamous epithelium it may lead to vulval warts, VIN, and squamous cell carcinoma. The finding of any of these HPV-related conditions in the vulva should prompt a thorough examination of the lower genital tract to look for HPV-related diseases of the vagina and cervix, and for other sexually transmitted diseases.

Vulval warts are caused by infection with low risk HPV

Vulval warts are caused by persistent infection with low risk types of HPV, usually type 6. Warts may be flat (**flat condyloma**) or frond-like papillary growths (**condyloma acuminatum**). Whilst vulval warts are benign neoplasms with no capacity for malignant transformation, the presence of warts is important as a marker of sexually transmitted disease.

Vulval intraepithelial neoplasia is a pre-malignant condition

Vulval intraepithelial neoplasia (VIN) is a neoplastic disorder in which the squamous epithelium of the vulva shows evidence of dysplasia microscopically, i.e. disordered maturation with nuclear abnormalities of keratinocytes. Two distinct types of VIN are recognized: undifferentiated VIN and differentiated VIN.

Undifferentiated VIN is related to HPV infection

Undifferentiated VIN is by far the more common type of VIN. It is seen in women of reproductive age in whom it is strongly related to persistent infection of the squamous epithelium of the vulva by high risk types of HPV, particularly type 16. Almost all women with this form of VIN are smokers.

It is thought that VIN develops in women who fail to mount an appropriate immune response to HPV infection. This theory is corroborated by the fact that immunosuppressed women (e.g. those with HIV) are at particular risk of developing VIN.

Undifferentiated VIN is divided into three grades of increasing severity (VIN 1, 2, and 3) according to the severity of the changes in the epithelium on a biopsy in the same way as is used for cervical intraepithelial neoplasia (CIN) in the cervix.

Differentiated VIN is related to chronic inflammatory skin disease

Differentiated VIN is characterized microscopically by atypical squamous cells confined to the basal region with normal differentiation above it. This form is much less common than the undifferentiated form and differs in several respects from it: differentiated VIN occurs in older women, is usually unifocal, and is not associated with HPV infection. Instead differentiated VIN usually arises on a background of lichen sclerosus.

Note that despite the name suggesting a lower grade lesion, differentiated VIN is actually associated with a significantly greater risk of progression to squamous cell carcinoma than even the severe forms of undifferentiated VIN.

VIN may present with persistent vulval itching or a visible lesion

Women with VIN may present with persistent vulval itching and irritation or may observe the lesions and seek medical assistance. Visible VIN lesions may be flat (macules) or raised (papules), and may look white, red, or pigmented. A biopsy is essential to confirm the diagnosis and to rule out the presence of invasion (i.e. a squamous cell carcinoma).

VIN is usually treated with local excision. This is not a problem if the disease is localized, but widespread disease may necessitate removal of larger areas of vulval skin with skin grafting. Patients found to have undifferentiated VIN associated with HPV must also have a thorough vaginal and cervical examination to look for co-existing HPV-related dysplasia at these sites.

Vulval squamous cell carcinomas develop from VIN

Vulval carcinoma represents only a small percentage of tumours of the female genital tract, but is important to be aware of. The vast majority are squamous cell carcinomas which develop when an area of VIN breaches the underlying basement membrane and becomes invasive. Note, however, that only a small minority of all cases of VIN ever progress into a squamous cell carcinoma.

The aetiology and epidemiology of vulval squamous carcinomas is similar to that of VIN, developing either in young smokers with persistent HPV infection or in older women on a background of lichen sclerosus.

The first symptom attributable to a vulval squamous cell carcinoma is often persistent pruritus. As the tumour grows, an obvious mass becomes apparent which may ulcerate and bleed. Vulval carcinoma typically spreads by direct extension and via lymphatics to the inguinal lymph nodes. Recurrence after surgical excision tends to be local, with distant metastases being less common.

Key points: Vulval neoplasms

- Important vulval neoplasms include vulval warts, vulval intraepithelial neoplasia (VIN), and vulval squamous cell carcinoma.

- Most vulval neoplasms are related to persistent infection with HPV and are a marker for other sexually transmitted diseases.

- Vulval warts are benign neoplasms caused by low risk HPV types.

- VIN is a pre-malignant condition which may present with vulval itching or a visible lesion.

- Undifferentiated VIN occurs in younger women (30–40 years of age), is associated with persistent HPV infection, and is usually multifocal. Undifferentiated VIN is divided into three grades according to the extent of dysplasia in the epithelium.

- Differentiated VIN occurs in older women (50–60 years of age), is usually associated with lichen sclerosus, and is usually unifocal. Differentiated VIN is always high grade.

- Treatment of VIN is usually by surgical excision of the involved area.

- A minority of cases of VIN progress to invasive squamous cell carcinoma which causes vulval pruritus and eventually a palpable lump which may ulcerate and bleed.

Vagina

The vagina is a muscular tube which extends from the vestibule to the uterus, where it attaches to the vaginal portion of the cervix. It is lined by non-keratinized stratified squamous epithelium.

Infections are the most common and important diseases of the vagina. Although HPV can infect the vagina much like the vulva and cervix, the development of vaginal intraepithelial neoplasia and squamous cell carcinoma of the vagina is extremely rare.

Vaginal infections

Vaginal infection is one of the most common problems in clinical medicine

The normal vagina is colonized predominantly with lactobacilli. These are Gram positive bacilli which convert glucose to lactic acid, thereby maintaining the normal vaginal pH at under 4.5. The acidic environment helps inhibit the growth of many pathogens.

The factors that alter the normal vaginal 'ecosystem' and predispose to vaginal infections are not well understood. The three most common infections are bacterial vaginosis, candidiasis, and trichomoniasis. Trichomoniasis is the only one known to be sexually transmitted.

Bacterial vaginosis is caused by overgrowth of anaerobic bacteria in the vagina

Bacterial vaginosis is the most common cause of an abnormal vaginal discharge. It does not appear to be caused by a single organism. Instead there is a loss of the normal lactobacilli with overgrowth of anaerobic bacteria such as *Gardnerella vaginalis* and *Bacteroides* species. The metabolic products of these bacteria include volatile amines which gives the discharge a distinctive fishy odour. There is no actual inflammation in the vaginal wall unlike in trichomoniasis and candidiasis, which is why the term vaginosis (as opposed to vaginitis) is used.

Candidal infection of the vulva and vagina is a common problem

Vulvovaginal candidiasis (yeast infection, or 'thrush') is a common infection, particularly in young women. The most common fungal organism implicated is *Candida albicans*. Candidiasis presents with vulvovaginal itching and burning, together with pain on intercourse (dyspareunia), and stinging on urination (dysuria). A thick white discharge is common, often likened to cottage cheese. Recurrent *Candida* infections are often seen in patients with an underlying disorder such as diabetes or immunosuppression.

Trichomoniasis is a sexually transmitted disease

Trichomonas vaginalis is a flagellate protozoan which is sexually transmitted. The male partner is usually asymptomatic and half of infected women are also asymptomatic. Women with symptoms usually complain of vaginal pruritus and a thin, frothy, offensive discharge. Dyspareunia and dysuria may also occur. Treatment with metronidazole is usually effective, although reinfection can be a problem, especially if the male partner is not treated at the same time.

Simple microbiological tests can help determine the cause of a vaginal infection

A sample of vaginal discharge can be tested in a number of ways to help determine the cause of a vaginal infection (Table 12.2):

- Microscopy of a wet mount slide. A sample of the discharge is placed on a glass microscope slide and mixed with normal saline. The prepared slide is then examined under the microscope for pseudohyphae, trichomonads, and clue cells. Trichomonads are usually easy to spot because their flagellae enable

TABLE 12.2 Diagnostic features of vaginal infections

	Bacterial vaginosis	Trichomoniasis	Candidiasis
pH	>4.5	>4.5	<4.5
Whiff test	Positive	Positive	Negative
Wet prep	Clue cells	Motile trichomonads	Pseudohyphae

them to move. Clue cells are squamous epithelial cells coated with adherent bacterial colonies which are seen in bacterial vaginosis.

- Whiff test. A further sample of the discharge is placed on a slide and mixed with a few drops of 10 per cent potassium hydroxide. The presence of a strong fishy odour is noted in bacterial vaginosis and trichomoniasis.

- pH testing. The pH of the discharge should be determined using pH paper. The normal vaginal pH is between 3.8 and 4.5. A pH higher than 4.5 suggests either bacterial vaginosis or trichomoniasis, though note that recent unprotected sexual intercourse may also cause a high pH value as semen is alkaline.

- Culture. *Candida albicans* can be cultured in the laboratory.

Key points: Vaginal infections

- The most common vaginal infections are bacterial vaginosis, trichomoniasis, and candidiasis.

- Bacterial vaginosis is caused by loss of the normal lactobacilli flora and overgrowth of a mixture of organisms. There is a thin discharge with a characteristic fishy odour.

- Vulvovaginal candidiasis is usually caused by *Candida albicans* and manifests with vulval and vaginal itching and a thick white discharge.

- Trichomoniasis is a sexually transmitted disease caused by a protozoan which gives a foul-smelling thick yellow discharge.

- Examination of a sample of vaginal discharge by a combination of microscopy, the whiff test, pH measurement, and culture helps determine the underlying cause of the infection.

Cervix

The cervix is the inferior portion of the uterus. Its upper end communicates with the endometrial cavity via the **internal os** and the lower end opens into the vagina at the **external os**.

By far the most important disease of the cervix is cervical carcinoma and its precursor lesions. Other common diseases of the cervix which we will discuss are infections and endocervical polyps.

Cervicitis

Significant inflammation of the cervix is usually caused by sexually transmitted infections

Some degree of cervical inflammation is seen in nearly all adult women in the absence of infection and is usually of no significance. More severe inflammation is usually the result of infection of the cervix. The responsible organisms are usually *Chlamydia trachomatis* and *Neisseria gonorrhoeae*, both of which are sexually transmitted bacteria. In the UK, chlamydial cervicitis is much more common than gonococcal cervicitis.

If symptoms occur from cervicitis they may include vaginal discharge (derived from the cervix), pain during intercourse, or intermenstrual bleeding. Asymptomatic patients may present because their partner has been found to have a sexually transmitted infection.

Women with symptoms suggestive of cervicitis must have their cervix examined using a vaginal speculum. The cervix appears swollen and red, often with a plug of pus exuding from the external os (Fig. 12.3). The mucus covering the vaginal surface of the cervix should be cleaned away with a fresh cotton swab. A sterile swab is then used to obtain a sample from the endocervix for microscopy and culture. *Chlamydia trachomatis* can be cultured in the laboratory, though it is difficult and unreliable. PCR testing on urine is now the preferred way to identify this organism.

Many cases of cervicitis go undiagnosed with a danger of developing pelvic inflammatory disease

Because women with cervicitis are often asymptomatic, many of them go undiagnosed. The danger of untreated cervicitis is ascending infection into the upper female genital tract. Infection of the upper genital tract is usually termed **pelvic inflammatory disease** and can have significant consequences such as infertility (see later).

> ## Key points: Cervicitis
>
> - Minor degrees of inflammation are common in the cervix and are of no clinical significance.
>
> - Severe cervicitis is usually due to sexually transmitted infection with *Chlamydia trachomatis* or *Neisseria gonorrhoeae*. Chlamydial cervicitis is more common in the UK.
>
> - Most cases of cervicitis are asymptomatic and go undiagnosed. The danger of untreated cervicitis is ascending infection and the development of pelvic inflammatory disease which can cause infertility.
>
> - Women who are diagnosed with cervicitis either do so because their partner has been found to have a sexually transmissible infection, or they have symptoms due to the cervicitis such as discharge, dyspareunia, or intermenstrual bleeding.
>
> - In cervicitis, the cervix appears red and swollen, often with mucopurulent discharge exuding from the external os. A sterile swab should be used to obtain an endocervical sample to identify the causative organism.

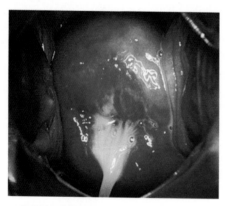

Fig. 12.3 Cervicitis. The cervix is inflamed and there is mucopurulent material exuding from the external os.

Endocervical polyps

Endocervical polyps are a common cause of intermenstrual bleeding

Endocervical polyps are benign overgrowths of the endocervix which project into the endocervical canal.

They probably represent polypoid areas of inflamed endocervix rather than true neoplasms. Endocervical polyps are important because the tip can erode or ulcerate, giving rise to intermenstrual bleeding and concern for sinister pathology such as cervical carcinoma. Endocervical polyps appear to have no significant risk of malignant transformation, and simple curettage is usually curative.

Cervical squamous neoplasia

Cervical squamous neoplasia arises in the transformation zone of the cervix

In order to understand cervical neoplasia, it is essential to appreciate the normal microanatomy of the cervix (Fig. 12.4). Before puberty, the cervix consists of the ectocervix and the endocervix. The ectocervix is covered by squamous epithelium and the endocervix is covered by mucin-secreting glandular epithelium. The ectocervix meets the endocervix at the external os.

Around puberty, the rise in female sex steroid hormones causes the cervix to change shape such that the lower part of the endocervix comes to lie on the vaginal portion of the cervix where it is visible as a roughened, red area. It appears red because the underlying blood vessels are visible through the thin single layer of columnar epithelial cells and looks rough because the endocervix is thrown into villous folds. The presence of visible endocervix is known as an ectropion (derived from the word 'ectopic').

Exposure of the sensitive columnar epithelium to the acidic environment of the vagina induces squamous metaplasia, i.e. the fragile columnar epithelium undergoes a change to a tougher and thicker squamous type of epithelium better equipped to protect the area from the acidic environment. The area of the cervix that becomes covered by this new squamous epithelium, between the original squamous-lined ectocervix and the columnar-lined endocervix, is known as the **transformation zone**. *The transformation zone is of utmost importance as it is within this metaplastic epithelium that virtually all cervical neoplasia arises.*

Note that the formation of the transformation zone is an entirely physiological process which occurs in all women at puberty. The development of neoplasia within the transformation zone, however, is a pathological event associated with persistent infection with HPV.

JARGON BUSTER

Cervical erosion

The term 'cervical erosion' has become engrained in medical terminology as people thought the raw red area of an ectropion represented an area of epithelial loss or erosion. There is no evidence that this is the case, and the term cervical erosion should not be used when describing an ectropion.

Infection with high risk HPV is the main cause of cervical neoplasia

In the presence of HPV infection, the physiological metaplastic process which gives rise to the transformation zone may be diverted into a neoplastic process (Fig. 12.5). Important epidemiological evidence supports the key role of high risk HPV (particularly types 16 and 18) in cervical neoplasia.

Cervical neoplasia has a low incidence in virgins, and a high incidence in people who have multiple sexual partners and became sexually active at an early age. Furthermore, high risk HPV types can be detected using molecular techniques in virtually all cases of cervical cancer.

INTERESTING TO KNOW

HPV vaccines

One of the first trials of a genetically engineered vaccine against HPV types 6, 11, 16, and 18 has shown extremely promising results. In a prospective, randomized, double-blind, placebo-controlled trial, none of the women given the vaccine developed high grade CIN!

The E6 and E7 proteins of HPV are known to be crucial in cervical carcinogenesis

The high risk HPV types associated with cervical carcinogenesis produce two proteins which have been shown to be oncogenic. The E6 protein is capable of binding to p53 and targeting it for degradation. Without p53, cells are unable to halt cell division in the presence of DNA damage, allowing genetic mutations

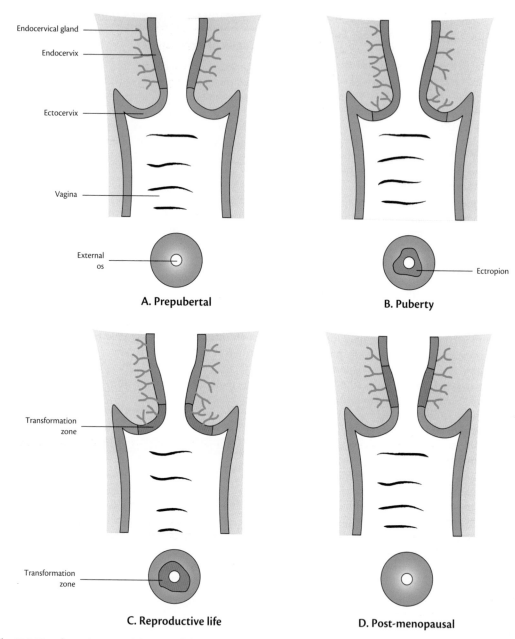

Fig. 12.4 Transformation zone of the cervix. (A) Before puberty, the ectocervix covered by squamous epithelium meets the endocervical epithelium at the external os. (B) At puberty, the lower endocervix becomes exposed to the vagina and is visible as a rough red area (ectropion). (C) The endocervical epithelium undergoes squamous metaplasia in response to the acidic environment of the vagina, creating the transformation zone where squamous epithelium overlies endocervical glands. It is this process which is diverted into a potentially neoplastic pathway by persistent infection with high risk types of human papillomavirus. The transformation zone is visible and must be completely sampled when taking a cervical smear. (D) After the menopause, the cervix involutes such that the transformation zone is drawn up into the endocervical canal.

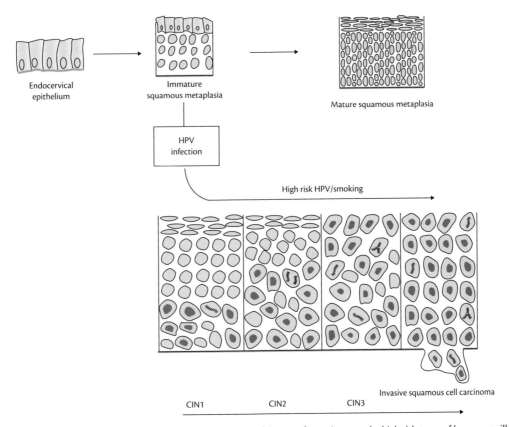

Fig. 12.5 Infection of immature squamous metaplastic epithelium of the transformation zone by high risk types of human papillomavirus (HPV) diverts the metaplastic process into a neoplastic process. Persistent infection in some women leads to the development of increasing degrees of cervical intraepithelial neoplasia (CIN). In a small minority of untreated women, an invasive squamous cell carcinoma develops.

to accumulate. The E7 protein has a similar effect on the Rb protein. As the Rb protein normally blocks cell cycling, degradation of Rb stimulated by E7 leads to permanent cell cycling.

Cervical squamous neoplasia progresses through increasing degrees of CIN into squamous carcinoma

The earliest recognizable neoplastic change in the cervix is the presence of microscopic dysplasia of the metaplastic squamous epithelium of the transformation zone, known as **cervical intraepithelial neoplasia** or CIN.

CIN is a continuous disease process with varying degrees of nuclear abnormality and extent of involvement of the squamous epithelium (Fig. 12.5). For practical

purposes, this continuous process is divided into three grades of increasing severity known as CIN 1, 2, and 3 according to how much of the metaplastic squamous epithelium is dysplastic.

CIN 1 involves only the lower third of the epithelium, CIN 2 extends into the middle third, and CIN 3 involves the full thickness of the epithelium. If an area of CIN 3 breaches the underlying basement membrane, the neoplastic lesion is called a squamous cell carcinoma.

Only a small percentage of women infected with high risk HPV develop dysplasia or carcinoma

It is very important to appreciate that of all the people infected with HPV, only a very small proportion develop CIN, and only a very small proportion of people with CIN go on to develop invasive carcinoma.

We do not know why infection persists in some women or what factors determine who will go on to develop cervical carcinoma, but the nature of an individual's immune response to the virus is likely to be key. Women who are immunosuppressed for any reason are known to be at greater risk of developing invasive carcinoma. Women who smoke are also known to be at greater risk of high grade CIN and invasive carcinoma, and this is probably also related to effects on the immune system.

> ◆ Only a small proportion of women infected with high risk HPV develop CIN, and of these only a small proportion develop squamous cell carcinoma. Our knowledge about why certain women go on to develop high grade CIN and squamous cell carcinoma and others do not is minimal, though the nature of the immune response to HPV is likely to be crucial.

Key points: Cervical squamous neoplasia

◆ Cervical squamous neoplasia arises in the transformation zone of the cervix which develops in all women at puberty when the lower part of the endocervix comes into contact with the acidic environment of the vagina and undergoes squamous metaplasia.

◆ Cervical squamous neoplasia occurs when high risk types of HPV persistently infect the metaplastic squamous epithelium of the transformation zone, diverting the metaplastic process into a neoplastic process.

◆ The high risk types of HPV have transforming properties by virtue of two viral proteins known as E6 and E7 which inhibit the actions of the tumour-suppressor genes p53 and retinoblastoma, respectively.

◆ The earliest recognizable lesion in cervical squamous neoplasia is cervical intraepithelial neoplasia or CIN.

◆ CIN has three grades of severity depending how much of the metaplastic squamous epithelium is dysplastic.

◆ If high grade CIN breaches the basement membrane, the lesion is called a squamous cell carcinoma.

Cervical screening

Our knowledge that cervical squamous carcinoma arises from CIN means that potentially we could prevent all cases of cervical squamous carcinoma if we could pick up and treat every women with CIN. This theory has led to the development of cervical screening programmes which aim to do just that.

Diagnosing CIN requires careful inspection of the cervix to identify any abnormal areas, followed by biopsy. Clearly it is impractical to invite every woman in the at-risk age group for this investigation. Instead, we have a screening test known as a **cervical smear** which selects out those women who should have further examination of the cervix.

The cervical smear samples cells from the entire transformation zone for cytological examination

In the UK, the NHS cervical screening programme invites all women aged between 25 and 64 for regular cervical smears. The test involves visualizing the cervix and sampling the entire transformation zone of the cervix by scraping cells off its surface and smearing them on to a glass slide. The cells are immediately doused in fixative and then sent to the pathology laboratory.

On receipt in the laboratory, the slides are stained with the Papanicolaou ('Pap') stain and examined microscopically. As individual cells are being examined rather than whole cores of tissue, this is known as cervical *cytology*.

Cervical cytology looks for cervical squamous epithelial cells showing dyskaryosis

In the pathology laboratory, the stained slides are scrutinized for squamous epithelial cells showing dyskaryosis. **Dyskaryosis** is a term used in cytology which refers to abnormalities of the nucleus of a cell.

Dyskaryotic cells tend to have enlarged, irregularly shaped nuclei with dark chromatin.

Dyskaryosis in cervical smears is graded into low, moderate, or severe dyskaryosis depending on how severe the nuclear abnormalities are. Generally speaking, there is a good correlation between the grade of dyskaryosis found on cytology with the grade of CIN seen on a cervical biopsy.

If dyskaryosis is present the woman will be referred for colposcopy

The presence of high grade dyskaryosis or persistent low grade dyskaryosis on cervical smears should prompt referral of the woman to a colposcopy clinic. Colposcopy is usually performed in the gynaecology outpatient department in a hospital, either by a gynaecologist or a specialist nurse trained in colposcopy.

The cervix is visualized in detail with the help of a binocular microscope called a colposcope and an intense light source. Abnormalities in the appearance of the cervical epithelium can be identified which are not visible to the naked eye. Application of acetic acid to the cervix coagulates proteins in the superficial squamous cells and helps atypical areas stand out. Any suspicious areas are then biopsied for histopathological examination.

Microscopic examination of a cervical biopsy is required to confirm the presence of dysplasia

Histopathological examination of a cervical punch biopsy allows the examination of a small core of cervix with the tissue architecture intact. This confirms the presence of dysplasia and allows definitive grading of the level of CIN.

Patients with confirmed CIN 2 or 3 return to colposcopy where the entire transformation zone is removed using an electrical excision device, a technique known as **large loop excision of the transformation zone** (LLETZ) or **diathermy loop excision** (DLE). This cures the patient of CIN, preventing the chance of progression to invasive cancer.

The management of women with CIN 1 is controversial. Some may advise excision even though it is likely that most cases will regress. Others will simply monitor these women with follow-up smears and colposcopy.

Future developments in cervical screening

In the near future, the routine cervical smear may be supplemented, or even replaced, by DNA tests for high risk HPV strains in cells from the smear, with a smear or colposcopy reserved for those patients who test positive.

Key points: Cervical screening

- Cervical screening aims to detect and treat women with cervical abnormalities which if left untreated could progress into cervical carcinoma.

- The NHS cervical screening programme in the UK invites all women aged between 25 and 64 for regular cervical smears.

- Taking an adequate cervical smear involves sampling of the entire transformation zone by scraping cells from its surface and spreading them on to a glass slide.

- The slide is sent to a pathology laboratory where it is stained with the Papanicolaou stain and examined under a light microscope for squamous epithelial cells showing dyskaryosis.

- Dyskaryotic cells are graded into mild, moderate, or severe according to how abnormal their nuclei appear.

- Women with moderate or high grade dyskaryosis on a single smear, or persistent low grade dyskaryosis on multiple consecutive smears, are referred to colposcopy for close examination of the cervix. Any abnormal areas are biopsied for histological examination.

- If CIN is present in a cervical biopsy, the degree of dysplasia is graded into three categories of increasing severity: CIN 1, 2, and 3.

- Women with CIN 2 or 3 undergo a loop excision of the transformation zone to remove the CIN.

Continued

Key points: Cervical screening—cont'd

♦ Women with CIN 1 may also undergo excision or be monitored with follow-up smears and colposcopy.

♦ Dyskaryosis is a *cytological* term for nuclear abnormalities in cells on a cervical smear, whereas dysplasia is a *histological* term for abnormalities in the squamous epithelium seen on a cervical biopsy.

Squamous cell carcinoma of the cervix

The NHS cervical screening programme has been successful at substantially reducing the number of cases of cervical carcinoma in the UK. However, some 2000 women still present with an established cervical squamous carcinoma each year. These are women who either failed to attend for screening or who rapidly developed a squamous carcinoma in the period between screening tests.

Patients with invasive squamous carcinomas usually present with vaginal bleeding, particularly after intercourse (post-coital bleeding). Abnormal bleeding between menstrual periods may also occur (intermenstrual bleeding).

Treatment of cervical carcinoma involves surgery or radiotherapy, or a combination of both. Tumours that are amenable to surgery require radical hysterectomy (removal of the uterus and upper third of the vagina) and pelvic lymph node dissection. In older women, the fallopian tubes and ovaries are also removed. The two principle factors that determine the prognosis of cervical carcinoma are the size and depth of invasion of the tumour and the presence of lymph node metastases.

INTERESTING TO KNOW

Microinvasive cervical carcinoma

Sometimes very small carcinomas which show minimal invasion are picked up in a cervical biopsy carried out as part of the screening programme. These tiny microscopic carcinomas are so small that they do not produce a visible growth.

Microinvasive carcinomas have such a low risk of metastatic spread that cure is achievable without hysterectomy by removing a large proportion of the cervix (cone biopsy) or the entire cervix (trachelectomy). Avoidance of hysterectomy allows these women to preserve their fertility.

Glandular neoplasia of the cervix

Neoplasia of the cervical glandular epithelium is much less common than squamous neoplasia

So far we have concentrated on squamous neoplasia of the transformation zone of the cervix. Neoplasia can also develop in the glandular epithelium of the cervix, though this is much less common than squamous neoplasia.

A pre-invasive lesion is also recognized in glandular neoplasia, known as **cervical glandular intraepithelial neoplasia** (CGIN), which can develop into invasive adenocarcinoma. As HPV is implicated in glandular neoplasia, it is not uncommon for women with high grade CIN also to have CGIN.

Note that whilst abnormalities in glandular cells may be seen in cervical smears, the cervical screening programme is *not* designed to diagnose CGIN nor impact on the incidence of adenocarcinoma of the cervix.

JARGON BUSTER

Adenocarcinoma in situ

In some countries, particularly the USA, the term **adenocarcinoma in situ** is used instead of cervical glandular intraepithelial neoplasia.

Uterine body

The function of the uterus is to protect and nourish the developing fetus, and expel it at the end of gestation. The uterine wall has two layers: the endometrium and the myometrium. The **myometrium** is composed of smooth muscle and is the thicker layer. The **endometrium**, which lines the uterine cavity, is composed of endometrial glands set within endometrial stroma.

The endometrium is hormonally responsive and undergoes a series of changes during the reproductive years with each menstrual cycle. During the first half of the cycle, the endometrium comes under oestrogenic stimulus and enters a **proliferative phase** in which the glands become elongated. After ovulation, the corpus luteum in the ovary begins to secrete progesterone which causes the endometrium to change from a proliferative state into a **secretory phase**. In the secretory phase, the endometrial glands become tortuous and engorged with thick secretions intended to nourish a blastocyst arriving in the uterine cavity. The endometrial stromal cells also swell in the secretory phase, ready to nourish the embryo as it implants.

In the absence of an implanted blastocyst, the corpus luteum involutes, progesterone levels fall, and the endometrium disintegrates and is shed (menstruation). After the menopause, ovulation ceases entirely. Oestrogen and progesterone levels fall, resulting in a permanently thin atrophic endometrium. Bleeding related to endometrial atrophy is a very common cause of post-menopausal vaginal spotting or bleeding.

The vast majority of important diseases of the uterus are endometrial disorders. The only common disease of the myometrium is the leiomyoma, a benign neoplasm of smooth muscle. The dynamic nature of the endometrium during reproductive life makes it particularly prone to overgrowths such as endometrial polyps, endometrial hyperplasia, and endometrial carcinomas. The continuous shedding and regrowth of endometrium also makes it liable to ectopic growth, and endometrium is often found burrowed deep in the myometrium (adenomyosis) and even outside the uterus itself (endometriosis), conditions which commonly cause severe pain during menstruation.

Endometrial infections

Infections of the endometrium are much less common than infections of the lower genital tract. This is largely because regular shedding of the endometrium makes establishment of infection difficult. The two main settings in which endometrial infections do occur are post-partum women and as part of pelvic inflammatory disease.

Endometrial infection in the post-partum period is related to retention of placental remnants in the uterus which allow bacteria from the vaginal flora to gain access to the endometrium and establish infection. The typical clinical picture is fever, an offensive vaginal discharge originating from the endometrium, and pelvic pain in a post-partum woman.

Endometrial infection unrelated to pregnancy is part of the clinical syndrome of pelvic inflammatory disease due to ascending infection by *C. trachomatis* or *N. gonorrhoeae*, both of which are sexually transmitted bacteria. Pelvic inflammatory disease is discussed further later in the chapter.

Adenomyosis

Adenomyosis refers to the presence of endometrial tissue deep in the myometrium

Adenomyosis is a condition in which endometrial glands and stroma extend deep into the myometrium. The endometrial glands appear to remain in continuity with the endometrial surface, suggesting that they arise from downgrowths of endometrial glands into the myometrium. It is thought that the lowest portions of the endometrial glands are pushed through into the myometrium during periods of high intrauterine pressure, e.g. menstruation and parturition.

Adenomyosis is believed to be a common cause of dysmenorrhoea around the menopause

The lowermost parts of the endometrial glands which give rise to adenomyosis are usually non-functional glands, meaning that they do not cycle like the rest of the endometrium with fluctuating hormone levels. The symptoms resulting from adenomyosis are thought to be related to hypertrophy of the smooth muscle cells of the myometrium which are stimulated by the presence of endometrial glands in the myometrium. This leads to enlargement of the myometrium, and the uterus as a whole, which may be appreciated on transvaginal ultrasound scan.

Endometriosis

Endometriosis refers to the presence of functional endometrium outside the uterus

Endometriosis is a common disorder in which functional endometrium is found outside the confines of the uterus. Strictly speaking, the diagnosis requires the presence of not only endometrial glands, but also endometrial stromal cells surrounding the endometrial glands—a scenario which can only be recognized microscopically. Thus although endometriosis may be strongly suspected by the typical location and appearance of the deposits, definitive diagnosis can only be made histologically.

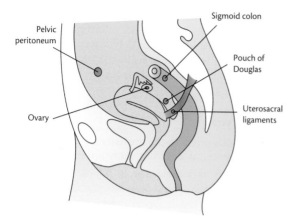

Fig. 12.6 Common sites of endometriosis in the pelvis.

Endometriosis may be found in many locations in the pelvis

Endometriosis has been reported in virtually every site in the body, but almost all cases are found in the pelvis (Fig. 12.6). The two most common sites for endometriosis are the ovaries and the uterosacral ligaments. Other common sites include the pouch of Douglas and areas of pelvic peritoneum. Endometriosis has been reported in sites outside the pelvis such as surgical scars and even the lungs, but this is rare.

Implantation, metaplasia, and 'metastasis' are the main theories behind endometriosis

Most cases of endometriosis are probably explained by the implantation theory. This theorizes that endometriotic deposits arise when viable endometrial glands are regurgitated into the peritoneal cavity during menstruation and subsequently implant in the peritoneal surface. Credence to this theory is lent by successful experimental induction of endometriosis in animals by placing endometrial tissue in the peritoneal cavity.

The metaplastic theory states that endometriosis arises due to metaplasia of the peritoneal surface epithelium into endometrial-type epithelium. Given that the peritoneum and the female genital tract both arise from the same embryological cells (the **coelomic epithelium**), the possibility of areas of peritoneum undergoing metaplasia towards female genital tract epithelium seems plausible. Indeed the metaplastic theory is highly likely to account for endometriotic deposits in areas in which implantation is unlikely.

Cases of endometriosis arising in locations where both implantation and metaplasia are improbable, such as the lung, are thought to arise by haematogenous spread of endometrial tissue, which presumably manages to enter the circulation at menstruation. Note that despite being called the 'metastatic' theory of endometriosis, the endometrial tissue is *not* malignant.

Endometriosis is a common cause of dysmenorrhoea

Endometriotic deposits cycle like normal endometrium, typically giving rise to cyclical symptoms which depend on the site of the deposits. The most common complaint is dysmenorrhoea, caused by swelling of endometriotic deposits during menstruation. However, symptoms of endometriosis correlate poorly with the actual extent of disease. Women with minimal disease may have marked pain, and, at the other extreme, extensive disease may be found in an asymptomatic woman.

Endometriosis often comes to light during investigation of infertility

Subfertility is a well recognized problem in women with endometriosis. Very often endometriosis is diagnosed when laparoscopy is performed as part of the investigation of subfertility. The exact mechanisms by which endometriosis gives rise to subfertility is far from clear. The most obvious explanation would be a mechanical effect due to obstruction of the fallopian tubes, but there is little evidence to support this. Only a small minority of subfertile women with endometriosis can be shown to have tubal distortion or blockage. The underlying reason appears to be much more subtle and may involve endocrine dysfunction, immune dysfunction, and implantation failure.

INTERESTING TO KNOW

Implantation failure and endometriosis

Recent work has shown that some subfertile women with endometriosis have abnormal expression of adhesion molecules in their endometrium, preventing attachment to the blastocyst. These observations suggest that there may be something wrong with all the endometrial tissue in endometriosis.

Key points: Endometriosis

- Endometriosis refers to the presence of endometrial glands and stroma outside the uterus.

- Deposits of endometriosis may be found anywhere in the pelvis, the most common sites being the pouch of Douglas, the uterosacral ligaments, and the ovaries.

- Endometriosis can be found outside the pelvis, but this is rare.

- The implantation theory of endometriosis suggests that the deposits arise from fragments of shed endometrium which enter the pelvis and implant. The metaplasia theory suggests that endometriosis develops as a result of metaplasia into endometrial tissue.

- Endometriosis cycles like normal endometrium, giving rise to symptoms when the deposits swell. Severe pelvic pain during menstruation is a common symptom.

- Infertility is associated with endometriosis and may be related to a defect in the endometrium as a whole which leads to failure of implantation of the embryo.

- Endometriosis is usually diagnosed at laparoscopy where the characteristic deposits are identified. Proving the presence of endometrial glands and stroma can only be achieved histologically on a tissue specimen, but this is not usually necessary to make the diagnosis.

Endometrial polyps

Endometrial polyps are small overgrowths of endometrium

Endometrial polyps are thought to arise from small areas of endometrium that do not cycle with the rest of the endometrium. They grow but do not slough during menstruation, eventually forming a polyp which projects into the endometrial cavity.

The tip of the polyp often ulcerates and bleeds, resulting in intermenstrual bleeding in younger women or post-menopausal bleeding in older women.

They can therefore mimic more sinister conditions such as cervical or endometrial carcinoma. Endometrial polyps are benign lesions with no potential for malignant transformation.

Endometrial hyperplasia

Endometrial hyperplasia refers to an increase in endometrial glands relative to stroma

The normal endometrium has a roughly equal ratio of endometrial glands relative to the surrounding endometrial stroma. **Endometrial hyperplasia** is defined by an increase in the number of endometrial glands relative to the endometrial stroma. The process usually diffusely affects the endometrium.

Endometrial hyperplasia is related to unopposed oestrogen stimulation of the endometrium

The single most important stimulus leading to endometrial hyperplasia is *prolonged unopposed oestrogen stimulation of the endometrium* which leads to persistence of proliferative phase activity of the endometrial glands.

Hyperplasia is most commonly seen in perimenopausal women where falling numbers of follicles lead to a failure in ovulation. Anovulatory cycles do not produce a corpus luteum, so there is no progesterone to stimulate a switch from proliferative phase to secretory phase in the endometrium. Most cases of hyperplasia in perimenopausal women spontaneously evolve into cystic atrophy of the endometrium, with no long-term consequences once the menopause becomes established and both oestrogen and progesterone levels are permanently low.

Post-menopausal women who develop hyperplasia are usually taking oestrogen hormone replacement therapy; some may be found to have an oestrogen-producing tumour of the ovary such as a granulosa cell tumour (see later). Hyperplasia is relatively uncommon in women of reproductive age where it is usually associated with an underlying condition leading to oestrogen excess, particularly the **polycystic ovarian syndrome**.

Endometrial hyperplasia usually presents with abnormal bleeding

Endometrial hyperplasia can be asymptomatic, but may present with abnormal bleeding. Prolonged periods of bleeding occur as a result of the flourishing endometrium outgrowing its blood supply and breaking down. The thickened endometrium may be appreciated on transvaginal ultrasound, but making a diagnosis requires sampling of the endometrium and histological examination to confirm the increase in endometrial glands.

Hyperplasias are divided into those with or without cytological atypia

The pathologist examining the endometrial sample will classify the hyperplasia into two broad categories: **hyperplasia without cytological atypia** and **hyperplasia with cytological atypia** (or **atypical hyperplasia**). The distinction is made depending on whether or not the nuclei of the endometrial epithelial cells look abnormal (Fig. 12.7).

The reasoning behind this classification is that the presence of cytological atypia confers a significant risk of progression to endometrial carcinoma. Fewer than 2 per cent of hyperplasias without cytological atypia progress to carcinoma, whereas about 25 per cent of atypical hyperplasias progress to carcinoma.

> ### JARGON BUSTER
> ## Simple and complex hyperplasia
> Some classifications of endometrial hyperplasia further subdivide hyperplasias into simple or complex according to the extent of the crowding and complexity of the endometrial glands. This generates four possibilities: simple hyperplasia, complex hyperplasia, simple atypical hyperplasia, and complex atypical hyperplasia. It is worth knowing this as some doctors still prefer to use these terms, the main rationale being that the complex forms of hyperplasia appear to have a higher risk of progression to carcinoma, though not to the extent that cytological atypia does.

Hyperplasia without atypia can be managed conservatively

Hyperplasia without atypia has an extremely low risk of progression to carcinoma. Simple observation or treatment with progestagens to suppress the hyperplasia is quite adequate.

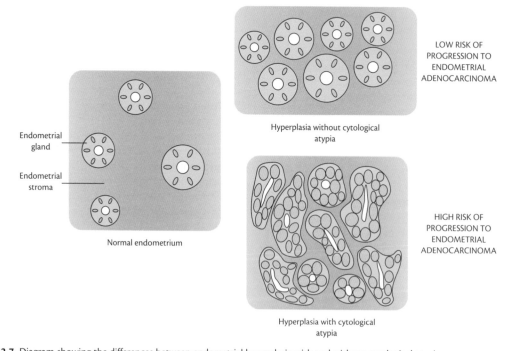

Fig. 12.7 Diagram showing the differences between endometrial hyperplasia with and without cytological atypia.

Atypical hyperplasia should be treated with hysterectomy unless the woman is young

Atypical hyperplasia carries a significant risk of progression to endometrial adenocarcinoma, and indeed there is a chance that the uterus already harbours an invasive adenocarcinoma which was not sampled. The recommended treatment for atypical hyperplasia is therefore hysterectomy.

As most women with atypical hyperplasia are menopausal, hysterectomy is usually an acceptable treatment. Managing younger women who may not have completed a family is more difficult, requiring balancing of the risk of developing carcinoma against preventing the ability to have future children.

Key points: Endometrial hyperplasia

- Endometrial hyperplasia is defined by an increase in the ratio of endometrial glands relative to endometrial stroma.

- Overgrowth of the endometrium with subsequent breakdown of the tissue leads to abnormal bleeding.

- Thickening of the endometrium may be appreciated on a transvaginal ultrasound scan.

- Diagnosis of hyperplasia requires microscopic examination of endometrial samples by a histopathologist.

- There are two main types of endometrial hyperplasia: hyperplasia without cytological atypia and hyperplasia with cytological atypia (atypical hyperplasia)

- Hyperplasia without cytological atypia carries an almost negligible risk of progression to carcinoma. Conservative management with either simple observation or treatment with progestagens to suppress the hyperplasia is acceptable.

- Hyperplasia with cytological atypia carries a significant risk of progression to endometrial carcinoma. Treatment with hysterectomy is necessary unless the woman is young and wants to preserve her fertility, in which case careful conservative treatment may be warranted.

Endometrial carcinoma

Endometrial carcinoma presents with post-menopausal bleeding

Endometrial carcinoma is the most common cancer in the female genital tract. The vast majority of endometrial carcinomas are adenocarcinomas which develop from the glandular epithelium of the endometrium. Carcinomas of the endometrium usually produce symptoms because they bleed. Since most of these tumours are seen in post-menopausal women, the most common presentation is vaginal bleeding after the onset of menopause. Post-menopausal bleeding is a serious symptom which should prompt immediate investigation.

Post-menopausal bleeding should be investigated with endometrial sampling

Any women suspected of having endometrial carcinoma requires microscopic examination of a sample of the endometrium. Retrieval of a sample of endometrium may be achieved by visualizing the endometrium at hysteroscopy and taking **curettings** of the endometrium, or taking random samples of the endometrium through a small suction device called a **pipelle**. The advantage of the pipelle sampler is that it can be used in the outpatient department without need for an anaesthetic and appears to produce entirely adequate specimens for histopathological examination.

There are two main types of endometrial adenocarcinoma

The most common type of endometrial adenocarcinoma arises in women soon after the menopause (aged 55–65 years) and is linked to conditions associated with prolonged oestrogen stimulation, particularly *unopposed* oestrogen exposure, i.e. a high oestrogen: progesterone ratio, a situation known to occur in obesity, nulliparity, and the polycystic ovarian syndrome. The endometrium first develops hyperplasia without atypia, then progresses through hyperplasia with cytological atypia into an invasive adenocarcinoma. These tumours, known as **endometrioid endometrial adenocarcinomas** because the malignant glands resemble normal endometrial glands, tend to carry a better prognosis than other types of endometrial adenocarcinoma.

The second type arises in older women and appears to be unrelated to oestrogen exposure; the background endometrium is usually atrophic rather than hyperplastic. These tumours are generally more poorly differentiated and have a worse prognosis. Two tumour types worth knowing about are the **papillary serous carcinoma** and the **clear cell carcinoma**, which resemble the ovarian tumours of the same name.

Endometrial carcinoma can spread locally, to lymph nodes, and to distant sites

Endometrial carcinomas can spread locally into the myometrium (Fig. 12.8) and cervix, via lymphatic channels to regional lymph nodes, or in the blood to distant sites.

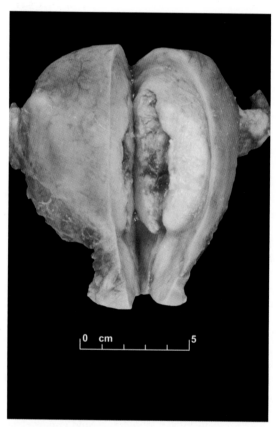

Fig. 12.8 Endometrial carcinoma. This is a uterus from a post-menopausal women who presented with vaginal bleeding. Endometrial sampling showed an endometrioid carcinoma and so she underwent hysterectomy. The uterus has been sliced open to reveal the white endometrial carcinoma seen infiltrating the underlying myometrium.

Patients with tumours apparently confined to the uterus undergo hysterectomy and bilateral salpingo-oophorectomy. Postoperative radiotherapy is also administered if examination of the hysterectomy specimen by the pathologist shows that the tumour is poorly differentiated, if there is deep spread into the myometrium, if the cervix is involved, or if there are any lymph node metastases.

Carcinosarcoma is a special type of endometrial carcinoma

Carcinosarcoma is the name given to an endometrial carcinoma in which some of the malignant epithelium takes on the appearance of malignant mesenchyme. In the uterus, it is also sometimes known as a malignant mixed Müllerian tumour (MMMT). The tumour has a mixed appearance when examined microscopically, with both malignant epithelial and malignant mesenchymal elements.

Carcinosarcomas are very aggressive tumours with a considerably worse prognosis than other endometrial carcinomas. Post-menopausal bleeding is the usual mode of presentation, but by this time there is invariably deep myometrial invasion and spread outside the uterus.

Key points: Endometrial carcinoma

- Endometrial carcinoma usually presents with post-menopausal bleeding.

- Transvaginal ultrasound is a simple investigation to image the endometrium.

- Endometrial curettings are a useful way of sampling the endometrium.

- Almost all endometrial carcinomas are adenocarcinomas which arise in two main settings.

- The first group is seen in the setting of prolonged oestrogen exposure, leading to endometrial hyperplasia and progression to a well differentiated endometrioid adenocarcinoma.

Key points: Endometrial carcinoma—cont'd

- The second group arises in much older women and is unrelated to oestrogen exposure. These tumours are much more aggressive, with a poor prognosis.
- Carcinosarcoma is a special type of endometrial carcinoma which is extremely aggressive.

Smooth muscle tumours of the uterus

Leiomyoma is the most common tumour of the female genital tract

A **leiomyoma**, or 'fibroid', is a very common benign tumour of smooth muscle origin which arises in the myometrium. They are often multiple and can vary in size considerably from just a few millimetres to huge tumours (>20 cm) distorting the uterus (Fig. 12.9).

Oestrogen promotes the growth of leiomyomas, making them most common during the reproductive years. Most stop growing after the menopause, and often calcify into hard masses. Leiomyomas may be asymptomatic, even if large, but can produce a variety of symptoms including abnormal vaginal bleeding and painful periods.

The malignant counterpart of a leiomyoma is known as a **leiomyosarcoma**. These are much rarer than their benign counterparts and tend to be larger tumours occurring in older women over 50 years of age.

Dysfunctional uterine bleeding

Dysfunctional uterine bleeding (DUB) is a clinical term used to describe bleeding in which no underlying pathological cause can be found. DUB is therefore a diagnosis of exclusion which can be used only when known causes of abnormal bleeding have been ruled out, e.g. endometritis, endometrial polyps, adenomyosis, hyperplasia, carcinoma, and leiomyomas.

DUB is thought to be the result of subtle derangements in hormonally mediated effects on the endometrium. DUB is therefore different from *menorrhagia* (prolonged heavy bleeding at menses) which is generally thought to be due to local abnormalities in coagulation in the endometrium.

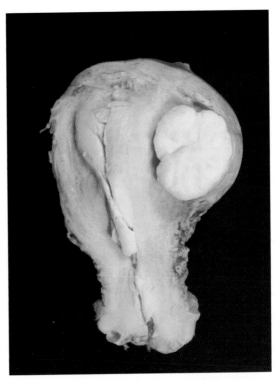

Fig. 12.9 Leiomyoma. This uterus was removed due to severe menorrhagia. On bisecting the uterus, a well circumscribed white mass is seen in the myometrium which bulges from the cut surface. This is the typical macroscopic appearance of a leiomyoma (fibroid) and this was confirmed on microscopic examination.

Fallopian tubes

The fallopian tubes provide a link between the ovaries and the uterus. They are the site of fertilization and help deliver the zygote to the uterine cavity for implantation. Diseases of the fallopian tube are not common; the most important are infections as part of pelvic inflammatory disease, and ectopic pregnancy (see later). Neoplasms of the fallopian tube are exceedingly rare.

Pelvic inflammatory disease

Pelvic inflammatory disease is infection of the upper genital tract

Pelvic inflammatory disease occurs when there is an infection of the upper genital tract. The infection may involve the endometrium, fallopian tubes, ovaries, and pelvic peritoneum. Infection occurs by ascending infection from the lower genital tract.

The two most common responsible microorganisms are *C. trachomatis* and *N. gonorrhoea*, both of which are sexually transmitted bacteria. *Chlamydia* appears to be the major aetiological agent, responsible for over 80 per cent of all cases of pelvic inflammatory disease.

Pelvic inflammatory disease has a very wide spectrum of clinical manifestations

The spectrum of presentation of pelvic inflammatory disease is extremely wide ranging. Many cases are probably asymptomatic. Most women with symptoms present with varying degrees of lower abdominal pain and dyspareunia. There may also be post-coital or intermenstrual bleeding. These symptoms may not immediately prompt consideration of pelvic inflammatory disease, and the diagnosis is often missed as non-infective causes are pursued. Tenderness on pelvic examination is often found in pelvic inflammatory disease and should always raise one's suspicion.

Severe cases of pelvic inflammatory disease present with an acute abdomen. There is severe abdominal pain, often with signs of peritonism, and high fever. The differential diagnosis in a young woman includes appendicitis, ectopic pregnancy, or a torted or ruptured ovarian cyst.

Pelvic inflammatory disease should be treated with appropriate antibiotics

Treatment for pelvic inflammatory disease is with a combination of antibiotics which should cover *Chlamydia*, *N. gonorrhoeae*, and anaerobes. The specific choice will depend on local sensitivities, though possible combinations include ofloxacin and metronidazole.

Mild to moderate cases can be treated in the community, but severe cases require hospital admission with intravenous therapy. An endocervical swab should first be taken and sent to microbiology to identify the causative organism. Treatment should be started pending the result.

Pelvic inflammatory disease may result in a number of sequelae including infertility

Undiagnosed or inadequately treated pelvic inflammatory disease can have a number of sequelae including:

- Infertility. The risk of infertility increases with each episode of infection. Women with three or more

episodes of pelvic inflammatory disease have a 40 per cent chance of being infertile.

- Ectopic pregnancy. There is a sixfold increase in the risk of ectopic pregnancy, presumably related to fallopian tube distortion.

- Chronic pelvic pain and dyspareunia.

Given these potentially serious complications, it is important not to miss a diagnosis of pelvic inflammatory disease. The huge variation in possible presentations and lack of specific features can make this seem difficult, but the flip side is simply to consider pelvic inflammatory disease in any young woman presenting with symptoms that may be related to the genital tract!

Key points: Pelvic inflammatory disease

- Pelvic inflammatory disease is a clinical syndrome due to infection of the upper genital tract.

- The infection is the result of ascending spread from the lower genital tract and may involve the endometrium, fallopian tubes, ovaries, and the pelvic peritoneum.

- The two major causative organisms are *Chlamydia trachomatis* and *Neisseria gonorrhoeae*, both of which are sexually transmitted bacteria. *Chlamydia* is the more common infection and appears to be increasing in frequency.

- The clinical spectrum of pelvic inflammatory disease is extremely wide, ranging from asymptomatic infection to a severe illness with high fever and abdominal pain with peritonism.

- Correctly diagnosing and adequately treating pelvic inflammatory disease is important as it has a number of serious sequelae including infertility and ectopic pregnancy.

Ovary

The ovaries are the female gonads and have two main functions: the monthly release of mature ova and the secretion of steroid hormones. Both of these functions are controlled by the hormones **follicle-stimulating hormone** (FSH) and **luteinizing hormone** (LH) from the anterior pituitary, hormones which are in turn regulated by **gonadotrophin-releasing hormone** (GnRH) from the hypothalamus.

Each ovary is covered by a single layer of specialized mesothelial cells derived from embryonic coelomic epithelium. This layer is important because the epithelial tumours of the ovary are thought to arise from it. Underneath the serosal layer is a thick fibrous zone often termed the tunica albuginea of the ovary.

Beneath this fibrous layer is the ovarian **cortex** which contains the developing follicles. The ovarian cortical stroma consists of spindled cells from which the theca cells which form the outer part of maturing follicles develop. The centre of the ovary is the **medulla** which contains the blood vessels supplying the ovary. In young women, the medulla also contains developing follicles. In older women, the medulla becomes occupied by corpora albicantia.

Each ovulatory cycle is divided into two halves: the **follicular phase** and the **luteal phase**. Ovulation occurs midcycle and marks the switch from follicular phase to luteal phase. In the follicular phase, FSH from the anterior pituitary stimulates the enlargement of several primordial follicles. The primordial follicles consist of a germ cell surrounded by a layer of granulosa cells. The granulosa cells surrounding the ovum proliferate, and stromal cells from the ovarian cortical stroma condense around the granulosa cell layer of the follicles to form thecal cells. Androgens synthesized in the thecal cells diffuse into the follicles where they are converted by granulosa cells into oestrogens. During the follicular phase, oestrogen levels rise.

Of all the maturing follicles, only one becomes dominant and ruptures midcycle to release its ovum. The others are sadly doomed to a process of degeneration called **atresia**. After ovulation, the collapsed dominant follicle becomes a **corpus luteum** which starts secreting large amounts of progesterone as well as oestrogen. During the second half of the cycle, the luteal phase, plasma oestrogens and progesterone rise dramatically.

Unless stimulated by human chorionic gonadotrophin (HCG) from trophoblast of a fertilized zygote, the corpus luteum undergoes a programmed involution after about 9 days (i.e. day 23 of a 28 day cycle), and oestrogen and progesterone levels plummet. After several months, the corpus luteum turns into a collapsed white scar called a **corpus albicans** which persists in the ovary (Fig. 12.10).

The most common ovarian lesions are functional cysts and tumours. The polycystic ovarian syndrome is a complex metabolic disorder with many manifestations, but is considered here because it is usually managed by gynaecologists. Recall also that the ovary is one of the most common sites of endometriosis. Infections of the ovary are rare, probably because bacteria cannot easily penetrate the dense tunica albuginea.

Functional cysts

Functional cysts are usually asymptomatic and are discovered incidentally

Functional cysts arise from ovarian follicles which become abnormally cystic during their development. They are most common in women of reproductive age, particularly around the menopause. Most are discovered by chance when pelvic ultrasound, laparoscopy, or laparotomy is performed for unrelated reasons. Some functional cysts may be detected as a palpable adnexal mass. Uncommonly, functional cysts present with the sudden onset of abdominal pain, due either to torsion of the ovary or rupture of the cyst into the peritoneal cavity.

Follicular cysts and corpus luteum cysts are the two most common types of functional cyst

Follicular cysts are one of the two most common types of functional cyst. They are lined by granulosa cells and result from non-rupture of a dominant follicle or failure of involution of a non-dominant follicle. By definition, they are greater than 2 cm in size to distinguish them from normal physiological cystic follicles.

Corpus luteum cysts are thought to arise from a corpus luteum which fails to collapse and resolve.

Functional cysts usually spontaneously resolve

Functional cysts usually resolve by spontaneous resorption of the fluid contained within them. Women found to have a solitary cyst thought to be a functional cyst should be monitored over a period of 2–3 months. If the cyst does not resolve, then further investigation is warranted to rule out a neoplastic cyst. Some gynaecologists will proceed straight to surgical removal of the cyst to allow a definitive histological diagnosis to be made. Others may prefer to aspirate the cyst fluid first

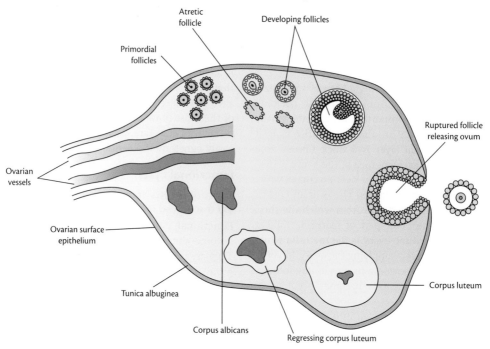

Fig. 12.10 Follicular development and ovulation.

and send it for cytological examination, proceeding to surgical removal only if the cytology is suspicious.

Polycystic ovarian syndrome

Polycystic ovarian syndrome, or PCOS, is a very common condition believed to affect up to 10 per cent of women. The fundamental problem in PCOS appears to be over-production of androgens by the ovaries. The excess androgens cause impaired maturation of developing follicles, leading to a failure in ovulation (Fig. 12.11). In some women, the multiple poorly developed follicles are large enough to become visible cysts.

The diagnosis of polycystic ovarian syndrome requires at least two of the following three features:

- *Ovulatory failure*, usually manifest by oligomenorrhoea (fewer than nine menstrual periods per year) or amenorrhoea (complete cessation of menstruation).

- *Androgen excess*, either by finding elevated levels of circulating androgens in the blood or by clinical manifestations of excess androgens, e.g. hirsutism or acne.

- *Polycystic ovaries* seen on ultrasound.

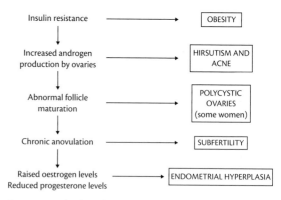

Fig. 12.11 Pathophysiology and clinical features of polycystic ovarian syndrome.

Note that despite the name of the syndrome, the presence of polycystic ovaries is *not* essential to make the diagnosis! Furthermore the presence of polycystic ovaries alone does not equate to a diagnosis of PCOS.

Polycystic ovarian syndrome is characterized by the excess production of androgens

In the normal ovary, the theca cells of the follicle are responsible for the synthesis of androgens under the influence of LH from the anterior pituitary. The granulosa cells are able to convert androgens to oestrogens under the control of FSH from the pituitary. The balance of LH and FSH is therefore crucial in determining the relative amounts of androgens and oestrogens produced by the developing follicle.

It is well established that the theca cells in women with PCOS are more efficient at making androgens than normal theca cells. It is still not entirely clear why women with PCOS have ovaries that produce excess androgens. It was always thought to be a primary ovarian problem, but recently there has been much interest in the role of insulin resistance in the pathogenesis of PCOS. The high level of circulating insulin in women with insulin resistance is believed to be important in upsetting the balance of androgen and oestrogen production by the ovaries.

Anovulation may cause subfertility and endometrial hyperplasia

Chronic anovulation in PCOS often means these women have problems conceiving, and many cases are diagnosed following investigation for subfertility. Anovulatory cycles are also a cause of unopposed oestrogen stimulation to the endometrium which may lead to endometrial hyperplasia (see earlier).

Women with polycystic ovarian syndrome also have metabolic abnormalities

It is increasingly recognized that PCOS is not only an ovarian disease. Metabolic abnormalities are also an important component of the syndrome. Obesity in particular is a common problem in PCOS, with weight gain beginning in adolescence. Insulin resistance also appears to be a critical feature of the disease, which leads to a tendency to further weight gain. This provokes additional insulin resistance and hypersecretion of insulin, and a vicious cycle is established. Weight reduction in obese women with PCOS is therefore an essential part of managing the condition.

> ## Key points: Polycystic ovarian syndrome
>
> - Polycystic ovarian syndrome is a very common metabolic disorder in women.
> - Overproduction of androgens by the ovaries leads to failure of ovulation and to symptoms related to excess circulating androgens.
> - Ovulatory failure causes subfertility and endometrial hyperplasia.
> - PCOS is also strongly associated with other metabolic abnormalities. Insulin resistance is thought to be critical in the pathogenesis of PCOS, leading to the increased androgen production by the ovaries and a tendency to obesity.

Ovarian neoplasms

Ovarian neoplasms are common. About 80 per cent of all ovarian neoplasms behave in a benign fashion, and these occur mostly in young women aged 20–45 years. The malignant ovarian tumours are seen in older women aged 45–65 years.

Ovarian tumours tend to present late

Although some ovarian tumours are hormonally active, most are non-functional and therefore produce minimal symptoms until they have grown to a large size. Unfortunately, most malignant neoplasms have spread outside the ovary by the time the diagnosis is made, making prognosis poor. Malignant ovarian tumours are therefore a leading cause of cancer-related death in women.

The ovary has a formidable list of neoplastic entities

The ovaries have more types of neoplasms than any other organ in the body (well over 100!). Thankfully, there is a convenient method of categorizing the tumours based on their presumed cell of origin (Fig. 12.12):

- **Epithelial** tumours, derived from the mesothelial lining of the ovary.
- **Sex cord stromal** tumours, derived from cells originating from the sex cords of the primitive gonad.

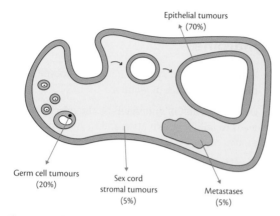

Fig. 12.12 Diagram showing the origin of common ovarian tumours.

- **Germ cell** tumours, derived from the germ cells in the ovary.

- **Metastatic** tumours from primary malignancies elsewhere in the body.

Epithelial tumours

Epithelial tumours are the most common type of ovarian tumour

Epithelial tumours are the most common neoplasms of the ovary. They are believed to originate from small mesothelial-lined inclusion cysts which become incorporated into the substance of the ovary following rupture and repair of ovulation sites.

An origin from pelvic peritoneum goes some way to explain why there are so many different types of ovarian epithelial neoplasms. You may remember from embryology that the mesothelial cells of the peritoneum and the epithelial cells lining the entire female genital tract are all derived from the **coelomic epithelium** of the embryo.

The current theory is that the mesothelial cells lining the inclusion cysts become neoplastic and differentiate into epithelial cells which resemble the lining of the endocervix, endometrium, and fallopian tube.

Epithelial tumours are classified according to their cell type and behaviour

Epithelial tumours are named according to the type of cell they differentiate towards:

- **Serous**: cells resembling fallopian tube epithelium.

- **Mucinous**: cells resembling endocervical epithelium.

- **Endometrioid**: cells resembling endometrial epithelium.

- **Clear cell**: cells with no obvious normal counterpart, but with strikingly clear cytoplasm.

In addition, epithelial ovarian tumours are classified according to their behaviour and microscopic features into benign, borderline, and malignant (Fig. 12.13). Benign tumours are usually cystic and are therefore termed **cystadenomas**. Malignant tumours are often partly cystic and may be called **cystadenocarcinomas** but often are just termed **adenocarcinomas**. Borderline tumours, as we shall see, are a slightly grey area and are just called 'borderline tumours' to reflect a degree of uncertainty over their malignant potential.

The most common epithelial ovarian tumours are listed in Table 12.3. As can be seen, the serous and mucinous types account for most epithelial ovarian tumours. Tumours with cells resembling endometrial epithelium (i.e. endometrioid tumours) are not as common. Most endometrioid tumours are malignant and are therefore termed ovarian endometrioid adeno-carcinomas. Virtually all clear cell tumours are malignant, i.e. clear cell carcinomas. Benign and borderline clear cell tumours are very rare.

Benign ovarian epithelial tumours are cystic neoplasms which lack a significant solid component

The benign epithelial ovarian tumours are cystic neoplasms which are often called benign cystadenomas. Microscopically, the cyst(s) are lined by a single layer of epithelial cells with no evidence of increased proliferation or invasion of the underlying stroma. The two most common benign epithelial tumours are the benign mucinous cystadenoma and the benign serous cystadenoma.

Benign mucinous cystadenomas may grow to a very large size: tumours weighing over 20 kg have been reported! They are multiloculated tumours, each locule being filled with thick gelatinous fluid. Microscopically, they are composed of numerous cysts lined by tall columnar epithelial cells containing mucin, resembling the cells of normal endocervical epithelium.

Benign serous cystadenomas tend to be unilocular and filled with clear watery serous fluid (Fig. 12.14). Microscopically the cyst is lined by columnar ciliated

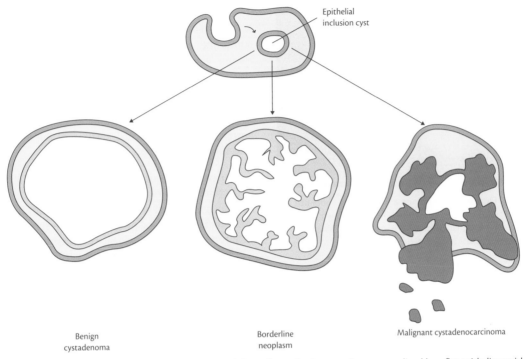

Fig. 12.13 Benign, borderline, and malignant ovarian epithelial neoplasms. Benign cystadenomas are lined by a flat epithelium with no invasion. Borderline neoplasms show proliferative activity, creating complex infoldings of the cyst epithelial lining but without invasion. Malignant neoplasms show invasive behaviour.

epithelial cells which resemble the epithelium lining the normal fallopian tube.

Malignant ovarian epithelial tumours invade the underlying stroma

Ovarian carcinomas are partly cystic but tend to have a significant solid component to them. By the time they become symptomatic, many have metastasized to other organs and the peritoneum. The survival for patients with ovarian carcinoma is therefore poor.

TABLE 12.3 Common ovarian epithelial neoplasms
Benign mucinous cystadenoma
Benign serous cystadenoma
Malignant serous adenocarcinoma
Borderline serous tumour
Borderline mucinous tumour

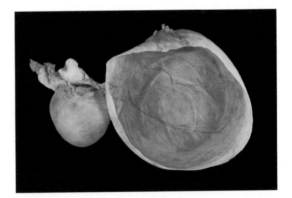

Fig. 12.14 This ovarian tumour was removed from a woman who presented with abdominal discomfort and was found to have a pelvic mass. The ovary has been replaced by a cystic tumour containing thin clear fluid. Microscopic examination of the cyst wall showed the lining to be composed of bland epithelial cells resembling normal fallopian tube, making this a serous cystadenoma.

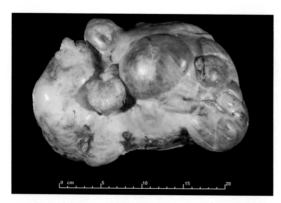

Fig. 12.15 Ovarian adenocarcinoma. This tumour contained a mixture of solid and cystic elements when sliced open, raising suspicion of a malignant tumour. Microscopic examination showed a high grade serous adenocarcinoma.

Serous adenocarcinoma is the most common type of malignant epithelial ovarian tumour (Fig. 12.15). Mucinous adenocarcinomas also occur, but metastasis from a mucin-producing tumour from elsewhere in the body (particularly the gastrointestinal tract) is much more likely than an ovarian primary and so should be rigorously excluded first. Clear cell carcinomas are not common but are important because they behave particularly aggressively and have a very poor prognosis, rather like their counterparts arising in the endometrium.

Ca125 is a tumour marker often found in patients with ovarian carcinoma

Ca125 is a large glycoprotein which is found in normal tissues derived from coelomic epithelium, including the epithelium lining the ovary, fallopian tubes, endometrium, and endocervix. Ca125 is found circulating in the serum of more than 80 per cent of patients with ovarian carcinomas. Unfortunately the marker is not very specific, being elevated in other malignancies (endometrial, pancreatic, lung, breast) and some non-malignant conditions.

LINK BOX

BRCA1 and ovarian carcinoma

Although more famous in relation to breast cancer (p. 291), patients with inherited mutations of the BRCA1 gene also have a high risk of developing ovarian carcinomas, usually serous adenocarcinomas.

Borderline tumours are a distinct subset of ovarian epithelial tumours

Borderline epithelial ovarian tumours lie between benign and malignant tumours both in their appearance and in their prognosis. The neoplastic cells show evidence of increased proliferation, with heaping up of the cells and the formation of numerous papillae within the tumour. Unlike the malignant tumours, however, there is no actual invasion of the neoplastic cells into the underlying stroma.

Implants are a curious feature of borderline tumours

A curious feature of some borderline ovarian tumours is the remarkably good prognosis seen in some women with tumours showing evidence at surgery of apparent widespread 'metastases' in the peritoneum. These latter lesions have come to be referred to as **implants**. Implants are most commonly found in association with borderline serous tumours of the ovary, but have been described in association with borderline mucinous tumours.

The concept of implants and borderline tumours is one of the most contentious issues in ovarian pathology. Many people believe that implants reflect multi-focal neoplasia arising *de novo* from the peritoneal surface, rather than being true metastases from the ovarian tumour.

When examined microscopically, implants may appear to be 'non-invasive' or 'invasive'. Current best practice is to consider further adjuvant treatment for patients with peritoneal implants which are of the invasive category. Those with non-invasive implants have careful clinical follow-up only. There is no evidence that further treatment offers any survival advantage in these patients who generally do very well.

Sex cord stromal tumours

Sex cord stromal tumours recapitulate the cells of the ovarian stroma which in turn are derived from the sex cords of the primitive gonad. There are three main elements that they may be composed of:

+ **Fibroblasts**

+ **Thecal cells**, which synthesize androgens and oestrogens

+ **Granulosa cells**, which do not synthesize oestrogens from scratch but can convert other steroid hormones into oestrogens.

These elements can occur in various combinations and so a wide variety of tumour types have been described. Usually the tumours are known by the predominant cell type within them, and this gives rise to three important tumours: fibromas, thecomas, and granulosa cell tumours. *The importance of the last two tumours is that they are often functional tumours which produce excess oestrogen.*

Unlike the epithelial ovarian tumours which are often completely cystic, or have a cystic component, the sex cord stromal tumours are usually completely solid tumours (Fig. 12.16).

Fibromas are the most common type of sex cord stromal tumour

Fibromas are by far the most commonly encountered sex cord stromal tumour. Fibromas are composed of cells recapitulating the fibroblasts of the normal ovarian stroma. Unlike many of the other ovarian tumours, fibromas are solid and firm, rather than cystic. Many of these tumours present due to abdominal pain and/or a pelvic mass. An odd, but well recognized further feature of ovarian fibromas is their association with ascites which may be found in up to half of all cases and may be the presenting feature.

Thecomas are benign tumours that usually present with symptoms of oestrogen excess

Thecomas are benign tumours that recapitulate the thecal cells of the developing follicle. Most cases present with symptoms related to the production of excess

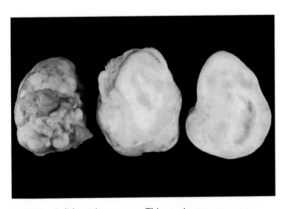

Fig. 12.16 Solid ovarian tumour. This ovarian tumour was completely solid when it was transected by the pathologist, raising suspicion of a sex cord stromal type tumour. This tumour was shown histologically to be a fibroma.

oestrogen, usually abnormal uterine bleeding as a result of endometrial hyperplasia. Endometrial carcinoma may also occur. Only about 10 per cent of cases are associated with manifestations of androgen excess. Thecomas are typically solid tumours with a bright yellow cut surface due to the high steroid content of the cells.

Granulosa cell tumours are potentially malignant tumours with a tendency to late recurrence

Granulosa cell tumours may occur at any age and, like thecomas, often produce excess oestrogen and give rise to concomitant endometrial pathology. Unlike fibromas and thecomas which are benign tumours, granulosa cell tumours are all potentially malignant, with a characteristic propensity to very late recurrence, often more than 10 years after removal of the original tumour. Granulosa cell tumours usually have a cystic element when examined macroscopically.

Germ cell tumours

Germ cell tumours of the ovary resemble those seen in the testis. Although the classification of ovarian and testicular germ cell tumours is very similar, the incidence and behaviour of each type is different.

Mature cystic teratoma is the most common germ cell tumour of the ovary

Teratomas are germ cell tumours which differentiate toward normal somatic structures. Most teratomas contain elements derived from all three embryonic layers (ectoderm, mesoderm, and endoderm).

Mature cystic teratomas, or 'dermoid cysts', are the most common type of germ cell tumour. They are cystic tumours lined by skin with underlying sebaceous glands and hair follicles. The cyst becomes filled with thick greasy sebaceous material and hair (Fig. 12.17). It is not unusual to find teeth buried within the cyst contents. On microscopic examination, the tumours usually also contain mesodermal derivates such as cartilage and smooth muscle, and endodermal derivates such as respiratory and intestinal epithelium. Mature cystic teratomas are entirely benign neoplasms which do not recur.

Dysgerminomas are the ovarian counterpart of testicular seminomas

Dysgerminomas are tumours composed of primordial germ cells which tend to arise in young women, usually younger than 20 years old. They are identical to

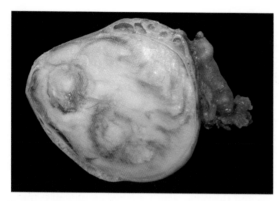

Fig. 12.17 Mature cystic teratoma. Typical appearance of a mature cystic teratoma (dermoid cyst) filled with greasy yellow material and hair.

seminomas arising in the male testis, and like seminomas are malignant tumours capable of local invasion and metastasis. Fortunately dysgerminomas are responsive to chemotherapy and radiotherapy, and prognosis following treatment is generally excellent.

Ovarian metastases

The ovaries are common sites of metastasis from other malignant neoplasms

Malignancies which often give rise to metastases in the ovary include stomach, colon, and breast. The ovaries may also be the site of metastatic spread from other malignancies of the female genital tract such as the endometrium and the opposite ovary. Metastatic deposits vary considerably in size, from small microscopic foci to large masses which completely replace the ovary. Clues to the metastatic nature of an ovarian tumour are bilateral involvement and multinodularity.

JARGON BUSTER

Krukenberg tumour

The **Krukenberg tumour** refers specifically to the presence of *bilateral* infiltration of the ovaries by *metastatic* adenocarcinoma with a signet ring cell appearance microscopically. The most common primary tumour giving rise to a Krukenberg tumour is the diffuse type of gastric adenocarcinoma (p. 148).

Key points: Ovarian neoplasms

◆ The ovaries can give rise to a very large number of neoplasms.

◆ The main types of ovarian neoplasms are epithelial, sex cord stromal, germ cell, and metastases.

◆ Epithelial tumours are the most common subtype and are thought to be derived from inclusion cysts lined by mesothelial cells that form following rupture of the ovarian cortex at ovulation.

◆ The mesothelial cells lining the cysts become neoplastic and can differentiate into epithelium appearing like any part of the female genital tract, i.e. mucinous, serous, or endometrioid.

◆ Ovarian epithelial tumours are usually cystic and may be benign (cystadenomas), malignant (adenocarcinomas), or an intermediate category known as borderline.

◆ Sex cord stromal tumours include fibromas, thecomas, and granulosa cell tumours. The importance of the latter two tumours is their ability to secrete oestrogens, which may lead to endometrial hyperplasia and endometrial carcinoma.

◆ Germ cell tumours of the ovary are similar to germ cell tumours of the testis. The two most common types are the benign mature cystic teratoma (dermoid cyst) and the malignant dysgerminoma, which is the ovarian counterpart of the testicular seminoma.

Disorders of pregnancy

Ectopic pregnancy

An ectopic pregnancy results when implantation occurs outside the uterine cavity

Ectopic pregnancy affects about 12 per 1000 pregnancies in the UK. Nearly all ectopic pregnancies occur in the fallopian tubes, usually in the ampullary region. Other sites include the ovaries and abdominal cavity, but these are rare.

Tubal ectopics are more likely if there is a structural abnormality of the tube which delays transit of the fertilized ovum. The most common predisposing factor is tubal scarring from previous episodes of pelvic inflammatory disease; however, about half of all cases occur for no apparent underlying reason.

Ectopic pregnancy should be considered in any woman of reproductive age with abdominal symptoms

Ectopic pregnancy usually presents with the sudden onset of severe abdominal pain. The pain is due to intense haemorrhage into the lumen of the affected tube, caused by trophoblast of the implanting blastocyst eroding into large blood vessels in the submucosa of the fallopian tube. There may also be associated vaginal bleeding due to shedding of the decidualized endometrium (rather than bleeding from the ectopic pregnancy itself).

Often the woman will not realize she is pregnant, so the diagnosis may catch out the unwary. Any woman of reproductive age presenting with abdominal symptoms should be routinely asked if there is any possibility of her being pregnant, and consent gained for a pregnancy test.

A positive pregnancy test together with absence of an intrauterine gestation on ultrasound scan confirms the diagnosis. Surgical treatment is required, which may be removal of the fallopian tube (salpingectomy) or aspiration of the ectopic pregnancy through an incision in the wall of the fallopian tube (salpingotomy).

Rupture of an ectopic pregnancy is a surgical emergency

If the implanting embryo invades through the entirety of the tubal wall, there is rupture into the peritoneal cavity with bleeding into the pelvis. Haemorrhage into the lower abdominal cavity causes an acute abdomen with the rapid development of hypovolaemia and shock. Aggressive fluid resuscitation is required followed by immediate transfer to theatre for ligation of the bleeding point and removal of the fallopian tube.

Key points: Ectopic pregnancy

♦ Ectopic pregnancy occurs when a blastocyst implants outside the uterine cavity.

♦ Almost all ectopic pregnancies occur in the fallopian tube. The most common predisposing factor is tubal distortion following previous episodes of pelvic inflammatory disease.

♦ Most ectopic pregnancies present with lower abdominal pain due to bleeding into the tube. Any woman with abdominal symptoms should be consented for a pregnancy test to exclude an ectopic pregnancy.

♦ The diagnosis of ectopic pregnancy is confirmed if a pregnancy test is positive and an ultrasound scan fails to demonstrate a gestational sac in the uterus.

♦ Urgent surgical treatment is required, either removal of the fallopian tube or aspiration of the ectopic pregnancy.

♦ Rupture of an ectopic pregnancy presents with acute abdominal pain and hypovolaemic shock. Aggressive fluid replacement and immediate transfer to theatre is required.

Gestational trophoblastic disease

Gestational trophoblastic diseases are a group of diseases related to abnormal development and behaviour of trophoblast. Trophoblast is a fetal tissue which surrounds the developing embryo and forms the interface between maternal and fetal tissues. Trophoblast has a number of vital functions:

♦ Formation of *chorionic villi* where exchange of material between mother and fetus occurs.

♦ Acting as an *immunological barrier* which prevents rejection of the fetus by the mother.

♦ *Hormone production*, notably HCG. This hormone is a useful serological marker of trophoblast activity and is very useful in the diagnosis and follow-up of some types of gestational trophoblastic disease.

Although a number of conditions come under the remit of gestational trophoblastic disease, only two are important. One is a non-neoplastic condition called hydatidiform mole and the other is a neoplasm called a choriocarcinoma.

Hydatidiform mole

Hydatidiform mole is characterized by exuberant proliferation of trophoblast

Hydatidiform moles are essentially abnormal placentas which arise as a result of cytogenetic abnormalities in a conceptus. The chorionic villi become swollen and oedematous ('hydropic') such that the mole appears like a cluster of grapes to the naked eye. Hydatidiform moles occur in about 1 in 1000 pregnancies in the western world. For completely unknown reasons, they are much more frequent in the Far East.

Hydatidiform moles are usually diagnosed when bleeding occurs in early pregnancy

Hydatidiform moles usually declare themselves when vaginal bleeding occurs in early pregnancy. If bleeding does not occur, or is trivial, the diagnosis may be suspected on physical examination because the size of the uterus on palpation is larger than would be expected for the gestational date. Definitive diagnosis is made following histopathological examination of the evacuated products of conception, which reveals the abnormal trophoblastic proliferation.

Hydatidiform moles may be partial or complete

There are two types of hydatidiform mole: partial and complete. A **complete mole** has hydropic change in all of the villi. No normal placental villi are present and no fetal parts are present. The chromosomal make up of a complete mole is 46XX but all the chromosomes are paternally derived. This is most likely to arise following fertilization of an 'empty' ovum with no maternal genetic material by a 23X spermatozoon which then duplicates its genetic material.

In **partial moles**, the abnormal hydropic villi affect only some of the chorionic villi. Some normal placental villi remain, and fetal parts are present. The genetic makeup of partial moles is different from that of complete moles. Most partial moles are triploid containing one maternal and two paternal sets of chromosomes, i.e. 69XXY, 69 XXX, or 69 XYY.

Hydatidiform moles that extend deeply into myometrium are called invasive moles

A small proportion of both partial and complete moles may show deep extension of the abnormal villi into the myometrium. Moles showing this behaviour are known as **invasive moles** and are unlikely to be cured by simple evacuation. Chemotherapy, however, is extremely effective at treating them.

Despite their name and the fact that chemotherapy is used to treat them, invasive moles are *not* true neoplasms, they are simply collections of abnormal trophoblast which show marked invasive behaviour.

Gestational choriocarcinoma

Choriocarcinoma is a highly malignant neoplasm of trophoblast

Trophoblast can undergo malignant change, and the resulting tumour is known as a **choriocarcinoma**. About half of gestational choriocarcinomas develop from a preceding hydatidiform mole, with the remainder following either a normal pregnancy or a miscarriage.

Choriocarcinomas are extremely vascular tumours which have a great propensity for invading blood vessels. Early, widespread dissemination to distant sites is a typical feature of choriocarcinomas. Such behaviour is not surprising considering that normal trophoblast is programmed for spread through the uterus into maternal blood vessels. Fortunately, gestational choriocarcinomas respond extremely well to chemotherapy, and the prognosis for most women with these neoplasms is good.

INTERESTING TO KNOW

Non-gestational choriocarcinomas

Although most choriocarcinomas complicate some form of pregnancy, choriocarcinomas can also arise from germ cells in the ovaries and testes. Non-gestational choriocarcinomas carry a much worse prognosis than gestational choriocarcinomas, with a 5 year survival of only 60 per cent.

Key points: Gestational trophoblastic disease

- Gestational trophoblastic disease is an umbrella term for diseases associated with abnormal trophoblast.

- Hydatidiform moles form when there is excess trophoblastic proliferation due to cytogenetic abnormalities of a conceptus.

Key points: Gestational trophoblast disease—cont'd

- Complete moles are diploid. All of the villi are abnormal and no fetal parts develop.

- Partial moles are triploid. Only some of the chorionic villi undergo hydropic change and fetal parts may be present.

- Hydatidiform moles usually present with bleeding early in pregnancy or with a uterus that is large for the gestational date.

- Most patients with hydatidiform moles are cured by simple evacuation of the contents of the uterus.

- Hydatidiform moles which show deep spread into the myometrium are called invasive moles.

- Invasive moles are recognized by persistent elevation of HCG after evacuation of a mole and usually require chemotherapy to eradicate them fully.

- Choriocarcinomas are highly malignant neoplasms derived from trophoblast which may follow a molar pregnancy or a normal pregnancy. Choriocarcinomas tend to produce marked rises in serum HCG levels.

- Choriocarcinomas show a marked tendency to invade blood vessels and spread widely in the blood to distant sites.

- Fortunately, choriocarcinomas respond well to chemotherapy and the prognosis is generally good.

Pre-eclampsia

Pre-eclampsia is a disorder of pregnancy which can become extremely serious

Pre-eclampsia is a common disorder which affects about 5 per cent of all pregnancies and is more frequent in women carrying their first child. The underlying problem in pre-eclampsia is widespread damage to the mother's vascular endothelial cells, leading to organ damage. The most susceptible organs are the liver, kidneys, and brain.

Placental ischaemia seems to be the key problem in pre-eclampsia

Although there remain many unanswered questions in the aetiology and pathogenesis of pre-eclampsia, current evidence strongly suggests that abnormal placentation is crucial to its development.

In normal placentation, fetal trophoblast deeply penetrates into the myometrium where it surrounds and infiltrates the maternal spiral arteries, destroying their muscular walls and converting them into large low resistance conduits adequate for the increasing demands of the fetus.

Placentas from pre-eclamptic pregnancies are abnormal. The trophoblast shows very shallow invasion of the myometrium with failure to convert the maternal spiral arteries. Whether this is due to an intrinsic defect of the invading trophoblast or some problem with the interaction between the trophoblast and the maternal immune cells in the placenta is unclear. The net effect, though, is placental ischaemia as the demand of the increasing placental bulk is not met by the supply from the maternal spiral arteries. The spiral arteries may also become thrombosed, leading to areas of placental infarction.

An ischaemic placenta releases large quantities of toxic substances into the mother's circulation

The link between the clinical manifestations of pre-eclampsia and placental ischaemia is thought to be the release of toxic substances from the ischaemic placenta. These substances enter the maternal circulation and damage endothelial cells throughout the mother's vascular system, leading to organ damage (Fig. 12.18). Intense research efforts have been directed at finding the agent(s) responsible for pre-eclampsia, but as yet none has been found to be causative.

INTERESTING TO KNOW

sFlt-1 and pre-eclampsia

Recent gene expression profiling has been used to search for candidate genes expressed by the placenta in pre-eclampsia in an attempt to track down the nature of the toxic substances released by the ischaemic placenta. These studies have flagged the gene sFlt-1 (soluble fms-like tyrosine kinase 1) as being upregulated in pre-eclampsia.

Pre-eclampsia is defined by hypertension and proteinuria

Pre-eclampsia is defined clinically by pregnancy-induced hypertension (>140/90 mmHg) developing after 20 weeks gestation in a previously normotensive woman, together with proteinuria (>300 mg/l). Oedema is no longer considered to be a diagnostic feature as most pregnant women are oedematous.

Most women are asymptomatic when diagnosed with pre-eclampsia, the diagnosis being made when routine antenatal screening picks up an elevated blood pressure with proteinuria on stick testing of the urine.

The clinical features of pre-eclampsia are extremely variable and unpredictable

One of the big problems with pre-eclampsia is its notoriously unpredictable clinical course. There is no one symptom, sign, or investigation that reliably predicts disease progression, and patients can become extremely ill very quickly.

In severe pre-eclampsia, there is increasing end-organ damage. Women with severe pre-eclampsia are therefore at risk of hepatic failure, renal failure, and convulsions. Disseminated intravascular coagulation (DIC) often develops as a result of widespread small vessel damage, and the resulting coagulopathy is a further grave complicating factor.

The fetus is also in danger in pre-eclampsia

The fetus itself is also affected in pre-eclampsia. Most show evidence of intrauterine growth restriction and they are at increased risk of sudden intrauterine death. As delivery is the one way to cure severe pre-eclampsia, many fetuses suffer the consequences of a pre-term delivery.

The only curative treatment of pre-eclampsia is delivery of the placenta

Pre-eclampsia may be *controlled* by using antihypertensive agents and antiplatelet drugs; however, the only definitive treatment is delivery of the placenta. Managing women with pre-eclampsia can be extremely challenging and involves difficult decisions. The only effective cure is delivery of the baby and the placenta, so the risks of pre-term delivery must be weighed up against the danger to the mother and the baby of the pre-eclampsia.

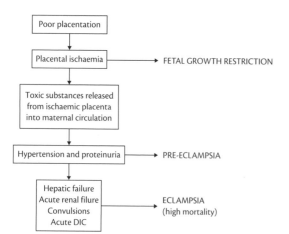

Fig. 12.18 Postulated pathogenesis of pre-eclampsia.

Key points: Pre-eclampsia

- Pre-eclampsia is a common and important disorder of pregnancy in which there is damage to the mother's endothelial cells leading to end-organ damage. The liver, kidneys, and brain are particularly susceptible organs.

- Pre-eclampsia is defined by the onset of hypertension and proteinuria in the second half of pregnancy.

- The danger of pre-eclampsia is the unpredictable risk of progression to severe organ damage with liver failure, renal failure, convulsions, and acute DIC, which carries a grave prognosis for both mother and baby.

Key points: Pre-eclampsia—cont'd

+ Pre-eclampsia is thought to develop due to the release of a substance from an ischaemic placenta into the maternal circulation which causes widespread damage to the mother's endothelial cells.

+ The only effective treatment for pre-eclampsia is delivery of the placenta. Managing pre-eclampsia is therefore challenging, involving balancing the risks to the mother and fetus of ongoing pre-eclampsia against the benefits to the fetus of further intrauterine maturation.

Further reading

www.cancerscreening.org.uk/cervical, NHS Cervical Screening Programme.

Breast disease

Introduction

The breast is essentially a large sweat gland which has become modified to produce milk instead of sweat. The organ consists of a complex network of glands and ducts embedded in connective tissue and padded with fat. Except for its deep surface, the breast is not a well defined organ; it has no capsule, and breast glands can often be found extending beyond its obvious boundaries.

The basic functional unit of the breast is known as the **terminal duct lobular unit** (TDLU) which consists of a grape-like cluster of acini (the actual secretory portions) known as a **lobule** with its attached **terminal duct**. Each lobule drains via its terminal duct into the main duct system of the breast, which eventually opens out at the nipple. The whole of the normal duct and lobular system is two cell layers thick, being composed of an inner glandular epithelial cell layer and an outer myoepithelial cell layer and surrounded by a basement membrane (Fig. 13.1).

The breast is a hormonally responsive organ, although there is a marked difference in response by different parts of the breast. The large and intermediate sized ducts of the breast are unaffected by the changing hormone levels of the menstrual cycle or pregnancy. The TDLUs, however, are dynamic structures which undergo marked changes in response to cyclical hormonal fluctuations. This almost certainly explains why virtually all of the important breast diseases arise from the TDLU.

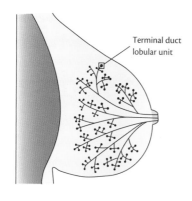

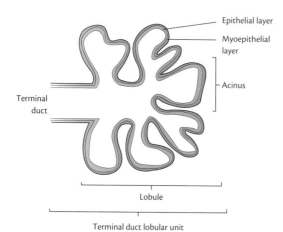

Fig. 13.1 Structure of the adult female breast. Note how the normal acini and ducts are made up of two cell layers (inner epithelial cells and outer myoepithelial cells) surrounded by a basement membrane.

Of all the diseases of the breast, by far the most important is breast carcinoma and virtually all of the workload of a breast surgeon revolves around either treating proven breast carcinoma, or ruling it out as a cause of a breast problem.

Inflammatory disorders of the breast

Inflammatory disorders of the breast are not common, but they are important because they can give rise to symptoms and signs that may mimic breast carcinoma.

The two most common inflammatory conditions of the breast are acute mastitis and fat necrosis.

Acute mastitis

Acute mastitis is a bacterial infection of the breast usually seen in lactating women

Acute mastitis is a bacterial infection of the breast which invariably develops in a breast-feeding mother. Presumably it occurs when a duct becomes blocked by secretions, with stasis and secondary infection. The offending microbe is usually *Staphylococcus aureus*.

The breast appears swollen, tender, and red. Usually treatment with antibiotics is successful, though occasionally infection may progress to abscess formation which requires surgical drainage. One very important point to be aware of is that the clinical picture of acute mastitis may be exactly mimicked by a breast carcinoma inciting an inflammatory response, a clinical condition known as **inflammatory carcinoma**. Vigilance is key: *remember that a swollen red breast is not always due to infection alone.*

Fat necrosis

Fat necrosis is an inflammatory response to spilled fat which can give rise to a palpable lump

Fat necrosis in the breast is usually caused by trauma (car seat belts are well recognized culprits!) leading to an inflammatory response to lipid spilled from adipocytes. A solid irregular mass may form which can be quite firm to palpation. This may raise suspicion of a carcinoma, especially if the woman cannot recall any previous trauma. Fat necrosis is entirely benign and usually spontaneously resolves.

Duct ectasia

Duct ectasia is characterized by dilation of large ducts which become filled with secretions. A nipple discharge is often the presenting feature. If the contents of the ducts spill out, the inflammation and fibrosis that are elicited may form a firm lump, causing concern for a breast carcinoma.

The nipple discharge should be sent for cytological examination. Provided this does not show any malignant cells and a mammogram is normal, the patient can be reassured. If the discharge is very troublesome, excision of the involved duct system can be performed.

TABLE 13.1	Common benign breast lesions
Fibrocystic change	
Fibroadenoma	
Papilloma	

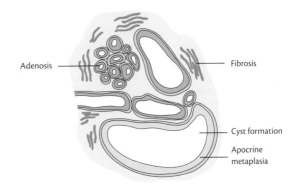

Fig. 13.2 Fibrocystic change. Typical changes in a terminal duct lobular unit seen in fibrocystic change, including adenosis, fibrosis, cyst formation, and apocrine metaplasia.

Benign breast disease

A wide variety of benign diseases occur in the breast (Table 13.1). Some of these present with palpable lumps, but many are now being discovered when mammography is performed as part of the breast screening programme.

Fibrocystic change

Fibrocystic change is the most common alteration seen in the breast

Fibrocystic change is a term used to cover a variety of entirely benign changes in the breast which are the result of minor aberrations in the normal response to cyclical hormonal changes. In the past it was known as fibrocystic 'disease', but the term fibrocystic change is now used to reflect the fact that most people see it almost as a variant of normal. Some have argued that, albeit common and completely benign, it is still an aberration from normal and therefore a disease.

You may also come across the term **ANDI**, which is an acronym for the rather cumbersome name 'aberrations of normal development and involution'. Again this is synonymous with fibrocystic change. Whichever term one uses is really only of personal interest. What is important to appreciate is that fibrocystic change is an umbrella term for a variety of changes in the breast *which have no association with the future development of breast carcinoma.*

Fibrosis, cyst formation, and adenosis are the major alterations associated with fibrocystic change

The alterations seen in fibrocystic change all affect the TDLU and comprise three main patterns of change, which may occur in isolation or in any combination (Fig. 13.2):

- **Fibrosis**
- **Cyst formation**
- **Adenosis.**

Fibrosis refers to the deposition of scar tissue. This often gives the breast tissue a firm feeling which may cause concern. The reason for the development of fibrosis is not entirely clear, but the most plausible explanation is that it follows organization of inflammation in response to ruptured cysts.

Cysts are dilated ducts which are filled with a watery fluid. They are often a prominent component of fibrocystic change and range in size from those detectable only by microscopy to large palpable lesions. Frequently the epithelial cells lining the cysts undergo **apocrine metaplasia**, meaning they change into cells which look like the epithelium of apocrine sweat glands. The presence of apocrine metaplasia appears to have no clinical significance.

Adenosis is an extremely common benign change in the breast. It simply means an increase in the number of acini within some of the lobules. This gives the lobules a crowded appearance histologically, but the acini themselves are completely benign and normal. In simple adenosis, the ducts may be slightly distended but they are not deformed or compressed.

Sclerosing adenosis can mimic an invasive carcinoma clinically and microscopically

One important variant of adenosis is **sclerosing adenosis**, in which the adenosis is accompanied by marked fibrosis which stretches and distorts the crowded glands. Sclerosing adenosis is important because large areas can cause firm lumps which may be suspicious to palpation, and even down the microscope can be alarming because the distortion caused by the fibrosis can mimic the appearance of an invasive carcinoma.

Sclerosing adenosis on its own appears to have no clinical significance, although often areas of sclerosing adenosis show proliferative changes within them which may be significant.

Fibroadenoma

Fibroadenoma is a common benign tumour of the breast in young women

Fibroadenoma is a benign tumour of the breast and is the most common breast tumour occurring in young women aged 20–35 years. Fibroadenomas are interesting because they are made up of overgrowths of both the epithelial and the stromal component of the terminal duct lobular unit. Pathologists sometimes call such tumours 'biphasic' because they have two distinct components to them. In essence, they can be considered as overgrowths of a whole breast lobule.

Fibroadenomas usually present as a painless, discrete, firm, rubbery, round lump. The surrounding breast tissue is compressed but there is no tethering, so the mass is very mobile, accounting for the endearing alternative name of a 'breast mouse'.

The epithelial component of a fibroadenoma is hormonally responsive (remember it is derived from the TDLU) and so there is often enlargement of these lesions at the end of each menstrual cycle. During pregnancy, fibroadenomas may enlarge markedly. Fibroadenomas usually regress after the menopause, though may enlarge in post-menopausal women taking hormone replacement therapy.

Fibroadenomas do not transform into a malignancy if left alone and so do not have to be excised unless there are any worrying features or the woman requests removal. The only exception is a palpable fibroadenoma occurring in a woman over 40 years of age; these are usually removed to exclude a more worrying lesion, particularly a phyllodes tumour (see later).

Papilloma

Papillomas are benign epithelial tumours which arise in large ducts close to the nipple

A **papilloma** is a benign epithelial tumour composed of multiple branching fronds of tissue lined by a normal double layer of breast epithelial and myoepithelial cells. Papillomas usually arise in large ducts close to the nipple, making them unlike most other breast lesions which arise from the TDLU.

Papillomas are most common in middle-aged women, and most present with nipple discharge. The remainder present as small palpable masses within the breast, or as densities on a mammogram. Malignant transformation of a papilloma is extremely rare and no increased risk for invasive breast carcinoma has been demonstrated.

Proliferative breast disease

Proliferative breast disease is associated with an increased risk of subsequent carcinoma

Proliferative breast disease encompasses a number of lesions which are separated out of the spectrum of fibrocystic change because they appear to be markers for an increased risk of cancer. A few important points should be stressed at this point about the lesions of proliferative breast disease:

- They rarely produce lumps. The vast majority are detected either incidentally in breast tissue examined for another reason, or on mammography. As such they have been increasingly recognized since the advent of the breast screening programme.

- They are associated with an increased risk, of greatly varied magnitude, for subsequent development of invasive carcinoma. The lesions themselves are *not* necessarily the direct precursors of breast cancer, but are markers that suggest the breast in general has become genetically unstable and therefore more prone to developing carcinoma.

- They can be seen within an area of otherwise typical fibrocystic change. If this occurs, then the presence of proliferative breast disease 'trumps' the diagnosis of fibrocystic change. Terms such as 'proliferative fibrocystic change' used to refer to proliferative breast disease within an area of fibrocystic change should be avoided. The term fibrocystic change should be reserved only for lesions which are composed *entirely* of elements known to have no association with an increased risk of carcinoma.

Proliferative breast diseases are characterized by epithelial proliferation

At the beginning of this chapter, we briefly described the normal microanatomy of the breast. Recall that the walls of normal ducts and acini are two cell layers

TABLE 13.2	Proliferative breast diseases
Usual epithelial hyperplasia	
Atypical ductal hyperplasia	
In situ lobular neoplasia	
Ductal carcinoma in situ (DCIS)	

thick, made up of an inner epithelial cell layer and an outer myoepithelial cell layer.

The most common proliferative change is an increase in the number of epithelial cells lining the TDLU. Rather than a simple two cell layer, the affected ducts and acini show multilayering such that the epithelial cells start to grow into and fill the affected duct or acinus.

The different types of proliferative diseases are distinguished by their microscopic appearance

Several different types of epithelial proliferation are recognized (Table 13.2). Distinguishing between each type of proliferative breast disease can only be made *morphologically*, i.e. what they look like down the microscope when biopsied. Do not worry about knowing the details of each proliferative lesion; leave that to a pathologist!

Note that the distinction between 'ductal' and 'lobular' proliferative lesions is decided purely on the appearances of the proliferating cells and is nothing to do with where the cells may have originated. In fact, it is likely that all ductal and lobular lesions are derived from the same type of cell, but depending on their subsequent genetic mutations take on different appearances.

Usual epithelial hyperplasia

Usual epithelial hyperplasia has a very low risk of future invasive carcinoma

Usual epithelial hyperplasia is currently the preferred term for a type of epithelial proliferation which is also known as 'usual ductal hyperplasia' and 'hyperplasia of usual type'. This type of proliferative breast disease is a marker which is associated with a very small increased risk of future invasive carcinoma. It is extremely unlikely that usual epithelial hyperplasia becomes malignant; its presence is merely a marker that the breast epithelium has become unstable in general. As such, women found to have areas of usual epithelial proliferation in

a breast biopsy are simply monitored. No specific treatment is required.

Atypical ductal hyperplasia

Atypical ductal hyperplasia is usually managed by a wider excision of the involved area

Atypical ductal hyperplasia is a lesion which lies somewhere between the features of usual epithelial hyperplasia and ductal carcinoma in situ (DCIS), i.e. it has some of the features of DCIS but the changes are not marked enough to be able to apply the label of DCIS. Deciding what to call atypical ductal hyperplasia and what to call DCIS can be very difficult, and indeed many pathologists disagree on the more challenging cases.

In situ lobular neoplasia

In situ lobular neoplasia carries a risk of developing invasive carcinoma at any site in either breast

In situ lobular neoplasia is a term which has recently replaced two entities known as atypical lobular hyperplasia and lobular carcinoma in situ. Traditionally these two lesions were considered separately, but recent molecular studies have shown that these lesions have similar genetic profiles and that biologically they are in fact the same. As such, they are now grouped together as 'in situ lobular neoplasia'.

In situ lobular neoplasia is defined by a proliferation of cells with similar morphological features to invasive lobular carcinoma but which is confined to the ducts and acini. The majority of cases of in situ lobular neoplasia do not produce a lump and are not associated with calcifications on mammography. The diagnosis is therefore often made as an incidental microscopic finding in a breast biopsy performed for other indications. For these reasons, many asymptomatic women presumably go undiagnosed, and the true incidence of in situ lobular neoplasia in the general population remains unknown.

The important point about in situ lobular neoplasia is that the disease is usually found in many different locations in both breasts, i.e. it is *multifocal* and *bilateral*. The presence of in situ lobular neoplasia is therefore associated with an increased risk of developing invasive carcinoma at *any site in either breast*. Because of this, patients who are diagnosed with in situ lobular neoplasia on a biopsy are usually simply monitored closely. A wide local excision is not warranted because the disease is likely to be widespread and bilateral.

Ductal carcinoma in situ

DCIS carries a high risk of progression to an invasive breast carcinoma in that area of the breast

Ductal carcinoma in situ (DCIS) is a proliferation of neoplastic cells with appearances similar to invasive ductal carcinoma but which remain confined to the duct and lobular system. It is therefore distinguished from invasive ductal carcinoma by the absence of invasion through the myoepithelial cell layer and basement membrane surrounding the ducts and lobules.

Most cases of DCIS cannot be detected by palpation, so it is usually picked up on mammography as small areas of calcification. The number of cases of DCIS has therefore increased markedly since the introduction of the national breast screening programme. It is possible for extensive DCIS to distend ducts to such a degree that a palpable mass occurs, but this is very rare.

Very extensive DCIS can track all the way up to the nipple via the duct system and fill the epidermis of the skin. The presence of DCIS cells in the epidermis causes an itchy eczematous lesion called **Paget's disease of the nipple**. Although this is a manifestation of extensive DCIS, in most cases there is also an underlying invasive carcinoma.

DCIS is classified into three grades (high, intermediate, and low) on the basis of how abnormal the nuclei of the cells look. High grade DCIS shows more aggressive features than intermediate or low grade disease and is more likely to develop into an invasive carcinoma.

DCIS is different from all the other types of proliferative breast diseases in that there is good evidence that DCIS is a genuine precursor lesion which carries a risk of developing into an invasive carcinoma *at that site*. In addition (unlike in situ lobular neoplasia), DCIS is almost always a unifocal lesion concentrated in one area of the breast. Surgical removal of DCIS is therefore curative, and prognosis is excellent if excision is complete. Thus, although only a minority of cases of DCIS ever become invasive, all cases should be surgically removed.

Genetic studies are helping us work out how the proliferative lesions may relate to one another

There was a long-held notion that invasive breast carcinoma developed via a linear progression from normal epithelium, through usual epithelial hyperplasia, atypical hyperplasia, and carcinoma in situ. Recent studies, however, have shown that this stepwise theory is far too simplistic and the relationship between these entities is in fact far more complex. Certainly it now seems that usual epithelial hyperplasia is biologically distinct from all the other types of epithelial proliferations, and atypical ductal hyperplasia is genetically very similar to low grade DCIS.

Key points: Proliferative breast disease

- Proliferative breast diseases encompass a number of entities associated with an increased risk of the future development of breast carcinoma. The level of risk varies considerably depending on the precise type of change.

- There are four main types of proliferative breast disease: usual epithelial hyperplasia, atypical ductal hyperplasia, in situ lobular neoplasia, and ductal carcinoma in situ.

- All of these entities arise from the terminal duct lobular unit. The terms 'ductal' and 'lobular' merely reflect the appearances of the proliferating cells and do not imply a site of origin.

- The distinction between the types of proliferative changes can only be made by microscopic examination of the affected area of breast tissue.

- Usual epithelial hyperplasia is associated with a very low risk of future breast carcinoma and these women are just followed-up.

- Atypical ductal hyperplasia is usually treated with a wider excision of the area to exclude an adjacent more sinister lesion.

- In situ lobular neoplasia is a multifocal bilateral disease associated with an increased carcinoma risk in both breasts. Patients with in situ lobular neoplasia are managed with careful monitoring.

Key points: Proliferative breast disease—cont'd

- DCIS is a unifocal lesion which is a recognized precursor lesion of invasive carcinoma and so must be excised in its entirety.

- Molecular studies analysing the specific genetic aberrations in proliferative breast disease is starting to help us work out how each of the lesions may or may not relate to one another, and to invasive breast carcinoma.

Breast carcinoma

Breast carcinomas are a group of malignant epithelial tumours arising in the breast which invade adjacent tissues and have a marked tendency to spread to distant sites. Almost all breast carcinomas are adenocarcinomas derived from the glandular epithelial cells lining the terminal duct lobular unit.

Invasive breast carcinoma is the most common cancer in women, with about 1 in 9 developing it during their life. Although it is no longer the number one cause of cancer-related death in women (lung cancer has now overtaken it), it justifiably remains the most feared malignancy in women.

Breast cancer is a hormone-driven disease

There is overwhelming epidemiological evidence that sex steroid hormones play an important role in the development of breast cancer. Many of the known risk factors for breast cancer can be explained by their effects on hormone levels.

- Reproductive lifestyle. Breast cancers occur more commonly in women who had an early menarche, do not have children, and had a late age at menopause. These are all associated with an increased lifetime exposure to oestrogens.

- Exogenous hormones. The use of oral contraceptives and hormone replacement therapy have both been associated with a small increase in the relative risk of breast cancer.

- Body weight. Adult weight gain is a strong and consistent predictor of post-menopausal breast cancer risk.

The mechanisms are not clear; the risk may be mediated by the elevations in endogenous oestrogen production among heavier women.

Inherited mutations of BRCA1 and BRCA2 predispose to breast cancer

In about 5 per cent of breast cancers, there is clear evidence of an inherited mutation. Two of the best known genes in this regard are BRCA1 and BRCA2. Women with mutations in these genes have a lifetime risk of breast cancer up to 85 per cent and are more likely to develop the disease at a younger age. Mutations in BRCA1 also markedly increase the risk of ovarian carcinoma.

Both BRAC1 and BRCA2 are tumour suppressor genes which appear to function by halting the cell cycle and stimulating DNA repair. In hereditary carcinomas, one mutated allele is inherited and the second allele is inactivated during life.

The two most common types of invasive breast carcinoma are ductal and lobular carcinoma

Many different types of breast cancer have been described (Table 13.3) but only two are commonly seen: invasive ductal carcinoma and invasive lobular carcinoma. Yet again, we stress the point that the distinction between 'ductal' and 'lobular' is made purely on the appearances of the malignant cells and the terms do not imply a particular site of origin.

Invasive ductal carcinoma is the most common type of breast carcinoma

Invasive ductal carcinoma accounts for 80 per cent of all breast carcinomas. It is a heterogeneous group of tumours that fail to exhibit sufficient characteristics to achieve classification as one of the special types of breast carcinoma, such as lobular or tubular carcinoma. Invasive ductal carcinomas are often accompanied by areas of DCIS. The grade of the DCIS often correlates with the grade of the invasive carcinoma.

TABLE 13.3 Types of invasive breast carcinoma

Invasive ductal carcinoma	80%
Invasive lobular carcinoma	10%
Tubular carcinoma	5%
Mucinous carcinoma	2%
Medullary carcinoma	2%

Invasive lobular carcinoma is characterized by loss of cohesion of the cells

Invasive lobular carcinoma represents some 10–15 per cent of all invasive breast cancers. It is composed of small cells which lack cohesion and appear individually dispersed or arranged in single-file linear cords that invade the surrounding breast tissue. Over 90 per cent are associated with areas of adjacent in situ lobular neoplasia.

Breast carcinomas infiltrate locally and metastasize to distant sites via lymphatics and the blood

Direct local spread of a breast tumour may lead to involvement of the overlying skin and underlying muscles. Fixation of a breast lump to the underlying muscles or tethering of the skin over the lump are both worrying features which are highly suspicious of a breast carcinoma.

Lymphatic spread from the breast occurs into the axillary and internal mammary node groups. The axillary lymph nodes are the most common initial site of metastasis. By the time a breast lump is palpable, there is a 50 per cent chance of axillary node involvement. Clinical palpation of lymph nodes is not reliable for detecting metastases, so histological examination is required.

Blood-borne metastasis can lead to widespread dissemination of the tumour to distant sites. The lungs and bones are most frequently involved, but spread often occurs to liver, brain, and the adrenal glands.

Breast carcinoma usually presents as a palpable breast lump

Most breast carcinomas come to clinical attention when the patient discovers a lump in the breast. Other possible methods of presentation include a mammographic abnormality picked up by the breast screening programme or a manifestation of metastatic disease.

All breast lumps should be fully investigated to rule out the possibility of malignancy. Currently a so-called 'triple' assessment is carried out, which involves *clinical* assessment of the lump by palpation, *radiological* assessment with mammogram and/or ultrasound, and *pathological* assessment with fine needle aspiration cytology or core biopsy of the lump. Together, these modalities are very good at correctly diagnosing or ruling out a breast carcinoma.

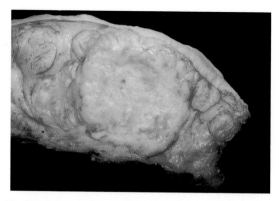

Fig. 13.3 Breast carcinoma. This is a slice from a mastectomy specimen showing a large white tumour mass which felt firm to palpation. Microscopy showed this to be an invasive ductal carcinoma.

Surgical resection is the primary mode of treatment for breast carcinoma

In the absence of demonstrable evidence of metastatic disease, all patients with a breast carcinoma should be considered for surgical resection. Adequate resection can be obtained in most cases by a **wide local excision** ('lumpectomy') of the tumour together with sampling of the axillary lymph nodes.

A wide local excision involves removing the entire tumour mass with a complete margin of normal breast tissue. In some circumstances a full mastectomy is required, particularly if the tumour is so large that performing a wide local excision with adequate margins becomes difficult (Fig. 13.3). Following wide local excision, most patients also have a course of postoperative radiotherapy to the chest wall to treat any tiny amounts of residual disease that have escaped resection.

INTERESTING TO KNOW

Sentinel lymph node sampling

Sentinel lymph node sampling is rapidly evolving as a less invasive method of assessing axillary lymph node status. Rather than removing a large proportion of the axillary nodes, only the 'sentinel' lymph nodes are sampled and examined.

INTERESTING TO KNOW—cont'd

Because the 'sentinel' nodes stand sentry to the rest of the nodal basin, malignant cells must first pass through the sentinel nodes to enter the lymph node region. Theoretically, then, the nodal basin will contain malignant cells only if the sentinel node is first involved. Patients with sentinel nodes free of malignant cells are therefore assumed to have completely clear axillary lymph nodes and can be spared the additional burden of undergoing axillary node removal.

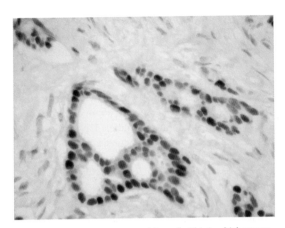

Fig. 13.4 Oestrogen receptor positive cells. This is a high power microscopic image of a breast carcinoma that has been stained with an antibody to the oestrogen receptor. The nuclei of the malignant cells have stained brown, marking them as positive for oestrogen receptor.

Survival of a patient with breast carcinoma can be predicted from a host of prognostic factors

There is great variation in survival following treatment of breast carcinoma. It is important that patients are made fully aware of their prognosis, which can be predicted from a number of features including the histological type of carcinoma, the stage of the tumour, and the grade of the tumour. These three vital pieces of information are all provided by the pathologist examining the surgical resection specimen.

Each tumour type tends to be associated with a different prognosis. For instance, the special types of invasive carcinoma (tubular, mucinous, and medullary) tend to have a more favourable outcome than the ductal and lobular types.

The stage of the tumour reflects the extent of spread, including local spread within the breast, the status of the regional lymph nodes, and if there are any distant metastases. Staging of breast cancer is performed using the TNM system, similar to other tumours.

The grade of the tumour is assessed by the pathologist by examining the tumour cells microscopically. On the basis of how well differentiated the tumour appears, it is assigned a grade between 1 (well differentiated) and 3 (poorly differentiated). High grade tumours are associated with a poorer prognosis.

The receptor status of a breast carcinoma is important in guiding further treatment

As well as typing and grading the tumour and assessing the extent of spread, the pathologist will also assess the receptor status of the tumour. This entails staining a sample of the tumour to see if the malignant cells express certain receptors on their surface (Fig. 13.4). Three receptors are usually investigated: **oestrogen receptor**, **progesterone receptor**, and Her2.

Oestrogen is mitogenic in the breast, stimulating cellular growth by binding to oestrogen receptors. Carcinomas which express oestrogen receptors appear to be slower growing than negative tumours, although they are still capable of metastasizing. The presence of oestrogen receptors is also important in predicting a response to treatment with tamoxifen.

Tamoxifen is an oestrogen receptor antagonist which should be given to all women with oestrogen receptor positive breast carcinoma. Treatment with tamoxifen has been shown to delay the growth of metastases, increase survival, and reduce the risk of developing carcinoma in the other breast.

Progesterone receptors are useful to investigate because they are induced by oestrogens via the oestrogen receptor. The presence of progesterone receptors on the tumour cells therefore indicates that the oestrogen receptors are actually working. Patients with a carcinoma which is positive for oestrogen receptors but negative for progesterone receptors typically show a much poorer response to treatment with tamoxifen than patients positive for both receptors.

Her2 (human epidermal growth factor 2) is a normal glycoprotein involved in the control of cell growth. In some cases of breast cancer, the gene encoding Her2 becomes *amplified* as part of the process of malignant transformation and tumour progression. Instead of the normal two copies of the gene, the malignant cells may contain numerous (>20) copies of the gene.

An abundance of the Her2 protein on the surface of the malignant cells causes them to divide very rapidly. Overexpression of Her2 is seen in about a quarter of all breast cancers, and many studies have shown that these tumours have a poor prognosis. Evaluation of the Her2 status is important because a monoclonal antibody against the Her2 receptor has been developed. The antibody, known as **trastuzumab**, has been shown to improve outcome when given with chemotherapy in patients with Her2-amplified carcinomas.

INTERESTING TO KNOW

Oestrogen receptor positive carcinomas

It may seem counterintuitive that cancers with oestrogen receptors are slower growing, when oestrogen stimulates growth in the breast. The explanation for this is that oestrogen receptors are really just a marker that suggest that the malignant cells are in general still expressing receptors that control their growth in some fashion. Thus the presence of oestrogen receptors should be thought of more as a marker suggestive that the malignant cells are still under some sort of growth control, albeit highly dysregulated.

Genetic studies suggest there are two distinct pathways in the development of breast carcinoma

Studying the genetics of breast cancers is having a massive impact on our understanding of the development of breast cancers. One of the most striking findings is the difference in genetic profiles between cancers designated as low grade or high grade on microscopic appearance. This suggests that low and high grade cancers represent quite distinct molecular pathways, and that progression from a low grade cancer to a high grade cancer is rare (Fig. 13.5).

Key points: Breast carcinoma

- Breast carcinoma is the most common cancer in women and the second most common cancer killer in women.

- Breast carcinoma is a hormone-driven disease strongly related to lifetime oestrogen exposure.

- Virtually all breast carcinomas are adenocarcinomas derived from the glandular epithelial cells lining the terminal duct lobular unit.

- The most common types of breast carcinoma are invasive ductal carcinoma and invasive lobular carcinoma.

- Breast carcinoma spreads locally within the breast, via lymphatics to axillary nodes, and haematogenously to distant sites such as the liver, lungs, and brain.

- Most breast cancers present with a palpable lump, but may also be picked up on mammography as part of the breast screening programme.

- All breast lumps should be investigated with a triple assessment involving clinical examination, radiological imaging, and pathological examination (either fine needle aspiration cytology or core biopsy).

- The standard treatment for breast carcinoma is surgical excision of the lesion with a margin of normal breast tissue, and removal of the axillary lymph nodes on the same side as the tumour.

- The pathologist will examine the resection specimen and provide important prognostic information including the grade and stage of the tumour and the receptor status of the tumour. This determines any further treatment postoperatively.

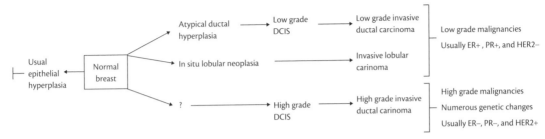

Fig. 13.5 Postulated pathways in the development of breast carcinomas. ER, oestrogen receptor; HER2, human epidermal growth factor 2 receptor; PR, progesterone receptor.

Breast cancer screening

The UK has a national screening programme for breast cancer

The NHS Breast Screening Programme invites all women aged between 50 and 70 for a screening mammogram every 3 years. Women under 50 years of age are not offered routine screening because the density of the breast tissue in pre-menopausal women makes it more difficult to detect abnormalities on the mammogram. As women go past the menopause, the glandular tissue in their breast involutes, and the breast tissue is increasingly made up of only fat. Fat is clearer on the

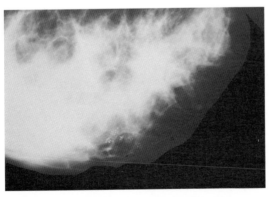

Fig. 13.6 Mammogram showing calcification. This mammogram, performed as part of the breast screening programme, shows numerous flecks of calcification, most obvious at the bottom of the mammogram. Other flecks can also be seen at the top of the image. Core biopsy of the calcification revealed high grade ductal carcinoma in situ.

mammogram, making interpretation more reliable. Breast cancer is also far more common in post-menopausal women and the risk continues to increase with rising age.

The aim of the screening programme is to identify pre-invasive lesions (mainly DCIS) or small invasive carcinomas before they have spread widely. Suspicious features on mammograms include small areas of calcification (Fig. 13.6) and densities, which are directed for further investigations such as ultrasound, fine needle aspiration cytology, or core biopsy of the area. If DCIS or small invasive carcinomas are diagnosed in this way, often a guide wire has to be placed into the lesion by a radiologist under guidance so that the surgeon knows which area to excise.

Other breast neoplasms

Phyllodes tumour

Phyllodes tumour is distinguished from fibroadenoma by the degree of stromal cellularity

A **phyllodes tumour** is best considered as a 'worrying fibroadenoma'. Like fibroadenoma, a phyllodes tumour is a biphasic tumour composed of an epithelial and a stromal component, but the stromal component is more atypical than a fibroadenoma. Phyllodes tumours usually present with a palpable mass, but in older women (10–20 years later than the average presentation age for a fibroadenoma). The majority are low grade tumours that may recur locally unless widely excised. Metastases to lymph nodes or distant sites are extremely rare.

Phyllodes tumours are distinguished from fibroadenomas by their microscopic appearance. The stromal cellularity is greater and there is more atypia within the cells. The stromal overgrowth leads to the formation of bulbous protrusions due to nodules of proliferating stroma covered by epithelium.

Male breast disease

The male breast is a rudimentary structure, consisting of small numbers of large ducts but no terminal duct lobular units. The ducts of the male breast are, however, responsive to hormonal stimuli—oestrogen stimulates the breast tissue and androgens inhibit it.

Gynaecomastia

Gynaecomastia is an enlargement of the male breast

Gynaecomastia is an enlargement of the male breast. It is the result of an imbalance between hormone levels, leading to relative excess of oestrogens. The most common cause of gynaecomastia is chronic liver disease, as the liver is responsible for metabolizing oestrogens. Drugs which alter oestrogen or androgen levels are also common causes of gynaecomastia and include therapeutic drugs such as spironolactone and recreational drugs such as marijuana and anabolic steroids. Gynaecomastia is also often seen in elderly men as oestrogens produced by the adrenal glands increase and androgens from the testis fall with age.

Carcinoma of the male breast

Carcinoma of the male breast is rare

Breast carcinoma in men can occur, but is rare. The only well recognized risk factor for male breast carcinoma is **Klinefelter syndrome**. The tumours typically present with a lump. As the tumours arise in large ducts close to the nipple, nipple discharge and retraction often occur. The spread of breast carcinoma in the male is identical to that in the female, and the treatment and prognosis are also the same.

Further reading

Hartmann LC, Sellers TA, Frost MH *et al.* (2005). Benign breast disease and the risk of breast cancer. *New England Journal of Medicine* 353: 229–237.
www.cancerscreening.nhs.uk/breastscreen, NHS Breast Screening Programme.

Endocrine disease

Introduction

An **endocrine gland** is an organ that produces hormones (Fig. 14.1). **Hormones** are molecules secreted into the blood which act on specific target cells throughout the body. Endocrine glands are therefore distinguished from *exocrine* glands which release their secretions into the bowel, respiratory tract, or skin.

Most hormones are either proteins/peptides or steroids. Protein/peptide hormones interact with receptors located on the surface of their target cells. Binding to the receptor triggers a complex sequence of signalling pathways in the cell, leading to changes in cell function that mediate the response to the hormone. Examples of protein hormones include insulin, growth hormone, follicle-stimulating hormone, luteinizing hormone, and adrenocorticotrophic hormone.

Steroid hormones are synthesized from cholesterol and travel in the blood bound to transporting proteins. They act by crossing through the cell membrane and binding directly to receptors located within their target cell, usually in the nucleus. Examples of steroid hormones include cortisol, oestrogen, progesterone, and testosterone.

Most endocrine diseases can be divided into conditions of hormone excess and hormone deficiency. Tumours of endocrine glands, as well as potentially causing increased or decreased hormone production, may also produce problems by virtue of their mass effect.

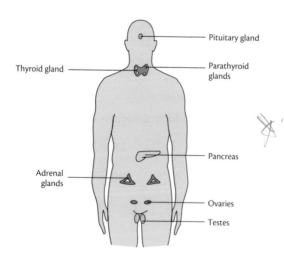

Fig. 14.1 Endocrine organs.

Because most hormones have multiple actions at multiple sites, hormonal excess or deficiency can lead to a multitude of clinical symptoms and signs. Often the clinical features are subtle and appear gradually, meaning the diagnosis may be missed for some time. Endocrinology can therefore be an immensely satisfying speciality to practice: if you make the correct diagnosis, the treatment is often simple yet extremely effective.

Anterior pituitary

The pituitary gland consists of the anterior pituitary and the posterior pituitary

The **pituitary gland** is an endocrine organ located at the base of the brain where it attaches to the hypothalamus. It is composed of two parts which, though closely related anatomically, are embryologically and functionally distinct. The anterior pituitary comprises glandular tissue derived from an upgrowth from the developing oral cavity, whilst the posterior pituitary is a downgrowth from the developing brain and is therefore of neural origin.

The **anterior pituitary** secretes six hormones: growth hormone (GH), prolactin, follicle-stimulating hormone (FSH), luteinizing hormone (LH), thyroid-stimulating hormone (TSH), and adrenocorticotrophic hormone (ACTH). The last four hormones are known as **trophic hormones** because they stimulate the activity of other endocrine organs (the gonads, thyroid, and adrenal glands). The secretion of all six anterior pituitary hormones is in turn regulated by hormones from the hypothalamus, which reach the pituitary through a portal system of blood vessels.

Pituitary adenoma

Pituitary adenoma is the most common disease of the anterior pituitary

Pituitary adenoma is a benign neoplasm derived from the glandular tissue of the anterior pituitary. The aetiology of pituitary adenomas is not known. Symptoms related to a pituitary adenoma may include the following:

◆ *Endocrine effects.* Functional adenomas can produce syndromes related to excess hormone secretion. In addition, both functional and non-functional adenomas may also cause hypopituitarism (see later) by compressing adjacent normal pituitary tissue.

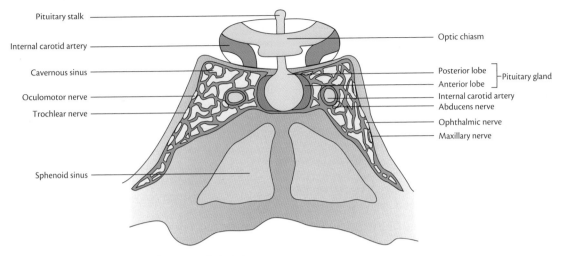

Fig. 14.2 The pituitary gland and its close anatomical relations.

◆ *Mass effects*. The anterior pituitary has a number of important nearby anatomical relations which may be compressed by an expanding pituitary adenoma (Fig. 14.2). Impingement on the optic chiasm just above the pituitary causes a *visual field disturbance* known as a **bitemporal hemianopia** in which the lateral halves of each visual field are lost. Diplopia (double vision) may also occur from compression of cranial nerves III, IV, or VI by lateral extension of a tumour into the cavernous sinus. Non-specific symptoms related to any intracranial mass, such as headache and nausea, may also occur with pituitary adenomas. The headaches, which are thought to be related to stretching of the dura, tend to be worse in the morning on waking.

Pituitary adenomas may be functional or non-functional

Many non-functional adenomas remain tiny and never come to clinical attention. Small non-functional incidental adenomas appear to be common, found in about 25 per cent of pituitary glands examined at autopsy and in some 20 per cent of people having pituitary magnetic resonance imaging (MRI). Patients with larger tumours present with mass effects, i.e. headache and a visual field disturbance. Surgical excision is the mainstay of treatment which may be followed by postoperative radiotherapy in patients with incompletely excised tumours.

Functional tumours tend to present earlier than non-functional tumours, because of the effects of excessive hormone secretion. Despite producing profound effects throughout the body, functional tumours can be extremely small. The most commonly secreted hormones from functional pituitary adenomas are prolactin, GH, and ACTH, in that order. Functional pituitary adenomas secreting FSH, LH, or TSH are extremely rare.

Prolactinoma is the most common type of functional adenoma

Prolactinomas are pituitary adenomas which originate from the prolactin-producing cell in the anterior pituitary. The presentation depends on the patient's age and sex. Men and post-menopausal women usually come to medical attention because of symptoms of a pituitary mass with headache and visual disturbance. Women of reproductive age commonly present earlier because of menstrual disturbance (oligomenorrhoea and amenorrhoea) or galactorrhoea. These patients often have extremely small tumours.

Most small prolactinomas respond to medical therapy with a dopamine agonist, e.g. cabergoline or bromocriptine. These agents activate dopamine D2 receptors on the neoplastic cells, leading to inhibition of prolactin production and a reduction in prolactin levels. Treatment dramatically shrinks tumour size, with disappearance of headaches and improvement in visual fields. The success rate of treatment with dopamine agonists in prolactinomas avoids the need for surgery in most patients.

Growth hormone-secreting adenomas present with acromegaly

GH is a peptide hormone essential for normal growth. It also has a number of metabolic effects such as increasing protein synthesis and increasing hepatic glucose production. In adults, excessive GH secretion causes increased growth of the hands, feet, jaw, and internal organs. The clinical result is **acromegaly**, which has a number of features (Fig. 14.3). Common features which lead patients to seek medical attention include the following:

♦ Facial changes. The skin and lips thicken, and the frontal sinuses expand resulting in protrusion ('frontal bossing'). Growth of the lower mandible leads to protrusion of the lower jaw.

♦ Enlargement of the hands and feet. Patients notice rings becoming tighter and their shoe size increases.

♦ Excessive sweating, which is a very prominent symptom.

♦ Carpal tunnel syndrome, due to the increased soft tissue mass compressing the median nerve at the wrist.

The insidious onset of acromegaly means that the diagnosis is easily missed, and often delayed for 10 years or so. Although the cosmetic features are the most obvious features of acromegaly, the condition is serious, associated with a doubling in mortality compared with normal populations. This is mainly due to the high incidence of cardiovascular disease due to left ventricular

hypertrophy and hypertension, which is common in acromegaly. Acromegaly is also a diabetogenic state because GH antagonizes the effects of insulin. Twenty-five per cent of patients with acromegaly have impaired glucose tolerance and 10 per cent have frank diabetes mellitus, both of which are strong risk factors for cardiovascular disease.

A clinical diagnosis of acromegaly should be confirmed biochemically by performing an **oral glucose tolerance test**, in which GH concentrations are measured following ingestion of a glucose drink (p. 325). In normal subjects, plasma GH concentration falls to an undetectable level. In acromegaly, *GH fails to suppress normally* and may even rise.

The treatment of choice in the majority of cases is trans-sphenoidal resection of the pituitary tumour. If there is ongoing evidence of excessive GH secretion after surgery, medical therapy can be used. The most widely used drug is octreotide, a long-acting analogue of somatostatin which inhibits GH secretion.

ACTH-secreting adenomas cause Cushing's disease

ACTH-secreting pituitary adenomas lead to bilateral hyperplasia of the adrenal cortices with resulting excess secretion of glucocorticoids. Prolonged exposure to elevated levels of glucocorticoids causes **Cushing's syndrome** which is discussed in the section on the adrenal cortex. When Cushing's syndrome is caused by an ACTH-secreting pituitary adenoma, it is known as Cushing's *disease* or pituitary-dependent Cushing's syndrome.

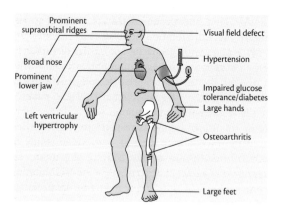

Fig. 14.3 Clinical features of acromegaly.

> # Key points: Pituitary adenomas
>
> ♦ Pituitary adenomas are benign neoplasms of the anterior pituitary.
>
> ♦ Symptoms resulting from pituitary adenomas are related to mass effects and/or endocrine disturbances.
>
> ♦ Non-functional adenomas are very common and many remain small and subclinical. Large tumours cause symptoms due to their size, such as headaches and visual field disturbances.

Key points: Pituitary adenomas—cont'd

- Prolactinomas are the most common functional pituitary adenoma. In men and post-menopausal women, they usually present with mass effects, whereas in pre-menopausal women they present much earlier due to menstrual disturbances and galactorrhoea.

- GH-secreting adenomas lead to acromegaly in adults. Acromegaly has a number of cosmetic manifestations as well as an associated doubling in cardiovascular risk. A clinical diagnosis of acromegaly is confirmed by demonstrating a failure of the normal suppression of plasma GH concentration in response to a glucose load.

- ACTH-secreting pituitary adenomas cause bilateral adrenal cortical hyperplasia and elevated circulating glucocorticoid levels, resulting in Cushing's syndrome. Cushing's syndrome due to an ACTH-secreting pituitary adenoma is known as Cushing's disease or pituitary-dependent Cushing's syndrome.

Hypopituitarism

Hypopituitarism is usually due to a destructive process involving the anterior pituitary. The most common causes are as follows:

- Pituitary adenomas. These are the most common cause.

- Metastatic deposits in the pituitary.

- Iatrogenic, as a complication of pituitary surgery or irradiation.

- Severe head injury may also cause traumatic damage to the anterior pituitary.

Partial hypopituitarism is seen much more frequently than complete hypopituitarism (panhypopituitarism). The classic finding is progressive loss of pituitary hormone secretion in the following order: LH, GH, TSH, ACTH, and FSH. Prolactin deficiency is very uncommon.

The clinical features of hypopituitarism are often subtle, and most cases are in fact picked up when tests of anterior pituitary function are performed in a patient known to be at risk of a deficiency, e.g. during the investigation of a patient found to have a pituitary adenoma, or as part of the routine follow-up of a patient who has had previous pituitary surgery or irradiation.

Posterior pituitary

The posterior pituitary secretes two hormones: **antidiuretic hormone** (ADH, or vasopressin) and **oxytocin**. Both hormones are actually synthesized in the hypothalamus but travel down through nerve axons into the posterior pituitary where they are released into the blood.

ADH has a vital role in controlling the tonicity of the extracellular fluid. It acts on the collecting ducts of the kidney, leading to water reabsorption (hence its 'antidiuretic' name). The major stimulus to ADH release is an increase in plasma osmolality which is sensed by the hypothalamus, leading to increased ADH secretion. Oxytocin stimulates contraction of the smooth muscle cells of the myometrium during labour, and stimulates the release of milk from the lactating breast.

Diseases of the posterior pituitary are rare, and the clinically relevant ones involve ADH. Disorders of oxytocin secretion are uncommon and not clinically important.

Syndrome of inappropriate ADH secretion

Excess secretion of ADH causes water retention by the kidneys leading to dilutional hyponatraemia

Continued and inappropriate production of ADH is known as the **syndrome of inappropriate ADH secretion** (SIADH). There is excessive reabsorption of water by the kidneys, leading to water overload. The condition is usually asymptomatic, the diagnosis being first considered when a patient is found to have unexplained hyponatraemia. Symptoms related to water excess such as confusion, drowsiness, and convulsions do not normally develop unless there is profound water intoxication. Of particular note, peripheral oedema is not a feature of SIADH because excess water alone (as opposed to excess water and sodium) is shared between the extracellular and intracellular fluid compartments, and the increase in extracellular fluid volume is insufficient to cause oedema.

SIADH has been associated with many conditions. Head injuries, encephalitis, and brain tumours have all been associated with SIADH, presumably by disrupting normal hypothalamic function. The most common extracranial cause of SIADH is ectopic ADH secretion by tumours, particularly small cell carcinomas of the lung.

As a brief aside, it is important to stress that hyponatraemia is a very common electrolyte abnormality with numerous causes. SIADH is not a common cause of hyponatraemia, and it is crucial to exclude more common causes of hyponatraemia before considering SIADH.

Diabetes insipidus

Decreased secretion of ADH causes uncontrollable water loss through the kidneys

Failure of ADH production causes uncontrollable water loss through the kidneys, a condition known as **diabetes insipidus**. The patient develops polyuria and thirst, and is in danger of severe dehydration.

TABLE 14.1 Causes of diabetes insipidus
Idiopathic
Head injury
Pituitary tumour
CNS infection (meningitis, encephalitis)

Virtually any type of intracranial pathology may lead to failure in ADH secretion (Table 14.1). Most cases are due to hypothalamic or pituitary stalk damage as a result of head injury or a pituitary tumour. Of note, no specific cause can be found in about one-third of cases, although some of these patients may have circulating autoantibodies to the ADH-synthesizing neurones, suggesting a possible autoimmune aetiology.

Adrenal cortex

The adrenal glands are composed of two distinct parts: the cortex and medulla. The adrenal cortex produces three steroid hormones: **glucocorticoids**, **mineralocorticoids**, and **androgens**.

Glucocorticoids, of which the most important is **cortisol**, are secreted in response to ACTH from the anterior pituitary. Cortisol is essential to life: it is involved in the response to stress and regulates many pathways of metabolism.

The most important mineralocorticoid is **aldosterone**. Aldosterone plays a central role in the control of extracellular fluid volume. It is secreted in response to a decreased blood volume through activation of the renin–angiotensin–aldosterone system (Fig. 14.4). The main action of aldosterone is to stimulate sodium and water reabsorption in the distal convoluted tubules of the kidney.

Adrenocortical diseases are relatively rare but are important nonetheless as they can be easy to diagnose and simple to treat. The diseases are most readily considered on the basis of whether they lead to hormone excess (adrenocortical hyperfunction) or hormone deficiency (adrenocortical hypofunction).

Adrenocortical hyperfunction

The outcome of hyperfunction of the adrenal cortex depends on whether the dominantly produced hormones are glucocorticoids or mineralocorticoids. Unregulated secretion of glucocorticoids from the adrenal cortex

---

Key points: Posterior pituitary disease

- Diseases of the posterior pituitary are much rarer than those of the anterior pituitary.

- Virtually all posterior pituitary diseases are disorders of ADH secretion.

- Excess ADH secretion leads to water retention by the kidneys, a condition known as syndrome of inappropriate ADH secretion. The diagnosis is usually made when a patient is found to have unexplained hyponatraemia. The underlying cause is usually intracranial pathology affecting pituitary function or ectopic ADH from a tumour, usually a small cell carcinoma of the lung.

- Decreased secretion of ADH leads to uncontrollable water loss through the kidneys, a condition known as diabetes insipidus. The patient presents with polyuria and polydipsia. Diabetes insipidus may be caused by any intracranial disease affecting ADH secretion. Up to one-third of cases are idiopathic.

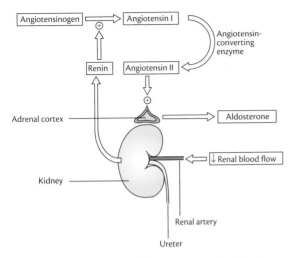

Fig. 14.4 Renin–angiotensin–aldosterone system. A reduction in renal blood flow stimulates release of renin from the kidney, which leads to the production of angiotensin II. Angiotensin II stimulates the release of aldosterone from the adrenal cortex, which causes reabsorption of sodium and water by the kidneys to restore circulating volume.

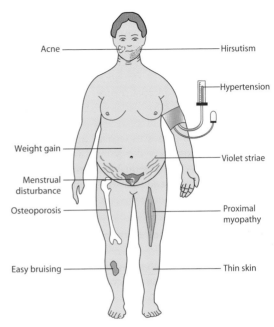

Fig. 14.5 Clinical features of Cushing's syndrome.

leads to Cushing's syndrome. Unregulated secretion of mineralocorticoids from the adrenal cortex causes Conn's syndrome.

Cushing's syndrome

Cushing's syndrome is the result of persistent excess circulating glucocorticoids

Cushing's syndrome refers to a constellation of symptoms and signs caused by prolonged exposure to inappropriately high levels of circulating glucocorticoids. Similarly to other endocrine disorders, the features of Cushing's syndrome are extremely varied (Fig. 14.5) and the early manifestations can be subtle.

Weight gain and muscle weakness are common presenting symptoms of Cushing's syndrome

One of the earliest symptoms that patients with Cushing's syndrome become aware of is *weight gain*. Over time, a typical pattern of fat deposition becomes apparent, with marked truncal obesity and a 'moon' face. Weakness of muscles, particularly in the proximal limbs, is another common symptom (proximal myopathy). Patients will often describe problems tackling stairs and

getting up from a sitting position. Gonadal dysfunction is common, with menstrual irregularities in women and loss of libido in men. Hirsutism is often seen in women with Cushing's syndrome, as is acne.

LINK BOX

Proximal myopathy

A proximal myopathy is also seen in thyrotoxicosis (p. 312), osteomalacia (p. 405), and polymyositis (p. 446).

The most common cause of Cushing's syndrome is therapeutic administration of synthetic glucocorticoids

In everyday practice, Cushing's syndrome is most often seen as a troublesome side effect of synthetic glucocorticoids given in large doses as immune-suppressing agents. Strictly speaking, of course, Cushing's syndrome due to exogenous glucocorticoids is not the result of adrenocortical hyperfunction. In fact, patients taking synthetic glucocorticoids have *hypofunctional* adrenal cortices because the exogenous glucocorticoids suppress secretion of ACTH from the anterior pituitary by negative feedback. In the absence of the trophic effects of ACTH, the adrenal cortices undergo atrophy. This is the reason why patients should always be weaned off glucocorticoid treatment gradually to allow their own adrenal glands to recover function. Sudden withdrawal is extremely dangerous, as the patient's own adrenal glands will be unable to provide sufficient glucocorticoid output and they will go in acute adrenal failure.

There are three common causes of endogenous Cushing's syndrome

In patients with Cushing's syndrome who are not taking exogenous steroids, there are three common underlying causes:

- *ACTH-secreting pituitary adenoma.* Cushing's syndrome caused by a functional pituitary adenoma producing ACTH is also known as Cushing's *disease*, or pituitary-dependent Cushing's syndrome. This is the most common cause of endogenous Cushing's syndrome. The adrenal glands show bilateral cortical hyperplasia due to stimulation by high levels of ACTH.

- *Hypersecretion of cortisol by an adrenal cortical tumour.* Both adrenal adenomas and carcinomas may cause Cushing's syndrome if they produce cortisol. Adrenal carcinomas tend to be inefficient at producing cortisol, meaning that they are often quite large by the time Cushing's syndrome becomes clinically apparent.

- *Secretion of ACTH by a non-pituitary tumour.* This is known as ectopic ACTH production and is most well described in association with a small cell carcinoma of the lung. In reality, it is unusual for patients with small cell carcinoma of the lung and ectopic ACTH production to develop full-blown Cushing's syndrome, as unfortunately most are dead before this can happen.

Cushing's syndrome can be confirmed by finding a raised 24 h urinary free cortisol level

Any patient suspected of having endogenous Cushing's syndrome should have the diagnosis confirmed before any investigations into the underlying cause are attempted. Confirming the presence of Cushing's syndrome can be achieved biochemically by measuring 24 h urinary free cortisol which is raised in most patients with endogenous Cushing's syndrome.

Plasma ACTH measurement helps distinguish between the causes of Cushing's syndrome

Once Cushing's syndrome has been confirmed, investigations should then aim to determine the cause. This is usually achieved with a combination of biochemical tests and imaging studies. Plasma ACTH measurements are useful to differentiate between causes. In Cushing's disease, ACTH will be either inappropriately normal or mildly elevated. ACTH levels in cases of ectopic ACTH are usually markedly elevated. In patients with adrenal tumours, ACTH is invariably undetectable due to normal negative feedback mechanisms.

INTERESTING TO KNOW

Blood samples for ACTH measurement

To be sure of a meaningful value for plasma ACTH, the blood sample must be drawn into a *plastic* EDTA tube (ACTH sticks to glass) and delivered immediately to the biochemistry laboratory on ice to prevent natural degradation of ACTH.

Imaging of the pituitary or adrenals should be performed depending on the results of biochemical tests

If biochemical tests suggest pituitary-dependent Cushing's syndrome, then imaging of the pituitary with MRI is indicated to confirm the presence of a pituitary adenoma. If biochemical tests suggest pituitary-independent disease, then a CT scan of the abdomen is indicated to image the adrenals to look for the presence of an adrenal tumour.

Key points: Cushing's syndrome

- Cushing's syndrome refers to a collection of symptoms and signs caused by prolonged exposure to high levels of circulating glucocorticoids.

Key points: Cushing's syndrome—cont'd

- Weight gain, proximal myopathy, and menstrual abnormalities are common presenting symptoms. Common clinical signs include hypertension, violet abdominal striae, and bruising.

- The most common cause of Cushing's syndrome is therapeutic administration of glucocorticoids.

- In patients with endogenous Cushing's syndrome, there are three main causes: an ACTH-producing pituitary adenoma (Cushing's *disease*), a cortisol-producing adrenal tumour, and ectopic ACTH production by a non-pituitary tumour.

- Patients suspected of having endogenous Cushing's syndrome should have biochemical confirmation by measuring urinary free cortisol in a 24 h urine collection.

- Once endogenous Cushing's syndrome has been confirmed, the underlying cause can usually be determined by a combination of biochemical tests (such as plasma ACTH) and imaging studies of the pituitary or adrenal glands.

- Treatment of endogenous Cushing's syndrome is usually surgical, with trans-sphenoidal hypophysectomy for a pituitary adenoma or adrenalectomy for an adrenal tumour.

Primary hyperaldosteronism

Primary hyperaldosteronism is caused by excessive production of aldosterone by the adrenal cortex

Primary hyperaldosteronism, or **Conn's syndrome**, is characterized by excessive production of aldosterone from the adrenal cortex. The most common cause of this is a unilateral functional adrenal cortical adenoma. Most of the other cases are due to unexplained bilateral hyperplasia of the aldosterone-producing zone of the adrenal cortex. Adrenal cortical *carcinomas* leading to Conn's syndrome are vanishingly rare.

Hyperaldosteronism leads to sodium retention and potassium wasting by the kidneys

Excess aldosterone in Conn's syndrome stimulates reabsorption of sodium and water by the distal collecting tubules and collecting ducts of the kidneys. The extracellular fluid volume expands and blood pressure rises. When the extracellular fluid volume reaches a certain point, however, excretion of sodium and water by the kidneys *resumes* despite the raised aldosterone levels. This so-called 'escape phenomenon' is the result of increased secretion of atrial natriuretic peptide which overcomes the effect of aldosterone at the level of the collecting ducts. The escape phenomenon explains why patients with Conn's syndrome do not become oedematous. Escape does not occur at the level of the distal collecting tubules, however, where the high circulating aldosterone levels stimulate continued exchange of sodium for potassium, leading to hypokalaemia.

Patients with Conn's syndrome usually come to medical attention due to hypertension

Patients with Conn's syndrome are usually asymptomatic. The diagnosis is usually first suspected when hypokalaemia is found during investigation of a patient with mild to moderate hypertension. A minority of patients will have symptoms related to the hypokalaemia such as muscle weakness and polyuria.

LINK BOX

Conn's syndrome and hypertension

Conn's syndrome is one of the causes of secondary hypertension (p. 73). Although accounting for only 1 per cent of all cases of hypertension, it is important since it is potentially curable by excision of the adrenal adenoma.

A high plasma aldosterone:renin ratio is diagnostic of primary hyperaldosteronism

When a diagnosis of Conn's syndrome is suspected, confirmation requires evidence of high plasma aldosterone levels in the absence of an elevated renin level. Measuring renin levels excludes secondary hyperaldosteronism where the high aldosterone levels are a normal physiological response to a high renin concentration (see later). A high aldosterone:renin ratio should prompt imaging of the adrenal glands to determine if the underlying cause is an aldosterone-secreting adrenal adenoma or bilateral adrenal cortical hyperplasia.

Adrenal adenomas should be excised, whereas bilateral hyperplasia should be treated with spironolactone

Patients found to have a unilateral adrenal cortical adenoma should undergo adrenalectomy. Because the tumours are always small, they can usually be easily removed by laparoscopic surgery. Surgery is usually curative and most patients can stop all antihypertensive medications.

Patients found to have bilateral hyperplasia are managed medically with spironolactone, a competitive antagonist of the aldosterone receptor. Most patients treated with spironolactone have a substantial reduction in blood pressure with normalization of electrolytes after about 1 month of therapy.

INTERESTING TO KNOW

Conn's syndrome—more common than we think?

The incidence of Conn's syndrome has always been stated as being in the region of 1–2 per cent of all hypertensives based on cases with the typical electrolyte pattern. Recently, however, as many as 5 per cent of all hypertensives without the typical electrolyte abnormalities have been shown to have Conn's syndrome on the basis of aldosterone:renin ratios.

The take-home message is that a diagnosis of Conn's syndrome should still be considered in a hypertensive patient who appears resistant to conventional treatment and whose electrolytes are heading in the direction of a Conn's picture even if they are not actually outside the normal range (i.e. sodium at the high end of normal and potassium at the low end of normal).

Key points: Primary hyperaldosteronism (Conn's syndrome)

- Conn's syndrome describes a state in which the adrenal cortex autonomously produces excess aldosterone.

- The two main underlying causes of Conn's syndrome are a unilateral adrenal cortical adenoma and bilateral hyperplasia of the adrenal cortices.

- The majority of patients with Conn's syndrome are asymptomatic and are diagnosed following investigation of hypertension.

- Hypertensive patients should be suspected of having Conn's syndrome if they are found to have hypokalaemia and hypernatraemia, or if hypertension is difficult to treat and the patient's sodium is at the high end of normal and their potassium is at the low end of normal.

- Patients suspected of having Conn's require measurement of plasma aldosterone and renin to seek evidence of a raised aldosterone:renin ratio.

- Imaging can then be used to determine if the patient has a unilateral adenoma or bilateral hyperplasia.

- Surgical removal is the treatment of choice for an adrenal cortical adenoma.

- Spironolactone, an aldosterone antagonist, is the treatment of choice for patients with Conn's syndrome due to bilateral adrenal hyperplasia.

Secondary hyperaldosteronism

Secondary hyperaldosteronism refers to the presence of high aldosterone concentrations in the context of raised renin levels. In contrast to Conn's syndrome, the adrenal glands are responding appropriately to their normal stimulus. *Secondary hyperaldosteronism is therefore not a disease of the adrenal glands; it is a biochemical manifestation of a non-adrenal disease causing raised renin levels.* This is similar to the situation in the parathyroid glands, where secondary hyperparathyroidism is a biochemical manifestation of a disease causing low calcium levels; the parathyroid glands are responding appropriately to their normal stimulus.

Secondary hyperaldosteronism is most commonly the result of conditions that cause a reduction in effective renal blood flow, and hence stimulate renin release. Such conditions include chronic left ventricular failure, end-stage chronic liver disease, and the nephrotic syndrome. The precise mechanisms which lead to the reduction in renal blood flow in these conditions is complicated and not fully understood.

Hypertension is not necessarily a feature of secondary hyperaldosteronism as the underlying condition often modifies blood pressure of its own accord. For instance, end-stage liver disease tends to cause systemic vasodilation which lowers blood pressure.

Adrenocortical hypofunction

Adrenocortical insufficiency is seen in two clinical settings: chronic insufficiency and acute insufficiency. Chronic adrenal insufficiency (Addison's disease) is due to gradual destruction of the adrenal cortex with the progressive onset of symptoms. Acute adrenal insufficiency is a life-threatening situation caused by a sudden total loss of adrenocortical function.

Addison's disease

Chronic adrenal insufficiency is also known as Addison's disease

Addison's disease is an uncommon disorder resulting from progressive destruction of the adrenal cortex. The most common cause of Addison's disease in developed countries is **autoimmune adrenalitis**, in which the adrenal cortices are slowly destroyed by autoreactive T lymphocytes. Autoantibodies can be detected in almost all cases, but these are thought to be markers of the autoimmune process rather than the underlying cause of the tissue destruction. The major autoantibody is targeted against the enzyme 21-hydoxylase.

Caseous necrosis of the adrenal glands from tuberculosis once accounted for most cases of Addison's disease; however, this has become less common since the introduction of effective antituberculous therapy. However, tuberculosis should still be considered as a possible cause especially in areas of resurgence. Other causes of Addison's disease (such as metastatic infiltration of both adrenal glands) are very rare.

By the time symptoms of Addison's disease appear, both adrenal cortices have been destroyed

The clinical features of Addison's disease are a result of a significant lack of both glucocorticoids and mineralocorticoids. There is insidious onset of non-specific symptoms such as tiredness, lethargy, and weakness. Gastrointestinal disturbances such as anorexia, nausea, vomiting, and diarrhoea are common. Loss of weight is also common, and may be prominent. Indeed many cases of Addison's disease have been initially misdiagnosed as anorexia nervosa.

Increased skin pigmentation, particularly in skin creases and old surgical scars, occurs due to high concentrations of ACTH which has some melanocyte-stimulating activity. The high ACTH levels occur due to the lack of negative feedback on the anterior pituitary. Blood pressure is usually normal when patients are lying down, but almost invariably falls on standing. This postural drop in blood pressure is an extremely useful pointer to the underlying depletion in extracellular fluid volume.

Measurement of plasma electrolytes typically shows hyponatraemia and hyperkalaemia. The blood urea concentration is usually elevated, reflecting the dehydration. Up to half of all patients have hypoglycaemia.

The diagnostic test to confirm adrenocortical insufficiency is the ACTH stimulation test

Measurement of a random cortisol level is only of value in diagnosing adrenal failure if the value is found to be exceedingly low. In reality, most patients have intermediate values which are not low enough to diagnose adrenal failure confidently.

Any patient suspected of having adrenocortical hypofunction should therefore have dynamic testing of the adrenal cortex using an ACTH stimulation test. This involves measuring plasma cortisol levels in response to an intramuscular injection of synthetic ACTH (Synacthen). The normal response to an injection of Synacthen is a rise in plasma cortisol. In adrenal failure, there is either no cortisol rise or only a minimal rise.

Patients with adrenal failure require lifelong replacement therapy

Replacement therapy for Addison's disease is usually given in the form of hydrocortisone (a synthetic glucocorticoid) and fludrocortisone (a synthetic mineralocorticoid). It is vital for patients to be educated about their disease and the treatment. *The importance of increasing their dose of hydrocortisone during any intercurrent illness must be stressed to them.* Long-term follow-up is essential to ensure adequacy of replacement therapy and to check for the development of other autoimmune diseases.

Acute adrenal failure is a medical emergency

Acute adrenal insufficiency is associated with a sudden total loss of adrenocortical function. Patients rapidly develop a deadly combination of hypovolaemic shock, hypoglycaemia, hyperkalaemia, and hyponatraemia. This grave condition may develop in the following settings:

- Patients with overwhelming bacterial infection. A catastrophic complication of severe septicaemia, particularly meningococcal, is sudden haemorrhagic destruction of the adrenals. The adrenals are completely destroyed by bleeding into the glands as a result of the severe coagulopathy related to the septicaemia.

- A complication of chronic adrenal insufficiency. Patients with Addison's disease who have critically failing adrenal cortical function can be pushed into complete adrenal failure as a complication of any co-existing illness. This scenario may occur in patients with previously undiagnosed Addison's disease, or in patients known to have Addison's disease who fail to increase their replacement dose when they become unwell.

- Patients taking therapeutic glucocorticoids. If patients taking exogenous glucocorticoids suddenly stop taking the drug or fail to increase their dose in response to an acute illness, acute adrenal failure may occur due to the inability of the atrophic adrenals to provide steroid support.

Acute adrenal failure is rapidly fatal unless promptly treated with aggressive supportive measures and corticosteroids, and even then carries a poor prognosis.

Key points: Adrenal insufficiency

- Adrenal insufficiency refers to inadequate circulating levels of glucocorticoids and mineralocorticoids.

- Adrenal insufficiency may present as an insidious chronic disease (Addison's disease) or acute adrenal failure.

- Most cases of chronic adrenal insufficiency are due to autoimmune adrenalitis, in which the adrenal cortices are destroyed by autoreactive T cells. Circulating antiadrenal autoantibodies are often found in the serum of these patients.

- Chronic adrenal failure presents with fatigue, loss of appetite, and gastrointestinal upset. On clinical examination, there is usually hypotension and there may be pigmentation of skin creases. Electrolyte measurements typically reveal hyperkalaemia and hyponatraemia.

- Confirming a diagnosis of adrenal insufficiency requires a Synacthen test in which synthetic ACTH is administered. In adrenal failure, there is a failure to stimulate a significant rise in cortisol levels.

- Patients with adrenal failure require lifelong replacement therapy with synthetic glucocorticoids and mineralocorticoids.

- Acute adrenal failure is a medical emergency. Patients are extremely unwell with severe hypovolaemic shock, hypoglycaemia, hyperkalaemia, and hyponatraemia. Acute adrenal failure may arise as a complication of septicaemia, in patients known to have Addison's disease, or in patients taking synthetic glucocorticoids who suddenly stop taking their treatment.

Adrenal medulla

The adrenal medulla is embryologically distinct from the adrenal cortex. It is composed of cells called chromaffin cells which are derived from the neural crest. Functionally the adrenal medulla is part of the sympathetic nervous system, producing **catecholamines** (adrenaline and noradrenaline) which are secreted directly into the blood.

Catecholamines have very diverse roles in the body, reflected by the wide distribution of adrenergic receptors on which they act. They act on the heart to cause increased rate and strength of contraction, and have numerous metabolic actions including stimulation of glycogenolysis and lipolysis.

There is only one important disease of the adrenal medulla, which is a tumour of the chromaffin cells known as a phaeochromocytoma.

Phaeochromocytoma

A **phaeochromocytoma** is a tumour of the chromaffin cells of the adrenal medulla which produces excess amounts of catecholamines. The term phaeochromocytoma ('dusky coloured tumour') came about because of the colour change the tumour tissue underwent when immersed in oxidizing agents such as chromate salts. Sporadic phaeochromocytomas are generally solitary tumours which present in people 30–50 years old.

Hypertension is the most common presentation of a phaeochromocytoma

Most patients with phaeochromocytoma first come to medical attention when they are found to have hypertension. Usually they are asymptomatic, but some patients may report symptoms related to episodic increases in circulating catecholamines such as throbbing headache, sweating, and palpitations.

The possibility of an underlying phaeochromocytoma should be suspected if hypertension is severe, occurs in a young person, and is refractory to treatment or requires multiple drugs to control it. Although phaeochromocytomas account for a tiny proportion of cases of hypertension (0.1 per cent), the possibility should always be considered as it has the best chance of cure out of all the secondary causes of hypertension.

Rarely patients may present with a hypertensive complication due to very high uncontrolled blood pressure, such as hypertensive encephalopathy or aortic dissection.

Patients suspected of having a phaeochromocytoma require 24 h urine collection and imaging of the adrenals

Confirmation of the diagnosis of phaeochromocytoma first involves biochemical confirmation of raised catecholamine levels. The best investigation is a 24 h urine collection to measure urinary catecholamines and their metabolites, a normal result being extremely rare in a patient with a functional phaeochromocytoma. CT imaging of the adrenals is then required to localize the tumour.

Surgical removal of a phaeochromocytoma is usually curative

The definitive treatment for phaeochromocytoma is surgical removal. The role of the physician, however, is just as crucial as the surgeon in preparing the patient for surgery to ensure the operation will be safe. The main objective is to control the blood pressure and also to restore blood volume, which is always reduced in patients with phaeochromocytomas. The agent of choice is phenoxybenzamine which is an irreversible α-blocker.

Most phaeochromocytomas are benign tumours which remain confined to the adrenal gland, and surgery is curative. About 10 per cent of all phaeochromocytomas are malignant. Unfortunately there are no reliable microscopic features of a malignant phaeochromocytoma. Even the benign tumours can have cells which look horrendous. *The only way to prove that a phaeochromocytoma is malignant is the presence of metastases.*

INTERESTING TO KNOW

Phaeochromocytoma and inherited syndromes

Phaeochromocytomas are well known to be associated with a number of inherited syndromes, including multiple endocrine neoplasia type 2, neurofibromatosis type 1, and von Hippel–Lindau syndrome. A phaeochromocytoma is often the first clinical manifestation of the syndrome.

Although it has been estimated that 10 per cent of all phaeochromocytomas are part of a syndrome, recent evidence suggests that this proportion is actually considerably higher. Familial cases tend to present at a younger age and the tumours are more likely to be bilateral.

Key points: Phaeochromocytoma

- Phaeochromocytomas are tumours of the catecholamine-secreting chromaffin cells of the adrenal medulla.

Continued

Key points: Phaeochromocytoma—cont'd

♦ Phaeochromocytomas usually present with asymptomatic hypertension. Some patients may report paroxysms of headache, sweating, and palpitations due to episodic rises in circulating catecholamines.

♦ A phaeochromocytoma should always be considered if hypertension occurs in a young person or is difficult to control.

♦ Patients suspected of having a phaeochromocytoma should have a 24 h urine collection to measure the concentrations of urinary catecholamines and their metabolites.

♦ CT or MRI scanning of the abdomen should then be performed to localize the tumour.

♦ Most phaeochromocytomas are benign, and surgical excision is curative.

♦ The only reliable indicator of malignancy in a phaeochromocytoma is the presence of metastases.

♦ An increasing proportion of phaeochromocytomas are known to be associated with inherited syndromes such as multiple endocrine neoplasia type 2, neurofibromatosis type 1, and von Hippel–Lindau syndrome. Tumours arising in patients with these syndromes are more likely to be bilateral and occur in younger people than the sporadic tumours.

Thyroid gland

The thyroid gland is situated just below the thyroid cartilage in the anterior neck and consists of two lobes joined by an isthmus. Microscopically, it is made up of numerous tightly packed thyroid **follicles**. These are spherical structures lined by a single layer of thyroid follicular epithelial cells and filled with **colloid**, a proteinaceous material containing thyroglobulin and stored thyroid hormones.

Thyroglobulin is a large glycoprotein containing many tyrosine residues which are iodinated and then coupled to one another to make the two thyroid hormones **thyroxine** (T4) and **triiodothyronine** (T3). Scattered between the follicles are smaller numbers of epithelial cells called parafollicular, or 'C', cells which secrete **calcitonin**, a hormone of uncertain function in humans.

The thyroid hormones are essential for normal growth and development. They also control basal metabolic rate and stimulate many metabolic processes. Over 90 per cent of secreted thyroid hormone is T4, but most of it is metabolized in peripheral tissues to T3, which is the more active hormone.

Synthesis and release of thyroid hormones is stimulated by another hormone, thyroid-stimulating hormone (TSH). TSH is released from the anterior pituitary under the control of thyrotropin-releasing hormone (TRH) derived from the hypothalamus. T3 and T4 exert negative feedback on TSH release, in order to maintain normal circulating thyroid hormone levels (Fig. 14.6).

Thyroid disease presents in four main ways

Thyroid disease is common and often overlooked. This is a shame as it is often very easy to treat. There are

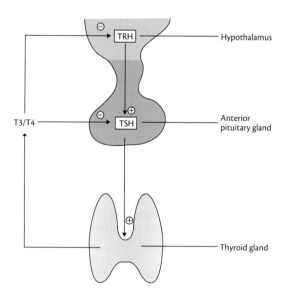

Fig. 14.6 Control of thyroid hormone release. TRH from the hypothalamus stimulates release of TSH from the anterior pituitary which drives T3 and T4 production in the thyroid gland. The thyroid hormones then provide negative feedback on release of TRH and TSH to maintain normal levels of thyroid hormones.

four common ways in which thyroid disease presents:

♦ Enlargement of the whole thyroid gland (goitre).

♦ Symptoms due to overactivity of the thyroid gland.

♦ Symptoms due to underactivity of the thyroid gland.

♦ A solitary nodule in the thyroid gland.

It is important to realize that there may be a combination of these patterns. A patient with a goitre could have symptoms of hyperthyroidism (e.g. Graves' disease), hypothyroidism (Hashimoto's disease), or have normal thyroid function (e.g. simple goitre). Note that a patient with normal thyroid status is said to be **euthyroid**.

Goitre

Goitre is a clinical term for an enlarged thyroid

The normal thyroid gland is impalpable. The term **goitre** is used to describe a *generalized* enlargement of the whole thyroid gland. Careful palpation is needed to distinguish a true goitre, which moves with swallowing, from a prominent pad of fat over the front of the neck. A goitre may be associated with features of hyper- or hypothyroidism; these will be discussed later. Patients who have a goitre with normal thyroid status are said to have a simple goitre.

JARGON BUSTER

Goitre

The term goitre when used unqualified just means an enlarged thyroid gland. It is therefore a clinical sign and not a disease. Simple goitre and multinodular goitre refer to actual disease entities, both of which cause a goitre.

Simple goitre

Simple goitres are sporadic goitres of unknown aetiology

Simple goitre is a term used to describe an enlargement of the thyroid gland which occurs sporadically and is of unknown aetiology. Many of these cases are thought to be caused by mild genetic defects in components of the hormone synthetic machinery ('dyshormonogenesis'), a theory supported by familial clustering of simple goitres.

The reduced levels of circulating thyroid hormones stimulate the release of TSH from the anterior pituitary, which stimulates the thyroid to undergo hyperplasia in order to increase the output of thyroid hormones to a normal level.

Simple goitres usually first present with a diffuse goitre in a young person

The typical clinical picture of a simple goitre is a diffuse goitre in a young patient with normal thyroid status. Often the goitre is noticed by friends and relatives rather than the patient. The diagnosis of a simple goitre is usually straightforward. The patient presents with a painless goitre which moves freely on swallowing. No treatment is necessary and many cases regress spontaneously.

Some simple goitres evolve over many years into multinodular goitres

In some patients with simple goitres, the stimulus to thyroid enlargement persists and, over a period of many years, repetitive cycles of stimulation and involution eventually result in the formation of numerous nodules within the thyroid, forming a **multinodular goitre**. Patients usually present in middle age with a goitre with palpable nodules which are often visible. Most patients are otherwise asymptomatic and do not require treatment. The major concern is compression of the trachea by a large multinodular goitre, and this is an indication for operation (Fig. 14.7). Surgery may also be performed for cosmetic reasons.

LINK BOX

Dominant nodules

Occasionally a single large dominant nodule forms in a multinodular goitre, with the remainder of the nodules remaining impalpable. This is a common cause of a solitary thyroid nodule and can raise concern by mimicking a thyroid neoplasm (p. 318).

Subacute thyroiditis is a self-limiting condition which causes a painful goitre

Subacute, or de Quervain's, thyroiditis is due to an acute viral infection of the thyroid which causes a painful enlargement of the gland. It is often seen in

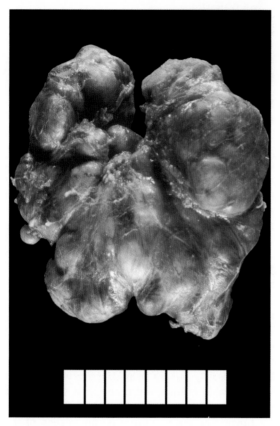

Fig. 14.7 Multinodular goitre. This massive multinodular goitre was removed from an elderly lady because it was compressing her trachea.

association with a systemic viral illness with malaise and fever. The diagnosis is usually straightforward and requires no specific treatment, with spontaneous resolution over 1–2 months. Sometimes there may be mild symptoms of thyrotoxicosis related to release of thyroid hormones from the inflamed gland.

Key points: Goitre

- Goitre is a clinical sign referring to a generalized enlargement of the whole thyroid gland.

- A simple goitre refers to an enlargement of the thyroid gland which occurs sporadically for unknown reasons.

- Simple goitres are thought to be due to subtle inherited defects in thyroid hormone synthesis.

- The earliest manifestation of simple goitre is a diffuse enlargement of the thyroid in a young patient. The goitre is often noticed by friends or relatives. The thyroid status is normal; there are no symptoms and often the goitre regresses spontaneously.

- In some patients with simple goitre, the goitre enlarges over many years and evolves into a multinodular goitre with numerous palpable and visible nodules. Most people are asymptomatic, but large multinodular goitres may cause discomfort and symptoms due to compression of other neck structures, in which case surgical removal is indicated.

- Subacute thyroiditis is an acute viral infection of the thyroid which leads to painful enlargement of the thyroid.

Hyperthyroidism

Hyperthyroidism refers to overactivity of the thyroid gland, which leads to the clinical state known as **thyrotoxicosis**. Hyperthyroidism and thyrotoxicosis are often incorrectly used interchangeably, but there is a difference between them; although most types of thyrotoxicosis are due to hyperthyroidism, thyrotoxicosis can also be caused transiently by destruction of thyroid tissue leading to release of stored thyroid hormones (e.g. subacute thyroiditis), or by accidental ingestion of too much thyroid hormone.

Thyrotoxicosis is associated with many different symptoms and signs, most of which are a consequence of a raised metabolic rate (Fig. 14.8). The precise clinical presentation depends on the severity and duration of the thyrotoxicosis, as well as the age of the patient.

Typical symptoms of thyrotoxicosis include weight loss (despite an increased appetite), sweating, palpitations, fatigue, and muscle weakness. In elderly patients, the development of atrial fibrillation is particularly common.

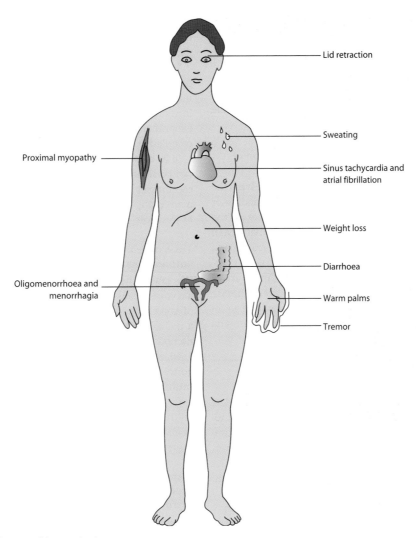

Fig. 14.8 Clinical features of thyrotoxicosis.

Patients suspected of having thyrotoxicosis should have biochemical confirmation

If thyrotoxicosis is suspected clinically, the diagnosis should be confirmed biochemically. Thyrotoxicosis is confirmed by the presence of a low or undetectable TSH level, together with elevated T3 and T4 levels. It is usual to check both T3 and T4 as sometimes T3 is elevated but T4 is not, particularly in the early stages of hyperthyroidism.

There are three common causes of thyrotoxicosis

Having established that a patient has thyrotoxicosis, the next stage is to determine the underlying cause. There are three common causes that you should know about:

- **Graves' disease**. This is by far the most common cause of hyperthyroidism. The peak age of onset is between 20 and 50 years.

- **Toxic multinodular goitre**. This is seen in patients older than those with Graves' disease.

- **A functional follicular adenoma.**

The diagnosis is often straightforward based on the clinical features. In cases of uncertainty, a thyroid radioisotope scan may be helpful in establishing the diagnosis.

Radioisotope scanning allows the distribution of activity in the thyroid gland to be visualized

Radioisotope scanning of the thyroid involves the administration of a low dose of radiolabelled iodine or technetium which is taken up by active areas of the thyroid. Scanning the thyroid for radioactivity then allows the distribution of activity in the thyroid gland to be visualized.

By localizing active ('hot') and inactive ('cold') areas, the scan can distinguish between Graves' disease (uniformly increased uptake), a toxic multinodular goitre (multiple patches of uptake), or a functional adenoma (a single hot spot).

Graves' disease is caused by circulating TSH receptor-stimulating antibodies

Graves' disease is the result of the production of an IgG autoantibody that mimics the effects of TSH. The autoantibody binds to the TSH receptor and activates it, stimulating hyperplasia of the thyroid follicular epithelium and unregulated secretion of thyroid hormones. The result is a diffuse symmetrical goitre and thyrotoxicosis.

The autoantibody in Graves' disease goes by many different names, including thyroid-stimulating immunoglobulin (TSI), long-acting thyroid stimulator (LATS), and TSH receptor-stimulating antibody. The last one is currently the preferred term. Exactly why patients with Graves' disease produce the TSH receptor-stimulating antibody is uncertain. Although it is possible to measure TSH receptor-stimulating antibodies to make a diagnosis of Graves' disease in a thyrotoxic patient, the test is expensive and is not widely used.

In addition to thyrotoxicosis and a diffuse goitre, patients with Graves' disease may also develop a type of orbital disease known as Graves' ophthalmopathy. It is thought that the soft tissues behind the eye also bear antigens which bind the TSH receptor-stimulating antibody. Swelling of the retroorbital tissues leads to protrusion of the orbit, a clinical sign known as

exophthalmos or proptosis. Note that lid lag and lid retraction may occur in *any* thyrotoxic state, but exophthalmos is characteristic of Graves' disease.

Typical symptoms of Graves' ophthalmopathy include pain and watering of the eyes. Double vision (diplopia) may also develop due to swelling of the orbital muscles. In more severe cases of Graves' ophthalmopathy, the exophthalmos may impair the ability to close the eyes completely, leading to corneal damage.

In its most devastating form, Graves' ophthalmopathy can be sight threatening if severe retro-orbital swelling compresses the optic nerve. The development of optic neuropathy necessitates urgent surgical decompression of the orbit.

Toxic multinodular goitre is due to an autonomous nodule within a multinodular goitre

We saw earlier how a simple multinodular goitre is a common cause of thyroid enlargement in the absence of any change in thyroid hormone levels. If, however, a nodule within a multinodular goitre begins to autonomously secrete thyroid hormones (independently of TSH), thyrotoxicosis can occur. When a multinodular goitre causes thyrotoxicosis, it is called a **toxic multinodular goitre**. This usually occurs in people over 50 who have had a long-standing multinodular goitre. Thyroid hormone production is usually much less marked than in Graves' disease and so the clinical presentation is less dramatic.

A small proportion of follicular adenomas produce enough thyroid hormone to cause thyrotoxicosis

Patients with functional follicular adenomas typically present with thyrotoxicosis and a readily palpable solitary thyroid nodule. About half of all functional follicular adenomas are due to an activating mutation in either the gene encoding the TSH receptor or its associated signalling proteins, leading to persistent stimulus to thyroid hormone production. It is important to appreciate that the vast majority of thyroid follicular adenomas are not functional; only about 1 per cent produce enough hormone to cause thyrotoxicosis.

Treatment of thyrotoxicosis aims to reduce thyroid hormone output

Reducing thyroid function in thyrotoxicosis can be achieved in a variety of ways, including antithyroid drugs, surgery to remove part of the thyroid, and radioactive iodine which destroys functioning thyroid follicular cells. The choice depends on the underlying cause of the thyrotoxicosis and other factors such as the age of the patient. Whichever treatment is chosen, it is essential to continue long-term follow-up of patients. Some patients may relapse and become hyperthyroid again, whilst others may become hypothyroid as a result of destructive treatment to the gland.

Key points: Hyperthyroidism

- Hyperthyroidism refers to overactivity of the thyroid gland, which leads to the clinical state known as thyrotoxicosis.

- Thyrotoxicosis causes many symptoms including restlessness, sweating, palpitations, weight loss, and diarrhoea. Important clinical signs include sinus tachycardia (often atrial fibrillation in the elderly), tremor, warm skin, lid retraction, and lid lag.

- Thyrotoxicosis is diagnosed biochemically by the presence of low TSH and high T3 and T4.

- There are three common causes of thyrotoxicosis: Graves' disease, toxic multinodular goitre, and a functional follicular adenoma.

- Graves' disease is characterized by thyrotoxicosis, a diffuse goitre, and Graves' ophthalmopathy. Graves' disease is caused by TSH receptor-stimulating antibodies which continuously activate the thyroid follicular epithelial cells.

- Toxic multinodular goitre occurs in older patients when a long-standing multinodular goitre develops an autonomous functional nodule which releases thyroid hormones.

- A functional follicular adenoma presents with thyrotoxicosis and a readily palpable solitary thyroid nodule.

- Often the clinical picture is sufficiently characteristic to enable the cause of the thyrotoxicosis to be determined. Where there is uncertainty, a thyroid radioisotope scan is helpful in determining the diagnosis.

- The treatment of thyrotoxicosis depends on the underlying cause, but the principle is to reduce thyroid hormone output. Options include antithyroid drugs, surgery, and radioactive iodine.

Hypothyroidism

Hypothyroidism refers to underactivity of the thyroid gland. The reduction in circulating thyroid hormones causes a wide variety of symptoms and signs which are mostly the result of a reduction in metabolic rate (Fig. 14.9). Patients typically suffer from tremendous fatigue with mental slowing, often mistaken for depression. Other common symptoms include weight gain, cold intolerance, constipation, drying and thinning of the hair, and menstrual disturbances in women.

JARGON BUSTER

Myxoedema

The term **myxoedema** was originally coined to refer to the non-pitting oedema of the skin seen in patients with hypothyroidism due to accumulation of ground substance in the dermis. Since then, the term has come to be used for the clinical effects of hypothyroidism in general.

Any patient with symptoms suggestive of hypothyroidism should have thyroid function tests

The ready availability of reliable biochemical tests of thyroid function means that one should have a low threshold for excluding hypothyroidism in a patient with any suggestive features, particularly middle-aged women with fatigue or depression.

Hypothyroid patients have a high plasma TSH concentration and a low T4 concentration. The high TSH level is an appropriate physiological response to the low T4 levels. In fact, measurement of serum TSH is a more sensitive test for early hypothyroidism than serum T4. Note that measurement of T3 is of no value in the diagnosis of hypothyroidism as it is often normal in hypothyroidism due to increased formation from T4.

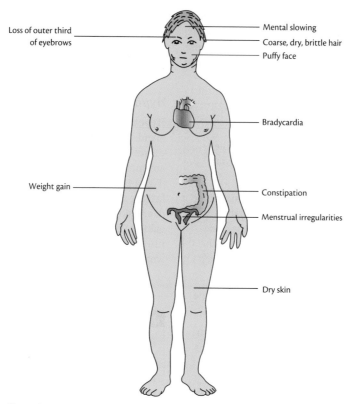

Fig. 14.9 Clinical features of hypothyroidism.

Most cases of hypothyroidism are due to problems in the thyroid gland itself

Failure of the thyroid gland itself accounts for 95 per cent of cases of hypothyroidism. This is termed **primary hypothyroidism** and the most common causes are:

♦ Autoimmune thyroid disease (Hashimoto's thyroiditis).

♦ Previous destructive therapy to the thyroid, particularly radioiodine treatment.

♦ Certain drugs, particularly lithium and amiodarone.

Note that hypothyroidism due to hypopituitarism causing a reduction in TSH (**secondary hypothyroidism**) is rare, and hypothyroidism due to hypothalamic disease causing a reduction in TRH (**tertiary hypothyroidism**) is even rarer!

Hashimoto's thyroiditis is caused by autoimmune destruction of the thyroid

Hashimoto's thyroiditis is an example of an organ-specific autoimmune disease. The exact underlying mechanism remains unclear. For some reason, T helper lymphocytes become sensitized to antigens on thyroid follicular cells and stimulate an autoimmune attack by cytotoxic T lymphocytes, leading to destruction of the gland. If the thyroid is examined microscopically, it is packed with lymphocytes which infiltrate and destroy thyroid follicles.

Patients with Hashimoto's typically present with symptoms of hypothyroidism and a goitre

Patients with Hashimoto's disease will usually present with symptoms related to hypothyroidism. Most patients also have a diffuse firm goitre due to the massive lymphocyte infiltration of the thyroid gland. Patients presenting late in the natural history of the disease may not have a goitre as the thyroid has become atrophic and shrunken following widespread destruction of the follicles.

Circulating antithyroid autoantibodies are present in most patients with Hashimoto's thyroiditis

Hashimoto's is typically associated with high levels of circulating antithyroid autoantibodies, of which the most important are the following:

- Thyroglobulin antibody.
- Thyroid peroxidase antibody. Thyroid peroxidase is an enzyme in follicular epithelial cells which catalyses the oxidation and iodination of tyrosine residues on thyroglobulin.
- TSH receptor-blocking antibody. Note that this is different from the TSH receptor-stimulating antibody which *activates* the TSH receptor, leading to Graves' disease.

These autoantibodies may contribute to the thyroid destruction by fixing complement and stimulating thyroid follicular cell killing and by blocking the action of TSH, but the majority of thyroid destruction appears to be due to antithyroid cytotoxic T lymphocytes rather than the autoantibodies.

Development of non-Hodgkin lymphoma is an important complication of Hashimoto's thyroiditis

Patients with Hashimoto's thyroiditis are at increased risk of developing a particular type of low grade non-Hodgkin B cell lymphoma called marginal zone lymphoma. This is presumably related to persistent stimulation of autoreactive B lymphocytes in the thyroid, eventually leading to malignant transformation.

Hypothyroidism is treated by replacement of thyroid hormones

Patients with hypothyroidism require lifelong replacement therapy with thyroxine. The effect of the treatment is easily monitored by measuring plasma TSH. Ideally the replacement dose should be sufficient to maintain a normal TSH.

Key points: Hypothyroidism

- Hypothyroidism refers to underactivity of the thyroid gland.
- The reduction in circulating thyroid hormone levels leads to a reduction in basal metabolic rate.
- Typical symptoms of hypothyroidism include fatigue, mental slowing, weight gain, and cold intolerance. It is often mistaken for depression.
- A diagnosis of hypothyroidism is confirmed biochemically by demonstrating a high TSH level and a low T4 level.
- The most common cause of hypothyroidism is Hashimoto's thyroiditis which is due to autoimmune destruction of the thyroid gland. Circulating antithyroid autoantibodies are present in the serum.
- Most patients with Hashimoto's thyroiditis present with hypothyroidism and a goitre, although patients presenting later in the course of the disease may have a shrunken thyroid due to complete destruction of the gland.
- Hypothyroidism may also be iatrogenic due to drugs which interfere with thyroid hormone production, such as amiodarone, and following treatment for hyperthyroidism.
- Hypothyroid patients usually require lifelong treatment with thyroxine at a dose sufficient to maintain a normal TSH level.

LINK BOX

Marginal zone lymphomas and chronic inflammatory diseases

The development of marginal zone lymphoma in the thyroid as a complication of Hashimoto's thyroiditis is similar to the development of marginal zone lymphoma in the stomach as a complication of chronic inflammation caused by *Helicobacter pylori* infection (p. 149) and marginal zone lymphoma of the salivary gland in Sjögren's syndrome (p. 455).

Solitary thyroid nodule

A solitary nodule in the thyroid is a palpable discrete swelling in an otherwise apparently normal thyroid. It is a common clinical problem which has three common causes:

- A large dominant nodule within a multinodular goitre.
- A benign follicular adenoma.
- A malignant thyroid tumour.

Fortunately the vast majority of solitary nodules are due to dominant nodules and follicular adenomas. However, because of the possibility of a malignant tumour, they require very careful investigation.

Fine needle aspiration is a quick, useful initial investigation of solitary nodules

Fine needle aspiration cytology is the initial investigation of choice for solitary thyroid nodules. The technique involves passing a thin needle (usually a blue 23 gauge) into the lump and aspirating cells into the needle and needle hub. The contents of the aspirate are then immediately smeared onto a slide and allowed to dry. The slide can then be stained and immediately examined by a cytopathologist.

The answer from the pathologist will usually be one of five options: inadequate specimen (repeat), benign process (no need for surgery but keep an eye on the patient), a follicular neoplasm (excise), a lesion suspicious for malignancy (excise), or a definitely malignant lesion (excise). The term 'follicular neoplasm' means the nodule is either a follicular adenoma or a follicular carcinoma, but fine needle aspiration cytology is unable to distinguish between the two.

Thus, although a precise diagnosis is not always possible, fine needle aspiration cytology is handy as a triaging process to divide patients into those who can be reassured and those who should have surgical excision of the nodule for a definitive histological diagnosis.

A benign follicular adenoma is the most common tumour of the thyroid

A **follicular adenoma** is a benign, encapsulated tumour of the thyroid. Most follicular adenomas are non-functional and present with a solitary lump in the neck in a euthyroid patient. Occasionally haemorrhage into the adenoma may cause sudden pain and enlargement in the thyroid.

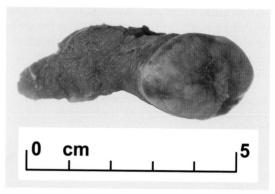

Fig. 14.10 Follicular neoplasm. This patient presented with a solitary thyroid nodule. A fine needle aspiration cytology preparation diagnosed a 'follicular neoplasm' so the tumour was removed. Macroscopically, a well circumscribed tumour is seen surrounded by a thin capsule. This is likely to be a follicular adenoma, however microscopic examination of the edge of the tumour at the capsule must be carefully carried out to detect evidence of capsule invasion or vascular invasion diagnostic of a follicular carcinoma.

A fine needle aspirate from a follicular adenoma will produce large numbers of follicular cells which produce characteristic small follicle structures called microfollicular aggregates. Because this pattern may also be seen in aspirates from follicular carcinomas, the final conclusion from the pathologist will be 'follicular neoplasm' and the nodule will be excised. A diagnosis of a follicular adenoma can only be made once the lesion is excised and examined histologically to rule out a follicular carcinoma (see below). Thus although adenomas are benign tumours, most will be removed surgically (Fig. 14.10).

Thyroid carcinomas are malignant epithelial tumours

Thyroid carcinomas are malignant tumours arising from thyroid epithelial cells. Although thyroid cancers account for only 1 per cent of all malignancies, they are the most common endocrine malignancies and occur primarily in young adults. Thyroid carcinomas rarely interfere with the functional capacity of the thyroid gland, so most patients present with a solitary lump in the thyroid and with a normal thyroid hormone status.

There are four common types of thyroid carcinoma:

- Papillary carcinoma (80 per cent)
- Follicular carcinoma (10 per cent)
- Anaplastic carcinoma (5 per cent)
- Medullary carcinoma (5 per cent).

Papillary carcinoma is defined by specific features of the nuclei of the malignant cells

Papillary carcinoma of the thyroid is defined as a malignant epithelial tumour arising from thyroid follicular cells which shows distinctive nuclear features (Fig. 14.11). Although papillary carcinomas of the thyroid often show a papillary architecture microscopically, this is not necessary to make the diagnosis; *it is the characteristic features of the nuclei of the malignant cells that are diagnostic regardless of the architecture of the tumour.* Fine needle aspiration cytology is therefore excellent at unequivocally diagnosing papillary carcinoma as the characteristic nuclei can be identified in the aspirate.

Papillary carcinoma is the most common type of thyroid carcinoma. It occurs in young adults aged 20–50, with a female to male ratio of 4:1. Papillary carcinoma has a tendency to spread into the lymphatics (in contrast to follicular carcinomas which usually spread in the blood), and many patients have regional lymph node metastases at the time of diagnosis. Despite this,

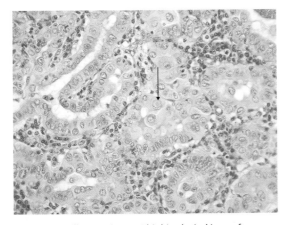

Fig. 14.11 Papillary carcinoma. This histological image from a papillary carcinoma of the thyroid shows the diagnostic nuclear features of nuclear clearing, nuclear grooving, and intranuclear inclusions (arrow).

papillary carcinoma is a well differentiated tumour which is slow growing and has an excellent prognosis.

Follicular carcinoma can only be diagnosed by histological examination of the thyroid nodule

Follicular carcinoma of the thyroid is a well differentiated invasive neoplasm which arises from the thyroid follicular epithelial cells but which lacks the diagnostic nuclear features of papillary carcinoma. Follicular carcinomas are distinguished from follicular adenomas purely by the presence of invasive behaviour, i.e. evidence of invasion through their capsule, or vascular invasion.

The only way to distinguish a follicular adenoma from a follicular carcinoma of the thyroid is by excising the lump and submitting it for complete histological examination. The appearances of the cells themselves are of no help in deciding if a lesion is a follicular adenoma or carcinoma. This is why fine needle aspiration (where dispersed cells are examined) can only diagnose a 'follicular neoplasm' and cannot tell you if the nodule is an adenoma or a carcinoma.

The incidence of follicular carcinoma peaks slightly later than that of papillary carcinoma, and is more common in women. Metastases occur mainly via the blood stream, and it is one of the tumours that characteristically spreads to bone. Whilst most patients present with a solitary thyroid nodule, some patients may present with symptoms related to metastases, for instance a pathological fracture in a bone containing metastatic disease. The prognosis is generally very good in follicular carcinoma, even in patients with metastatic disease, as therapy with radioactive iodine is a highly specific way of targeting the tumour cells.

Anaplastic carcinoma is an undifferentiated epithelial tumour with a dismal prognosis

Anaplastic carcinoma of the thyroid is an extremely deadly malignancy which is confined to the elderly. Patients present with a rapidly enlarging thyroid mass which extensively invades adjacent tissues in the neck, leading to dysphagia and breathlessness. The prognosis is very poor.

Medullary carcinoma is an endocrine tumour that is derived from parafollicular cells

Medullary carcinoma is derived from the parafollicular or 'C' cells of the thyroid which produce calcitonin.

Although patients with medullary carcinomas have high circulating levels of calcitonin, this appears to produce no clinical effects, and so patients present with a solitary thyroid nodule. Of note, up to one-quarter of all medullary carcinomas are seen in patients with the condition **multiple endocrine neoplasia type 2**, caused by inherited mutations in the RET proto-oncogene (see later). The aetiology of sporadic medullary carcinoma is unknown.

Key points: Solitary thyroid nodule

- A solitary nodule in the thyroid is a common clinical problem. Most are due to a dominant nodule in a multinodular goitre or a follicular adenoma. A small proportion are due to a thyroid carcinoma.

- Excluding a malignant nodule is the aim of investigating thyroid nodules. The most helpful test is fine needle aspiration cytology, in which cells from the nodule are aspirated into a needle and examined microscopically.

- Although fine needle aspiration cannot always provide a precise diagnosis, it is good at triaging patients into those with completely benign features who can be reassured and monitored, and those patients with potentially suspicious nodules which should be surgically removed.

- Follicular adenomas are the most common thyroid neoplasms. They are benign encapsulated tumours which, by definition, show no evidence of invasive behaviour.

- Papillary carcinoma is a malignant epithelial tumour defined by the presence of characteristic features of the nuclei of the malignant cells. It is a slow growing tumour with an excellent prognosis.

- Follicular carcinoma is a malignant epithelial tumour which lacks the nuclear features of papillary carcinoma and by definition shows invasive behaviour, i.e. invasion through its capsule, vascular invasion, or evidence of distant metastases.

- Anaplastic carcinoma is a malignancy of the elderly composed of undifferentiated epithelial cells. It presents as a rapidly growing mass in the neck with extensive local invasion into adjacent structures. The prognosis is very poor.

- Medullary carcinoma is derived from the calcitonin-producing parafollicular cells of the thyroid. Up to a quarter of cases are associated with the inherited disorder multiple endocrine neoplasia type 2.

Sick euthyroid syndrome

Abnormalities of thyroid function tests are common in hospitalized patients without thyroid disease

It is important to be aware that many ill patients without thyroid disease may have abnormal thyroid function tests, typically a low serum T3 with a normal TSH. This is sometimes known as the 'sick euthyroid syndrome'. The underlying mechanism is thought to be a depression in the action of the deiodinase enzyme that converts T4 into T3. The resultant reduction in T3 levels is thought to be an adaptive response to allow the sick patient to conserve energy and protein.

Common conditions known to depress deiodinase function include major surgery, trauma, advanced cancer, and myocardial infarction. Unless one strongly suspects thyroid disease, it is therefore best to perform thyroid function tests when the patient is well.

Parathyroid glands

The parathyroid glands are tiny glands about the size of a grain of rice which occupy a variable position behind the thyroid gland. Most people have four glands, but the number can vary from just one to as many as 12.

Most of the parathyroid gland is composed of **chief cells** responsible for the synthesis of **parathyroid hormone**. A small number of **oxyphil cells** are also present in the parathyroid glands, whose function is uncertain. Parathyroid hormone is secreted in response to a fall in plasma calcium, and acts to increase blood calcium levels by increasing reabsorption of calcium from the gut and kidneys, and increasing osteoclastic activity in bone.

Like other endocrine organs, abnormalities of the parathyroid glands present because of hyperfunction or hypofunction.

Hyperparathyroidism

Hyperparathyroidism refers to overactivity of one or more parathyroid glands, leading to excess production of parathyroid hormone. Hyperparathyroidism may be seen in two distinct situations:

♦ An inappropriate, pathological release from one or more abnormal parathyroid glands, known as primary hyperparathyroidism.

♦ An appropriate, physiological response to prolonged hypocalcaemia by normal parathyroid glands, known as secondary hyperparathyroidism.

It is important to emphasize here that primary and secondary hyperparathyroidism are quite distinct disorders. Primary hyperparathyroidism is due to a specific abnormality of the parathyroid glands themselves, whereas secondary hyperparathyroidism is the biochemical consequence of a non-parathyroid disease that has caused hypocalcaemia. The two are only related by the presence of raised parathyroid hormone levels.

Prolonged hyperparathyroidism of any cause leads to bony disease because parathyroid hormone stimulates osteoclasts, leading to bone resorption. In its earliest stages, hyperparathyroid bone disease is asymptomatic but may be readily diagnosed radiologically. The typical radiological feature is subperiosteal bone resorption, best seen on the radial side of the middle phalanges of the hands (Fig. 14.12).

As the disease progresses, bone mass is reduced and the patient may become osteopenic or even osteoporotic. The most florid form of hyperparathyroid bone disease, osteitis fibrosa cystica, in which large holes appear in the bones, is now rarely seen because hyperparathyroidism is diagnosed and treated well before these changes develop.

Primary hyperparathyroidism

Primary hyperparathyroidism is one of the most common endocrine disorders

Primary hyperparathyroidism is a common endocrine condition which affects about 1 in 1000 people. The disorder occurs when an abnormality within one or more of the parathyroid glands leads to uncontrolled release of parathyroid hormone with resultant hypercalcaemia.

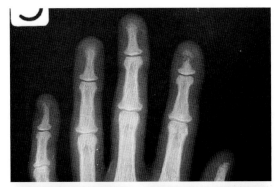
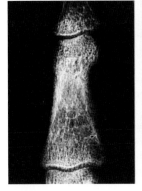
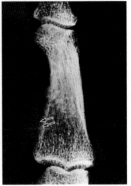

Fig. 14.12 Hyperparathyroid bone disease. Radiographic features of hyperparathyroid bone disease in a patient with chronic renal failure. There is erosion of the edges of the bones, most marked in the middle phalanges.

The calcium rise is predominantly due to enhanced absorption from the gut and kidneys, with a minor contribution from mobilization of calcium out of bone.

Primary hyperparathyroidism is due to either a single parathyroid adenoma or four gland hyperplasia

Parathyroid adenomas are benign neoplasms composed of a mixture of chief cells and oxyphil cells. They are almost always solitary tumours and, in contrast to primary hyperplasia, the other three unaffected parathyroid glands are normal in size.

Primary parathyroid gland hyperplasia refers to a situation where all four parathyroid glands undergo hyperplasia. All of the glands are enlarged, although often asymmetrically. In most cases, this happens sporadically for unknown reasons. A minority of cases of parathyroid hyperplasia are associated with the inherited multiple endocrine neoplasia syndromes (see later).

Primary hyperparathyroidism is a common cause of asymptomatic hypercalcaemia

Most patients with hyperparathyroidism are diagnosed whilst asymptomatic due to the incidental finding of hypercalcaemia on a blood test. Patients may have vague symptoms of fatigue and weakness on specific questioning, but most feel completely well. Only patients with severe hypercalcaemia develop symptoms such as renal stones, polyuria, and constipation. In a hypercalcaemic patient, the diagnosis of primary hyperparathyroidism is clinched by finding a raised, *or inappropriately normal*, parathyroid hormone level.

Patients with primary hyperparathyroidism should be checked for hyperparathyroid bone disease

Bone disease in primary hyperparathyroidism is unusual nowadays as most patients are diagnosed early in the course of the disease. Nonetheless, all patients diagnosed with primary hyperparathyroidism should have radiographs of the hands to look for evidence of hyperparathyroid bone disease, and measurement of bone density to check for osteopenia or osteoporosis.

Primary hyperparathyroidism can be managed conservatively or with surgery

Many patients with primary hyperparathyroidism can be safely managed with close follow-up and do not develop progressive disease. Surgery is the only curative therapy and is indicated for patients aged less than 50, symptomatic patients, those with a calcium level above 3.0 mmol/l, and those found to be osteopenic or osteoporotic on bone densitometry. However, many endocrine surgeons have a low threshold for recommending surgery, as many apparently asymptomatic patients retrospectively claim to derive benefit after surgery.

Before the operation, the parathyroid glands can be localized by injecting a radioactive dye that selectively stains the parathyroid glands blue. The radioactivity allows activity to be assessed, enabling distinction between adenoma and four gland hyperplasia to be made before the operation.

In the case of an adenoma, that gland can be removed using minimally invasive surgery. In four gland hyperplasia, all of the glands are enlarged and active, in which case most of the parathyroid tissue is removed, leaving a small remnant no larger than the size of a normal parathyroid gland.

INTERESTING TO KNOW

Calcium receptor agonists

A novel method of treating patients with primary hyperparathyroidism is with calcium receptor agonists which increase the sensitivity of the parathyroid calcium-sensing receptors, leading to a reduction in parathyroid hormone secretion. Trials with these agents have resulted in a substantial reduction in parathyroid hormone levels with normalization of serum calcium concentrations. These agents may offer an effective medical treatment for primary hyperparathyroidism in the future.

Key points: Primary hyperparathyroidism

- Primary hyperparathyroidism is a sporadic or familial disorder characterized by hypercalcaemia due to elevated (or inappropriately normal) parathyroid hormone levels.

- Almost all cases of primary hyperparathyroidism are due to either a single parathyroid adenoma (80 per cent) or four gland hyperplasia (20 per cent).

- Most patients with primary hyperparathyroidism are diagnosed following the incidental finding of a mildly raised blood calcium level. Symptomatic primary hyperparathyroidism is less common.

- Many cases of primary hyperparathyroidism can be managed conservatively with close monitoring of serum calcium and parathyroid hormone levels, and annual bone densitometry.

- Surgery is the only curative therapy, and is indicated in young patients, symptomatic patients, and patients with markedly raised calcium levels.

Secondary hyperparathyroidism

Secondary hyperparathyroidism is quite different from primary hyperparathyroidism

Secondary hyperparathyroidism is caused by any condition associated with persistently low calcium levels, the most common being chronic renal failure. All four of the parathyroid glands enlarge, in a similar way to the primary hyperplasia we described earlier. In contrast to primary hyperplasia, the glands are reacting *appropriately* to prolonged hypocalcaemia by producing parathyroid hormone

The chronically raised parathyroid hormone level acts to try to raise calcium levels back to normal, but *hypercalcaemia does not occur*. The clinical picture of secondary hyperparathyroidism is therefore dominated by the bony manifestations of prolonged hyperparathyroidism, together with features of the underlying cause.

The most common disease leading to secondary hyperparathyroidism is chronic renal failure. Hyperparathyroid bone disease is the main component of the complex bony disorders encountered in patients with chronic renal failure known as renal osteodystrophy.

Hypoparathyroidism

Hypoparathyroidism is usually iatrogenic following surgery in the neck

Hypoparathyroidism, which results from decreased secretion of parathyroid hormone, is much less common than hyperparathyroidism. Most cases of hypoparathyroidism are complications of surgery in the neck due to accidental removal of parathyroid tissue. Common operations where this is a risk include thyroidectomy, lymph node dissection in the neck, and parathyroid surgery for primary hyperparathyroidism.

Hypoparathyroidism leads to hypocalcaemia, and thus the hallmark of hypoparathyroidism is neuromuscular irritability due to low serum calcium levels. The earliest symptom is numbness and tingling of the fingers and toes, and around the mouth. These symptoms should always be specifically asked about, in addition to measuring calcium, in patients recovering from the operations listed above.

Endocrine pancreas

The pancreas is a mixed exocrine and endocrine organ. The exocrine portion consists of secretory cells which secrete digestive enzymes into the duodenum via the pancreatic duct system. Diseases of the exocrine pancreas are discussed in Chapter 9.

The endocrine component of the pancreas consists of small groups of cells called **islets** scattered throughout the organ. The islets are in a distinct minority compared with the number of exocrine glands, making up only 2 per cent of the mass of the pancreas. The islets contain a number of different cell types, each of which synthesizes and releases one or more hormones. The most important are the alpha cells which release **glucagon** and the beta cells which release **insulin**.

Far and away the most important disorder of the endocrine pancreas is diabetes mellitus. Neoplasms of the endocrine pancreas can occur, but these are rare.

Diabetes mellitus

Diabetes mellitus is a very common metabolic disorder characterized by chronic hyperglycaemia which leads to long-term damage to many organs. Over 2 per cent of the population of the UK are diabetic (equating to >1 million people) and the disease is rising in incidence. Diabetes therefore carries an immense clinical burden to health services and has been estimated to absorb some 5–10 per cent of the total health budget.

Two main types of diabetes are recognized: type 1 and type 2

Primary diabetes mellitus is divided into type 1 and type 2 (Table 14.2). Type 1 diabetes is also known as insulin-dependent diabetes mellitus (IDDM) and type 2 diabetes is also known as non-insulin-dependent diabetes mellitus (NIDDM). Although the two types have a different underlying pathogenesis, the long-term complications of both are similar.

Diabetes may also occur secondary to disorders which destroy islet cells such as chronic pancreatitis or haemochromatosis, or conditions associated with

TABLE 14.2   Type 1 and type 2 diabetes mellitus

Type 1 diabetes mellitus	Type 2 diabetes mellitus
Onset in childhood or adolescence	Onset in adulthood
Thin	Obese
Complete lack of insulin	Relative lack of insulin and insulin resistance

excessive levels of hormones which antagonize the effects of insulin, e.g. Cushing's syndrome and acromegaly. Secondary diabetes accounts for only 1 per cent of cases of diabetes, but should not be missed as the underlying cause may be treatable.

Type 1 diabetes is due to autoimmune destruction of insulin-secreting cells

Type 1 diabetes presents suddenly in young people over a period of days or weeks. By the time the patient presents, virtually all of their insulin-producing beta cells have been destroyed by an autoimmune attack that started many years before. Beta cell destruction appears to be the result of a combination of the actions of CD4+ T lymphocytes which activate macrophages, CD8+ cytotoxic T lymphocytes which directly kill beta cells, and autoantibodies against beta cells and insulin. Together, these mechanisms progressively destroy beta cells until there is a complete lack of insulin.

Type 2 diabetes is due to cellular resistance to the actions of insulin

Type 2 diabetes is by far the more common type of diabetes, accounting for about 85 per cent of cases in white populations. It tends to present more chronically,

in middle-aged people, with symptoms developing over months or longer. Often the diagnosis is made when routine blood or urine testing in an asymptomatic patient reveals hyperglycaemia or glycosuria.

A key feature of type 2 diabetes is *insulin resistance*, which is a decreased ability of peripheral tissues to respond to insulin. Initially the pancreas can compensate for insulin resistance by increasing insulin secretion, but over time the beta cells suffer 'secretory exhaustion' and insulin levels then become inappropriately low. Type 2 diabetes is therefore characterized by a combination of insulin resistance and inadequate insulin secretion.

The development of insulin resistance is complex, but is strongly linked to obesity. The risk of developing type 2 diabetes increases as body mass index rises. The escalating incidence of diabetes in the developed world parallels the similar explosion in obesity levels.

Polyuria and polydipsia are the classic symptoms of uncontrolled diabetes

Lack of insulin drives the mobilization of energy stores from muscle, fat, and the liver, leading to the production of glucose (Fig. 14.13). Glucose accumulates in the

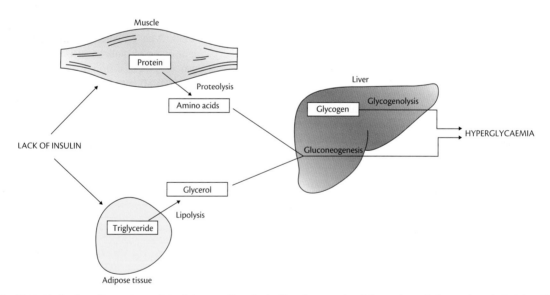

Fig. 14.13 Mechanism of hyperglycaemia in diabetes mellitus. Lack of insulin causes breakdown of protein in muscle and of triglyceride in fat, providing substrates for gluconeogenesis in the liver. This, together with glucose formed from glycogen in the liver, causes hyperglycaemia.

blood, causing hyperglycaemia. In the kidneys, filtered glucose is normally completely reabsorbed in the proximal tubules, but at high blood glucose concentrations, the reabsorption mechanism becomes saturated and glucose appears in the urine (glycosuria). Glucose in the renal tubules draws water in by osmosis, leading to increased water loss in the urine (osmotic diuresis). The raised plasma osmolality due to water loss stimulates the thirst centre. Polyuria and polydipsia together are the classic symptoms of diabetes.

Hyperglycaemia also predisposes diabetics to infections, as organisms grow easily in sugary environments. Recurrent vulvovaginal candidiasis is common in diabetic women and should prompt testing for diabetes. Skin infections and urinary tract infections, sometimes complicated by severe renal damage, are also common in diabetics.

LINK BOX

Acute pyelonephritis in diabetics

Diabetes is a well recognized predisposing factor to ascending infection into the kidney and the development of acute pyelonephritis. Diabetics with acute pyelonephritis may also develop papillary necrosis (p. 220).

The diagnosis of diabetes mellitus requires the demonstration of hyperglycaemia

A diagnosis of diabetes mellitus should not be made lightly as it has serious lifelong implications for the patient. The World Health Organization has laid down criteria for the diagnosis of diabetes mellitus to allow standardization across the world. The diagnosis requires a fasting plasma glucose exceeding 7.0 mmol/l or a random plasma glucose greater than 11.1 mmol/l. These values are used because they have been shown to be associated with a risk of significant long-term complications if sustained over many years.

Patients who have a borderline value in the fasting or random glucose sample should have an **oral glucose tolerance test**. After an overnight fast, the patient drinks 75 g of glucose dissolved in 250 ml water (usually given as 394 ml of Lucozade!) and venous blood is sampled at baseline and after 2 h. Diabetes mellitus is diagnosed if the fasting glucose is greater than 7.0 mmol/l or if the 2 h value is greater than 11.1 mmol/l.

INTERESTING TO KNOW

Impaired glucose tolerance

The oral glucose tolerance test also defines a further category of hyperglycaemia called **impaired glucose tolerance** in which the fasting glucose is less than 7.0 mmol/l and the glucose tolerance test value at 2 h is between 7.8 and 11.1 mmol/l.

Although impaired glucose tolerance does not cause complications such as retinopathy and nephropathy, it is associated with a doubling of cardiovascular mortality (e.g. myocardial infarction), so regular follow-up is required.

Most of the long-term complications of diabetes are due to its effect on blood vessels

Long-term chronic tissue damage is the major burden of diabetes, much of which is due to the severe damage diabetes inflicts upon blood vessels of all sizes. The vascular damage appears to be directly related to the degree of hyperglycaemia, and trials have shown that tight control of blood glucose levels delays the onset and severity of chronic complications.

Large and medium sized arteries of diabetes are prone to accelerated atherosclerosis. Diabetics are extremely susceptible to the development of severe, florid atherosclerosis, and this is the major reason for their high risk of myocardial infarctions, stroke, and peripheral vascular disease.

The most consistent change in capillaries of diabetics is a *diffuse thickening of the basement membrane*. Although the basement membrane is thickened, diabetic capillaries are more leaky than normal to plasma proteins. The microvascular changes are particularly prominent in the capillaries supplying the retina, glomerulus, and nerves.

Virtually every organ system may be damaged by the effects of diabetes (Fig. 14.14), but the most important conditions are ischaemic heart disease, chronic renal failure, retinopathy, and foot ulceration.

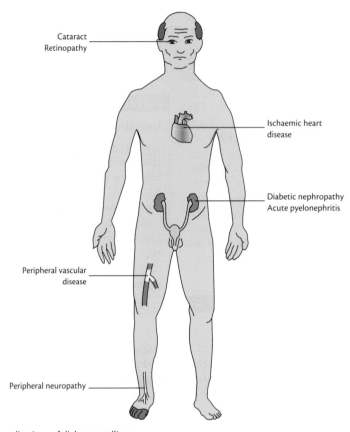

Cataract
Retinopathy

Ischaemic heart
disease

Diabetic nephropathy
Acute pyelonephritis

Peripheral vascular
disease

Peripheral neuropathy

Fig. 14.14 Long-term complications of diabetes mellitus.

Diabetics have a high risk of ischaemic heart disease

Diabetics have a greater than double the risk of significant ischaemic heart disease than non-diabetics. This is due to severe coronary artery atherosclerosis. Angina and chronic heart failure are common long-term problems. Acute myocardial infarction is the most common cause of death in diabetics, and may be harder to diagnose as they are often 'silent' (p. 90).

Diabetes is a leading cause of chronic renal failure

Diabetes mellitus is one of the most common causes of chronic renal failure. The renal damage is predominantly due to a type of glomerular injury known as **diabetic nephropathy**, though other factors such as ischaemia

due to atherosclerosis affecting the origins of the renal arteries and infections in the urinary tract may also contribute.

The hallmark of diabetic nephropathy is thickening of the glomerular basement membrane and expansion of the mesangium. The very first manifestation of this structural change in the glomeruli is leakage of tiny amounts of protein into the urine, known as **microalbuminuria**. Over time, the glomeruli become completely sclerosed with loss of the whole nephron. Proteinuria becomes more marked, the kidneys begin to shrink due to loss of renal mass, and there is biochemical evidence of renal impairment. Ultimately, there is end-stage renal failure requiring renal replacement therapy.

Diabetes is a leading cause of blindness in the developed world

Diabetic eye disease is a potentially serious problem which can be sight threatening. The two main eye problems seen in diabetics are **cataract formation** and **diabetic retinopathy**.

Cataract formation in diabetics is the same as the more common senile type, but is accelerated. It is thought that hyperglycaemia leads to cross-linking of the proteins within the lens of the eye, which distorts the normal transmission of light through it.

Diabetic retinopathy is the result of damage to retinal capillaries and is discussed more fully on p. 474. The earliest changes, known as background retinopathy, are not sight threatening. However, pre-proliferative or proliferative retinopathy both require urgent ophthalmological referral as they are potentially sight threatening. The risk of developing retinopathy progressively increases with increasing duration of diabetes. Nearly all type 1 diabetics will have some evidence of retinopathy (i.e. background changes at least) 15 years following diagnosis, and half will have proliferative changes 20 years after diagnosis.

Footcare is extremely important in diabetics

The feet can be involved by a number of diabetic complications. Chronic ulceration and ischaemia are the main problems. Ulceration usually begins with minor trauma which goes undetected due to peripheral neuropathy. Poor blood supply as a result of vascular disease makes healing difficult. Infection commonly complicates diabetic foot ulcers, often penetrating deep into the soft tissues and even into bone. The development of osteomyelitis requires urgent treatment.

Uncontrolled type 1 diabetes can lead to diabetic ketoacidosis

Diabetic ketoacidosis is a complication of type 1 diabetes in which a severe lack of insulin leads to gross hyperglycaemia and a systemic acidosis due to the generation of ketone bodies in the liver. **Ketone bodies** are moderately strong organic acids whose formation is driven in hepatocytes by the large quantities of free fatty acids generated from rapid lipolysis in adipocytes stimulated by the lack of insulin.

Diabetic ketoacidosis may be the presenting feature of type 1 diabetes or may develop in a patient known to be diabetic if they omit their insulin. An error which commonly leads to ketoacidosis is omission of insulin by patients because they feel unable to eat due to nausea or vomiting. *Insulin should never be stopped.*

Diabetic ketoacidosis usually presents with malaise, vomiting, and often abdominal pain. There is tachypnoea as the lungs attempt to compensate for the metabolic acidosis generated by the ketones. There is profound dehydration due to massive osmotic diuresis stimulated by glucose and ketones filtered by the kidneys. The diagnosis of ketoacidosis requires a combination of marked hyperglycaemia, ketonuria, and acidosis.

Diabetic ketoacidosis is a medical emergency. Without treatment, there is circulatory collapse, coma, and death. The immediate danger to patients is the profound hypovolaemia. There are considerable deficits of fluid (>5 l) and this must be immediately replaced with intravenous fluids. The metabolic disturbance can then be reversed with intravenous insulin. Subcutaneous insulin is not sufficient as subcutaneous blood flow is very low in hypovolaemic patients. If there is an underlying trigger such as an infection, this should also be treated.

Uncontrolled type 2 diabetes causes non-ketotic hyperglycaemia

Patients with uncontrolled type 2 diabetes can develop severe hyperglycaemia (>50 mmol/l) with extreme dehydration due to osmotic diuresis, but they do *not* become ketotic or acidotic. This is because the small amount of circulating insulin they do have is sufficient to prevent the formation of ketone bodies. The management is similar to that for diabetic ketoacidosis.

> # Key points: Diabetes mellitus
>
> - Diabetes mellitus is a very common metabolic disorder characterized by a lack of insulin or resistance to its actions.
>
> - In type 1 diabetes, there is a severe absolute lack of insulin due to autoimmune destruction of the insulin-secreting beta cells in the pancreas. Type 2 diabetes is due to insulin resistance which is strongly linked with obesity.

Continued

Key points: Diabetes mellitus—cont'd

- The typical presenting symptoms of diabetes are polyuria and polydipsia. Recurrent skin and genital infections are also common and should prompt testing for diabetes.

- Diagnosing diabetes requires demonstration of a fasting glucose level >7.0 mmol/l or a random glucose level >11.1 mmol/l. Borderline cases should be formally tested for diabetes using the oral glucose tolerance test.

- The long-term complications of diabetes are related to the effects of hyperglycaemia on blood vessels.

- Diabetes is a leading cause of ischaemic heart disease, chronic renal failure, and blindness.

- Severely uncontrolled diabetes leads to diabetic ketoacidosis in type 1 diabetes and to non-ketotic hyperglycaemia in type 2 diabetes.

Neoplasms of the endocrine pancreas

Pancreatic endocrine neoplasms are far less common than neoplasms of the exocrine pancreas, but generally have a better prognosis. Pancreatic endocrine neoplasms may be functional or non-functional (Table 14.3).

Non-functional tumours which remain small are usually benign and remain subclinical. Large non-functional tumours are more likely to behave in a malignant fashion and present late with symptoms related to their size, usually abdominal pain.

Functional endocrine pancreatic tumours may produce a number of different hormones. The two most common functional tumours are insulinomas and gastrinomas.

TABLE 14.3 Pancreatic endocrine neoplasms

Non-functional	40%
Insulinomas	30%
Gastrinomas	12%
Glucagonomas	8%

Insulinomas

Insulinomas are functional beta cell neoplasms which autonomously release insulin

Insulinomas are functional beta cell neoplasms which release insulin in an unregulated fashion. Insulinomas are the most common islet cell neoplasm but are still rare tumours (annual incidence 2 per million). The presenting features of an insulinoma are related to episodic hypoglycaemia caused by release of insulin from the tumour. Common symptoms related to hypoglycaemia include confusion, incoordination, sweating, and palpitations.

Diagnosis of an insulinoma requires proof of insulin-related hypoglycaemia

Hypoglycaemia has many causes, of which insulinoma is only one. The path to diagnosing an insulinoma first requires demonstration that the hypoglycaemia is insulin mediated. This requires demonstration of inappropriately raised plasma insulin levels in the setting of hypoglycaemia. Elevation of the proinsulin and C peptide levels (two peptides produced during natural production of insulin) makes it possible to distinguish an insulinoma from hypoglycaemia due to administration of exogenous insulin.

Surgical removal of an insulinoma is usually curative

Patients with proven insulin-mediated hypoglycaemia should undergo surgical exploration to identify the pancreatic tumour. The tumours are often very small, and use of an ultrasound probe during the operation is helpful to localize the tumour. Most insulinomas behave in a benign fashion, and surgical removal is curative.

Gastrinomas

Gastrinomas are functional pancreatic endocrine neoplasms which autonomously secrete gastrin

Gastrinomas are functional pancreatic endocrine neoplasms which release gastrin in an unregulated fashion. Gastrinomas are the second most common functional pancreatic endocrine neoplasm (annual incidence 1 per million), most of which occur in the head of the pancreas. Note that gastrinomas can occur at other sites, such as the duodenum. Approximately one-quarter of patients with pancreatic gastrinomas have multiple endocrine neoplasia 1 (MEN 1).

Gastrin is a potent stimulus to acid secretion by the stomach. Patients with gastrinomas typically present with abdominal pain from severe gastro-oesophageal reflux disease and/or peptic ulcer disease. The high gastric acid output into the duodenum neutralizes pancreatic enzymes, leading to malabsorption and diarrhoea. When these effects are due to inappropriate gastrin secretion, it is known as the **Zollinger-Ellison syndrome**. Zollinger-Ellison syndrome should always be considered in young patients with peptic ulcer disease, especially if the ulceration is poorly responsive to treatment or if ulcers occur in unusual locations such as the jejunum.

Gastrinomas are much more likely to behave aggressively than insulinomas. About 50 per cent of gastrinomas are locally invasive or have already metastasized by the time of diagnosis (i.e. they are malignant).

Key points: Pancreatic endocrine neoplasms

- Pancreatic endocrine tumours are rare and may occur sporadically or as part of the inherited syndrome MEN 1.

- The most common pancreatic endocrine tumours are insulinoma and gastrinoma.

- Insulinoma is a functionally active and usually benign pancreatic endocrine tumour with clinical symptoms of hypoglycaemia due to inappropriate secretion of insulin.

- Diagnosis of an insulinoma requires demonstration of abnormally elevated plasma insulin, proinsulin, and C peptide in the setting of hypoglycaemia.

- Surgical removal of the insulinoma is curative.

- A gastrinoma is a functionally active and usually malignant pancreatic endocrine tumour with clinical symptoms due to inappropriate secretion of gastrin (Zollinger-Ellison syndrome). Gastrinomas are much more likely to behave aggressively than insulinomas.

Multiple endocrine neoplasia syndromes

Multiple endocrine neoplasia syndromes are inherited cancer disorders

The **multiple endocrine neoplasia** (MEN) syndromes are classic examples of inherited tumour syndromes which manifest with the development of proliferative lesions (hyperplasias and neoplasms) affecting multiple endocrine organs.

Two MEN syndromes are recognized, MEN 1 and MEN 2, which are both inherited in an autosomal dominant pattern and arise due to inheritance of a germline mutation of the MEN1 and RET genes respectively.

MEN 1 involves the parathyroid, pancreas, and pituitary

MEN 1 is characterized by parathyroid hyperplasia, pancreatic islet cell neoplasms, and pituitary adenomas ('the three Ps'). MEN 1 may therefore lead to a number of clinical problems including renal calculi (parathyroid hyperplasia), recurrent hypoglycaemia (insulinoma), intractable peptic ulcers (Zollinger–Ellison syndrome), and amenorrhoea and galactorrhoea (prolactinoma).

The MEN 1 gene is a tumour suppressor gene, but its precise role is not yet well established. For individuals with a parent affected with MEN 1, DNA testing before the development of any symptoms that might be attributable to the syndrome is now being recommended. If a MEN 1 mutation is detected, appropriate intermittent biochemical screening and imaging studies are suggested.

MEN 2 is characterized by medullary carcinoma of the thyroid

MEN 2 is characterized by the almost inevitable development of medullary carcinoma of the thyroid. Phaeochromocytoma is also common. For those individuals known to have MEN 2, a total prophylactic thyroidectomy is recommended. Phaeochromocytoma should intermittently be screened for with imaging and appropriate urine studies in people with MEN 2.

The definitive diagnosis of MEN 2 relies on germline RET mutation analysis. Such analysis should be carried out on anyone who develops medullary carcinoma of the thyroid, and it is suggested that people who have a phaeochromocytoma should also have it done. RET is a proto-oncogene that encodes a growth-stimulating receptor.

> ## Key points: Multiple endocrine neoplasia syndromes
>
> ◆ The MEN syndromes are autosomal dominant syndromes which predispose to the development of hyperplasias and neoplasms of endocrine organs.
>
> ◆ MEN 1 is due to mutation of the MEN1 tumour suppressor gene and is characterized by parathyroid hyperplasia, pancreatic islet cell neoplasms, and pituitary adenomas.
>
> ◆ MEN 2 is due to mutation of the RET proto-oncogene. Virtually all MEN 2 patients develop medullary carcinoma of the thyroid and many develop phaeochromocytomas.

Haematological disease

Introduction

The blood is a vital transport medium which consists of a fluid called **plasma** in which the cellular elements of the blood are suspended. Plasma is made up of mostly water in which a number of substances are held in solution, including mineral ions (e.g. sodium, potassium), small organic molecules (e.g. amino acids, glucose), plasma proteins (e.g. albumin, immunoglobulins, clotting factors), and hormones. If a blood sample is allowed to stand, it separates into a clot and a clear yellow fluid called **serum**.

The cellular elements of the blood include the **red blood cells** (erythrocytes), **white blood cells** (leukocytes), and **platelets**. All of the cells of the blood are derived from pluripotential stem cells in the bone marrow. These stem cells proliferate into two distinct cell lines: the lymphoid stem cells, which mature into B and T lymphocytes, and the myeloid stem cells which differentiate into all the other cell types of the blood (Fig. 15.1).

Red blood cells are the most numerous cells in the blood. They are small non-nucleated cells whose chief function is to deliver oxygen to the tissues of the body. The oxygen-carrying molecule in red cells is **haemoglobin**. Haemoglobin is composed of four polypeptide **globin** chains, each of which has a **haem** group which binds oxygen (Fig. 15.2). In fetal and neonatal life, red blood cells make fetal haemoglobin (HbF) which has two α-globin chains and two γ-globin chains ($\alpha_2\gamma_2$). By 2 months of age, red cells begin synthesizing predominantly adult haemoglobin, HbA, made up of two α- and two β-globin chains ($\alpha_2\beta_2$). A small proportion of adult haemoglobin is HbA$_2$ which has an $\alpha_2\delta_2$ configuration. Note that developing red cells in the bone marrow are nucleated, allowing them to synthesize proteins including haemoglobin. Prior to release into the circulation,

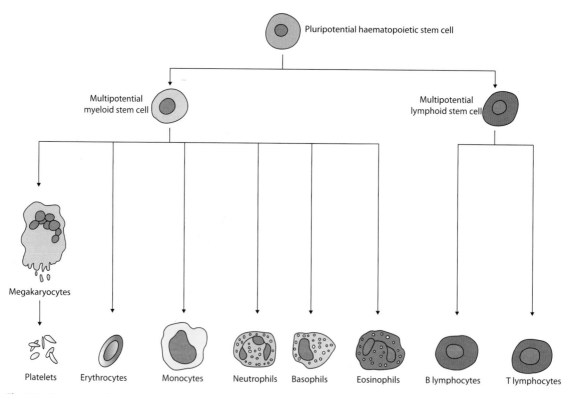

Fig. 15.1 Haematopoiesis.

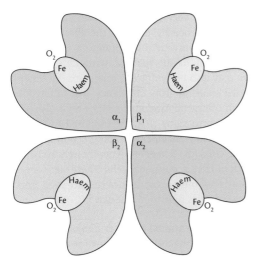

Fig. 15.2 Haemoglobin molecule composed of four polypeptide globin chains, each of which contains a haem molecule. The iron atom at the centre of the haem group binds to oxygen.

mature red blood cells lose their nucleus and are thus unable to make new proteins.

Leukocytes, or white blood cells, are the nucleated cells of the blood. Their main role is protection against infection. Five varieties of white cells are recognized: neutrophils, lymphocytes, monocytes, eosinophils, and basophils. **Neutrophils** are the most numerous leukocyte in the blood. They have a segmented nucleus with up to five lobes and their cytoplasm has granules containing enzymes used to destroy engulfed organisms and particles. **Lymphocytes** are small leukocytes divided into B and T subtypes which are crucial to the adaptive immune response. **Monocytes** are the largest leukocyte in the blood. Monocytes enter tissues where they become tissue macrophages (histiocytes). Macrophages have phagocytic and antigen-presenting functions. **Eosinophils** have a bilobed nucleus and large cytoplasmic granules. They are important in defence against parasitic infections and are associated with allergic reactions. **Basophils** are the least common leukocyte in the blood. They contain very large granules which contain histamine.

Platelets are small cells about one-fifth the size of a red blood cell. They are cell fragments derived from the megakaryocytes of the bone marrow and they play a crucial role in haemostasis. Platelets form the primary haemostatic plug at sites of vascular injury and provide a suitable surface on which the coagulation cascade can occur, leading to the formation of a fibrin clot.

Virtually every disease causes some kind of haematological alteration, and measurement of simple haematological parameters forms an important part of routine clinical assessment. In this chapter, we concentrate predominantly on primary disorders of the blood managed by haematologists.

Anaemia

Anaemia is defined as a haemoglobin level below the normal range

Anaemia is a very common clinical disorder and is defined by a haemoglobin concentration below the reference range for the sex of the individual (<13.5 g/dl in men and <11.5 g/dl in women). Anaemia should not be considered a final diagnosis; it is a manifestation of an underlying problem that should be investigated.

Many patients with anaemia are asymptomatic. There may be symptoms related to the underlying cause of the anaemia, but symptoms directly related to anaemia usually only become apparent if it occurs suddenly or if other disorders impairing tissue oxygenation co-exist (typically some form of chronic heart or lung disease). Such symptoms include lethargy and breathlessness on exertion. The main physical sign of anaemia is pallor.

In the simplest sense, anaemia may be due to either *reduced production of red blood cells or increased loss of red blood cells*. There are many possible causes of anaemia, but only a handful are common (Table 15.1).

Anaemia due to reduced production of red blood cells

Impaired red blood cell production may be due to an actual reduction in erythropoietic tissue due to bone marrow disease (**insufficient erythropoiesis**) or to a high death rate of the developing red cell precursors (**ineffective erythropoiesis**). Ineffective erythropoiesis is the more common mechanism causing anaemia, and is usually the result of a haematinic deficiency. Haematinics are essential molecules required for normal red cell production such as iron, vitamin B12, and folate.

TABLE 15.1	Causes of anaemia

Reduced production of red cells

   Iron deficiency

   Anaemia of chronic disease

   Vitamin B12 and folate deficiency

   Myelodysplasia

   Marrow infiltration

Increased loss of red cells

   Hereditary spherocytosis

   Glucose-6-phosphate dehydrogenase deficiency

   Sickle cell disease

   Thalassaemia

   Immune haemolysis

   Mechanical haemolysis

Iron deficiency anaemia

Iron deficiency is the most common cause of anaemia

Iron is an essential constituent of the haem group of haemoglobin. When there is chronic iron deficiency, the final step in haem synthesis is interrupted, leading to reduced haemoglobin synthesis. Haemoglobin levels fall slowly and, by the time anaemia develops as a result of iron deficiency, body iron stores are completely exhausted.

Chronic blood loss is the most common cause of iron deficiency anaemia

About two-thirds of total body iron is found within the haemoglobin of red blood cells. Persistent blood loss can therefore lead to profound depletion of body iron stores and hence iron deficiency anaemia. The most common site of chronic blood loss is the gastrointestinal tract. Important causes of gastrointestinal blood loss include bleeding related to peptic ulcers, carcinoma of the stomach, sigmoid diverticular disease, and colorectal carcinoma. Worldwide, the most common cause of iron deficiency anaemia is gastrointestinal bleeding related to hookworm infestation. Women with heavy menstrual blood loss may develop iron deficiency anaemia.

Iron deficiency may also result from gastrointestinal diseases that lead to malabsorption of iron. Iron deficiency anaemia is a very common presentation of gluten-sensitive enteropathy, often in the absence of any significant gastrointestinal symptoms (p. 153).

In addition to the general symptoms of anaemia, there may also be symptoms related to the underlying disorder causing iron deficiency (e.g. altered bowel habit in colorectal carcinoma). Many texts also describe other physical signs that are supposed to be seen in iron deficiency anaemia including spoon-shaped nails (koilonychia) and a beefy tongue, thought to be related to lack of iron in epithelial cells. These signs are rarely seen as they only occur in severe untreated iron deficiency which is uncommon today.

Iron deficiency anaemia causes a microcytic hypochromic anaemia with a low serum ferritin

A full blood count in a patient with iron deficiency anaemia reveals a low haemoglobin concentration, a low mean cell volume, and a low mean cell haemoglobin concentration, i.e. *microcytic hypochromic anaemia*. A blood film will confirm the small pale red cells and also show variation in the size and shape of the red cells (Fig. 15.3).

Confirming iron deficiency as the cause of a microcytic hypochromic anaemia requires measurement of serum ferritin levels. **Ferritin**, a combination of iron and the protein apoferritin, is the main form in which iron is stored in the body and is low in iron deficiency anaemia.

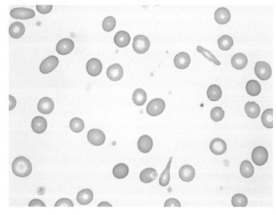

Fig. 15.3 Blood film in iron deficiency anaemia showing pale and distorted red blood cells.

Older patients with iron deficiency anaemia must have investigation of the gastrointestinal tract

Once iron deficiency anaemia has been established, it is essential to find the underlying cause. Unless the patient is young and there is a clear cause for the iron deficiency (e.g. heavy menstrual bleeding), it is mandatory to investigate the gastrointestinal tract for a source of bleeding or a cause of malabsorption. *Excluding a gastrointestinal malignancy is particularly important.* If gluten-sensitive enteropathy is suspected, measurement of serum endomysial antibodies and duodenal biopsy are indicated. Of note, no cause can be found in up to 20 per cent of cases of iron deficiency anaemia.

Key points: Iron deficiency anaemia

- Iron deficiency anaemia is the most common cause of anaemia and is due to depletion of body iron stores.

- Lack of iron interrupts the final stage of haem synthesis, impairing haemoglobin production and thus causing anaemia.

- The most common cause of iron deficiency is chronic gastrointestinal bleeding or menorrhagia.

- Iron deficiency anaemia causes a microcytic hypochromic anaemia with small, pale red cells on the blood film. A low serum ferritin confirms iron deficiency.

- Investigation of the gastrointestinal tract is mandatory in patients with iron deficiency anaemia unless they are young and have a clear underlying cause.

Anaemia of chronic disease

Anaemia of chronic disease has a complex pathogenesis

Anaemia is a very common manifestation of a variety of persistent diseases such as chronic infections, chronic inflammatory disorders, and malignancy. This type of anaemia is known as **anaemia of chronic disease** and is the second most common type of anaemia.

The pathogenesis of anaemia of chronic disease is complex and involves multiple factors including reduced sensitivity of the bone marrow to erythropoietin and failure to incorporate iron into developing red blood cells. These effects appear to be the result of persistent high levels of circulating cytokines in the body as a result of the ongoing inflammation. The anaemia is usually normocytic, i.e. the red cells have a normal size.

Megaloblastic anaemias

Megaloblastic anaemias are accompanied by megaloblastic erythropoiesis

Anaemia may result if developing red blood cells are unable to synthesize DNA efficiently. The cells become progressively larger because they continue to make protein and other cell components, but are unable to divide because they cannot make enough DNA to form two nuclei. They become arrested in their development as large immature cells called **megaloblasts**, many of which die in the bone marrow.

Megaloblasts which survive develop into abnormally large red blood cells called **macrocytes** which are released into the circulation. Other blood cell lineages are also affected by inadequate DNA synthetic ability, a typical feature being the production of **hypersegmented neutrophils** with more than five nuclear lobes (Fig. 15.4).

Anaemias associated with megaloblastic erythropoiesis are called megaloblastic anaemias. The most common causes of a megaloblastic anaemia are **vitamin B12**

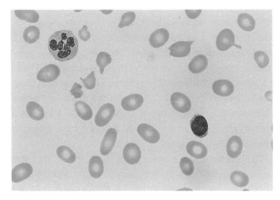

Fig. 15.4 Blood film in megaloblastic anaemia showing a hypersegmented neutrophil and oval macrocytes.

deficiency and **folate deficiency**, both of which are necessary to convert deoxyuridine monophosphate (dUMP) into deoxythymidine monophosphate (dTMP), a molecule required for DNA synthesis.

JARGON BUSTER

Macrocytosis

Red cells may be large in the absence of anaemia. This is known as macrocytosis and may be seen in heavy alcohol intake and hypothyroidism.

The most common cause of vitamin B12 deficiency is autoimmune gastritis

While most vitamins can be made by a wide variety of plants and animals, only microorganisms such as bacteria and yeast are capable of producing vitamin B12. Humans therefore rely entirely on vitamin B12 in the diet. Animal meat is the best source of B12 because animals ingest microorganisms containing the vitamin. Plant food may contain some B12 if they are contaminated with B12-containing bacteria. Vegetarians can also get B12 from milk and eggs. Dietary insufficiency is therefore a rare cause of vitamin B12 deficiency except in strict vegans who consume no animal produce of any kind.

Vitamin B12 deficiency is usually due to lack of **intrinsic factor**, which is necessary for the absorption of vitamin B12 by transporting it into the epithelial cells of the terminal ileum. Intrinsic factor is produced by the parietal cells of the gastric body (the same cells that produce hydrochloric acid). Severe atrophy of the specialized glands of the stomach due to autoimmune gastritis may therefore lead to a marked reduction in intrinsic factor secretion. In addition, many patients with autoimmune gastritis develop circulating antibodies to intrinsic factor which block its action. The reduced intrinsic factor levels, and the block to its action, means that vitamin B12 absorption from the gut is greatly impaired.

The presence of anaemia due to vitamin B12 deficiency in a patient with autoimmune gastritis is known as **pernicious anaemia**. Pernicious anaemia is common in northern Europeans, and the prevalence increases with age, possibly affecting as many as 2–3 per cent of

people aged over 70. It accounts for 80 per cent of all cases of megaloblastic anaemia.

Symptoms of pernicious anaemia develop slowly as the haemoglobin levels fall. Most patients present with symptoms of fatigue, weakness, and breathlessness on exertion, and are found to have a severe anaemia (haemoglobin often as low as 4–5 g/dl). The red cells are markedly enlarged, leading to a very high mean cell volume reading on the full blood count—values as high as 140 fl (normal 82–98) have been reported. The blood film shows macrocytes and hypersegmented neutrophils, indicative of a megaloblastic anaemia. Serum vitamin B12 is low.

Once vitamin B12 deficiency is established, the underlying cause must be investigated. The most likely causes will be pernicious anaemia or a small bowel disease leading to malabsorption of B12. The presence of **anti-intrinsic factor antibodies** is considered diagnostic of pernicious anaemia, though only about half of patients will demonstrate these. In the absence of intrinsic factor antibodies, a **Schilling test** can be considered to make the diagnosis.

In the Schilling test, vitamin B12 malabsorption is first confirmed by proving lack of urinary excretion of orally administered radiolabelled vitamin B12. Pernicious anaemia is confirmed if the malabsorption is then corrected by ingestion of recombinant intrinsic factor. If malabsorption remains following recombinant intrinsic factor, then another gastrointestinal disease is responsible for failure to absorb vitamin B12 (Fig. 15.5).

Patients with pernicious anaemia should be treated with intramuscular vitamin B12 injections. There is rapid normalization of haematological parameters, and patients usually feel better within 24 h of the first injection. Transfusion is usually not necessary unless the patient is severely compromised by the anaemia.

Long-term follow-up of patients with pernicious anaemia is essential, checking not only annual full blood counts, but also TSH levels as pernicious anaemia is associated with other organ-specific autoimmune diseases such as Hashimoto's thyroiditis. Patients with pernicious anaemia also have twice the risk of developing gastric adenocarcinoma compared with the normal population; recall the gastric atrophy, intestinal metaplasia, dysplasia, adenocarcinoma sequence (p. 147).

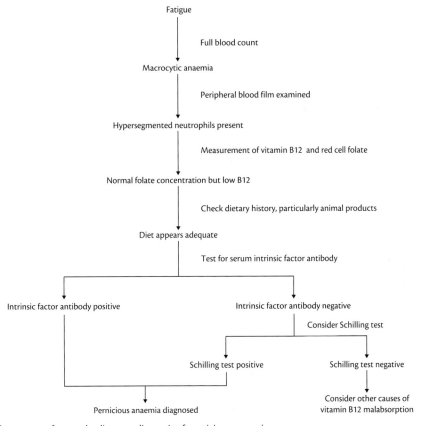

Fig. 15.5 Typical sequence of events leading to a diagnosis of pernicious anaemia.

LINK BOX

Vitamin B12 deficiency

In addition to the problem in making normal red blood cells, B12 deficiency may also be deleterious to the central nervous system. Demyelination of the posterior columns of the spinal cord is an early feature, and this leads to problems with sensation and proprioception. Loss of cortical neurones may also occur, causing dementia (p. 440).

Malnutrition is the most common cause of folate deficiency

Folate deficiency is the other major cause of megaloblastic anaemia. Whereas malnutrition is a very unusual cause of vitamin B12 deficiency, it is the most common cause of folate deficiency.

The main dietary sources of folate are leafy green vegetables such as broccoli, spinach, and lettuce, and fresh fruits. Folate deficiency is therefore typically seen in people who do not eat fresh fruit or vegetables (particularly alcoholics), and the elderly who may be unable to chew their food. Folate deficiency can also develop if absorption of folate from the jejunum is impaired, e.g. gluten-sensitive enteropathy.

The body only stores about 4 months supply of folate in reserve, so deficiency can develop quite quickly if folate intake or absorption is inadequate. Patients with folate deficiency develop a megaloblastic anaemia which is distinguished from B12 deficiency by finding a reduced red cell folate level.

Key points: Megaloblastic anaemia

- Megaloblastic anaemia refers to a macrocytic anaemia with megaloblastic erythropoiesis, caused by impaired DNA synthesis in developing red cells.

- Megaloblastic changes can be visualized on a blood film by the presence of hypersegmented neutrophils and macrocytes.

- The most common causes of a megaloblastic anaemia are vitamin B12 and folate deficiency.

- Vitamin B12 deficiency due to pernicious anaemia accounts for 80 per cent of all cases of megaloblastic anaemia. Other causes of vitamin B12 deficiency are rare in the UK.

- Pernicious anaemia results from autoimmune gastritis leading to severe lack of intrinsic factor, which is needed for the absorption of vitamin B12. Half of patients also have circulating antibodies against intrinsic factor which blocks its actions.

- Folate deficiency is usually due to inadequate dietary intake. It may also occur in gluten-sensitive enteropathy due to malabsorption of folate. Folate deficiency is distinguished from vitamin B12 deficiency by finding a reduced red cell folate.

Myelodysplasia

Myelodysplasia is a common cause of an isolated macrocytic anaemia in the elderly

Myelodysplasia is a type of haematological malignancy which we discuss in more detail later in this chapter. It is important to mention it here as the most common mode of presentation of myelodysplasia is with a persistent unexplained macrocytic anaemia.

The anaemia occurs because one of the early progenitor cells in the bone marrow becomes neoplastic, resulting in ineffective erythropoiesis. Many red cells do not survive the maturation process and are destroyed in the bone marrow, and those that do survive and enter the peripheral blood are abnormally large, hence the macrocytic anaemia.

Bone marrow infiltration

Bone marrow infiltration leads to a leukoerythroblastic anaemia

Infiltration of the bone marrow may lead to anaemia by destroying normal haemopoietic tissue, an example of insufficient erythropoiesis. Infiltration may occur due to metastatic disease in the bones (commonly from a breast, lung, prostate, thyroid, or kidney primary), multiple myeloma, or myelofibrosis.

When anaemia is due to marrow infiltration, immature red and white blood cells are squeezed out into the circulation and are seen in the peripheral blood smear. The presence of immature white and red blood cells in the blood of an anaemic patient is known as a **leukoerythroblastic anaemia** and strongly suggests marrow infiltration. There is often an associated neutropenia and thrombocytopenia as well.

Anaemia due to increased destruction of red blood cells

Pathological destruction of red blood cells is known as **haemolysis**. In response to ongoing haemolysis the bone marrow can increase red cell output sixfold, but if the rate of haemolysis exceeds the maximum erythropoietic capacity of the bone marrow, anaemia will occur.

Patients with haemolysis usually have a raised number of **reticulocytes** in the peripheral blood. Reticulocytes are immature red blood cells which still have large amounts of RNA in their cytoplasm. Normally reticulocytes are confined to the bone marrow where they lose their RNA and fully develop into mature erythrocytes. In haemolytic states, the increased productivity of the bone marrow leads to the premature release of reticulocytes into the peripheral blood. A raised reticulocyte count therefore provides good evidence that a haemolytic process is taking place.

Haemolysis may be due to structural abnormalities of red blood cells that make them fragile. Such disorders are usually inherited. Haemolysis may also occur if the red cells are normal but they are destroyed by an immune attack or by physical means.

is negative in spherocytosis and positive in immune haemolytic anaemia.

Patients with well compensated haemolysis and no transfusion requirements need no specific treatment but are usually given folate supplements.

Glucose-6-phosphate dehydrogenase deficiency

G6PD deficiency is another common inherited cause of haemolytic anaemia

Glucose-6-phosphate dehydrogenase (G6PD) is one of the enzymes required by red blood cells to maintain a source of reduced glutathione. Reduced glutathione protects the red cell membrane from oxidative damage by reducing compounds such as hydrogen peroxide to water.

G6PD deficiency is a disease in which the activity of the G6PD enzyme is reduced due to inherited mutations in the G6PD gene. Although uncommon in the UK, G6PD deficiency is common worldwide, affecting 10 per cent of the world's population, particularly African Americans, Asians, Italians, Greeks, and other Mediterranean people.

The G6PD gene is located on the X chromosome. Only a single mutated copy causes G6PD deficiency in men. Homozygous women are also affected, but such individuals are not often seen. Heterozygous women do not have clinical manifestations as the normal copy of the G6PD gene on the other X chromosome produces enough enzyme activity.

Most individuals with G6PD deficiency are asymptomatic and have normal haemoglobin levels. If, however, they are exposed to certain substances that cause oxidative stress to red blood cells, they suffer an acute haemolytic episode. They feel very unwell, have a fever, and pass dark urine due to haemoglobinuria. Haemoglobin levels decline rapidly, accompanied by a marked rise in the reticulocyte count. Common agents known to lead to haemolytic episodes include various drugs (including antimalarials) and fava beans, a common food in Mediterranean countries.

A useful screening test for G6PD deficiency indirectly assesses G6PD activity by testing the ability of red cells to reduce dyes. A low activity on a screening test should prompt direct assay of the enzyme for definitive diagnosis. Patients with G6PD deficiency should be counselled about avoiding known precipitants of haemolysis.

spleen, leading to their engulfment and premature destruction by splenic macrophages.

Patients with hereditary spherocytosis suffer from a chronic haemolytic anaemia with intermittent episodes of jaundice. The high levels of unconjugated bilirubin lead to the formation of pigment gallstones. In fact, gallstone-related disease can be what brings the underlying spherocytosis to clinical attention. The reticulocyte count will be raised, and the blood film will show easily recognizable spherocytes. Both of these features are also seen in an immune haemolytic anaemia, which is the main differential diagnosis. The two are distinguished by the **direct antiglobulin test** (p. 344) which

Sickle cell disorders

Sickle cell disorders are caused by a point mutation in the β-globin gene which causes a glutamate residue to be replaced with a valine molecule. The resultant haemoglobin molecule that is produced is known as haemoglobin S (HbS). Although HbS differs from HbA by only a single amino acid, HbS is 50 times less soluble than HbA. Under conditions of low oxygen tension, HbS polymerizes into rod-like aggregates which damage the red blood cell.

The gene for HbS is most prevalent in areas of tropical Africa and in parts of the Middle East and southern India. The distribution reflects areas of current or previous malaria endemicity. The mutant gene has survived because heterozygote carriers are protected against the effects of severe *P. falciparum* malaria through mechanisms that are still not clear.

Individuals with sickle cell trait are haematologically normal and usually asymptomatic

Heterozygotes for the sickle cell gene are said to have **sickle cell trait**. Sickle cell trait is not associated with sickling because the presence of a normal HbA gene reduces the formation of HbS aggregates. Individuals with sickle cell trait have a normal haemoglobin level and are usually asymptomatic, but nonetheless are genetically important as they are carriers of the sickle cell gene.

Patients with sickle cell disease have a chronic haemolytic anaemia

Patients homozygous for the sickle cell gene suffer from **sickle cell disease** or **sickle cell anaemia**. Once affected individuals reach about 2 years old, they have lost most of their HbF, and virtually all the haemoglobin in their red cells is HbS. Their red cells sickle at oxygen tensions typically seen in venous blood, causing repeated cycles of sickling and unsickling as the red cells pass through the circulation.

Repeated episodes of sickling ruins the red cell membrane and eventually the sickling becomes irreversible, leading to lysis of the red blood cell. The average life span of a red cell in sickle cell disease is shortened to just 16 days (normally 120 days).

The persistent haemolysis causes a chronic anaemia, usually with haemoglobin levels between 7 and 9 g/dl. Patients are generally not troubled by symptoms of

TABLE 15.2 Complications of sickle cell disease
Childhood
Hand and foot syndrome
Splenic sequestration crisis
Stroke
Later life
Chronic renal failure
Priapism
Lower limb ulceration
Pigment gallstones
Avascular necrosis of the femoral head
Pulmonary syndrome

anaemia in sickle cell disease, which are less than one would expect for the level of anaemia, because HbS releases oxygen more readily than HbA. The main threat to patients with sickle cell disease are episodes of so-called **vascular crises** (Table 15.2).

Sickle cell disease leads to occlusion of small vessels

Vascular crises occur because sickled cells tend to stick tightly to one another and to endothelium in areas of low oxygen tension. Nobody really knows precisely why this happens, but it is a big problem because the clumped cells occlude capillaries leading to episodes of acute tissue ischaemia.

The most common type of crisis, simply called a 'painful crisis', is associated with widespread bone pain and is usually self-limiting with good hydration and analgesia. In childhood, a typical manifestation is **dactylitis**, in which the vessels of the metacarpals and metatarsals become occluded. The hands and feet become swollen and painful. In older children and adults, larger infarcts of bones may occur, including avascular necrosis of the femoral head which is a serious complication that can lead to chronic disability and pain.

Pulmonary syndrome and stroke are two serious vascular crises in sickle cell disease

The **pulmonary syndrome** is a serious complication of sickle cell disease characterized by acute severe hypoxia due to red cell sickling in the pulmonary circulation.

Stroke in sickle cell disease occurs more commonly in children and is frequently due to occlusion of large arteries such as the internal carotid or the middle cerebral artery, leading to profound neurological deficits. The mechanism of occlusion of these vessels is not clear.

Both pulmonary syndrome and stroke in sickle cell disease are medical emergencies, requiring urgent **exchange transfusion** in which the patient's blood is removed and replaced with donated packed red cells.

Patients with sickle cell disease are at risk of bacterial infections

Patients with sickle cell disease suffer recurrent vaso-occlusion in the spleen which ultimately terminates in autoinfarction of the organ by the age of 6. This leaves patients at risk of overwhelming systemic infection, particularly by encapsulated bacteria such as *Streptococcus pneumoniae*, *Haemophilus influenzae*, and *Neisseria meningitidis*.

The diagnosis of sickle cell disease requires haemoglobin electrophoresis

The earliest suggestion of a diagnosis of sickle cell disease is often the presence of a few sickled cells on the blood film of a patient with a haemolytic anaemia. A simple screening test can then be performed such as the **sickle cell solubility test** in which a reducing agent is added to haemoglobin extracted from the red cells of a blood sample. The relative insolubility of HbS causes it to precipitate and the solution goes cloudy.

The sickle cell solubility test only demonstrates the presence of HbS-containing red cells and does not discriminate between sickle cell trait and sickle cell disease. Definitive diagnosis of sickle cell disease requires **haemoglobin electrophoresis**, which shows a single major HbS band and no normal HbA (Fig. 15.6). The parents will both have features of sickle cell trait.

Treatment of sickle cell disease is largely supportive

The treatment for sickle cell disease is supportive, and includes immunization against encapsulated bacteria, daily folate supplements, and education on how to avoid precipitating vascular crises by keeping well hydrated.

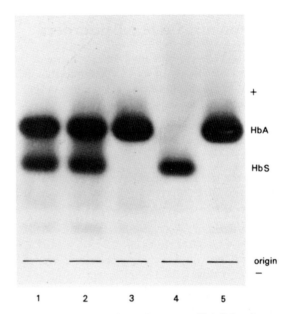

Fig. 15.6 Haemoglobin electrophoresis in sickle cell disorders. The following are shown from left to right: (1 and 2) sickle cell trait; (3) normal; (4) sickle cell anaemia; (5) normal.

Treatment of painful crises requires fluid replacement and analgesia, which may require high doses of opiates. Sadly, patients with sickle cell disease may become addicted to opiate medications and it is unfortunate that many of them become labelled by health care workers as drug seekers. The life expectancy of patients with sickle cell disease is about 40–50 years.

Sickle cell disorders can be a serious problem in surgery

Sickle cell disorders can be a serious problem in surgery as hypoxia, hypothermia, and dehydration all predispose to sickling. Even patients with sickle cell trait, who are normally asymptomatic, may sickle under conditions of severe hypoxia during anaesthesia. Any Afro-Caribbean patient undergoing general anaesthesia should therefore be screened for HbS using the sickle cell solubility test.

Patients with confirmed sickle cell disorder require strict anaesthetic care to minimize the risk of sickling. Patients with sickle cell disease having major operations may require pre-operative exchange transfusion.

Key points: Sickle cell disorders

- Sickle cell disorders result from inheritance of the sickle cell gene in which a point mutation in the β-globin chain leads to the formation of HbS molecules in red cells.

- HbS is less soluble than normal HbA and precipitates into rod-like aggregates in areas of low oxygen tension.

- Inheritance of a single sickle cell gene causes sickle cell trait which is an asymptomatic carrier state.

- Inheritance of two sickle cell genes causes sickle cell disease. All of the haemoglobin in the red cells is HbS which readily polymerizes in venous blood, causing the red cells to adopt a sickle shape.

- Recurrent episodes of sickling damage the red cell membrane until eventually the red cell irreversibly sickles and is removed in the spleen.

- Patients with sickle cell disease have a mild chronic haemolytic anaemia. The anaemia does not cause significant symptoms; the major morbidity in patients with sickle cell disease is related to episodes of vascular crises due to occlusion of small vessels by sickled red cells.

- The most common type of crisis is a painful crisis in which there is bony pain. Treatment is supportive with analgesia and hydration until the episode settles.

- More severe occlusive episodes include the pulmonary syndrome which causes severe hypoxia and stroke due to cerebral vessel occlusion. These require urgent exchange transfusion.

- Patients with sickle cell disease are at risk of infection as recurrent sickling in the spleen leads to autoinfarction of the organ.

- The diagnosis of sickle cell disease is first suspected when sickled cells are seen on a blood film in a patient with a haemolytic anaemia. The sickle cell solubility test is a widely used screening test for the presence of HbS-containing red cells and is positive in both sickle cell trait and sickle cell disease. Definitive diagnosis of sickle cell disease requires haemoglobin electrophoresis which demonstrates a single major band of HbS and near absence of HbA.

- There is no cure for sickle cell disease, and treatment is supportive with measures to reduce the risk of vascular crises.

Thalassaemias

Thalassaemias are inherited anaemias due to reduced production of α- or β-globin chains

The **thalassaemias** are a group of inherited anaemias associated with reduced production of a structurally normal globin chain. The thalassaemias are divided into α- and β-thalassaemia according to which globin chain is produced in reduced amounts. In α-thalassaemia, there is reduced production of α-chains with accumulation of excess β-chains. In β-thalassaemia, there is reduced production of β-chains with accumulation of excess α-chains.

Excess unpaired globin chains precipitate in red blood cells, leading to their destruction

The anaemia in thalassaemia is the result of accumulation of the excess unpaired globin chains in developing and mature red blood cells. Precipitation of excess globin chains in developing red blood cells leads to their destruction in the bone marrow. Excess globin chains in mature red blood cells distort their shape and lead to their premature removal in the spleen.

The anaemia in thalassaemia is therefore due to a combination of ineffective erythropoiesis in the bone marrow and haemolysis in the spleen. In β-thalassaemias, both mechanisms are responsible for the anaemia, whereas in α-thalassaemia, haemolysis makes the dominant contribution to the anaemia. The anaemia in thalassaemia is usually microcytic and hypochromic because the low haemoglobin content of the red cells makes them small and pale.

The clinical consequences of the thalassaemias depend on how many genes are affected, producing a wide range of disorders that range in severity from an extremely mild asymptomatic anaemia to death *in utero*.

β-Thalassaemias

The β-thalassaemias are the most important thalassaemias because they are the most common and produce the most severe anaemia. The prevalence of β-thalassaemia mutations is highest in the Mediterranean, South East Asia, and Africa. Rather like the HbS gene, it is thought that the β-thalassaemia genes have survived because they confer protection against falciparum malaria in heterozygote carriers.

There are two copies of the β-globin gene in each developing red blood cell. Abnormality of both β-globin genes results in β-thalassaemia major; if only one of the β-globin genes are mutated, the patient has β-thalassaemia minor.

β-Thalassaemia major

Patients with **β-thalassaemia major** have mutations which impair the output from both β-globin genes. The problem begins after a few months of life as HbF levels decline and excess α-chains begin to accumulate in red blood cells. As the anaemia worsens, there is an intense drive to red cell production, with expansion of the bone marrow compartment and resumption of haematopoiesis in the liver and spleen. Left untreated, β-thalassaemia major causes bony deformities, hepatosplenomegaly, and severe growth retardation.

The typical presentation of β-thalassaemia major is an infant that looks pale and is generally unwell with poor feeding. The diagnosis should always be considered in the differential diagnosis of an infant with failure to thrive, especially if the child is from an appropriate racial background. A full blood count will reveal a microcytic hypochromic anaemia, and the diagnosis is confirmed by demonstrating a near absence of HbA on haemoglobin electrophoresis.

The mainstay of the management of β-thalassaemia major is entry into a blood transfusion programme which aims to keep the haemoglobin level high enough to curtail the excess drive to red cell production. If the diagnosis is correctly made, and regular transfusions started, the bony complications are avoided and development is normal.

Unfortunately, the transfusions themselves cause secondary iron overload leading to cirrhosis, heart failure, and diabetes. These were major causes of death in teenagers and young adults with β-thalassaemia major until effective iron chelators were introduced. These have been a big help, but do have some disadvantages.

Desferrioxamine, the main chelator currently used, is ineffective orally, meaning it must be given by subcutaneous or intravenous infusions. As a consequence, there is a high incidence of non-compliance.

β-Thalassaemia minor

Patients with β-thalassaemia minor have lost the activity of only one of the two β-globin genes. They are silent carriers who are usually symptom free with a clinically insignificant mild microcytic anaemia. The key diagnostic feature is a raised HbA_2 ($\alpha_2\delta_2$) level on haemoglobin electrophoresis.

α-Thalassaemia

α-Chains are needed for both HbA ($\alpha_2\beta_2$) and HbF ($\alpha_2\gamma_2$), so defects in α-globin production result in defective fetal and adult haemoglobin. In the fetus, deficiency of α-chains leads to the production of excess γ-chains which form γ-tetramers known as Hb Bart's. In adults, excess β-chains form tetramers known as HbH.

There are two α-genes on each chromosome 16, making four in total. The various α-thalassaemias depend on how many are lost. Deletion of all four α-genes leads to complete absence of α-chains. As these are needed to make fetal-type haemoglobin, there is severe fetal anaemia leading to generalized oedema and massive hepatosplenomegaly. The disorder is incompatible with life, and death occurs *in utero*, usually between 28 and 40 weeks. Hb Bart's is a common cause of fetal loss in South East Asia.

Deletion of three α-globin genes leads to **haemoglobin H disease** due to accumulation of HbH. The excess β-chains do not precipitate extensively in developing red blood cells in the bone marrow and so erythropoiesis is mostly effective. HbH precipitates as the red cell ages, leading to haemolysis in the spleen. The anaemia of HbH disease is therefore mostly the result of haemolysis. The clinical picture of HbH disease is very variable, but most patients have a moderate chronic haemolytic anaemia throughout life (haemoglobin typically 7–10 g/dl) and splenomegaly. Unlike β-thalassaemia major, it is unusual to develop bony changes or growth retardation. Treatment is not usually required, but the disease requires monitoring.

Deletion of one or two genes leads to α-thalassaemia minor, which is usually asymptomatic. There may be a very mild microcytic anaemia.

Key points: Thalassaemias

- The thalassaemias are a group of inherited disorders in which there is a reduction in the amount of production of either α- or β-globin chains.

- Unbalanced globin chain production leads to accumulation of the unaffected globin chain in red cells. Anaemia is a result of a combination of ineffective erythropoiesis and haemolysis.

- The clinical consequences depend on which globin chain is affected and how many genes are mutated.

- β-Thalassaemia results from reduced synthesis of the β-globin chain with accumulation of α-chains in red cells.

- Mutations of both β-globin genes causes β-thalassaemia major which presents in the first few months of life with failure to thrive due to a severe haemolytic anaemia. Patients are transfusion dependent and require iron chelation therapy to prevent iron overload.

- Mutation of one of the two β-globin genes causes β-thalassaemia minor. Affected individuals are silent carriers with a clinically insignificant microcytic anaemia.

- α-Thalassaemia results from reduced synthesis of the α-globin chain with accumulation of γ-chains in the fetus and β-chains in post-natal life.

- There are four α-globin genes, and the clinical manifestations of α-thalassaemia depend on the number of genes affected by mutations.

- Deletion of all four α-globin genes causes severe fetal anaemia and intrauterine death.

- Loss of three α-globin genes causes α-thalassaemia major, in which unstable tetramers of β-chains known as haemoglobin H accumulate in red cells. Patients with HbH disease have a moderate chronic haemolytic anaemia throughout life. Treatment is not usually required.

- Loss of one or two α-globin genes causes α-thalassaemia minor which causes a very mild microcytic anaemia which is asymptomatic.

Acquired haemolytic anaemias

In acquired haemolytic anaemias, the red cells themselves are normal but are destroyed as a result of some defect 'outside' the red cell. This is usually due to *immune destruction* of red cells or *mechanical trauma* to red cells.

Immune haemolysis

Immune haemolytic anaemias are due to red cell destruction by the immune system. The red cells become coated with antibodies, stimulating their removal by phagocytes. In all cases of immune haemolytic anaemias, the antibody-coated red cells can be detected by performing the **direct antiglobulin test** in which red cells from the patient are mixed with a reagent containing antibody against human immunoglobulins. If the patient's red cells are coated with antibodies, the reagent will induce their agglutination and they will clump together.

Immune haemolytic anaemia may be **autoimmune**, where the individual makes antibodies against their own red cells, or **alloimmune**, where the antibody forms against foreign red blood cells. Examples of alloimmune haemolytic anaemias include haemolysis due to a mismatched blood transfusion and haemolytic disease of the newborn. Autoimmune haemolytic anaemia is often idiopathic, but sometimes it is precipitated by a drug or an underlying disease such as chronic lymphocytic leukaemia, systemic lupus erythematosus (SLE), or infections such as infectious mononucleosis and *Mycoplasma pneumoniae*.

Drug-induced autoimmune haemolytic anaemia may occur through a number of possible mechanisms:

- The drug binds to the red cell membrane, forming a complex which is antigenic leading to antibodies directed predominantly against the drug but which also destroy the red cell. Penicillins and cephalosporins are the most notorious examples of this mechanism.

- Antibodies form against the drug, producing immune complexes which then subsequently attach to the red cell surface and activate complement, resulting in haemolysis. Examples include quinine, quinidine, and sulphonylureas.

- The drug directly stimulates the production of red cell autoantibodies. Examples include levodopa.

Traumatic haemolysis

Anaemia may also result if red blood cells are destroyed within the circulation due to mechanical trauma. Such damage leads to the presence of red cell fragments (schistocytes) in the blood film. Red cell fragmentation may occur across prosthetic heart valves but more frequently is the result of trauma to red cells passing through a narrowed damaged microvasculature, a situation termed **microangiopathic haemolytic anaemia** (MAHA).

A microangiopathic haemolytic anaemia is usually just one component of conditions in which severe damage to endothelial cells leads to abnormal platelet aggregation and fibrin deposition in small vessels, e.g. disseminated intravascular coagulation (DIC) and the thrombotic microangiopathies **haemolytic uraemic syndrome** (HUS) and **thrombotic thrombocytopenic purpura** (TTP). DIC is distinguished from the thrombotic microangiopathies by the results of a clotting screen, which are markedly deranged in DIC but normal in HUS and TTP.

> # Key points: Acquired haemolytic anaemias
>
> - Acquired haemolytic anaemias may be due to immune destruction or mechanical trauma.
>
> - Immune haemolytic anaemias are caused by the formation of antibodies to red cells which lead to their destruction. They may be autoimmune or alloimmune.
>
> - Autoimmune haemolytic anaemia may be idiopathic or caused by drugs or underlying diseases such as chronic lymphocytic leukaemia and systemic lupus erythematosus.
>
> - Alloimmune haemolytic anaemia may be caused by a mismatched blood transfusion or haemolytic disease of the newborn.
>
> - Mechanical haemolysis is due to physical fragmentation of red cells within the circulation. This may occur across mechanical heart valves or when red cells are squeezed through a damaged microcirculation (microangiopathic haemolytic anaemia).

> - Microangiopathic haemolytic anaemia is one component of conditions such as disseminated intravascular coagulation and the thrombotic microangiopathies.

Haemostasis

Haemostasis is the mechanism through which fibrin clots are formed at sites of vessel injury. The haemostatic system is made up of a complex series of integrated mechanisms which ensure that coagulation is limited to an appropriate time and place.

Haemostasis begins with formation of a loose platelet plug which is stabilized by a fibrin clot

The first phase of haemostasis (primary haemostasis) is aggregation of platelets at the site of vascular injury. The platelets adhere to underlying collagen via a molecule called **von Willebrand factor**. The loose platelet plug is then stabilized by a more robust fibrin-rich scaffold (clot) generated by activation of the coagulation system. The coagulation system comprises a series of plasma proteins known as **clotting factors** which take part in a cascade of activation, terminating in the generation of large amounts of **thrombin** which converts fibrinogen to fibrin (Fig. 15.7).

The coagulation system requires something to set it off, a suitable 'work surface', and something to stop it

The main stimulator of the coagulation cascade is the protein **tissue factor** which is expressed on the surface of all cells not normally exposed to the blood. As soon as vascular integrity is disrupted, blood therefore comes into contact with tissue factor on the surface of cells, and coagulation is activated.

Stimulation of the coagulation cascade is useless unless there is a suitable surface on which the various coagulation factors can assemble (remember they are all floating free in the blood normally). This is provided by platelets which have already formed at the site of injury and have been activated. Activated platelets 'flip' particular phospholipids in their cell membranes, exposing critical binding sites for clotting factors.

Activation of the cascade by tissue factor generates a small amount of thrombin, the key molecule in the coagulation cascade. Normally natural anticoagulant

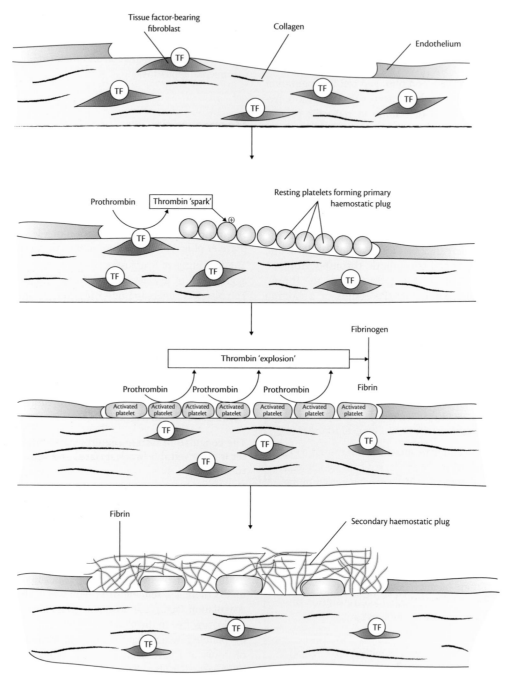

Fig. 15.7 Haemostasis. Following vascular injury, platelets bind to exposed collagen, forming the primary haemostatic plug. Simultaneously, the coagulation system is activated, leading to the deposition of fibrin on the platelets, forming the secondary haemostatic plug.

mechanisms act to destroy any thrombin rapidly. In the presence of activated platelets, this small thrombin 'spark' is just enough to ignite a powerful positive feedback loop which generates large volumes of thrombin (a thrombin 'explosion') on the surface of the platelets, which stimulates the conversion of fibrinogen to fibrin, forming a clot.

Almost as soon as the clot forms, the burst of thrombin activity is rapidly extinguished before it spreads and leads to inappropriate thrombus formation. The coagulation system is modulated by a number of natural anticoagulants found in plasma such as **antithrombin**, **protein C**, and **protein S**, all of which inactivate clotting factors.

The final stage is dissolution of the fibrin clot by the fibrinolytic system. In this system, an inactive plasma protein, **plasminogen**, is converted to active **plasmin** by plasminogen activators. Plasmin is a protease enzyme which breaks down fibrinogen and fibrin into **fibrin degradation products** (FDPs).

LINK BOX

Thrombolysis

Agents which break down fibrin clots are used in the treatment of myocardial infarctions due to occlusion of a coronary artery by thrombus, e.g. streptokinase and recombinant tissue plasminogen activator (p. 90).

Key points: Haemostasis

- Haemostasis is a complex physiological process which ensures appropriate and limited activation of the coagulation system.

- Haemostasis begins with the formation of a plug of aggregated platelets at the site of vessel injury.

- Exposure of tissue factor initiates the coagulation cascade, leading to the assembly of clotting factors on the surface of activated platelets at the site of injury and the generation of thrombin.

- A small thrombin spark then sets off an explosive amplification loop leading to the generation of large amounts of thrombin.

- Thrombin stimulates the conversion of soluble fibrinogen into insoluble fibrin, which stabilizes the loose platelet plug.

- Natural anticoagulants such as antithrombin, protein C, and protein S act to stop further thrombin production.

- The fibrin clot is then broken down by activation of the fibrinolytic system.

Bleeding disorders

Defects in haemostasis leading to bleeding may arise in a number of ways (Table 15.3). The most common cause is a deficiency of platelets (thrombocytopenia). The next most common cause is an abnormality in the clotting mechanism. Patients with low platelets tend to present with bleeding into the skin, whereas clotting defects usually present with mucosal bleeding or bleeding into deep tissues such as muscles or joints.

Thrombocytopenia

Thrombocytopenia presents with petechiae of the skin

The normal platelet count is $150–400 \times 10^9/l$. A low platelet count (thrombocytopenia) is a common cause of abnormal bleeding. Thrombocytopenia does not cause any symptoms or signs until the platelet count falls below $50 \times 10^9/l$ when petechiae appear.

Petechiae are tiny (<1 mm) impalpable red lesions found at sites of minor trauma, and represent collections of red blood cells which have extravasated from points of minor vessel injury. *Petechiae are specific*

TABLE 15.3	Bleeding disorders
Inherited disorders of clotting	
von Willebrand's disease	
Haemophilia A	
Haemophilia B	
Acquired disorders of clotting	
Thrombocytopenia	
Anticoagulant treatment	
Liver disease	
Disseminated intravascular coagulation	

for thrombocytopenia. Larger bruises (ecchymoses) may also be observed on the trunk or limbs, but these are less specific. If platelet levels fall below 20, spontaneous large bleeds may occur, causing haematemesis, melaena, or haematuria, and treatment is urgently required.

Thrombocytopenia may be due to reduced production or increased destruction of platelets

Thrombocytopenia may be caused by reduced production of platelets in the bone marrow or, more commonly, by increased destruction of circulating platelets (Table 15.4). In most of these disorders, other features are present which allow the underlying cause to be determined. For instance, marrow infiltration typically causes a pancytopenia, with anaemia and leukopenia as well as thrombocytopenia, and disseminated intravascular coagulation causes abnormalities in all clotting studies as well as thrombocytopenia. Thrombotic thrombocytopenia purpura is characterized by thrombocytopenia together with evidence of a microangiopathic haemolytic anaemia and a normal clotting screen.

The main disorders in which isolated thrombocytopenia is the main feature are idiopathic thrombocytopenic purpura, drug-related thrombocytopenia, and systemic lupus erythematosus (SLE).

TABLE 15.4 Causes of thrombocytopenia

Failure of production due to bone marrow disease
Bony metastases
Leukaemia
Lymphoma
Myeloma
Shortened life span
Idiopathic thrombocytopenic purpura*
Drugs*
Systemic lupus erythematosus*
HIV*
Sepsis
Disseminated intravascular coagulation
Thrombotic thrombocytopenic purpura

*Causes isolated thrombocytopenia.

Idiopathic thrombocytopenic purpura is due to autoimmune destruction of platelets

Idiopathic thrombocytopenic purpura (ITP) is an autoimmune disorder in which platelets become coated with antiplatelet antibodies, resulting in their destruction in the spleen. The aetiology of the disease remains obscure, and research has still to clarify why certain individuals develop antibodies to their platelets.

The clinical features merely reflect the thrombocytopenia, with cutaneous petechiae and a history of nose bleeds and bleeding from the gums. The clinical presentation of ITP differs between children and adults. ITP in children is often associated with a preceding viral infection, with the sudden onset of thrombocytopenia which typically resolves within 1–2 months. In adults, ITP occurs without an obvious precipitating event and usually persists as a chronic disease causing a mild to moderate bleeding tendency.

A diagnosis of ITP should be considered in patients who are otherwise well but present with petechiae. If a full blood count shows an isolated thrombocytopenia with a normal haemoglobin and white cell count, and physical examination is normal, then a diagnosis of ITP is highly likely. Tests for antiplatelet antibodies are not routinely available for diagnosis, and so ITP can only be diagnosed by excluding other causes of thrombocytopenia.

Drugs, SLE, and HIV are other important causes of an isolated thrombocytopenia

In adults, it is particularly important to exclude secondary causes of thrombocytopenia before making a diagnosis of ITP as some conditions may present with an isolated thrombocytopenia. Exclusion of SLE is particularly important, as this often presents with thrombocytopenia. Patients with latent HIV infection may develop an isolated thrombocytopenia long before developing other characteristic features.

Drugs are also a common cause of thrombocytopenia. If a drug binds to the platelet membrane and antibodies form to the drug–platelet complex, this leads to its destruction, and thrombocytopenia. The antibodies do not recognize platelets that have not bound the drug, so withdrawal of the offending drug leads to resolution of the thrombocytopenia. Many drugs have been associated with thrombocytopenia including penicillin, thiazides, diazepam, and heparin.

Heparin-induced thrombocytopenia predisposes to thrombosis

Heparin-induced thrombocytopenia develops between 5–8 days after starting heparin therapy, but may occur earlier if the patient has been exposed to heparin previously. Heparin binds platelet factor 4 on the surface of platelets, forming a highly antigenic complex. Individuals who develop antibodies to the complex coat their platelets in antibodies, stimulating their removal from the circulation in the spleen and the development of moderate thrombocytopenia (platelet counts typically $40–80 \times 10^9/l$).

The main problem in heparin-induced thrombocytopenia is not the low platelet count, but, paradoxically, a tendency to *thrombotic* complications such as deep venous thrombosis and pulmonary embolism because the heparin–platelet factor 4-IgG immune complexes cause platelet activation and initiation of coagulation. It is important to appreciate that heparin-induced thrombocytopenia may lead to devastating thrombotic complications in the absence of any clinical signs of thrombocytopenia (remember petechiae do not appear until platelet counts fall below $50 \times 10^9/l$).

> # Key points: Thrombocytopenia
>
> - Thrombocytopenia is a common cause of a bleeding tendency. Petechiae and ecchymoses are the typical presenting features, but these do not occur until platelet levels falls below $50 \times 10^9/l$.
>
> - Thrombocytopenia may be due to reduced production of platelets by the bone marrow or increased destruction.
>
> - Many of the diseases which cause thrombocytopenia have other useful diagnostic features. The main conditions which present with isolated thrombocytopenia are idiopathic thrombocytopenic purpura, drugs, SLE, and HIV.
>
> - ITP is an autoimmune disorder in which antiplatelet antibodies coat platelets, leading to their destruction. The typical presentation is with petechiae and bruising in an otherwise well patient. The physical examination is normal and a full blood count shows an isolated thrombocytopenia.

- In children, ITP typically follows a viral infection and resolves within 1–2 months.

- In adults, ITP has no obvious trigger and tends to persist, leading to a chronic mild bleeding disorder.

- ITP is a diagnosis of exclusion once other causes of thrombocytopenia have been excluded such as drugs, SLE, and HIV.

- Heparin-induced thrombocytopenia is an important cause of drug-induced thrombocytopenia because the platelets become activated, placing patients at risk of thrombotic complications such as deep venous thrombosis and pulmonary embolism.

Clotting disorders

Abnormalities in the coagulation cascade, which may be inherited or acquired, may lead to a bleeding tendency. The pattern of bleeding in clotting disorders differs from platelet abnormalities; petechiae are less common and instead the bleeding manifests by large bruises or haematomas following trauma or surgical procedures. Bleeding into the gastrointestinal tract, urinary tract, and into weight-bearing joints is particularly common.

Inherited clotting disorders
von Willebrand disease

von Willebrand disease is the most common inherited bleeding disorder

von Willebrand disease is an inherited bleeding disorder which leads to deficiency in the activity of von Willebrand factor. Unlike haemophilia, the defect is usually inherited in an autosomal dominant fashion, so both sexes may be affected.

The defect may be a reduction in the amount of von Willebrand factor synthesized or the amount produced may be normal but the factor itself is abnormal. There are three different types of von Willebrand disease: types 1, 2, and 3. Three-quarters of all patients with von Willebrand disease have type 1, the mildest form, in which the von Willebrand factor is normal but is produced in reduced amounts.

von Willebrand factor is required for normal platelet adhesion and acts as a carrier for factor VIII

von Willebrand factor has two functions. It acts as an adhesion molecule which allows platelets to bind to subendothelial tissues, and it acts as a carrier for factor VIII. The bleeding tendency in the disease is therefore due to a combination of failure of platelet adhesion and factor VIII deficiency.

Milder forms may not present until young adult life, but more significant disease presents earlier in childhood. As von Willebrand factor participates in the formation of the platelet plug at sites of vessel injury, patients with von Willebrand disease present with manifestations similar to reduced platelet function. Mucosal bleeding, particularly nose bleeds, and bleeding after injury or surgery are the main problems. Joint and muscle bleeds are rare.

von Willebrand disease causes a prolonged APTT and a prolonged bleeding time

Laboratory tests show a prolonged APTT (activated partial thromboplastin time) due to the reduced factor VIII activity, and a prolonged bleeding time. The bleeding time is a test in which a small superficial cut is made in the lower arm and blotting paper is touched to the cut every 30 s until the bleeding stops. The length of time it takes for the cut to stop bleeding is recorded. The bleeding time is a test of primary haemostasis and therefore assesses platelet number and function. An additional finding is that the glycopeptide **ristocetin** fails to induce platelet aggregation in platelet-rich plasma from people with von Willebrand disease, providing a useful diagnostic test.

The mainstay of treatment of von Willebrand disease is with desmopressin. Desmopressin causes the release of factor VIII and von Willebrand factor from endothelial cells, raising levels of plasma von Willebrand factor by up to 10 times.

Haemophilia

Haemophilia A and haemophilia B are clinically identical

Haemophilia describes an inherited bleeding tendency due to deficiency of either factor VIII (haemophilia A) or factor IX (haemophilia B). Because factor VIII and IX together form the factor VIII–factor IX complex which activates factor X, haemophilia A and B are clinically indistinguishable.

The factor VIII and factor IX genes are both located on the X chromosome, so haemophilia demonstrates a sex-linked inheritance pattern. Women are therefore rarely affected as the unaffected X chromosome can produce enough of the factor. Numerous mutations have been described in the factor VIII and IX genes, leading to a wide variation in the severity of haemophilia.

Haemophilia patients have a tendency towards easy bruising and massive bleeding after trauma or operative procedures. Spontaneous haemorrhages frequently occur in large weight-bearing joints (haemarthrosis). The main weight-bearing joints (knees, elbows, and ankles) are the most affected joints. It is not clear why bleeding in haemophilia shows a predilection for joints. Blood is highly irritant to synovium, and haemarthrosis causes synovial hypertrophy which has a tendency to rebleed, setting up a vicious circle.

Both disorders cause a prolonged APTT with a normal prothrombin time (PT) and a normal platelet count. Haemophilia A and B can only be discriminated by performing assays measuring the levels of each factor.

Replacement of the missing factor is the key to therapy of haemophilia. Because of the short half-lives of factors VIII and IX, freeze-dried factor concentrates are used. Because these are pooled from the blood of a large number of different donors, the risk of transmission of blood-borne viruses is increased. Infectivity risk has been reduced by improved donor selection and viral inactivation of the concentrates, but there remains a small risk. More recently there have been concerns about possible transmission of variant Creutzfeldt–Jakob disease by blood products. Although the real risk is unknown, the anxiety has fuelled the move towards the use of recombinant factors VIII and IX for the treatment of haemophilia. Since March 2006, all patients with haemophilia in the UK are now offered the option of synthetic factors rather than plasma-derived concentrates.

INTERESTING TO KNOW

Viral inactivation of factor concentrates

All of the significant blood-borne viruses such as HIV, hepatitis B, and hepatitis C are lipid-enveloped viruses which are extremely susceptible to membrane disruption by solvents and detergents.

Incubating plasma for 4 h with organic solvents and detergents inactivates the vast majority of the infectious units of these viruses without causing any functional change in plasma proteins such as clotting factors.

Since the introduction of viral inactivation of factor concentrates in 1985, there has not been a single report of transmission of HIV, hepatitis B, or hepatitis C to a haemophiliac from factor concentrate.

Acquired clotting disorders

Anticoagulant drugs are important causes of a bleeding tendency

Excess anticoagulant drug therapy is a common cause of a bleeding tendency, the main offender being warfarin. Warfarin is a vitamin K antagonist which acts as an anticoagulant by inhibiting the production of several clotting factors which are dependent on vitamin K for their activation. Nearly 500 000 people take warfarin in the UK, many of whom are elderly people with atrial fibrillation. It is very important to ensure that patients on warfarin are able to adhere to monitoring of their anticoagulation and are able to take the prescribed dosage correctly. Poor prescribing or compliance, intercurrent illness, or an interacting drug may significantly increase the anticoagulant effect with a risk of serious bleeding.

Severe liver failure is associated with a bleeding coagulopathy

The liver is vital to normal haemostasis as it produces most of the clotting factors of the coagulation cascade. Liver failure can therefore result in a severe coagulopathy, and indeed the PT (expressed as the international normalization ratio (INR)) is used as one of the criteria for assessing the severity of liver failure. Note that patients with *chronic* liver failure may also have thrombocytopenia due to pooling of platelets in an enlarged spleen caused by portal hypertension.

Acute DIC is a life-threatening coagulopathy associated with a severe bleeding tendency

Acute DIC is an explosive, life-threatening haemorrhagic tendency. DIC is not a disease in itself, but rather a severe complication of an underlying disorder that causes widespread damage to endothelial cells. Systemic activation of the coagulation cascade leads to rapid depletion of clotting factors and platelets, and a bleeding tendency.

A number of disorders may lead to acute DIC, the most common being severe sepsis (particularly with Gram negative bacteria and the meningococcus) and obstetric emergencies such as placental abruption and amniotic fluid embolism. Mismatched blood transfusions can also cause acute DIC.

Laboratory investigations in acute DIC reveal a very low platelet count, prolongation of the APTT, PT, and thrombin time (TT), together with a reduced fibrinogen level and increased levels of fibrin degradation products. The management of acute DIC is treatment of the underlying disorder and supportive haematological treatment by replacing clotting factors with fresh frozen plasma (FFP) and cryoprecipitate, and giving platelet transfusions.

Key points: Clotting disorders

- Disorders of clotting leading to a bleeding tendency may be inherited or acquired. They usually present with bruising and haematomas following surgical procedures or bleeding into deep tissues such as muscles and joints.

- The most common inherited clotting disorders are von Willebrand disease, haemophilia A, and haemophilia B.

- von Willebrand disease is due to reduced amounts of normal von Willebrand factor or production of a functionally abnormal von Willebrand factor. Because von Willebrand factor is important in platelet adhesion and as a carrier for factor VIII, it leads to a defect in primary haemostasis (prolonged bleeding time) and a defect in the coagulation cascade (prolonged APTT).

- There are three types of von Willebrand disease. Type 1 accounts for 75 per cent of all cases and is due to reduced production of normal von Willebrand factor. There is a mild bleeding tendency, and treatment with desmopressin is effective.

Continued

Key points: Clotting disorders— cont'd

- Haemophilia refers to an inherited bleeding tendency due to a deficiency in factor VIII (haemophilia A) or factor IX (haemophilia B). There is prolongation of the APTT and PT. Treatment requires replacement of the deficient clotting factor, either with factor concentrates from pooled donated blood or with synthetic recombinant factors.

- Acquired clotting disorders may be iatrogenic due to excess dosing with anticoagulant drugs such as warfarin, severe liver disease, and DIC.

Thrombotic disorders

Thrombosis (pathological clot formation) may occur anywhere in the circulatory system. *Arterial* thrombosis is almost always seen as a complication of an advanced atherosclerotic plaque and is discussed more fully in Chapter 6. *Venous* thrombosis, however, is usually the result of an increased tendency of the blood to clot and is therefore a primary haematological disorder.

Most venous thrombotic episodes occur in the deep veins of the leg. Deep vein thrombosis is common and important because of the risk of fatal pulmonary embolism. Deep venous thrombosis usually results from the interaction of multiple risk factors which may be inherited or acquired (Table 15.5).

INTERESTING TO KNOW

Thrombotic microangiopathies

Some thrombotic disorders are characterized by thrombi in small vessels, most notably in arterioles. Such disorders are known as **thrombotic microangiopathies** and are characterized by a combination of microangiopathic haemolytic anaemia, thrombocytopenia, and symptoms related to occlusion of arterioles by tiny platelet microthrombi.

The main thrombotic microangiopathy is **thrombotic thrombocytopenic purpura** (TTP) which is an idiopathic disease of adults dominated by neurological symptoms in addition to the anaemia and thrombocytopenia.

Haemolytic uraemic syndrome (HUS) is a related condition which is seen more often in children and is dominated by renal involvement. The pathogenesis of HUS is related to verocytotoxin-producing *Escherichia coli* acquired from eating undercooked meat.

Thrombophilia

There is no single universally accepted definition of thrombophilia, but the most useful definition is *an inherited predisposition to venous thrombosis*. A number of thrombophilias are recognized (Table 15.6).

Patients with thrombophilia typically present with thrombosis of the deep leg veins or pulmonary thromboembolism. Sometimes there may be venous thrombosis at an unusual site such as the axillary vein or the cerebral veins. Usually a second risk factor is present which tips the balance in favour of thrombosis, e.g. pregnancy, oral contraceptive pill use, a long period of immobility, or surgery.

Activated protein C resistance is the most common cause of thrombophilia

A point mutation in the factor V gene leads to the production of a factor V protein that has normal procoagulant activity but is not inhibited in the normal way by activated protein C. Activated factor V therefore persists, resulting in a tendency to thrombosis. This variant is called factor V Leiden and is present in as many as 5 per cent of people.

TABLE 15.5 Important risk factors for venous thromboembolism

Immobility
Dehydration
Pregnancy
Oestrogen therapy, e.g. oral contraceptives, hormone replacement therapy
Malignancy
Antiphospholipid syndrome
Surgery, particularly to abdomen, pelvis, or lower limb

TABLE 15.6 Inherited thrombophilias

Factor V Leiden	5–10%
Prothrombin G20210A	1–5%
Protein C deficiency	0.2%
Protein S deficiency	0.2%
Antithrombin deficiency	0.02%

The prothrombin G20210A mutation is the second most common cause of thrombophilia

The prothrombin G20210A mutation refers to a single nucleotide change of guanine for adenine at position 20 210 of the prothrombin gene. This has been shown to be associated with elevated prothrombin levels and an increased risk of venous thrombosis. How the mutation leads to raised thrombin levels and why the elevated prothrombin levels stimulate venous thrombosis is unclear. Higher concentrations of prothrombin may lead to increased rates of thrombin generation, excessive growth of fibrin clots, and possibly increased activation of platelets.

Mutations in the natural anticoagulants are rarer causes of thrombophilia

Inherited mutations in natural anticoagulant molecules such as antithrombin, protein C, and protein S have also been shown to predispose to venous thrombosis, although they are less common than the factor V Leiden and prothrombin G20210A mutations. There are almost certainly many other thrombophilic defects which have not yet been identified, as detailed tests often fail to detect an abnormality in patients who are clearly thrombophilic.

INTERESTING TO KNOW

Testing for thrombophilia

Increasing knowledge about the genetic alterations in thrombophilia has led to suggestions for routinely testing people with venous thrombosis for thrombophilia. At present, it is not recommended routinely as there is currently no clear long-term management plan for patients with thrombophilia. Although they predict first episodes of venous

---

thrombosis, the more common defects (factor V Leiden and prothrombin G20210A) do not appear to increase the risk of further episodes of venous thrombosis significantly enough to justify the risks associated with lifelong warfarin treatment.

Key points: Thrombophilia

♦ Thrombophilia refers to an inherited predisposition to venous thrombosis.

♦ Most patients present with deep vein thrombosis or pulmonary embolism at a young age, often when a further risk factor comes into play such as pregnancy or the oral contraceptive pill.

♦ The two most common genetic defects are the factor V Leiden and the prothrombin G20210A mutations.

♦ Inherited deficiencies of protein C, protein S, and antithrombin also occur, but these are rarer.

Acquired venous thrombosis

Malignancy is a major risk factor for venous thrombosis

Venous thrombosis is a major cause of mortality in patients with a malignancy. The risk of thrombosis varies with the type of cancer, being most common in colonic, lung, pancreatic, and breast carcinomas. The increased risk is due to the presence of molecules on the surface of malignant cells that activate coagulation ('tumour procoagulants'). Other important factors in cancer patients may include immobility and dehydration.

LINK BOX

Malignancy and thrombosis

As well as causing deep vein thrombosis and pulmonary embolism, malignancies may also cause thrombosis on the surface of heart valves—a condition known as non-bacterial thrombotic endocarditis (p. 98).

Immobility leads to venous stasis in the deep veins

Immobility is a risk factor for venous thrombosis as stasis of blood in veins allows the accumulation of clotting factors and platelets against the vessel wall. Immobility is almost certainly a significant factor in venous thrombosis in the elderly and in postoperative patients.

INTERESTING TO KNOW

Economy class syndrome

There has been much interest in the relationship between venous thrombosis and long-haul flights, a condition called 'economy class syndrome' because seating and leg room are particularly cramped for passengers in economy class. However, first class and business class passengers also get venous thrombosis, so other factors such as low cabin pressure, mild hypoxia, low humidity, and dehydration all probably contribute as these factors are constant throughout the aircraft.

The incidence of death from pulmonary embolism related to air travel is less than one in 1 million journeys. The duration of the flight is a factor, the risk increasing with flights longer than 4-5 h. Current thinking is that there is a low but increased risk of venous thrombosis with long-haul flights, and simple precautionary measures such as keeping well hydrated and performing calf exercises to maintain venous flow in the legs are recommended.

Surgical procedures stimulate a prothrombotic state

Postoperative patients are at risk of venous thrombosis independently of the effect of the immobility. Tissue trauma causes a procoagulant response, with increased concentrations of fibrinogen and a reactive increase in platelet numbers. The highest risk operations are orthopaedic procedures to the lower limb such as hip replacements and knee replacements. It is of utmost importance to use prophylactic anticoagulant treatment in surgical patients and be vigilant to the danger of venous thrombosis in postoperative patients.

Antiphospholipid syndrome is associated with arterial and venous thrombosis and recurrent miscarriage

Antiphospholipid syndrome is an important and common thrombotic disorder caused by circulating antiphospholipid antibodies. Precisely how antiphospholipid antibodies lead to thrombosis is not fully understood, but the simplest theory is that the antibodies bind to phospholipids on platelets and endothelial cells, causing platelet aggregation and thrombosis. This would also account for the thrombocytopenia often seen in these patients.

Antiphospholipid syndrome is seen mostly in young to middle-aged females. The principal manifestations are deep vein thrombosis and pulmonary embolism. Arterial thromboses may also occur and can cause ischaemic strokes. Recurrent miscarriage is also a feature due to placental thrombosis. A 'full house' presentation with arterial and venous thromboses and recurrent miscarriage is not often seen; women may have recurrent thrombotic episodes without fetal loss, whilst others may suffer from recurrent miscarriages without thrombotic manifestations.

Key points: Acquired venous thrombosis

- A number of factors may lead to an increased coagulability of the blood and predispose to venous thrombosis.

- Deep leg vein thrombosis is the most common site of venous thrombosis and is important because of the risk of fatal pulmonary thromboembolism.

- Malignancy is a major risk factor for venous thrombosis and is caused by prothrombotic molecules on the surface of the malignant cells.

- Immobility causes stasis of blood in the deep leg veins, allowing accumulation of clotting factors and platelets.

- Postoperative patients are at increased risk of venous thrombosis due to the procoagulant response to tissue trauma.

Key points: Acquired venous thrombosis—cont'd

♦ The antiphospholipid syndrome is a common thrombotic disorder characterized by episodes of arterial and venous thrombosis, recurrent fetal loss, and the presence of circulating antiphospholipid antibodies.

Haematological malignancies

The haematological malignancies are one of the most difficult areas of medicine to understand, probably second only to the glomerulopathies. The reason for this is the large number of different neoplasms and problems with changing terminology. It is important therefore first to stand back and explain some general concepts about haematological malignancies before launching into the finer details of the individual diseases further on in the chapter.

Many haematological malignancies result from a mutated haemopoietic stem cell in the bone marrow

A large number of haematological malignancies come about for the same basic underlying reason: a haemopoietic stem cell in the bone marrow acquires genetic mutations which disrupt the normal differentiation and maturation of its progeny. The specific disease that results depends on how the mutations affect the differentiation pathway of the daughter cells of the malignant stem cell.

If there is little or no differentiation, then immature undifferentiated blood cells ('blasts') accumulate in the bone marrow. Undifferentiated cells have a huge proliferative capacity and they rapidly overwhelm the normal haemopoietic cells, leading to the sudden onset of bone marrow failure. The malignant cells also spill into the blood, causing the white blood count to rise. The resulting disease is an **acute leukaemia**.

If differentiation does occur, the resulting diseases tend to be more indolent than the acute leukaemias (the more differentiated a cell becomes, the less proliferative capacity it has). The type of disease that results depends on whether the malignant cells differentiate down the lymphoid route or the myeloid route. If cells differentiate down the lymphoid lineage, then the marrow becomes filled with small, mature cells which resemble naïve resting lymphocytes. These cells also spill into the blood, and the resulting disease is called **chronic lymphocytic leukaemia**, which is a common indolent disease of elderly people.

If differentiation occurs down the myeloid line, there are two broad outcomes depending on whether the differentiation is normal or disordered. If differentiation is effective, then large numbers of normal myeloid cells are produced. Depending on which specific cell type is produced, there may be large numbers of neutrophils, red blood cells, or platelets. Together these diseases are called the **myeloproliferative disorders** and they typically present with high blood counts and enlargement of the liver and spleen.

If the differentiation is ineffective, then the developing myeloid cells are destroyed prematurely in the bone marrow. They never get out into the peripheral blood, so these diseases present with problems related to low blood counts. The red blood cells are preferentially affected first, so persistent anaemia is a common feature of these disorders, which are called **myelodysplastic syndromes**.

An important feature of the myeloproliferative disorders and the myelodysplastic syndromes is their tendency over time to get worse progressively. As mutations accumulate in the transformed progenitor stem cell, the degree of differentiation that the malignant cells undergo as they develop becomes less. Undifferentiated cells begin to accumulate in the bone marrow until eventually the patient develops an acute leukaemia, which may be of either myeloid or lymphoid type, and is usually poorly responsive to treatment and rapidly fatal.

The lymphomas are malignancies derived from lymphocytes that have left the bone marrow

The lymphomas are a large group of haematological malignancies which are different from the other haematological neoplasms. In contrast to the malignancies we have just discussed which arise from a transformed progenitor cell in the bone marrow, the malignant cells giving rise to lymphomas originate from lymphocytes that have left the bone marrow and taken up residence in lymph nodes or other organs. Lymphomas therefore tend to present with solid mass lesions, particularly enlargement of lymph nodes, rather than an abnormal blood count.

The vast majority of lymphomas are derived from B lymphocytes. The reason why mature B lymphocytes are particularly prone to undergoing malignant change is related to the further round of genetic instability they undergo when they rearrange their immunoglobulin genes in response to antigen stimulation. During the process of somatic hypermutation, they are at risk of acquiring mutations in growth-controlling genes which can give rise to malignant behaviour.

Lymphomas are divided into two broad groups, **non-Hodgkin lymphomas** and **Hodgkin lymphomas**, which differ in their clinical features, behaviour, and histological appearance.

Multiple myeloma is a malignant disorder of plasma cells

Plasma cells are terminally differentiated B cells that have encountered antigen and fully matured into immunoglobulin-secreting cells. Many plasma cells home back to the bone marrow where they secrete their antibodies. The most common type of plasma cell malignancy is **multiple myeloma**, which is characterized by bony lesions due to destructive growth in the bone marrow together with problems related to the large quantities of immunoglobulin the malignant plasma cells produce.

Examination of the bone marrow is central to the diagnosis of many haematological malignancies

Morphological examination of the bone marrow is vital to the diagnosis of many haematological malignancies. There are two main elements to a bone marrow examination: the bone marrow **aspirate** and the bone marrow **trephine**.

In a bone marrow aspirate, a small needle is used to aspirate 0.5 ml of marrow which is dropped on to a glass slide and spread. The aspirate is then stained and examined under a light microscope. Each cell type is counted and their morphological form is assessed.

The bone marrow trephine is taken after the aspirate has been performed. A larger hollow needle is pushed into the bone and a whole core of bone is removed, put into formalin, and sent to histopathology. The bone marrow trephine has to be decalcified in acid over several days before thin sections can be cut and stained with haematoxylin and eosin.

In most hospitals, the bone marrow aspirate is examined by a haematologist, whereas the bone marrow trephine is examined by a histopathologist. Good communication between the two specialties is therefore important as the two examinations are complementary—the trephine allows the overall architecture of the bone marrow to be examined, whereas the aspirate shows better individual cell detail.

Flow cytometry and cytogenetics are also important tests on bone marrow samples

At the time of bone marrow aspirate in suspected haematological malignancy, a further 5 ml of marrow may be aspirated and put into tissue culture medium for **cytogenetics**, and another 5 ml into an EDTA tube for **flow cytometry immunophenotyping**.

Flow cytometry immunophenotyping is a test which allows blood cells of different lineages and stages of maturation to be identified according to the cluster differentiation (CD) molecules they express on their surface. Antibodies to specific CD molecules that have been labelled with fluorescent markers that can be detected by a flow cytometer are added to the cell population being studied, enabling the number of cells with a given CD molecule to be counted. For example, the combination of CD13, CD33, and CD34 identifies a myeloid blast. If flow cytometry of a bone marrow aspirate shows 90 per cent myeloid blasts, the diagnosis is acute myeloid leukaemia.

Chromosomal abnormalities are common in haematological malignancies, and determination of the **karyotype** of the neoplastic cells may be helpful in the diagnosis of a haematological malignancy, and determining its prognosis. The marrow sample is incubated and cultured, and the chromosomes within the malignant cells are examined for deletions, breaks, and translocations. For example, identification of the Philadelphia chromosome t(9;22) is a helpful diagnostic feature in chronic myeloid leukaemia.

Acute leukaemias

Acute leukaemias are characterized by the presence of large numbers of undifferentiated blood cells ('blasts') in the bone marrow. The immature cells, which do not perform any useful function, rapidly overwhelm the normal developing blood cells in the marrow and spill out into the peripheral blood.

Acute leukaemias therefore present due to a sudden inability to produce any normal blood cells (bone marrow failure). Acute leukaemias are highly aggressive diseases which are rapidly fatal without urgent treatment. We really know very little about why particular individuals are suddenly struck down with this devastating condition.

Acute leukaemia presents abruptly due to severe lack of normal blood cells

Patients with acute leukaemia become suddenly very unwell with symptoms due to a severe lack of normal blood cells:

- Extreme fatigue and lethargy, due to the lack of red blood cells.
- Infections due to the lack of mature neutrophils.
- Petechiae and bleeding due to low platelet levels.

The expansion of the bone marrow space by the leukaemic cells often causes bone pain, particularly in children.

Acute leukaemia is divided into acute lymphoblastic leukaemia and acute myeloid leukaemia

Acute lymphoblastic leukaemia (ALL) is the familiar childhood leukaemia with a peak age of 4 years. In addition to symptoms related to bone marrow failure, infiltration of other organs by circulating blasts is common in ALL. There may be lymphadenopathy, hepatomegaly, and splenomegaly. Testicular involvement is common in male patients. The central nervous system may also be involved with symptoms such as headache, vomiting, and cranial nerve palsies.

Acute myeloid leukaemia (AML) may occur at any age, but is usually seen in adults. In older people, it is more likely to develop as a complication of previous chemotherapy for a different malignancy, or as a terminal phase of an existing chronic haematological malignancy such as a myelodysplastic syndrome. The clinical picture is related to the bone marrow failure. Infiltration of organs by circulating blasts is less common in AML than in ALL, although some variants of AML show a peculiar tendency to infiltrate the gums and skin.

A diagnosis of acute leukaemia requires the presence of more than 20 per cent blasts in blood or bone marrow

The diagnosis of acute leukaemia is made by examination of a peripheral blood film and a bone marrow aspirate. A differential count is made of 200 nucleated cells in the peripheral blood and 500 cells in the bone marrow film. A diagnosis of acute leukaemia requires the presence of more than 20 per cent blasts in the peripheral blood or bone marrow. Usually there is well in excess of 50 per cent.

Immunophenotyping by flow cytometry allows typing of the acute leukaemia

Sometimes the morphology of the blasts on the blood film or the marrow aspirate is characteristic enough to allow a diagnosis of AML or ALL to be made. However, immunophenotyping using flow cytometry is usually performed to confirm the presence of myeloid or lymphoid lineage-specific antigens on the blasts. Flow cytometry is also able to distinguish a B lymphoblastic leukaemia from a T lymphoblastic leukaemia.

Marrow samples should also be sent for cytogenetic analysis, as knowledge of the karyotype of the malignant cells is essential for determining prognosis and for choosing the best treatment.

Management of leukaemia requires treatment to stabilize the patient, followed by chemotherapy

Patients with acute leukaemia require urgent investigation and treatment. Initially they require aggressive supportive treatment with replacement of blood elements whilst the precise subtype of acute leukaemia is worked out. Once a specific diagnosis has been made, appropriate chemotherapy regimes may be started. ALL has an excellent prognosis in children, with the majority being cured of the disease. Cure rates in AML are lower than in ALL, around 35 per cent, and is harder to achieve with increasing age. Cure is rarely achievable in patients aged over 65 with AML.

> ## Key points: Acute leukaemias
>
> - Acute leukaemias arise due to the accumulation of immature undifferentiated blasts in the bone marrow and peripheral blood.
>
> - The malignant blasts rapidly overwhelm the normal haemopoietic cells of the bone marrow, leading to the abrupt onset of bone marrow failure.
>
> - Patients present with features of profound anaemia, neutropenia, and thrombocytopenia.

Continued

Key points: Acute leukaemias— cont'd

- ◆ A patient suspected of having acute leukaemia requires examination of a blood film and a bone marrow aspirate. More than 20 per cent blasts are needed to diagnose acute leukaemia.

- ◆ The morphology of the cells and their immunophenotype allows the distinction between acute myeloid leukaemia and acute lymphoblastic leukaemia.

- ◆ Cytogenetic analysis of the blasts is essential to look for karyotypic abnormalities which may help further define the precise type of leukaemia and provide prognostic information.

- ◆ Acute lymphoblastic leukaemia is typically seen in children aged 2–4 years. Symptoms are related to bone marrow failure. Infiltration of lymph nodes, liver, and spleen may cause lymphadenopathy and hepatosplenomegaly. CNS involvement is common and may cause cranial nerve palsies. The prognosis of ALL is excellent in children, with the vast majority achieving complete cure.

- ◆ Acute myeloid leukaemia is rare in children, with the incidence increasing with age. Older patients with AML are more likely to have secondary AML from previous chemotherapy or as a terminal complication of a pre-existing chronic haematological malignancy. Cure rates in AML are much lower than for ALL.

Chronic lymphocytic leukaemia

Chronic lymphocytic leukaemia is the most common leukaemia in adults

Chronic lymphocytic leukaemia (CLL) is a neoplastic disorder in which small mature B lymphocytes accumulate in the bone marrow and peripheral blood. CLL is a disease of older adults with a peak incidence between 60 and 80 years. Men are affected twice as often as women. The aetiology is unknown.

CLL is a slowly progressive disease with a predictable natural history

In most cases, CLL is a slowly progressive indolent disease which follows a typical natural course. Initially the bone marrow becomes filled with neoplastic cells which are released into the peripheral blood. Most patients are diagnosed at this early stage when an incidental full blood count reveals a high white cell count.

With progression, the neoplastic cells fill lymph nodes, causing lymphadenopathy. The liver and spleen are then involved, causing hepatosplenomegaly. Finally the bone marrow is completely overwhelmed and there is bone marrow failure with the onset of anaemia and thrombocytopenia.

A small minority of patients with CLL (<10 per cent) develop a high grade non-Hodgkin B cell lymphoma which occurs abruptly, is refractory to treatment, and has a poor prognosis (average survival just 4 months). Such transformation is known as **Richter's syndrome.**

Immune disorders are common in CLL

The neoplastic lymphocytes in CLL are functionally useless to the immune system, and impair the function of the normal B lymphocyte population. There are low levels of circulating immunoglobulins (hypogammaglobulinaemia) which predisposes patients to infections, particularly of the lower respiratory tract. Autoimmune phenomena are also common, such as autoimmune haemolytic anaemia and autoimmune thrombocytopenia. The autoantibodies are not thought to be produced by the neoplastic B cells.

Many patients with CLL are diagnosed on the chance finding of a raised white cell count

About half of all patients with CLL are diagnosed when a full blood count reveals a high white cell count due to a lymphocytosis. The remainder of patients present with the discovery of painless lymphadenopathy, or as a result of an autoimmune phenomenon, e.g. symptoms related to an autoimmune haemolytic anaemia or petechiae due to autoimmune thrombocytopenia.

A peripheral blood film reveals an excess of mature lymphocytes. A highly characteristic feature on the blood film is the presence of so-called 'smear cells' which occur when the neoplastic B cells are smudged during the preparation of the blood film (Fig. 15.8). In the absence of smear cells, an alternative diagnosis should be strongly considered. Immunophenotyping is

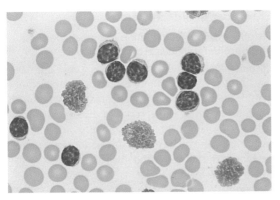

Fig. 15.8 Peripheral blood film from a patient with chronic lymphocytic leukaemia showing small neoplastic lymphocytes, some of which have formed smear cells.

essential to characterize the neoplastic cells, and the typical picture is a CD5, CD19, CD23 positive population.

A watch and wait policy is appropriate for many patients with CLL

CLL is an incurable disorder, but many patients follow an indolent course and die from an unrelated cause. Many do not require any treatment at all for many years, and a watch and wait policy is the recommended course of action for patients with early stage disease. Patients with more advanced disease may benefit from oral chemotherapy with agents such as chlorambucil.

INTERESTING TO KNOW

ZAP-70 and CLL

It has been observed that if the immunoglobulin gene of the neoplastic B cells in CLL has undergone somatic hypermutation the prognosis of the disease is much better than if it has not. This information may be useful in deciding who to treat early in the disease and who to monitor.

Reliably differentiating between 'mutated' and 'non-mutated' CLL currently requires gene sequencing of the heavy chain gene of the neoplastic B cells and comparing it with the germ line heavy chain gene. To perform this as a routine test for all patients is not feasible, so it would be useful to find other genes that are differentially expressed in mutated and unmutated CLL that are easy to test for. One such molecule is zeta-associated protein 70 (ZAP-70), an intracellular signalling molecule normally expressed in T cells but only very rarely in B cells. Several studies have shown that ZAP-70 is a potential surrogate marker for mutational status and prognosis, although the analysis of ZAP-70 is not straightforward.

Key points: Chronic lymphocytic leukaemia

- CLL is a haematological malignancy in which small mature neoplastic B lymphocytes accumulate in the bone marrow, blood, and lymphoid organs.

- CLL is a disease of older adults with a peak incidence between 60 and 80 years.

- CLL follows a predictable course. It starts with an isolated lymphocytosis, progresses through lymphadenopathy and hepatosplenomegaly, and finally terminates in bone marrow failure.

- Immune disorders are commonly seen in CLL, and include hypogammaglobulinaemia, autoimmune haemolytic anaemia, and autoimmune thrombocytopenia.

- Most patients with CLL are diagnosed with early stage disease following the chance finding of a raised white cell count. A watch and wait policy is often entirely appropriate, and many patients die of unrelated causes.

- Patients with more advanced disease may benefit from oral chemotherapy with agents such as chlorambucil.

Myeloproliferative disorders

The **myeloproliferative disorders** are a group of neoplastic disorders of haematopoiesis characterized by the overproduction of myeloid cells, occurring mostly in the elderly. The underlying cause is the acquisition of a genetic abnormality in a haematopoietic stem cell that bestows a proliferation advantage to one or more of the myeloid lineages.

Crucially, the excess proliferation is associated with *effective* maturation, resulting in increased numbers of normal neutrophils, red blood cells, and platelets in the peripheral blood. The genetic abnormality that initiates the myeloproliferative process may bestow a proliferative advantage to only one myeloid lineage or to all of them, but usually one is dominant and is used to name the disease:

♦ Chronic myeloid leukaemia when neutrophils dominate.

♦ Polycythaemia vera when red blood cells dominate.

♦ Essential thrombocythaemia when platelets dominate.

Definitive diagnosis of a myeloproliferative disorder may be difficult

One of the main difficulties in establishing a diagnosis of a myeloproliferative disorder is conclusively proving that the blood cell overproduction is a result of a neoplastic process and not a normal reactive response to some other stimulus. With the exception of chronic myeloid leukaemia, where a characteristic genetic translocation is usually present, such proof can be difficult to find. This explains why the diagnosis of a myeloproliferative disorder is usually based on a number of clinical criteria which aim to exclude reactive causes for the overproliferation.

Myeloproliferative diseases often terminate in bone marrow failure

Myeloproliferative disorders are often diagnosed when the patient feels quite well, due to the finding of a raised myeloid count on a full blood count. Hepatomegaly and splenomegaly are often present because the sinusoids of these vascular organs are distended by the excess cells.

Despite an often insidious clinical onset, all of the myeloproliferative diseases have potential to undergo evolution with a stepwise progression towards eventual bone marrow failure either due to fibrosis of the marrow or due to transformation into an acute leukaemia.

Chronic myeloid leukaemia

Chronic myeloid leukaemia is the most common myeloproliferative disease

Chronic myeloid leukaemia (CML) is a myeloproliferative disorder in which there is increased production of mature neutrophils. Many patients are asymptomatic when an elevated white count is discovered incidentally. The remainder present with symptoms of fatigue, weight loss, and night sweats. The patient may notice a swelling in the left upper abdomen due to splenomegaly, which can be massive.

Examination of the peripheral blood film shows the full spectrum of neutrophil precursors in significant numbers (Fig. 15.9). There is very often also an associated basophilia.

CML is associated with the Philadelphia chromosome

Of all the myeloproliferative disorders, CML is the easiest to diagnose. This is because in 95 per cent of cases there is a specific chromosomal translocation t(9;22) known as the Philadelphia chromosome which is present in all the leukaemic cells in CML. The translocation generates an abnormal fusion gene, **BCR–ABL**, which produces a protein with continuously active tyrosine kinase growth signalling properties. In patients suspected of having CML on the basis of the peripheral blood findings, the Philadelphia chromosome can usually be seen on karyotyping of the malignant cells.

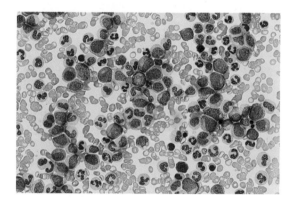

Fig. 15.9 Peripheral blood film from a patient with chronic myeloid leukaemia showing large numbers of neutrophils and neutrophil precursors.

CML begins in a chronic phase and progresses through an accelerated phase into a blast crisis

CML runs a predictable triphasic natural course. The first 'chronic' phase lasts for about 5 years (with treatment), during which the white cell count is controlled and the patient feels well. Eventually, the disease spontaneously transforms through an 'accelerated' phase, during which the blood count becomes difficult to control, into a 'blast' phase in which an acute leukaemia develops which is refractory to treatment.

Imatinib is a new tyrosine kinase inhibitor used in the treatment of CML

Most patients with CML are started on treatment soon after the diagnosis is made. The best agent for patients in chronic phase is imatinib, which works by binding to the Abl component of the aberrant Bcr–Abl oncoprotein and holding it in an inactive state.

Treatment with imatinib leads to a rapid reduction in splenic size and restoration of a normal white cell count. Provided the patient responds to imatinib, the drug should be continued indefinitely. The short-term results with imatinib are generally excellent, though the extent to which it prolongs life in the long term is not entirely clear because it is a new drug.

Polycythaemia vera

Polycythaemia vera results in increased red blood cell production

Polycythaemia is a haematological abnormality defined by a raised red cell mass, which has many causes. **Polycythaemia vera** is a myeloproliferative disorder dominated by increased red blood cell production. Excess proliferation of the other myeloid lineages is usually seen as well, leading to raised neutrophil and platelet counts. The cause is unknown.

The key to diagnosing polycythaemia vera is excluding a secondary erythrocytosis

A raised red cell mass may also occur as an appropriate response to a number of causes, the most common being persistent hypoxia and renal lesions producing erythropoietin (Table 15.7). Excluding a secondary cause is the main diagnostic challenge in polycythaemia vera. In the absence of a cause of secondary erythrocytosis, the presence of splenomegaly and raised neutrophil and platelet counts in addition to the

TABLE 15.7 Causes of secondary erythrocytosis
Chronic hypoxia
Chronic lung disease
Abnormal erythropoietin secretion
Renal cell carcinoma
Polycystic kidney disease

raised red cell mass is highly suggestive of polycythaemia vera.

Thrombosis is a serious risk in polycythaemia vera

Patients with polycythaemia vera have a dramatically increased risk of thrombosis, which may be arterial or venous. In some patients, the first manifestation of the disease is deep vein thrombosis or myocardial infarction. Thromboses in unusual locations such as the portal vein or mesenteric vein should always raise the suspicion of polycythaemia vera. Headache, dizziness, and visual disturbances are also major complaints.

The thrombotic risk is due to the raised red cell mass which increases blood viscosity; sluggish blood flow leads to increased interaction between platelets and endothelial cells. The raised platelet count often seen in polycythaemia vera is also contributory.

With treatment, patients with polycythaemia vera often survive for over 10 years. Most patients die from thrombosis or haemorrhage; some will succumb to bone marrow failure due to bone marrow fibrosis. Transformation into an acute leukaemia is rare in polycythaemia vera.

Essential thrombocythaemia

Essential thrombocythaemia leads to increased production of platelets

Essential thrombocythaemia is a myeloproliferative disorder characterized by increased proliferation largely confined to the megakaryocytic elements with the production of excess platelets.

The central feature of essential thrombocythaemia is persistent elevation of the platelet count to above $600 \times 10^9/l$. About a quarter of patients are asymptomatic when diagnosed. Most symptomatic patients present with symptoms relating to thrombotic episodes which may occur in arteries or veins of all sizes.

Essential thrombocythaemia is the hardest myeloproliferative disorder to diagnose, as all the myeloproliferative disorders can be associated with elevated platelet counts. To diagnose essential thrombocythaemia, any features typical of the other myeloproliferative disorders must be absent. It must also be distinguished from one of the many reactive causes of a raised platelet count, particularly infection or inflammation.

Essential thrombocythaemia is often an indolent condition with a median survival of 12–15 years. As it normally occurs in later life, life expectancy is therefore often normal. Transition to an acute leukaemia or development of bone marrow fibrosis occurs less frequently than in other myeloproliferative disorders.

Chronic idiopathic myelofibrosis

Chronic idiopathic myelofibrosis leads to bone marrow fibrosis

Idiopathic myelofibrosis is a myeloproliferative disorder with an incidence of only about 5 cases per 1 million people per year. There is overproliferation of megakaryocytes in the bone marrow which release fibroblast-stimulating factors such as platelet-derived growth factor, resulting in a reactive proliferation of marrow stromal cells and the laying down of fibrous tissue in the bone marrow.

The marrow space becomes obliterated by the fibrosis, and haematopoiesis occurs in organs outside the bone marrow such as the liver and spleen (extramedullary haematopoiesis). Immature red blood cells and neutrophils enter the peripheral blood from the marrow and from sites of extramedullary haematopoiesis, a pattern known as leukoerythroblastosis.

Chronic idiopathic myelofibrosis presents late with massive splenomegaly and anaemia

Because chronic idiopathic myelofibrosis does not lead to a significantly raised blood cell count, it rarely presents in its early stages. Most patients present late in the disease with a massively enlarged spleen and anaemia. A blood film shows red blood cells distorted by the fibrotic marrow, and numerous immature red blood cells and white blood cells. A bone marrow *aspirate* of a fibrotic marrow yields little material (a 'dry tap'), and so the bone marrow *trephine* is essential to diagnose chronic idiopathic myelofibrosis.

The only curative treatment for idiopathic myelofibrosis is bone marrow transplantation, but only a small number of patients are suitable. In most cases, treatment is supportive, aimed at alleviating symptoms related to bone marrow failure. Idiopathic myelofibrosis has the poorest prognosis of all the myeloproliferative disorders, with an average survival of 3–5 years.

> ## Key points: Myeloproliferative disorders
>
> - Myeloproliferative disorders are malignancies of haemopoietic stem cells in the bone marrow.
>
> - Uncontrolled proliferation and expansion of myeloid progenitors in the bone marrow results in increased numbers of mature neutrophils, red blood cells, and platelets in the peripheral blood.
>
> - Most patients present with raised blood counts and enlargement of the liver and spleen.
>
> - The main problem in diagnosing a myeloproliferative disorder is excluding for certain that the increased number of myeloid cells is due to a neoplastic disorder rather than representing a normal response to some other underlying problem.
>
> - Chronic myeloid leukaemia is the most common myeloproliferative disorder which usually presents with a raised neutrophil count. Almost all cases are associated with the Philadelphia chromosome. The disease typically passes through a stable chronic phase before terminating in an acute leukaemia.
>
> - Polycythaemia vera is a myeloproliferative disorder dominated by increased production of mature red blood cells. With treatment, survival is typically greater than 10 years. Most patients die from a thrombotic or haemorrhagic episode. Bone marrow failure due to fibrosis may also occur.

Key points: Myeloproliferative disorders—cont'd

- Essential thrombocythaemia is a myeloproliferative disorder dominated by increased production of mature platelets. Survival is good, and many elderly patients die with the disease rather than from it.

- Idiopathic myelofibrosis is a myeloproliferative disorder characterized by marrow fibrosis. Patients present late in the disease with marked splenomegaly and a leukoerythroblastic anaemia. Survival is poor.

Key points: Myelodysplastic syndromes

- Myelodysplastic syndromes are a group of haematological malignancies due to neoplastic transformation of a haemopoietic stem cell in the bone marrow.

- The malignant cells are unable to differentiate normally, so developing blood cells are destroyed in the bone marrow.

- Ineffective haematopoiesis may affect one or more of the myeloid cell lines.

- The majority of patients are elderly and present with fatigue due to refractory anaemia. Lymphadenopathy, hepatomegaly, and splenomegaly are rare.

- In myelodysplasia, blood cells in the peripheral blood and bone marrow look strange.

- It is important to rule out a non-neoplastic cause of the abnormality.

- The majority of patients with myelodysplasia suffer from progressive bone marrow failure, terminating in acute leukaemia.

Myelodysplastic syndromes

Myelodysplasia is another group of neoplastic haematopoietic disorders caused by mutations in a stem cell in the bone marrow. The malignant progenitor cells retain the ability to differentiate, *but do so in a disordered and ineffective manner*. As a consequence, the abnormal cells undergo apoptosis in the bone marrow leading to low peripheral blood counts (cytopenias).

The majority of patients present with symptoms related to anaemia. Organomegaly is not often seen in patients with a myelodysplastic syndrome. The hallmark of a myelodysplastic syndrome is the presence of weird looking ('dysplastic') blood cells and their precursors in the peripheral blood and bone marrow. Some of the changes in the blood cells can be extremely subtle and sometimes it is necessary to seek the opinion of an expert.

A further problem in diagnosing myelodysplastic syndromes is demonstrating that the dysplasia is due to a clonal disorder rather than some other cause. For instance, similar dysplastic changes in developing red blood cells can also be seen in a variety of metabolic and nutritional disorders, including vitamin B12 deficiency.

The ideal treatment for myelodysplastic syndrome would be a drug that could induce the differentiation of the immature myeloid cells into mature forms. Unfortunately such an agent does not exist, and so the treatment of myelodysplasia is largely supportive with appropriate use of red cell and platelet transfusions. Younger individuals who are fit and well motivated may derive some benefit from chemotherapy. Most patients die from bone marrow failure, usually due to transformation into an acute leukaemia.

Non-Hodgkin lymphomas

The **non-Hodgkin lymphomas** are a group of haematological malignancies derived from lymphocytes which have left the bone marrow. The aetiology of most non-Hodgkin lymphomas is obscure; however, a number of factors are known to be associated with an increased risk, including immunosuppression and chronic lymphoid stimulation (e.g. *Helicobacter pylori* gastritis and Hashimoto's thyroiditis).

Most non-Hodgkin lymphomas are of B lymphocyte origin

Although lymphomas may be derived from B or T lymphocytes, the vast majority of non-Hodgkin lymphomas are of B cell origin. This is due to the multiple rounds of genetic instability which B cells undergo when they are subjected to somatic hypermutation in germinal centres during which they are liable to acquire genetic abnormalities leading to malignant transformation.

T cells, however, once they have rearranged their T cell receptor and left the thymus, do not undergo any further genetic rearrangements and so are at lower risk of malignant transformation.

B cell non-Hodgkin lymphomas may arise at any stage of B lymphocyte development

B cell lymphomas may arise from B cells at any of the various stages of B cell development. This accounts for the large number of different types of B cell lymphoma. Getting to grips with B cell lymphomas therefore requires a basic knowledge of B cell development (Fig. 15.10).

Normal B cell differentiation begins in the bone marrow, where precursor B lymphoblasts undergo immunoglobulin gene rearrangement and differentiate into surface immunoglobulin-positive naïve B lymphocytes. Naïve B cells are small resting lymphocytes that

leave the bone marrow to circulate in the blood and occupy primary lymphoid follicles. Two lymphomas are thought to correspond to these naïve B cells: **small lymphocytic lymphoma** and **mantle cell lymphoma**.

On encountering antigen, naïve B cells undergo *blastic transformation*, forming larger cells called centroblasts which migrate into the centre of a primary follicle and fill the follicular dendritic cell meshwork, forming a germinal centre. Lymphomas composed of cells that resemble centroblasts are called **diffuse large B cell lymphoma** and tend to be clinically aggressive tumours.

Centroblasts mature into centrocytes which express surface immunoglobulin that has an altered antibody site because of the somatic mutations. **Follicular lymphomas** are tumours of germinal centre B cells (centrocytes and centroblasts) in which centrocytes fail to undergo apoptosis. Since follicular lymphomas are

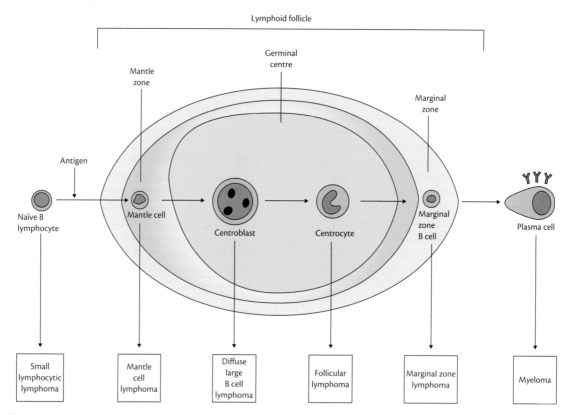

Fig. 15.10 Normal B lymphocyte development, showing postulated neoplastic counterparts.

composed of centrocytes, which are resting cells, they tend to be indolent.

Memory B cells reside at the edge of lymphoid follicles in lymph nodes in an area known as the marginal zone. Lymphomas that arise from memory cells in the marginal zone are called **marginal zone lymphomas**.

Non-Hodgkin lymphomas may be indolent or aggressive

The easiest way to subdivide non-Hodgkin lymphomas in clinical practice is into indolent lymphomas and aggressive lymphomas.

◆ Indolent lymphomas tend to present with widely disseminated disease at diagnosis involving several nodal and extranodal sites, but follow a slowly progressive course. Examples include follicular lymphoma, marginal zone lymphoma, and small lymphocytic lymphoma.

◆ Aggressive lymphomas tend to present with a short history of a rapidly growing destructive mass at a localized nodal or extranodal site. There may be additional features such as drenching night sweats, weight loss, and fever. The presence of these so-called 'B symptoms' implies rapidly progressing disease. Examples include diffuse large B cell lymphoma and mantle cell lymphoma.

Nodal disease means involvement of a lymph node by the lymphoma. Extranodal disease refers to involvement of any non-lymph node site by the lymphoma. Common extranodal sites involved by lymphomas include the gastrointestinal tract (including the oropharynx), the central nervous system, and the skin.

Excision of an involved lymph node or biopsy of an extranodal mass is mandatory for diagnosis

Diagnosis of a non-Hodgkin lymphoma requires histological examination of an involved site to define the precise type of non-Hodgkin lymphoma and to rule out an alternative diagnosis such as a Hodgkin lymphoma. If a lymph node is being sampled, it is best to excise the whole node for histopathological examination. In the case of extranodal disease, a biopsy of the mass is usually performed.

T cell lymphomas are much less common than B cell lymphomas, but more aggressive

T cell lymphomas are a group of malignancies derived from T lymphocytes which have left the bone marrow.

T cell lymphomas are uncommon, making up only 10 per cent of non-Hodgkin lymphomas. This is fortunate as they are amongst the most aggressive of all haematological malignancies; they respond poorly to treatment and the majority of patients die of their disease.

The T cell lymphomas are an extremely difficult group to categorize and, despite many attempts to create distinct and meaningful entities, most T cell lymphomas end up being called (somewhat unsatisfactorily) '**peripheral T cell lymphoma, unspecified**'. Of the small number of specific T cell lymphomas that are recognized, the most commonly seen are **anaplastic large cell lymphoma**, **enteropathy associated T cell lymphoma** which complicates gluten-sensitive enteropathy (p. 155), and the cutaneous T cell lymphoma **mycosis fungoides** (p. 383). All of these are rare.

> ## Key points: Non-Hodgkin lymphomas
>
> ◆ The non-Hodgkin lymphomas are a large group of haematological malignancies derived from mature lymphocytes.
>
> ◆ The vast majority of non-Hodgkin lymphomas are B cell lymphomas.
>
> ◆ B cell non-Hodgkin lymphomas usually present with solid masses in lymph nodes or at extranodal sites. Biopsy of an involved site for histopathological analysis is essential to categorize the type of lymphoma precisely.
>
> ◆ There are many different types of B cell lymphoma. For practical purposes, they are best considered as being either indolent or aggressive lymphomas.
>
> ◆ Indolent lymphomas typically present with widely disseminated disease but progress slowly. Examples include follicular lymphoma, marginal zone lymphoma, and small lymphocytic lymphoma.
>
> ◆ Indolent lymphomas can be controlled with treatment, but cure is rarely achievable. Survival is typically in the region of 8–10 years.

Continued

Key points: Non-Hodgkin lymphomas—cont'd

♦ Aggressive lymphomas typically present with rapidly enlarging nodal or extranodal masses and severe constitutional symptoms. Examples include diffuse large B cell lymphoma and mantle cell lymphoma.

♦ Although rapidly fatal if untreated, current therapy can lead to complete cure in diffuse large B cell lymphoma. Mantle cell lymphoma, however, shows a poor therapeutic response with a median survival of 3–4 years.

♦ T-cell non-Hodgkin lymphomas are much less common than B cell lymphomas. The two most common types are peripheral T cell lymphoma unspecified and anaplastic large cell lymphoma. T cell lymphomas are highly aggressive malignancies which respond poorly to treatment and have a poor outcome.

Hodgkin lymphomas

Hodgkin lymphomas are a special group of B cell lymphomas which account for about one-third of all lymphomas. They share the following characteristics:

♦ They usually arise in lymph nodes, particularly in the cervical region.

♦ The majority of them affect young adults, particularly males.

♦ The neoplastic tissue contains a small number of large tumour cells called **Hodgkin-Reed-Sternberg cells** residing amongst an abundant mixture of non-neoplastic inflammatory cells. Hodgkin–Reed-Sternberg cells are of B lymphocyte origin and have a variety of different appearances (Fig. 15.11).

There are two distinct entities within Hodgkin lymphoma: **classical Hodgkin lymphoma** and **nodular lymphocyte predominant Hodgkin lymphoma**. These two entities differ in their clinical features and behaviour as well as the features of the neoplastic Hodgkin-Reed-Sternberg cells found in each.

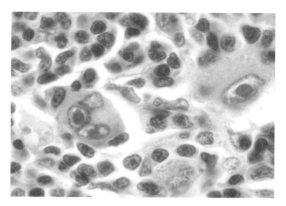

Fig. 15.11 Microscopic image of Hodgkin–Reed–Sternberg cells seen in Hodgkin lymphoma.

Classical Hodgkin lymphoma is subdivided into four subtypes

Based on the composition of the non-neoplastic inflammatory infiltrate and what the Hodgkin–Reed-Sternberg cells look like, four subtypes of classical Hodgkin lymphoma have been distinguished:

♦ Nodular sclerosis

♦ Mixed cellularity

♦ Lymphocyte rich

♦ Lymphocyte depleted.

Nodular sclerosis Hodgkin lymphoma is the most common form of classical Hodgkin lymphoma. It typically affects young adults, and involvement of nodes in the mediastinum is very common. Mixed cellularity classical Hodgkin lymphoma affects slightly older individuals and involves peripheral lymph nodes rather than mediastinal nodes. The lymphocyte rich and lymphocyte depleted subtypes of classical Hodgkin lymphoma are rare.

Nodular lymphocyte predominant Hodgkin lymphoma differs from classical Hodgkin lymphoma

Unlike classical Hodgkin lymphoma, nodular lymphocyte predominant Hodgkin lymphoma occurs in sites rarely involved by classical Hodgkin lymphoma such as the inguinal nodes. Involvement of mediastinal nodes is very unusual in nodular lymphocyte predominant Hodgkin lymphoma. The overall survival of patients with this subtype is excellent.

Diagnosis of Hodgkin lymphoma can only be made on microscopic examination of a lymph node

Like the non-Hodgkin lymphomas, the specific type of Hodgkin lymphoma can only be ascertained by histological examination of an involved lymph node. Do not worry about the microscopic features of each individual type of Hodgkin lymphoma: leave that to a histopathologist! In any event, what is important in predicting prognosis in Hodgkin lymphoma is how extensive the disease is rather than the specific type.

The cure rate is very good in Hodgkin lymphoma, even in patients with extensive disease

With modern treatment regimes, the cure rate of Hodgkin lymphoma is extremely good. Unfortunately, as the cure rate has improved, the late effects of the treatment have become apparent, particularly the development of second malignancies such as lung cancer and breast cancer. This is mainly attributable to the radiotherapy, and the hope for the future is that improved chemotherapy regimes will reduce the need for such intense courses of radiotherapy.

Key points: Hodgkin lymphoma

- Hodgkin lymphomas are a group of neoplasms arising from mature B lymphocytes.

- The disease typically affects young adults who present with lymph node enlargement, particularly in the neck.

- There are two main types: classical Hodgkin lymphoma and nodular lymphocyte predominant Hodgkin lymphoma.

- Classical Hodgkin lymphoma has four subtypes, the most common of which are the nodular sclerosis and mixed cellularity types. Involvement of mediastinal lymph nodes is common.

- Nodular lymphocyte predominant Hodgkin lymphoma involves node sites not normally seen in classical Hodgkin lymphoma such as the inguinal nodes.

- Cure rates are high for Hodgkin lymphomas, but long-term survivors are at risk of developing second malignancies as a complication of the treatment.

Multiple myeloma

Multiple myeloma is a malignant disease of plasma cells in the bone marrow

Multiple myeloma is a malignant disorder of plasma cells with a peak age of incidence between 50 and 60 years. The aetiology is unknown. Typically there is generalized bone marrow involvement, but the most prominent sites of involvement are the areas of most active haematopoiesis, i.e. the vertebrae, ribs, and skull in order of frequency.

The malignant plasma cells produce a single immunoglobulin in large quantities which accumulates in the blood. The monoclonal immunoglobulin is usually IgG and is also known as the M (myeloma) protein and is an example of a **paraprotein**. A paraprotein is any abundant, useless, monoclonal protein in the blood. Paraprotein formation is not unique to myeloma; monoclonal immunoglobulins are also sometimes seen in other haematological malignancies such as CLL and lymphomas.

The abnormal plasma cells may also churn out free immunoglobulin light chains. Unlike the complete immunoglobulin molecule, they do not accumulate in the blood as a paraprotein. Because of their small size, they pass readily through the glomerular filter in the kidneys and into the urine where they are called **Bence-Jones protein**. Most myeloma patients produce Bence-Jones protein.

INTERESTING TO KNOW

MGUS

A proportion of elderly people are found to have a paraprotein but without any of the other features of myeloma or lymphoproliferative disease. This is called a **monoclonal gammopathy of uncertain significance** (MGUS). Patients with MGUS do not have any symptoms, nor evidence of any organ damage, but they do have a small risk of developing myeloma.

Myeloma causes uncontrolled osteoclast activity which leads to severe bony destruction

In myeloma, there is a complex relationship between the malignant plasma cells, the bone marrow stromal

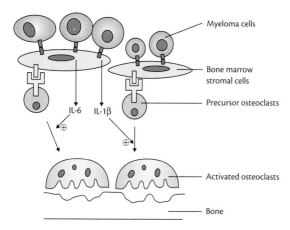

Fig. 15.12 Pathogenesis of bone disease in multiple myeloma. Lytic bony lesions in myeloma result from the interaction of myeloma cells with bone marrow stromal cells and the release of cytokines that stimulate osteoclast formation and activation.

cells, and osteoclasts (Fig. 15.12). The myeloma cells adhere to bone marrow stromal cells, leading to the release of cytokines such as interleukin-6 (IL-6) and IL-1β which stimulate uncontrolled osteoclast activity whilst inhibiting osteoblast formation. This uncoupling of bone resorption and formation leads to rapid bony loss. The extensive skeletal destruction results in severe persistent bony pain, pathological fractures, and hypercalcaemia.

Anaemia and a raised ESR are common haematological findings in myeloma

A normocytic anaemia is common in patients in myeloma. It is not directly related to marrow replacement, as neutropenia and thrombocytopenia are rarely seen. Instead, it seems to be due to a direct suppressive effect on red blood cell production by myeloma cell-derived cytokines such as IL-1.

A raised erythrocyte sedimentation rate (ESR) is also often present in myeloma. This occurs because the M protein in the blood coats red blood cells and causes them to group together in little clumps. This is called rouleaux formation, and causes the sedimentation rate to increase.

Myeloma patients are susceptible to infections

Production of large quantities of a single immunoglobulin by the neoplastic plasma cells has a suppressive effect on the production and release of other immunoglobulins by normal plasma cells ('immune paresis'). This defect in humoral immunity increases susceptibility to bacterial infections. Chest infections are a common problem in myeloma patients, and may be the presenting feature.

Renal impairment is very common in myeloma

Myeloma exacts a particularly nasty toll on the kidneys, the damage being caused predominantly by free immunoglobulin light chains. Free light chains filtered through the glomeruli form solid casts in the distal nephron, damaging the distal convoluted tubules and collecting ducts. Free light chains can also form amyloid, which deposits in the glomeruli leading to heavy proteinuria and the nephrotic syndrome (Fig. 15.13)

Renal impairment caused by light chains may be further impounded by the effects of hypercalcaemia and damage caused large quantities of non-steroidal anti-inflammatory drugs taken for the bony pain.

Definitive diagnosis of myeloma requires demonstration of excess plasma cells in the bone marrow

Patients suspected of having myeloma should first have simple screening tests to look for the paraprotein in the serum and urine using electrophoresis. Positive screening tests strongly suggest myeloma in the presence of a compatible history, but definitive diagnosis requires a bone marrow aspirate or trephine biopsy to demonstrate excess abnormal plasma cells in the bone marrow (Fig. 15.14).

> ## Key points: Myeloma
>
> ♦ Myeloma is a malignant proliferation of plasma cells which proliferate in the bone marrow and secrete large quantities of a monoclonal immunoglobulin known as an M protein.
>
> ♦ The proliferating plasma cells stimulate osteoclasts, leading to bony destruction. The production of immunoglobulins from normal B lymphocytes is impaired, leading to an immune paresis. Free light chains also produced by myeloma cells become stuck in the renal tubules and lead to renal damage.

Continued

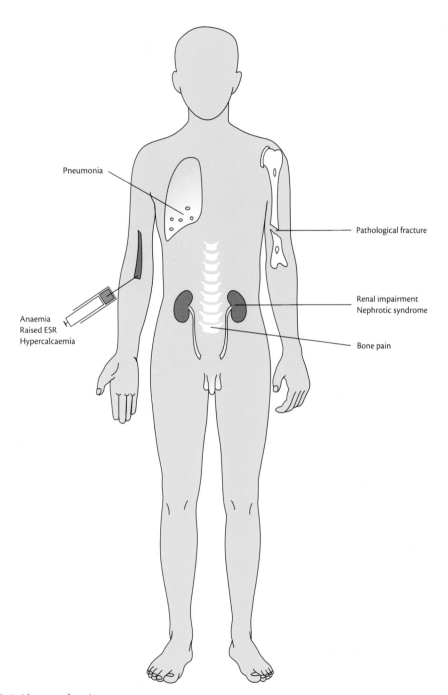

Pneumonia

Pathological fracture

Anaemia
Raised ESR
Hypercalcaemia

Renal impairment
Nephrotic syndrome

Bone pain

Fig. 15.13 Clinical features of myeloma.

Key points: Myeloma—cont'd

- Myeloma should be suspected in any patient aged over 50 with persistent bony pain, anaemia, recurrent infections, renal impairment, hypercalcaemia, or a raised ESR.

- Patients suspected of having myeloma should have serum electrophoresis to detect the serum paraprotein, and urine electrophoresis to detect Bence-Jones protein.

- Definitive diagnosis of myeloma requires a bone marrow aspirate to demonstrate excess plasma cell infiltration.

- Treatment is symptomatic, and chemotherapy aims to slow the progression of the disease. A small number of younger patients may be suitable for a bone marrow transplant which can be curative.

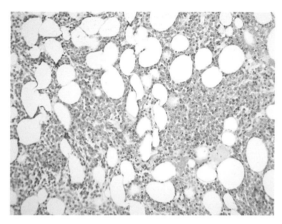

Fig. 15.14 A histological image of a bone marrow trephine biopsy taken from a patient with multiple myeloma. The white spaces represent fat cells in the bone marrow space which has been nearly completely replaced by large numbers of neoplastic plasma cells.

Bone marrow transplantation

Bone marrow transplantation is a form of treatment which is often the only hope of cure in haematological malignancies such as AML, CML, and multiple myeloma. However, only relatively fit young patients are normally suitable as it is a prolonged form of treatment with many of its own risks.

The aim of bone marrow transplantation is first to destroy the entirety of the patient's bone marrow using powerful drugs or radiation, and then transplant normal bone marrow cells from a suitably matched donor into the patient. The hope is that the patient's bone marrow will be repopulated with healthy cells which will proliferate and produce normal blood cells.

Patients undergoing bone marrow transplantation need very close careful monitoring. They are susceptible to a range of complications such as overwhelming infections due to their destroyed immune system, and a condition called **graft versus host disease** which results when immunologically competent immune cells from the donor mount a response against the patient's tissues (particularly the gut, liver, and skin) which the donor's immune cells recognize as foreign.

Further reading

www.bcshguidelines.com, British Committee for Standards in Haematology.
www.haemophilia.org.uk, UK Haemophilia Society.
www.tranfusionguidelines.org.uk, professional guidelines for blood transfusion in the UK.

CHAPTER 16

Skin disease

Chapter contents

Introduction

The skin is the largest organ in the body and forms the interface between the body and the environment. It acts as an important barrier, protecting the body from changes in external conditions and preventing loss of important body constituents such as water. The skin is also important in insulation, temperature regulation, and sensation.

The skin has three main layers. The outermost layer is the **epidermis**, which is firmly attached to the underlying **dermis**. Beneath the dermis is the **subcutis** which contains mostly fat (Fig. 16.1).

The epidermis is a keratinizing stratified squamous type of epithelium which contains **melanocytes** for protection against UV radiation, **Merkel cells** which play a role in sensation, and **Langerhans cells** which are the antigen-presenting cells of the skin.

The dermis is a tough connective tissue matrix which supports and nourishes the epidermis. The superficial dermis has upward projections called dermal papillae which interlock with downward ridges of the epidermis, the rete ridges. Collagen fibres make up 70 per cent of the dermis, imparting toughness and strength. Elastin fibres are loosely arranged in the dermis and provide elasticity to the skin. Embedded within the dermis are blood vessels, nerves, lymphatics, and the adnexal structures of the skin, namely the hair follicles, sebaceous glands, and sweat glands. The dermis also contains fibroblasts which synthesize the collagen and elastin, and cells of the immune system including mast cells, lymphocytes, macrophages (histiocytes), and dendritic cells known as dermal dendrocytes.

Diseases of the skin are common, and the prevalence of many skin disorders is increasing. Patients with skin disease account for about 15 per cent of all consultations in primary care in the UK, about half of whom are referred to a dermatologist. Although skin diseases rarely cause death, they can lead to significant discomfort and disability. Patients whose skin disease is on permanent display may also suffer tremendous psychological problems, with feelings of stigmatization and social isolation.

Dermatology can be a daunting subject to the newcomer, with a vocabulary of its own (Table 16.1). With the skin on permanent display for scrutiny, any change in its appearance, no matter how trivial, leads to the application of a diagnostic label. As such, dermatology has become an encyclopaedic subject with over 3000 named entities, many of which have peculiar

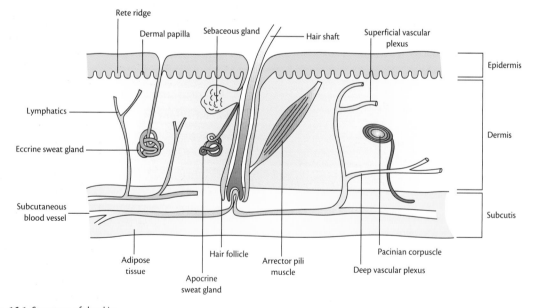

Fig. 16.1 Structure of the skin.

TABLE 16.1	Common terms in dermatology
Macule	Flat non-palpable lesion less than 10 mm
Patch	Flat non-palpable lesion greater than 10 mm
Papule	Raised palpable lesion less than 10 mm
Nodule	Raised palpable lesion greater than 10 mm
Plaque	Flat-topped elevated lesion greater than 10 mm
Pustule	Yellow white pus-filled lesion
Vesicle	Small fluid-filled blister
Bulla	Large fluid-filled blister

names based in Latin. The good news is that some 70 per cent of all dermatological practice is due to only a handful of common conditions, which we cover in this chapter. All of the remaining rarer conditions should be left firmly in the hands of dermatologists.

Benign skin neoplasms

Melanocytic nevi

Melanocytic nevi, or 'moles', are extremely common localized benign proliferations of melanocytes. Most Caucasian people have between 10 and 30 melanocytic nevi.

Melanocytic nevi begin when melanocytes in the basal layer of the epidermis proliferate, forming nests of cells at the dermoepidermal junction (Fig. 16.2). This lesion is called a **junctional nevus**. Junctional nevi are visible as flat brown macules which are round or oval in shape.

After a variable period of time, some of the melanocytes begin to migrate into the dermis, forming a **compound nevus** which has both a junctional and a dermal component. Compound nevi become raised lesions with a smooth surface (Fig. 16.3).

Eventually the junctional component disappears entirely; all of the melanocytes are within the dermis, and the lesion is termed an **intradermal nevus**. Intradermal nevi look like compound nevi but are less pigmented and often skin coloured (Fig. 16.4). Eventually melanocytic nevi disappear altogether.

Spitz nevus, blue nevus, and halo nevus are special types of melanocytic nevi

Spitz nevus is a melanocytic nevus which typically occurs on the face of a child and has a characteristic brick red colour. Although benign, they are often excised because of their rapid growth. Microscopically, Spitz nevi can be frightening lesions as the melanocytes can look very atypical, causing concern for a malignant melanoma.

Blue nevus is a melanocytic nevus found on the extremities and buttocks, with a characteristic steely blue colour. Blue nevi may develop at any age, but are usually noticed in the second decade or later. Although firm evidence is lacking, blue nevi are believed to represent collections of dermal melanocytes that failed to reach the epidermis during migration of embryonic neural crest cells. Their blue colour is due to the deep melanin absorbing long wavelengths of light and the overlying collagen bundles of the dermis scattering shorter wavelengths in the blue end of the spectrum.

Halo nevus is mainly found on the trunk of children or adolescents. A white halo of depigmentation

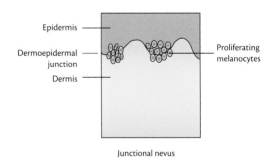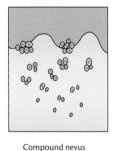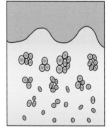

Fig. 16.2 Diagram of melanocytic nevi. Junctional nevi result from proliferating nests of melanocytes confined to the dermoepidermal junction. Some of the melanocytes then migrate into the dermis, forming a compound nevus. Once all of the melanocytes have migrated into the dermis, the lesion becomes an intradermal nevus.

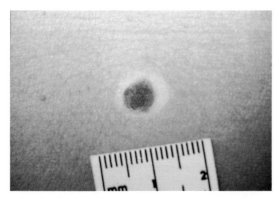

Fig. 16.3 Compound nevus on the neck of a young woman. The lesion is uniformly pigmented, slightly raised, and measures about 4 mm in diameter.

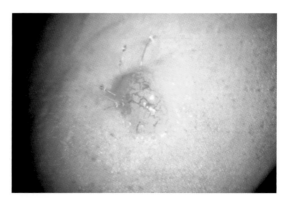

Fig. 16.4 Intradermal nevus. Note the lack of pigmentation.

surrounds the nevus due to immune destruction of the melanocytes. The nevus left in the centre usually involutes spontaneously and then the halo regains normal pigmentation.

Seborrhoeic keratoses

Seborrhoeic keratoses are common benign neoplasms of older people

Seborrhoeic keratoses (seborrhoeic warts) are extremely common benign skin neoplasms of older adults. They are often multiple, may occur anywhere on the body, and appear as dark brown greasy plaques composed of cells resembling the basal cells of the epidermis. They may occur anywhere on the body.

The diagnosis is usually straightforward, although a darkly pigmented seborrhoeic keratosis may cause concern for a malignant melanoma. Seborrhoeic keratoses have no potential for malignant transformation, but are often removed for cosmetic purposes.

Lipoma

Lipoma is the most common connective tissue neoplasm

Lipoma is a benign connective tissue neoplasm composed of mature adipocytes which frequently arises in the subcutaneous fat of the skin. Lipomas typically present in middle-aged adults as a slowly growing painless lump. The trunk and neck are common sites. Lipomas are entirely benign neoplasms and do not require excision unless they are a cosmetic nuisance.

Dermatofibroma

Dermatofibroma is a common benign cutaneous soft tissue tumour

Dermatofibroma (or **benign fibrous histiocytoma**) is a common benign soft tissue tumour of the skin which arises in the dermis. It typically occurs on the legs of young women as a firm light brown papule (Fig. 16.5).

Despite being common, the precise nature of the dermatofibroma remains unclear. The names dermatofibroma and benign fibrous histiocytoma were coined because the cell of origin of the tumour was thought to be either a dermal fibroblast or a histiocyte. It has also been proposed that the tumour arises from the dermal

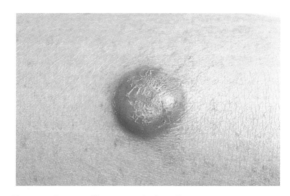

Fig. 16.5 Dermatofibroma on the leg of a young woman.

dendrocyte because some cells within the tumour stain positively for a marker, factor XIIIa, which is found on dermal dendrocytes. However, the cells in the tumour which stain for this marker are found mostly at the edge of the tumour and appear to be reactive cells rather than true tumour cells.

Whatever its histogenesis, simple excision of a dermatofibroma is usually curative. Local recurrence is very uncommon, with the exception of some of the variants (e.g. the **cellular dermatofibroma**) which have a higher recurrence rate.

Lobular capillary haemangioma

Lobular capillary haemangioma is a benign vascular tumour

Lobular capillary haemangioma is a mass composed of an organized proliferation of capillary sized blood vessels which appears rapidly, usually after a minor injury and often on a digit (Fig. 16.6). The lesion may cause concern if it resembles a squamous cell carcinoma or an amelanotic melanoma. If there is any doubt over the diagnosis, the lesion should be excised for histopathological examination.

Lobular capillary haemangiomas were once thought to be reactive conditions rather than true neoplasms, and are often still called by their original name of **pyogenic granuloma**. This is a rather unhelpful name as the lesion is neither pyogenic nor granulomatous!

Neurofibroma

Neurofibroma is a tumour composed of a mixture of cell types including Schwann cells, perineurial cells,

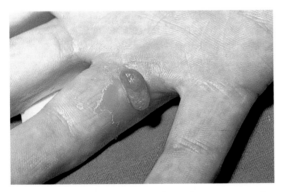

Fig. 16.6 Pyogenic granuloma. Typical vascular appearance of a pyogenic granuloma arising on a digit.

and fibroblasts. Neurofibromas are common and most occur as sporadic single tumours in the skin (localized cutaneous neurofibromas).

Multiple neurofibromas are typical of the inherited condition neurofibromatosis type 1 (p. 445). Other cutaneous manifestations of this condition include freckling and café au lait spots.

> ### Key points: Benign skin neoplasms
>
> ◆ Melanocytic nevi are extremely common benign skin neoplasms divided into junctional, compound, and intradermal types.
>
> ◆ Seborrhoeic keratoses are benign epithelial neoplasms composed of cells resembling the basal cells of the epidermis. They appear as dark brown, greasy lesions on the skin of elderly people.
>
> ◆ Lipoma is a benign connective tissue neoplasm composed of mature adipocytes which typically occurs on the trunk or neck of middle-aged adults. If excised for cosmetic reasons, they do not recur.
>
> ◆ Dermatofibroma is a benign soft tissue neoplasm of the skin which commonly occurs on the lower leg of young women. The precise cell of origin is uncertain.
>
> ◆ Lobular capillary haemangioma (pyogenic granuloma) is a benign vascular neoplasm composed of a mass of capillary sized blood vessels. They commonly occur on digits following minor trauma.
>
> ◆ Neurofibroma is a tumour composed of Schwann cells, perineurial cells, and fibroblasts which commonly occurs as a single sporadic tumour in the skin. Multiple neurofibromas are typical of neurofibromatosis type 1.

Pre-malignant skin neoplasms

Actinic keratoses

Actinic keratoses are areas of dysplastic epidermis in sun-exposed sites

Actinic keratoses, or **solar keratoses**, are common lesions seen on sun-exposed sites of the elderly. They are small, yellow brown, dry, scaly lesions which rarely

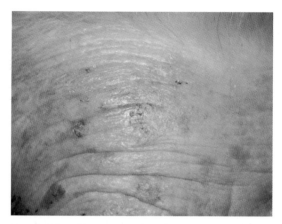

Fig. 16.7 Multiple actinic keratoses on the scalp of an elderly woman. These yellow scaly lesions on an erythematous base show the typical appearance of an actinic keratosis.

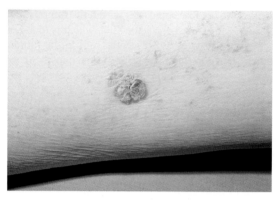

Fig. 16.8 Intraepidermal carcinoma. This scaly lesion on the lower leg of an elderly woman was excised. Microscopic examination showed full thickness dysplasia of the epidermis.

exceed 10 mm. Their rough surface is often more easily felt than seen (Fig. 16.7). Microscopically the keratinocytes of the epidermis show disarray and nuclear abnormalities (dysplasia), but there is no invasion.

Only a small percentage of actinic keratoses develop into an invasive squamous cell carcinoma, though patients often have multiple actinic keratoses and so overall may have a significant risk of eventually developing a squamous cell carcinoma. As actinic keratoses are the result of significant solar damage to the skin, patients are also at risk of other tumours related to UV exposure such as basal cell carcinoma.

Intraepidermal carcinoma

Intraepidermal carcinoma is an area of full thickness dysplasia of the epidermis

Intraepidermal carcinoma (**squamous cell carcinoma in situ**, **Bowen's disease**) is a lesion in which the full thickness of the epidermis contains neoplastic keratinocytes but there is no invasion through the basement membrane.

The lesion is usually a well defined solitary pink scaly plaque which slowly enlarges over many years (Fig. 16.8). Intraepidermal carcinoma may clinically resemble superficial basal cell carcinoma, discoid eczema, or an area of superficial fungal infection. Often, the diagnosis is suspected when a lesion originally thought to be a form of dermatitis fails to respond to topical steroid treatment.

Areas of intraepidermal carcinoma are usually excised to confirm the diagnosis microscopically and to prevent the chance of the development of an invasive squamous cell carcinoma.

Dysplastic nevus

Dysplastic nevi are melanocytic proliferations which show varying degrees of atypia

Dysplastic nevi are abnormal melanocytic lesions occupying an intermediate position between ordinary melanocytic nevi and malignant melanomas. They show a spectrum of changes, both clinically and microscopically, ranging from mild atypia in melanocytes to severe changes that look very similar to an in situ malignant melanoma.

Dysplastic nevi either occur as an isolated solitary lesion or at multiple sites. They may be located anywhere on the body, but are found most commonly on the trunk. Dysplastic nevi tend to be larger than ordinary melanocytic nevi and have an irregular edge and variable pigmentation (Fig. 16.9).

Most dysplastic nevi are stable and do not evolve into malignant melanoma

Dysplastic nevi are common, with a prevalence of up to 10 per cent reported in white populations. Although about one-third of melanomas appear to arise from a dysplastic nevus, it must be appreciated that dysplastic nevi are vastly more common than melanomas, and thus the overall percentage of dysplastic nevi which progress to melanoma is extremely small. *Most dysplastic*

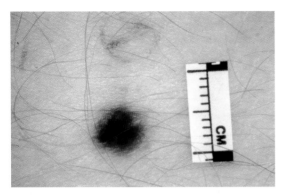

Fig. 16.9 Dysplastic nevus showing irregular borders and a diameter greater than 6 mm. Symmetry remains preserved and the pigmentation is even.

nevi remain stable or regress completely, and never evolve into malignant melanoma. However, many dermatologists tend to excise a dysplastic nevus and send it for histopathological examination to reassure the patient (and themselves!) that it is not a malignant melanoma.

Patients with a single dysplastic nevus do not normally need specialist follow-up

Patients with a single dysplastic nevus and no personal or family history of melanoma have an extremely low risk of developing a melanoma. Although some dermatologists may see these patients annually, this is almost certainly unnecessary and it is safe to educate the patient about self-examination and sun protection, leaving them to return if they are concerned.

Patients with multiple dysplastic nevi require follow-up

Patients with multiple dysplastic nevi and a personal or family history of melanoma must be kept under formal surveillance. There is a 100-fold increase in the incidence of melanoma in patients who have previously had melanoma, a 200-fold increase in those with at least two family members with melanoma, and a more than 1200-fold increase in those with both a personal and family history of melanoma.

These patients should have regular skin examinations by a dermatologist, together with serial photography of suspicious lesions to document any evolving changes. Studies have shown that people with dysplastic nevi under proper surveillance are very unlikely to die of melanoma.

Key points: Pre-malignant skin neoplasms

◆ Pre-malignant skin neoplasms are lesions which in some, but by no means all, people develop into invasive cutaneous malignancies.

◆ Actinic keratoses are rough scaly lesions seen on sun-exposed sites of elderly people which microscopically show dysplasia of the epidermis. Actinic keratoses are usually removed or destroyed to prevent the small chance of progression into a squamous cell carcinoma.

◆ Intraepidermal carcinoma is a slowly growing scaly plaque which microscopically shows full thickness severe dysplasia of the epidermis. The lesion is usually excised to prevent progression into squamous cell carcinoma.

◆ Dysplastic nevi are melanocytic lesions that show abnormal features both clinically and microscopically. A very small proportion of dysplastic nevi develop into malignant melanomas, and so they are usually excised.

Malignant skin neoplasms

Malignant skin neoplasms are the most common of all cancers, accounting for one-third of all cases of cancer but only 2 per cent of cancer deaths. Cutaneous malignancies are particularly common in fair-skinned people, and sunlight is a major aetiological agent.

A unique type of mutation has been identified in pre-malignant and malignant cutaneous neoplasms caused by UV radiation, namely the formation of *pyrimidine dimers* in DNA. Pyrimidine dimers may form between thymine and thymine, thymine and cytosine, or between cytosine and cytosine. Demonstrating such genetic changes in cutaneous tumours provides strong evidence that UV radiation is involved in their aetiology.

Basal cell carcinoma

Basal cell carcinoma is the most common cutaneous malignancy

Basal cell carcinoma is a common tumour, accounting for about 70 per cent of all malignant skin tumours.

They are thought to arise from an undifferentiated pluripotent epithelial stem cell.

Exposure to UV radiation is the major cause of basal cell carcinoma. The relationship between sun exposure and the risk of basal cell carcinoma is complex; the timing, pattern, and amount of exposure all appear to be important. Intense intermittent exposure to the sun carries a higher risk than a similar degree of continuous exposure.

Basal cell carcinomas are most common on the head and neck, followed by the trunk, and limbs. Interestingly, basal cell carcinomas often occur at sites slightly removed from direct sun exposure such as the nasolabial folds and the inner canthus of the eye.

Basal cell carcinoma has nodular, ulcerative, superficial, and diffuse subtypes

Basal cell carcinomas are divided clinically into nodular, ulcerative, superficial, and diffuse types:

* The **nodular** type begins as a small translucent papule with a pearly appearance. The epidermis is stretched over the lesion and a few small vessels are often visible on the surface (Fig. 16.10)

* The **ulcerative** type starts as a solid papule but, as the lesion enlarges, the centre ulcerates leaving characteristic rolled edges (Fig. 16.11). A history of an ulcer that does not heal is typical of a basal cell carcinoma.

* The **superficial** type arises most often on the trunk as slowly expanding pink scaly plaques which may be multiple. These may be confused with plaques of

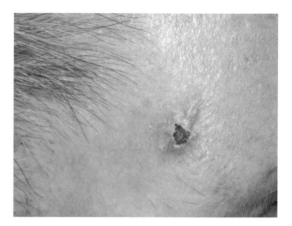

Fig. 16.11 Ulcerated basal cell carcinoma with characteristic rolled edges.

psoriasis, discoid dermatitis, and intraepidermal carcinoma. The importance of the superficial subtype is that it is notorious for being much more extensive than it appears to the naked eye.

* The **diffuse**, or infiltrating, type is a flat, pale pink plaque which slowly enlarges over several years. The margins of the lesion are poorly defined.

Basal cell carcinomas are composed of small neoplastic epithelial cells embedded in a delicate stroma

Microscopically, basal cell carcinomas are composed of neoplastic epithelial cells which resemble the normal basal cells of the epidermis and hair follicle (hence the term basal cell carcinoma), sitting in a delicate specialized tumour stroma (Fig. 16.12). The stroma proliferates along with the neoplastic epithelial cells and there appears to be an important mutual relationship between the epithelium and the stroma. In fact, survival of the epithelial component appears to rely on the presence of the stroma, a phenomenon known as 'stromal dependency'.

Basal cell carcinomas may show extensive local infiltration, but rarely metastasize

Basal cell carcinomas are slowly growing tumours with potential for extensive local infiltration, but distant metastases are extremely rare. Fewer than 0.1 per cent metastasize to regional lymph nodes. The low incidence of metastases is thought to be related to the stromal dependency of the tumour; only large tumour emboli

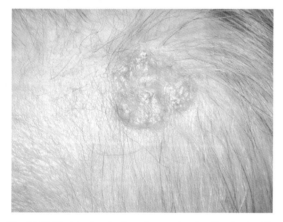

Fig. 16.10 Nodular basal cell carcinoma showing the characteristic telangiectatic vessels over the surface.

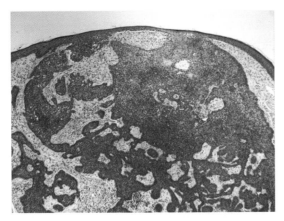

Fig. 16.12 Microscopic image of a basal cell carcinoma. The tumour, composed of nests of small blue neoplastic cells embedded in a loose stroma, is seen growing down from the epidermis at the top of the image.

* Clinically, basal cell carcinomas may be divided into nodular, ulcerated, diffuse, and superficial forms depending on their appearance.

* Histologically, basal cell carcinomas consist of neoplastic epithelial cells which resemble the basal layer of the epidermis and hair follicle in a specialized stroma.

* Although basal cell carcinomas may show extensive local infiltration, the incidence of metastases is extremely low.

* Complete surgical excision is the treatment of choice for a basal cell carcinoma. If this is difficult, other treatment methods include radiotherapy and curettage.

with attached stroma are likely to succeed in developing at a distant site.

Complete surgical excision of a basal cell carcinoma is curative, and is the treatment of choice. Sometimes the location or size of the tumour makes surgical excision difficult or impossible, in which case other treatment modalities such as radiotherapy or curettage may be employed.

Mutations in P53 and genes of the sonic hedgehog signalling pathway are common in basal cell carcinoma

About half of all basal cell carcinomas have mutations in the P53 tumour suppressor gene, many of which show the pyrimidine dimers typical of exposure to UV radiation. An additional pathway important in basal cell carcinomas is mutations that activate the hedgehog signalling pathway, such as gain-of-function mutations in PTCH (*patched*) and SMO (*smoothened*) oncogenes.

Key points: Basal cell carcinoma

* Basal cell carcinoma is the most common cutaneous malignancy and is related to sun exposure.

* It is commonly seen on the head and neck of elderly people.

Squamous cell carcinoma

Squamous cell carcinoma is the second most common cutaneous malignancy

Squamous cell carcinomas are invasive malignancies, most of which arise from actinic keratoses. The majority of cutaneous squamous cell carcinomas are related to UV radiation, with the majority occurring in areas of direct sun exposure such as the forehead, face, neck, and hands. The likelihood of developing actinic keratoses and squamous cell carcinoma seems to be related to cumulative total lifetime sun exposure.

The incidence of cutaneous squamous cell carcinoma is also significantly increased in immunosuppressed patients. In renal transplant patients, for example, the incidence has been found to be 18 times greater than in the general population. Squamous cell carcinomas also tend to be more aggressive in these patients.

Squamous cell carcinomas are irregular, keratotic tumours which ulcerate and crust (Fig. 16.13). Unlike basal cell carcinomas, squamous cell carcinomas grow rapidly over months rather than years. The risk of lymph node metastasis is higher than that for basal cell carcinomas, but is still only 1–2 per cent. Surgical excision is the treatment of choice.

Keratoacanthoma

Keratoacanthomas are curious lesions whose nature is controversial

Keratoacanthoma is an epidermal tumour which appears initially as a smooth, flesh coloured papule

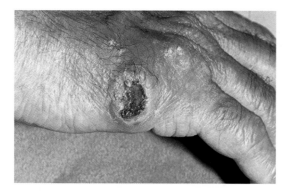

Fig. 16.13 Ulcerated squamous cell carcinoma of the skin.

which rapidly enlarges over a period of 6–8 weeks into a 10–20 mm nodule with rolled edges and a central keratin plug. Curiously the lesion then spontaneously shrinks until it disappears completely, leaving a small scar. The cause of keratoacanthoma is not known. Although a viral cause has been suggested, studies have not confirmed this.

The main problem with keratoacanthoma is distinguishing it from a squamous cell carcinoma, which it can closely mimic both clinically and histologically. Because of the close similarities between keratoacanthoma and squamous cell carcinoma, many authorities believe that keratoacanthomas should be considered as a variant of squamous cell carcinoma, largely as a result of reports of cases of keratoacanthomas that have behaved in a malignant fashion. Other people, however, believe that the two are quite distinct entities which should continue to be separated, arguing that cases of keratoacanthomas with malignant behaviour were squamous cell carcinomas misdiagnosed as keratoacanthomas in the first place.

If the history and appearance of a keratoacanthoma is characteristic, it is reasonable to monitor the lesion to see if it resolves, especially in cases where surgical removal would be difficult. If there is any doubt about the diagnosis, the lesion should be excised in its entirety and sent for histopathological examination. If there remains doubt about the diagnosis even on histology, it is always best to err on the side of caution and manage the lesion as if it were a squamous cell carcinoma.

Malignant melanoma

Malignant melanoma is a malignant tumour derived from melanocytes. The vast majority of melanomas arise in the skin, although it should be remembered that melanocytes in other sites such as the uveal tract of the eye can also give rise to melanomas.

Malignant melanomas are the most lethal of the skin tumours. A melanoma measuring as little as 1–2 mm thick has the potential to metastasize widely and kill, a chilling trait unrivalled by any other solid malignancy.

Intense sun exposure in childhood is an important risk factor in the development of melanoma

As with other cutaneous malignancies, the most important aetiological factor in melanoma is sun exposure. Two or more episodes of severe blistering sunburn before age 15 appear to be particularly important in the development of malignant melanoma.

Although some melanomas arise from pre-existing benign melanocytic nevi, the majority appear to arise *de novo.* This is probably because most of the cells in benign nevi are terminally differentiated and therefore unlikely to give rise to a malignancy. Whether or not all melanomas arise from a preceding dysplastic nevus remains controversial, although logically this seems likely.

Malignant melanomas may be in situ or invasive

Malignant melanomas may be entirely within the epidermis (in situ) or may extend into the dermis (invasive). Invasive melanomas usually, but not invariably, pass stepwise through two stages: radial growth phase and vertical growth phase (Fig. 16.14).

In the **radial growth phase**, most of the neoplastic melanocytes are located within the epidermis, with only a few present in the superficial dermis. The neoplastic cells in the dermis do not proliferate, and thus the growth of the melanoma is in a predominantly horizontal direction within the epidermis.

After about 1–2 years, the character of the growth of the melanoma begins to change. The dominant site of growth shifts from the epidermis to the dermis. The melanoma forms an expansile mass and the net growth of the lesion changes, such that it is perpendicular to the radial growth phase, i.e. **vertical growth phase**. The transition into vertical growth phase is heralded by the development of a nodule within a previously flat macule. Microscopically, the vertical growth phase is defined by the presence of large nests of malignant melanocytes within the dermis and/or the presence of mitoses within dermal melanocytes.

The radial and vertical growth phase model is useful as it has biological significance. A melanoma in radial growth phase has no metastatic potential and a 100 per cent survival rate if excised adequately. Vertical growth phase melanomas, however, have a much higher metastatic potential.

Four types of melanoma are recognized

There are four recognized patterns of malignant melanoma: superficial spreading, nodular, lentigo maligna, and acral lentiginous.

◆ **Superficial spreading malignant melanoma** is the most common form of melanoma, accounting for about 70 per cent of all cases. The leg is a common site in women, and the back in men. The lesion initially presents as a flat macule with irregular edges and a marked variation in colour. After a period of 1–2 years, a blue or black nodule develops within the macule, heralding the onset of the vertical growth phase (Fig. 16.15).

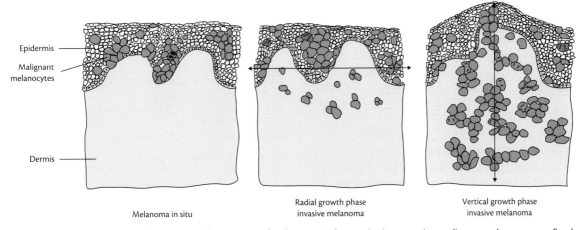

Epidermis

Malignant melanocytes

Dermis

Melanoma in situ

Radial growth phase invasive melanoma

Vertical growth phase invasive melanoma

Fig. 16.14 Diagrammatic representation of different stages of melanoma. Melanoma in situ comprises malignant melanocytes confined to the epidermis. In radial growth phase invasive melanoma, malignant melanocytes invade the dermis but the growth of the tumour is still confined to the epidermis. In vertical growth phase invasive melanoma, the growth of the tumour switches from the epidermis to the dermis.

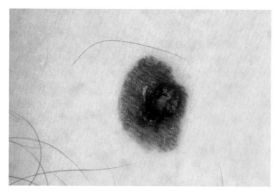

Fig. 16.15 Superficial spreading melanoma. Note the large nodule representing the vertical growth phase arising from a surrounding flat component of the preceding radial growth phase.

+ **Lentigo maligna** is a form of in situ melanoma which arises in sun-damaged skin, usually on the face of elderly people. The tumour presents as a variably pigmented, irregular macule or patch which gradually enlarges. The in situ form may be present for as many as 15 years before an invasive melanoma (**lentigo malignant melanoma**) develops within it.

+ **Nodular melanoma** accounts for about 5 per cent of all melanomas and is defined by direct entry into vertical growth phase with no obvious preceding radial growth phase. Clinically it appears as a pigmented nodule with no background flat macule around the nodule. Nodular melanomas generally have a poor prognosis as the majority are thick tumours by the time of presentation. The tumour also often lacks melanin pigment (**amelanotic melanoma**) and may be mistaken for a benign lesion such as a lobular capillary haemangioma.

+ **Acral lentiginous melanoma** is an unusual form of melanoma which occurs on the palms and soles of the feet and beneath the nails (subungual melanoma). Acral melanoma accounts for about 10 per cent of all melanomas in Caucasians, though it is the dominant form of melanoma seen in darker individuals. The tumour is usually located on the feet, with the heel being the most frequently affected region.

Any suspicious pigmented skin lesion should be completely excised for histological analysis

The ABCD guidelines have been developed as a simple way of assessing pigmented lesions for the possibility of melanoma:

+ *Asymmetry.* Most melanomas are asymmetrical; a line through the middle of the lesion does not create matching halves.

+ *Border.* The borders of melanomas are often uneven and may have scalloped or notched edges.

+ *Colour.* Melanomas contain variable shades of pigmentation.

+ *Diameter.* Melanomas tend to be larger than benign nevi, generally at least 6 mm in diameter.

Any suspicious pigmented skin lesion should be surgically removed without delay. An excision biopsy, which removes the entire lesion down to subcutaneous fat with a 2 mm margin of clearance, is recommended. The specimen should be sent for histopathological examination to allow definitive diagnosis of the lesion.

The histopathology report provides a number of important prognostic data

In cases of melanoma, the histopathology report will provide several important prognostic features of the tumour (Table 16.2).

The most important prognostic feature of a melanoma is the **Breslow thickness** which is measured, in millimetres to one decimal point, from the granular layer of the epidermis to the deepest point of invasion by the tumour. The Breslow thickness determines the extent of any

TABLE 16.2 Important histopathological features in malignant melanoma

Histological subtype
In situ or invasive
Radial or vertical growth phase (if invasive)
Breslow thickness
Clark level
Perineural invasion
Vascular invasion
Mitotic activity
Excision margins

further surgical excision that should be performed at the site of the melanoma. Melanomas less than 1 mm thick require a 1 cm margin, whilst melanomas greater than 1 mm in depth should have 2 cm margins.

The **Clark level** of the melanoma relates to the deepest level of the skin that has been invaded by the melanoma. The Clark level is recorded from I to V with increasing depth of invasion. It is still uncertain whether the Clark level is a true prognostic variable independent of the Breslow thickness, but it is still currently included in pathology reports.

Malignant melanoma is capable of wide dissemination

Metastases from a malignant melanoma usually initially involve the regional lymph nodes. Later, haematogenous spread occurs, with widespread dissemination of the tumour. Virtually any organ may be involved by metastatic malignant melanoma, including the central nervous system. Metastatic malignant melanoma does not respond well to chemotherapy or radiotherapy, and carries a poor prognosis.

Key points: Malignant melanoma

- Malignant melanoma is a highly malignant neoplasm derived from melanocytes.

- Sun exposure is the main aetiological factor in melanoma, particularly blistering sunburn in childhood.

- Malignant melanomas may be in situ or invasive.

- Invasive melanomas are classified as being in either radial growth phase (no potential for metastatic spread) or vertical growth phase (metastatic potential).

- There are four main types of melanoma: superficial spreading, nodular, lentigo maligna, and acral lentiginous.

- The ABCD guidelines are helpful in the assessment of pigmented lesions for the possibility of melanoma.

- Any suspicious pigmented skin lesion should be excised completely and sent for histology.

- If histology confirms melanoma, the report will provide a number of important pieces of prognostic information including the Breslow thickness and Clark level.

- Metastatic malignant melanoma is capable of very wide dissemination and does not respond to treatment, making prognosis poor.

Dermatofibrosarcoma protuberans

Dermatofibrosarcoma protuberans is a low grade malignant soft tissue tumour of the dermis

Dermatofibrosarcoma protuberans is a soft tissue tumour of the dermis which behaves as a low grade malignancy. Originally, it was thought to be the malignant counterpart of the dermatofibroma due to their morphological similarities. Now that immunohistochemistry has allowed the derivation of cell type to be determined, it has become clear that the two tumours are quite different.

Dermatofibrosarcoma protuberans is a locally infiltrative tumour which rarely metastasizes. Recently, genetic studies have shown a chromosomal translocation t(17;22) which results in one of the collagen genes being fused next to the platelet-derived growth factor β (PDGF-β) gene. This leads to persistent activation of the PDGF-β receptor and growth stimulation. Of interest, anecdotal success has been achieved in some patients with metastatic dermatofibrosarcoma protuberans treated with the tyrosine kinase inhibitor imatinib, which antagonizes the PDGF-β receptor.

Cutaneous lymphomas

Mycosis fungoides is the most common cutaneous lymphoma and is derived from T lymphocytes

Primary cutaneous lymphomas are lymphomas arising in the skin in the absence of a lymphoma elsewhere that may have spread to the skin secondarily. Primary cutaneous lymphomas are rare, with an incidence of 1 in 100 000 people.

The most common primary cutaneous lymphoma is **mycosis fungoides**, a slowly progressive cutaneous lymphoma in which the neoplastic cells are CD3+, CD4+, CD8−T lymphocytes. Mycosis fungoides passes through three main stages. In the *patch stage*, there are small scaly erythematous patches that are often bizarre in shape, and varied in size and colour. The patch stage may persist for up to 10 years. Over time, the patches become indurated and palpable: the *plaque stage*. Eventually large nodules of tumour appear, heralding the *tumour stage* which has a mean survival of 2–3 years.

The patch stage of mycosis fungoides may be difficult to diagnose, as it mimics common inflammatory skin diseases such as psoriasis or seborrhoeic dermatitis. The plaque and tumour stages are usually more characteristic due to their bizarre shape and asymmetrical distribution. Treatment for mycosis fungoides is not curative, and is aimed at controlling the disease.

Inflammatory skin disorders

Dermatitis

The terms **eczema** and **dermatitis** are synonymous. When used unqualified, they refer to a non-specific reaction pattern of the skin which may develop in response to a wide variety of stimuli. It is convenient to divide dermatitis into **endogenous**, due to internal factors, and **exogenous**, where contact with an external agent is responsible (Table 16.3). In clinical practice, however, the distinction between the two is often blurred.

Clinically, acute dermatitis presents with erythema, papules, and vesicles. The principle symptom of dermatitis is *itching* (pruritus). The absence of itching makes a diagnosis of dermatitis highly unlikely. Continued rubbing and scratching of the skin leads to thickening of the skin (lichenification). Painful cracking and fissuring of the dry thickened skin may occur over joints.

TABLE 16.3 Common forms of dermatitis
Exogenous
Irritant contact dermatitis
Allergic contact dermatitis
Endogenous
Atopic dermatitis
Seborrhoeic dermatitis
Discoid dermatitis

Contact dermatitis

Contact dermatitis occurs when exposure to an external agent leads to loss of the normal barrier function of the skin, and hence an eczematous rash. Contact dermatitis may occur due to exposure to a direct skin irritant, or due to a hypersensitivity response to an environmental antigen.

Contact dermatitis may affect any part of the body, although the hands and face are common sites. The site of the rash is often a helpful clue to the likely agent, although the diagnosis is not often easy as a history of irritant or allergen exposure is not always forthcoming. It is therefore important to inquire exhaustively about the patient's occupation, hobbies, clothing, and use of any topical agents.

Irritant contact dermatitis is due to direct physical damage to the skin

Irritant contact dermatitis may occur acutely after only brief contact with a strong irritant or after prolonged exposure to weaker irritants. It is particularly common in housewives with young children, and in certain occupations. For example, hairdressers spending a large proportion of the day with their hands immersed in shampoo often develop irritant contact dermatitis. Treatment requires avoidance of the responsible irritant, though this may prove extremely difficult, and often all that can be achieved is a reduction in exposure, e.g. by wearing protective gloves.

Allergic contact dermatitis is a hypersensitivity reaction to an external antigen

Allergic contact dermatitis is an example of a type IV delayed hypersensitivity reaction. Exposure of the epidermis to the offending antigen causes to a specific T cell response after 48 h, leading to an inflammatory response in the skin. Previous contact with the antigen is needed to induce sensitivity and, once sensitivity has been established, any areas of skin that subsequently come into contact with the offending antigen will react, and sensitization persists indefinitely.

The most common cause of allergic contact dermatitis is nickel sensitivity, which affects some 10 per cent of women and 1 per cent of men. It often manifests with areas of dermatitis under jewellery, bra clasps, and jean studs. Despite many 'hypoallergenic' cosmetics, hypersensitivity contact dermatitis may still be seen from cosmetics.

Allergic contact dermatitis

The term allergic contact dermatitis is appropriate in European countries where 'allergy' is used to refer to any hypersensitivity reaction. In the USA, where the word 'allergy' is restricted to immediate (type I) hypersensitivity reactions, this can cause confusion because allergic contact dermatitis is due to a type IV hypersensitivity reaction.

Atopic dermatitis

Atopic dermatitis is an extremely common allergic disease of the skin

Atopic dermatitis is extremely common, occurring in up to 5 per cent of the UK population. It is particularly common in early life, with up to 15 per cent of children affected at some point. The prevalence of atopic dermatitis is increasing and now affects as many as 1 in 10 school children.

Atopic dermatitis causes an intensely itchy rash

Atopic dermatitis is thought to develop due to an immediate (type I) hypersensitivity reaction to unknown environmental antigens in the skin (i.e. a true allergic disease). Atopic individuals respond to environmental antigens by producing large amounts of IgE which leads to degranulation of mast cells in the skin and stimulation of inflammation. The histamine from the mast cells stimulates nerve endings, giving rise to an intensely itchy rash.

The distribution and character of the rash of atopic dermatitis changes with age

In infancy, the rash of atopic dermatitis is vesicular and weeping, involving the face and trunk. In childhood, the rash becomes dry and thickened and settles on the backs of the knees, the front of the elbows, wrists, and ankles.

Atopic dermatitis may be secondarily infected by *S. aureus* and herpes simplex

Skin involved by atopic dermatitis is liable to becoming secondarily infected, particularly by *Staphylococcus aureus*, which causes a worsening in symptoms. Infection of atopic dermatitis by herpes simplex virus ('eczema herpeticum') is the most important complication of atopic dermatitis. Crops of vesicles develop in areas of atopic dermatitis, together with fever and general malaise. The systemic upset can be severe, and before the availability of aciclovir could even be fatal.

The potential impact of atopic dermatitis should not be underestimated

Unfortunately, there is no specific treatment for atopic dermatitis. Treatment involves use of emollients to moisturize the skin and topical steroids to reduce the inflammation. Whilst this is often effective in milder cases, severe cases of atopic dermatitis can cause great distress. In older children, it may cause sleep disturbance and problems at school. Lack of sleep may even disturb growth as growth hormone levels rise during deep sleep. Fortunately, complete spontaneous remission of the disease occurs by age 15 in 75 per cent of cases.

Seborrhoeic dermatitis

Seborrhoeic dermatitis is a common skin disease which affects about 1–2 per cent of the population. The lesions of seborrhoeic dermatitis are well defined, dull red, and covered by a greasy scale, making them easily mistaken for psoriasis.

Seborrhoeic dermatitis particularly affects those areas where sebaceous glands are numerous, such as the scalp, forehead, eyelids, ears, and cheeks. Vulval involvement is well recognized in women. Seborrhoeic dermatitis is one of the most common skin disorders seen in patients with HIV.

The exact mechanisms leading to seborrhoeic dermatitis are unclear. Despite the distribution and name of the disease, there is no good evidence of any abnormality of the sebaceous glands in seborrhoeic dermatitis. Most cases of seborrhoeic dermatitis are associated with heavy colonization of the skin by a yeast called *Pityrosporum ovale*, but it is not clear if this is a causal relationship or merely a secondary infection.

Discoid dermatitis

Discoid dermatitis is a chronic recurrent type of dermatitis classically involving the lower limbs of middle-aged males. The cause is unknown. The lesions are well defined, circular or oval, crusted, itchy plaques about 5 cm in size distributed symmetrically on the lower limbs. Classical discoid dermatitis is generally easy to diagnose, but atypical cases may resemble psoriasis, contact dermatitis, and intraepidermal carcinoma. Topical steroids are the most effective means of controlling the condition.

Key points: Dermatitis

◆ Dermatitis, or eczema, are non-specific terms for a reaction pattern of the skin to a variety of stimuli that manifests with an itchy erythematous rash.

◆ Irritant contact dermatitis occurs due to contact with a skin irritant, e.g. shampoo.

◆ Allergic contact dermatitis occurs due to a delayed type hypersensitivity reaction to an exogenous agent, e.g. nickel.

◆ Atopic dermatitis is a common form of dermatitis which affects 10 per cent of children.

◆ Atopic dermatitis is due to an immediate hypersensitivity reaction to unknown environmental allergens in the skin.

◆ Atopic dermatitis starts on the face and trunk of infants and then affects the flexor surfaces of the knees and elbows of older children.

◆ Exacerbations of atopic dermatitis may occur due to secondary infection by *S. aureus* or herpes simplex virus.

◆ Seborrhoeic dermatitis causes well defined dull red lesions covered with greasy scale on the scalp, forehead, eyelids, ears, and cheeks. The cause of seborrhoeic dermatitis is not clear.

◆ Discoid dermatitis causes well defined crusty itchy plaques on the lower limbs of middle aged males.

Psoriasis

Psoriasis is one of the most common inflammatory skin diseases, affecting up to 3 per cent of the population. Psoriasis may start at any age, but most often appears between 15 and 40 years. Most people who develop psoriasis have the disease for the rest of their life.

Many people report the onset following an episode of acute illness or stress.

Psoriasis is characterized by erythematous plaques covered with adherent silvery scale

The typical lesion in psoriasis is the **psoriatic plaque**, a well circumscribed erythematous plaque with a silvery scale (Fig. 16.16). If a psoriatic plaque is biopsied, three key abnormalities are seen: epidermal thickening, vascular proliferation, and an inflammatory cell infiltrate dominated by neutrophils and T lymphocytes.

◆ *Epidermal thickening* is due to excessive epidermal proliferation, reflecting a shortening of the duration of the keratinocyte cell cycle and a doubling of the proliferative cell population. During normal keratinocyte maturation, nuclei are eliminated from cells as they enter the cornified layer. In psoriasis, truncation of the cell cycle leads to accumulation of cells within the cornified layer with retained nuclei, a pattern known as parakeratosis. The thick layer of parakeratotic keratinocytes accounts for the silvery scale of psoriatic plaques.

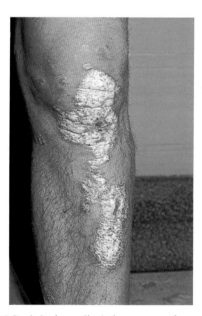

Fig. 16.16 Psoriatic plaque. Classical appearance of untreated psoriatic plaque topped with silvery scales.

+ *Endothelial cell hyperproliferation* in psoriasis yields pronounced dilation, tortuosity, and increased permeability of capillaries in the superficial dermis. These reach high up into the dermal papillae, very close to the skin surface. The vascular alterations contribute to the bright erythema seen clinically and account for the pinpoint bleeding seen when the scale is scraped off the top of a psoriatic plaque.

+ *Inflammatory cell infiltration* of the dermis and epidermis is dominated by neutrophils and T lymphocytes. The neutrophils often form collections in the epidermis called microabscesses or micropustules.

The precise cause of psoriasis remains unknown

Despite intense research, it is still not known why psoriasis develops. There is certainly a strong genetic component, and it is thought that some environmental trigger (infections, drugs, and stress have all been suggested) leads to the development of psoriasis in a genetically susceptible individual. Traditionally, the epidermal proliferation was thought to be the primary problem in psoriasis, but recent evidence has suggested that the primary problem is inflammatory in nature, and that the epidermal proliferation is a response to the inflammatory process driven by T lymphocytes.

There are a number of different patterns of psoriasis

Classical plaque psoriasis is the most common pattern of psoriasis, in which multiple red plaques with a silver scaly surface appear. The plaques may affect any part of the body, but they have a predilection for the extensor surfaces of the knees, elbows, and scalp. Plaque psoriasis usually begins in the teens and early adult life.

Flexural psoriasis may occur in combination with typical plaque psoriasis, but often occurs alone in older adults. The lesions occur in skin folds such as the groin, axillae, and submammary folds. The surface scale is lost, resulting in an erythematous lesion which can closely mimic other inflammatory skin disorders such as seborrhoeic dermatitis.

Guttate psoriasis is a variant which typically develops suddenly in young adults about 2 weeks after a streptococcal sore throat. Multiple small round coin-shaped lesions appear on the trunk and usually resolve rapidly. Guttate psoriasis can closely mimic pityriasis rosea (see later), though the two can usually be distinguished by closely examining the lesions, which are usually round and scaly in psoriasis and oval in pityriasis rosea.

The nails and joints may also be involved in psoriasis

About 50 per cent of patients with psoriasis have nail disease due to involvement of the skin of the nail bed. Common manifestations include pitting of nail (multiple small 0.5–1.0 mm depressions in the nail), onycholysis (separation of the nail edge from the nail bed), and yellow brown discoloration of the nail. Checking the nails for psoriatic involvement may be a very helpful pointer that a skin rash is due to psoriasis rather than some other skin disease.

Psoriatic joint disease, known as psoriatic arthropathy, occurs in about 5 per cent of patients with psoriasis. It may manifest in a variety of ways, but typically there is an asymmetrical swelling of the distal interphalangeal joints of the hands, with sparing of the metacarpophalangeal joints.

LINK BOX

Psoriatic arthropathy

Psoriatic arthropathy is an example of a **spondyloarthropathy** and is mostly seen in psoriasis patients carrying the HLA-B27 allele (p. 413).

Some types of psoriasis can be life threatening

There are some rarer forms of psoriasis which are important to be aware of as they can be extremely severe.

Generalized pustular psoriasis is characterized by the sudden eruption of widespread areas of fiery red skin studded with numerous small sterile pustules. The patient, who usually has no previous history of psoriasis, is systemically unwell with fever.

Erythrodermic psoriasis is most often seen in patients with known psoriasis that is difficult to control or has been neglected. It occurs when many psoriatic plaques merge, leading to confluent involvement of the skin and a state of erythroderma.

Erythroderma

Widespread confluent erythema involving more than 90 per cent of the skin surface is termed **erythroderma**. Erythroderma is life threatening due to complete loss of skin function, leading to fluid loss, temperature failure, and septicaemia. Pre-renal acute renal failure can develop rapidly. The first priority is therefore to stabilize the patient, who may be very unwell. The cause of the erythroderma can then be established. Severe forms of psoriasis and atopic dermatitis are the most common causes of erythroderma.

Key points: Psoriasis

- Psoriasis is a common chronic inflammatory skin disorder characterized by well demarcated erythematous plaques with a silvery scale.

- Psoriatic plaques are thought to develop from keratinocyte hyperproliferation driven by T lymphocytes activated by infections, drugs, and stress in genetically susceptible individuals.

- Plaque psoriasis is the most common pattern of psoriasis. Typical scaly plaques develop on the extensor surfaces of the elbows and knees. The scalp is also often involved. Plaque psoriasis typically develops in the teenage years and early adult life, fluctuating in severity throughout life.

- Flexural psoriasis tends to occur in later life, with well demarcated red plaques in the groins, natal cleft, and vulva. Scaling on top of the plaques is rarely seen, which may lead to difficulty in diagnosis.

- Guttate psoriasis is mostly seen in children and young adults. Numerous small circular plaques abruptly appear over the trunk following a streptococcal pharyngitis.

- About half of all patients with psoriasis develop nail changes which include pitting, onycholysis, and yellow brown discoloration.

- Up to 5 per cent of patients develop psoriatic arthropathy, characterized by asymmetric involvement of the joints of the fingers and toes.

Lichen planus

Lichen planus is a common inflammatory skin disease typically affecting middle-aged adults. The disease is characterized by the appearance of clusters of small, smooth, shiny, flat-topped papules measuring up to 1 cm and often having a violet colour (Fig. 16.17). On close inspection, the surface of the papules have a white streaky pattern (**Wickham's striae**).

The lesions are found most commonly on the flexor aspects of the wrists, the forearms, and the genitals. The lesions may be intensely itchy. Oral involvement is also very common and may be the sole manifestation. Hair follicles can be involved by the disease process and scalp involvement can lead to scarring alopecia.

Skin biopsy shows a tight band of lymphocytes at the dermoepidermal junction with damage to the basal layer of the epidermis. Lichen planus thus appears to represent a T cell-mediated attack on the epidermis, though the aetiology is unknown.

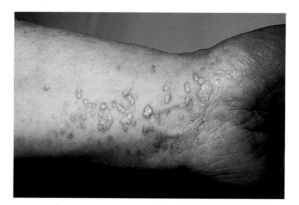

Fig. 16.17 The rash of lichen planus favouring the wrists. The lesions are flat topped, violet, and shiny.

Lichen planus is self-limiting and most cases slowly resolve over a period of 1–2 years. As they resolve, they become darker and flatter, leaving behind brown or grey macules. Management is aimed at relieving itching, and steroid creams are the most effective treatment.

Acne

Acne is an extremely common inflammatory skin disease, predominantly affecting adolescents. It is a cosmetically serious, potentially disfiguring condition which may be associated with considerable suffering in young people who are particularly conscious about their body image.

Acne is a disorder of the pilosebaceous unit

Acne is a disease which originates in the pilosebaceous unit (the hair follicle and its associated sebaceous gland), and the typical distribution on the face, upper back, and chest reflects the areas with the highest concentration of sebaceous glands.

Under the influence of rising levels of androgens in adolescence, the sebaceous glands increase in size and produce more sebum. Obstruction of the pilosebaceous duct by excess sebum allows overgrowth of the bacterium *Propionibacterium acnes*, a normal hair follicle resident, which cleaves triglycerides in sebum into irritant fatty acids, causing inflammation.

Note that there is no evidence to support any role of poor diet, bad hygiene, cosmetics, or lack of exercise in the aetiology or pathogenesis of acne.

Acne is characterized by comedones and inflammatory papules and pustules

The characteristic lesion of acne is the **comedone**, a non-inflammatory lesion which results from obstruction and dilation of the pilosebaceous unit. Closed comedones, or whiteheads, are the first stage of acne, seen as tiny white lesions beneath the skin surface. If they push open the mouth of the hair follicle, they form the open comedone, or blackhead. Inflammation caused by overgrowth of *P. acnes* then causes papules and pustules.

Severe forms of untreated acne may cause permanent scarring

In the most severe forms of acne, rupture of inflamed hair follicles leads to a foreign body-type granulomatous inflammation with the development of inflammatory

cysts, nodules, and scarring. Scarring in acne leads to permanent disfiguration, and prevention of scarring is the principal aim of acne treatment.

LINK BOX

Acne in adult women

It is thought that up to 85% of women with significant acne have the polycystic ovary syndrome (p. 272).

Key points: Acne

- Acne is an extremely common skin disorder of adolescence.

- The characteristic lesion of acne is the comedone, a non-inflammatory lesion caused by obstruction and dilation of a pilosebaceous unit.

- Inflammation within a comedone leads to inflammatory papules and pustules.

- In the most severe form of acne, rupture of inflamed pilosebaceous units leads to marked granulomatous inflammation and the development of nodules and cysts which heal with permanent scarring.

- Treatment of acne is tailored to the individual, though the principal aim is prevention of scarring.

Rosacea

Rosacea is a common inflammatory skin disorder affecting the face of middle-aged people

Rosacea is a common chronic inflammatory skin disease that affects the face of middle-aged people, especially females. Most patients present between ages 30 and 50. The convexities of the face such as the central forehead, nose, cheeks, and chin are most commonly affected, with sparing around the eyes and mouth.

Rosacea has vascular features and inflammatory features

The first manifestation of rosacea is intermittent flushing of the face. Fixed erythema and telangiectasia (prominent small blood vessels in the skin) then follow.

Inflammatory papules and pustules develop later. **Rhinophyma**, a disfiguring enlargement of the nose due to hyperplasia of the sebaceous glands and connective tissue, is a late complication of rosacea which occurs almost exclusively in men.

The diagnosis of rosacea is usually made clinically. Other skin disorders which can mimic rosacea include acne, contact dermatitis of the face, and seborrhoeic dermatitis. Acne may also have inflammatory papules and pustules, but can be distinguished by the presence of comedones which are absent in rosacea. In contact dermatitis, itch is the dominant symptom. Seborrhoeic dermatitis usually affects the nasolabial folds, eyebrows, and scalp.

The pathogenesis of rosacea is unknown. The strong flushing reaction seen in patients with rosacea suggests that there may be an underlying vascular disorder, although this may be a consequence rather than a cause of the condition. The mite *Demodex folliculorum* has also been implicated.

The natural course of rosacea is chronic, with remissions and relapses. As sunlight worsens the condition, daily use of sunscreen is advised, as is avoidance of any potentially irritating topical products on the face. Tetracycline antibiotics are the main mode of treatment, which may be followed by topical metronidazole gel to prolong the period of remission. Their mode of action in rosacea is uncertain, but they are good at controlling the inflammatory papules and pustules; the vascular features respond poorly. Note that topical steroids should not be used for rosacea; they make the condition worse.

Pityriasis rosea

Pityriasis rosea ('rose-coloured scale') is a relatively common disease seen mostly in young adults. The cause remains obscure but is probably related to a virus, the latest suspect being human herpes virus 7. The initial lesion is the 'herald patch', a pink plaque with its long axis along a skin tension line. After a while the herald patch fades, only to be replaced 1–2 weeks later by a widespread eruption of smaller plaques, with their long axes also oriented along skin tension lines. The rash may be asymptomatic, but in some people it may be itchy for a few weeks.

Granuloma annulare

Granuloma annulare is a common asymptomatic inflammatory skin disorder seen mostly in young adults. The lesion consists of several skin-coloured or

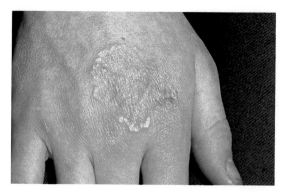

Fig. 16.18 Ring-like lesion of granuloma annulare on the dorsum of the hand.

red papules which coalesce into a ring-shaped plaque about 1–5 cm across. The hands and feet are the most common sites, in particular the knuckles and the dorsum of the hand (Fig. 16.18).

Microscopically, the characteristic appearance of granuloma annulare is the palisading granuloma. This structure has a central core of degenerate collagen surrounded by a radially arranged collection of lymphocytes, macrophages, and fibroblasts.

The cause of granuloma annulare is unknown; however, the presence of a granulomatous process suggests a delayed type hypersensitivity process similar to that seen in tuberculosis or sarcoidosis. There is no convincing evidence of an infectious aetiology, and presumably the lesion is the result of a reaction to an as yet unidentified antigen.

Granuloma annulare rarely requires treatment and has no significant consequences.

Erythema multiforme

Erythema multiforme is a skin reaction which may be provoked by many stimuli. The most commonly identifiable underlying causes are infections, particularly herpes simplex virus and *mycoplasma*, and drugs. In many cases, however, no precipitating factor can be identified.

The lesions of erythema multiforme are most commonly seen on the hands and feet. They start as raised erythematous plaques which expand to give the classic 'target lesion' appearance (Fig. 16.19).

Cases with severe involvement of the eyes and mucosal surfaces are known as erythema multiforme major, or Stevens–Johnson syndrome.

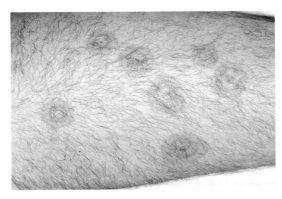

Fig. 16.19 Erythema multiforme on the leg showing typical target lesions.

Pyoderma gangrenosum

Pyoderma gangrenosum is a poorly understood destructive cutaneous disorder characterized by a large necrotic ulcerated lesion. About half of all cases of pyoderma gangrenosum are associated with an underlying disorder, most commonly inflammatory bowel disease and rheumatoid arthritis.

Pyoderma gangrenosum most commonly occurs on the lower legs and trunk. It usually begins as a tender papules and pustules that coalesce to form a large expanding ulcer with well demarcated, raised, violaceous edges.

The diagnosis of pyoderma gangrenosum is based primarily on the clinical history and the appearance of the lesion. Skin biopsy findings are non-specific, but are helpful to rule out a different cause of the ulceration, particularly an ulcerated neoplasm. Oral steroid therapy is the mainstay of treatment, leading to rapid relief of pain and healing of the lesion in most cases.

Erythema nodosum

Erythema nodosum is a clinical syndrome in which numerous tender, warm, bright red nodules suddenly appear over both lower legs. Erythema nodosum is often associated with an underlying cause, particularly infections, drugs, sarcoidosis, and inflammatory bowel disease. About 20 per cent of cases appear to be idiopathic.

Erythema nodosum typically affects young adults, with a marked predilection for women. General malaise and fever often accompany the lesions. As the lesions gradually fade over a period of 3–6 weeks, they may look very similar to bruises. If a lesion is biopsied and examined microscopically, the typical feature seen is chronic inflammation within the fibrous septae that separate lobules of fat in the subcutis, a pattern described as *septal panniculitis*.

The aetiology and pathogenesis of erythema nodosum are unknown. Currently it is thought that erythema nodosum represents a non-specific hypersensitivity reaction involving a mixture of immune complex-mediated and delayed type hypersensitivity patterns.

Blistering disorders of the skin

Blisters occur when fluid accumulates within or underneath the epidermis due to separation of keratinocytes from one another or from the underlying basement membrane. The clinical appearances of the blister depend on the level in the skin at which it forms. Intraepidermal blisters have thin roofs and so rupture easily, leaving an oozing surface, whereas subepidermal blisters have thicker roofs and tend to remain intact and tense.

Various skin diseases may have blistering as part of their clinical spectrum, but there are some skin diseases where blistering is the dominant feature, e.g. pemphigus, pemphigoid, and dermatitis herpetiformis.

Pemphigus

Pemphigus is a blistering disease caused by autoantibodies to intercellular bridges of keratinocytes

Pemphigus is a blistering skin disease affecting middle-aged to elderly adults. Pemphigus is caused by autoantibodies directed at components of the intercellular bridges which link neighbouring keratinocytes together. The epidermis crumbles, forming blisters.

There are several varieties of pemphigus depending on the level in the epidermis at which the blisters occur. In **pemphigus vulgaris**, the more common form, the blisters form deep in the epidermis, leading to persistent flaccid blisters in the skin and mouth. In **pemphigus foliaceus**, the blistering is very superficial, leading to fragile blisters prone to tearing; intact blisters are seldom seen.

Pemphigus is a serious disease which can be difficult to control. Patients should be treated in specialized units. The course is prolonged even with treatment, and the mortality rate remains significant due to a combination of the effects of erythroderma and side effects from the high doses of steroids and immunosuppressive drugs needed to control the disease.

Pemphigoid

Pemphigoid is a blistering disease caused by autoantibodies to the epidermal basement membrane

Pemphigoid is more common than pemphigus and is seen in older people. Pemphigoid is caused by autoantibodies to components of the epidermal basement membrane, leading to splitting of the epidermis from the dermis. Patients present with numerous tense blisters which start on the limbs and then spread to the trunk (Fig. 16.20). The mouth is normally not affected.

Skin biopsy shows blister formation at the dermoepidermal junction. The blisters are typically filled with eosinophils. Immunofluorescence shows a linear band of IgG and C3 along the basement membrane, highlighting where the autoantibodies have bound the basement membrane and activated complement.

Pemphigoid responds well to steroid treatment and requires lower doses than pemphigus. The disease is rarely persistent with treatment, and death is uncommon.

Dermatitis herpetiformis

Dermatitis herpetiformis is a blistering skin disease related to gluten-sensitive enteropathy

Dermatitis herpetiformis is a blistering skin disease in which crops of intensely itchy vesicles appear over the knees, elbows, and buttocks. Intact vesicles do not last for long as the intense pruritus leads to them being scratched away. Dermatitis herpetiformis affects a younger age group than pemphigus and pemphigoid, with most patients presenting in young adulthood.

The pathogenesis is thought to be related to the deposition of IgA in the dermal papillae of the skin which stimulates influx of neutrophils into that area. Release of enzymes from the neutrophils destroys the adhesion of the epidermis to the basement membrane, cleaving the epidermis from the dermis and forming a vesicle.

Often the clinical picture is characteristic enough to be diagnostic, but if the lesions are biopsied masses of fibrin and neutrophils are seen at the tops of the dermal papillae. If an intact vesicle is biopsied, the split at the dermoepidermal junction can be seen. Immunofluorescence reveals deposits of IgA in the superficial dermis.

It is thought that all patients with dermatitis herpetiformis have gluten-sensitive enteropathy (coeliac disease). Many will not be symptomatic, and so IgA endomysial antibodies should be measured and a duodenal biopsy taken.

The clinical response of dermatitis herpetiformis to **dapsone** is dramatic, and the drug is often administered for diagnostic as well as therapeutic purposes. Relief from itching occurs within hours of starting the drug and soon after the rash begins to clear. A gluten-free diet results in prolonged remission.

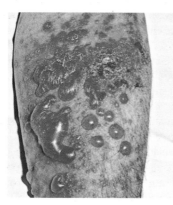

Fig. 16.20 Large, tense, raised blisters of pemphigoid.

LINK BOX

Dapsone-induced haemolysis

Dapsone is a known cause of drug-induced haemolysis, particularly when given at high doses, due to direct oxidant stress to red blood cells. Patients with glucose-6-phosphate dehydrogenase deficiency (p. 339) are at particular risk. Monitoring of the full blood count is therefore important in patients started on dapsone.

Key points: Blistering skin diseases

♦ Blisters are accumulations of fluid either within the epidermis or just beneath the epidermis due to separation of keratinocytes from one another or from the epidermal basement membrane.

Key points: Blistering skin diseases—cont'd

- The appearance of blisters depends on the level of the split. Superficial blisters tend to rupture leaving weeping erosions, whereas deep blisters remain intact and tense.

- Blistering may be a feature of a number of skin disorders, but there are three common skin diseases in which blistering is the dominant feature.

- Pemphigus is a severe, potentially life-threatening blistering disease caused by autoantibodies to adhesion molecules between keratinocytes within the epidermis. Patients present with numerous delicate blisters which often rupture. Involvement of the mouth is common. Treatment requires high doses of steroid and immunosuppressive drugs. Mortality remains high despite treatment.

- Pemphigoid is a blistering disease of the elderly due to autoantibodies to components of the dermoepidermal junction. Numerous tense intact blisters occur. The mouth is not involved. The disease responds well to low doses of steroids and typically resolves within 1–2 years. Death due to pemphigoid is not common.

- Dermatitis herpetiformis is a blistering skin disease in which crops of intensely itchy vesicles appear over the knees, elbows, and buttocks. All patients are thought to have underlying gluten-sensitive enteropathy, even if it is not symptomatic at the time of diagnosis. The skin disorder responds dramatically to dapsone, though continued remission usually requires a lifelong gluten-free diet.

Skin infections

Skin infections are common, as the skin is constantly exposed to microorganisms which may establish infection if the skin is broken through minor trauma. Infections may also complicate other skin disorders due to breakdown of normal skin defences. Bacteria, fungi, and viruses are all common causes of skin infections.

Impetigo

Impetigo is a highly infectious skin infection limited to the epidermis

Impetigo is a superficial skin infection seen most often in childhood. It occurs when minor skin abrasions become contaminated with *S. aureus*. Once extremely common, impetigo is now seen less often in the UK due to improved social conditions.

The infection causes groups of small vesicles which readily burst, leaving a thick yellow crust stuck to the skin with surrounding erythema. The mouth and nose are the most common sites of involvement. The lesions spread rapidly and are highly contagious. Localized impetigo is treated with saline soaks and application of a topical antibiotic such as fusidic acid. More widespread infection requires oral flucloxacillin or erythromycin.

Cellulitis

Cellulitis is a common infection of the subcutaneous tissue

Cellulitis is a bacterial infection of subcutaneous tissue, usually caused by *S. aureus* or *Streptococcus pyogenes*. Infection develops within hours to days following trauma to the skin, rapidly producing an area of hot, red, swollen skin. The edge of the lesion is usually ill defined. There may be signs of systemic infection such as fever and tachycardia.

Cellulitis commonly affects the lower leg as small breaks in the skin often occur here. Cellulitis of the lower leg can mimic the clinical picture of a deep venous thrombosis, and thrombosis should always be excluded before presuming that the diagnosis is cellulitis. Presumptive treatment of cellulitis in adults is with benzylpenicillin (targeting *S. pyogenes*) and flucloxacillin (targeting *S. aureus*).

Dermatophytoses

Dermatophytoses are the most common fungal skin infections

Dermatophytes are a group of related fungi capable of causing skin infection known as **dermatophytosis** or 'ringworm'. The infection is spread by direct contact and so often thrives in communal showers and public swimming pools.

The organisms are able to adhere to keratinocytes and penetrate between them, leading to an inflammatory response which gives rise to the skin lesion. Most patients with dermatophytosis are otherwise well, though immunosuppressed patients (e.g. those with HIV or those taking steroids) have a higher frequency of infection.

The type of dermatophytosis is named according to the location of the infection:

- **Tinea pedis** is the most common dermatophytosis and occurs between the toe clefts ('athlete's foot'). Infection is predisposed to by occlusion of the toe clefts by shoes, and by a moist environment. The skin appears white and macerated.

- **Tinea cruris** refers to dermatophytosis of the groin, which typically appears as well demarcated erythematous patches.

- **Tinea capitis** refers to scalp dermatophytosis, leading to scaling lesions associated with areas of hair loss.

- **Tinea corporis** occurs elsewhere on the body as a scaly erythematous patch (Fig. 16.21). This type may be confused with superficial basal cell carcinomas, intraepidermal carcinoma, discoid dermatitis, or psoriasis.

A clinical suspicion of dermatophytosis is usually confirmed by scraping the skin and sending the material for microscopy and culture. Milder dermatophyte infections may be self-limiting but can be treated with

Fig. 16.21 Scaling lesion of tinea corporis on the trunk.

a topical antifungal. The imidazole antifungals such as clotrimazole, ketoconazole, and miconazole are all effective treatments.

Candida albicans causes a variety of superficial skin infections

The yeasts, particularly *Candida albicans*, cause a number of superficial infections associated with moist surfaces subject to regular friction: most commonly the submammary folds in obese women and the groins and buttocks of babies.

Viral warts

Viral warts are caused by infection with human papillomavirus

Common warts (verrucae vulgaris) are caused by infection with human papillomavirus (HPV). Warts may occur anywhere on the skin, but are most common on the soles of the feet (plantar warts) and fingers. HPV types 1 and 4 tend to cause plantar warts, and types 2, 3, and 10 cause fingers warts. They are the result of epithelial overgrowth in response to viral infection of keratinocytes. They persist for a few months and then usually regress spontaneously as cell-mediated immunity to HPV develops.

Molluscum contagiosum

Molluscum contagiosum is caused by a pox virus

Molluscum contagiosum is a skin infection seen mainly in children or young adults caused by a pox virus. Spread occurs by contact with an infected individual, including sexually and on towels. The lesions are usually multiple and grouped, seen particularly on the face, neck, and trunk, appearing as pearly pink papules with a punctum on the surface. If the papules are squeezed, they liberate thick cheesy material full of viral particles.

Herpes simplex virus infection

Herpes simplex virus infection leads to recurrent vesicular eruptions

Herpes simplex is a very common viral infection caused by herpes simplex virus 1 (HSV-1) and HSV-2. Historically, HSV-1 was restricted to oral infections and HSV-2 to genital infections, but nowadays this distinction is very blurred due to the high frequency of orogenital contact.

Both viruses are highly contagious and are transmitted through traumatized skin by exposure to contaminated secretions. The virus replicates within epithelial cells, eventually destroying them and causing vesicles. The vesicles erode easily and may be very painful.

During the primary infection, the virus attaches to and enters cutaneous sensory nerves, followed by spread into the nucleus of the nerve cell in the dorsal root ganglion. The virus establishes latent infection in the dorsal root ganglion without expression of any viral proteins, allowing it to escape immune detection. Infection is lifelong and the virus may intermittently re-emerge and cause recurrent disease in the distribution of the sensory nerve.

Recurrent HSV attacks are usually less severe than the initial attack, and may be precipitated by intercurrent illness, stress, menstruation, and pregnancy. Repeated recurrences are almost inevitable with genital infection and common with oro-facial infection.

LINK BOX

HSV and erythema multiforme

Herpes simplex virus is the most common identifiable cause of erythema multiforme (p. 390).

Varicella zoster virus infection

Varicella zoster virus causes chickenpox and shingles

Varicella zoster virus (VZV) is a herpes virus which infects virtually every human during childhood. Infection is acquired either by inhalation of infected respiratory secretions or by direct skin contact from skin lesions of an infected person. Following infection, the virus infects macrophages and is then carried to lymphoid tissues where the virus slowly replicates.

After about 1 week, the virus enters the blood in monocytes, infecting multiple epithelial sites including the skin, respiratory tract, and mouth. In the skin, the characteristic vesicular rash of chickenpox appears, initially on the trunk, then on the face and scalp. The lesions are deeper than the vesicles of HSV, and scarring is more likely to occur.

During primary infection, VZV enters sensory nerve endings and establishes a latent infection in sensory neurones. Later in life, the virus may reactivate, travelling down the sensory nerve to the skin causing a painful vesicular rash to appear on the area of skin supplied by that nerve (shingles). The typical location for shingles is over the trunk. The vesicles occur in crops, crust over, and resolve over a period of 3–4 weeks. Some patients suffer from severe, persistent pain in the area after the rash has resolved (post-herpetic neuralgia).

Key points: Skin infections

- Impetigo is a highly infectious skin infection caused by *S. aureus* which usually occurs in children.

- Cellulitis is a subcutaneous skin infection caused by *S. aureus* or *S. pyogenes* that commonly affects the lower limb.

- Dermatophytoses are superficial fungal skin infections commonly occurring between the toes (tinea pedis), in the groin (tinea cruris), on the scalp (tinea capitis), or on the trunk (tinea corporis).

- *Candida albicans* commonly infects moist skin of the submammary fold of obese women and the groins of nappy-wearing babies.

- Viral warts are common lesions of the hands and feet caused by human papillomavirus.

- Molluscum contagiosum, caused by infection with a pox virus, manifests with crops of small pink papules with a surface punctum.

- Herpes simplex virus infection causes crops of vesicles around the mouth or genital tract. The virus establishes latent infection in dorsal root ganglia and can reactivate later in life, causing recurrent skin lesions.

- Varicella zoster causes a widespread vesicular rash following initial infection (chicken pox). The virus then establishes latent infection in sensory neurones and can reactivate in later life, manifesting with a painful vesicular rash in the distribution of a dermatome (shingles).

Common miscellaneous skin conditions

Fibroepithelial polyps (skin tags) are little wrinkled polypoid lesions which may appear anywhere on the body, but the neck is a favourite spot. Microscopically they are composed of soft fibrous tissue covered by unremarkable epidermis. They are often removed because they catch on clothing.

Epidermal cysts are common lesions which usually occur as firm lumps on the scalp, face, behind the ears, and on the trunk. They have a punctum which if squeezed yields cheesy material composed of keratin. They are often erroneously called 'sebaceous cysts', but they have nothing to do with sebaceous glands. Histologically, epidermal cysts are divided into epidermoid cysts which are lined by normal-appearing epidermis, and pilar cysts which are lined by hair follicle epithelium.

Campbell de Morgan spots are benign capillary proliferations, often seen as small red papules on the trunk of adults.

INTERESTING TO KNOW

Gardner's syndrome

Multiple deforming epidermoid cysts may be seen as part of **Gardner's syndrome**, an inherited condition in which there are also osteomas of the jaw and multiple polyps in the colon.

Drug-induced skin disease

The skin is one of the most common organs involved by side effects of drugs. Drug eruptions may mimic virtually any type of skin disease and are common, occurring in some 3 per cent of all hospital inpatients. A thorough drug history should be taken from any patient with a rash in an attempt to link an offending drug to the onset of the eruption. Particularly common offenders include antibiotics (especially penicillins) and non-steroidal anti-inflammatory drugs. A number of patterns of drug eruptions are recognized:

- **Maculopapular eruption**. This is the most common form of drug eruption, with a widespread itchy maculopapular rash which usually begins a few days after starting the drug and usually fades by 1 week after stopping the drug.

- **Erythema multiforme**. Drugs are one of the more common precipitating causes of erythema multiforme.

- **Urticaria** and **angiooedema**. An urticarial skin rash occurs due to degranulation of mast cells with the appearance of weals. Weals are pale pink, oedematous, itchy papules and plaques which always last less than 24 h and leave no mark. In up to half of all cases, there is also swelling of the face and mouth, known as angiooedema. The most severe forms may lead to an anaphylactic reaction which can be fatal if not treated rapidly.

- **Fixed drug eruption**. A fixed drug eruption is a curious phenomenon in which a solitary red macule or patch arises upon exposure to the drug, which then resolves when the drug is withdrawn. Upon re-exposure, the rash reappears *at the same site*, hence the term 'fixed' drug eruption.

Skin burns

Burns are important causes of skin injury. Most are minor and do not require medical intervention. Every year there are over 12 000 hospital admissions in the UK due to burns, and children under 5 years account for nearly half of all severe burns. About half of these occur in the kitchen, with scalds from hot liquids being the most frequent type of injury in children.

Burns can be categorized according to the depth of the damage:

- First degree: necrosis of epidermis only

- Second degree: necrosis of epidermis and superficial dermis

- Third degree: necrosis of full thickness of the skin including skin appendages

- Fourth degree: necrosis also involves subcutaneous fat or deeper.

First and second degree burns are collectively referred to as partial thickness burns and are painful. Third and fourth degree burns are called full thickness burns and are painless because the nerve endings have been destroyed.

Burns affecting more than 15 per cent of the total body surface area are serious, provoking massive loss of fluid with hypovolaemic shock and risk of secondary infection. Multiorgan failure due to sepsis is the leading cause of death in patients sustaining severe burns.

Partial thickness burns have the capacity to heal rapidly because of the presence of viable dermal components. Re-epithelialization occurs from both the base and the edge of the burn. Full thickness burns only heal from the edge and therefore healing is slow, with scar formation and impaired function.

Further reading

www.bad.org.uk, British Association of Dermatologists.

Bone, joint, and soft tissue disease

Introduction

Bone, joint, and soft tissue diseases are very common, particularly in primary care. In hospitals, these diseases are treated by rheumatologists and orthopaedic surgeons. This chapter will concentrate on common and important conditions seen in both primary and secondary care.

Bone disease

Normal bone

The bones of the skeleton have a number of important functions. As well as providing support and protection for the body, bones act as a reservoir for minerals such as calcium and phosphate, and provide a suitable microenvironment to support haematopoiesis.

Bone is composed of a basic protein scaffold ('matrix') called **osteoid** which is hardened by the deposition of **hydroxyapatite** ($Ca_{10}(PO_4)_6(OH)_2$) in a process called **mineralization**. Osteoid is composed predominantly of type 1 collagen, together with a number of proteins of uncertain function such as osteopontin, osteonectin, and osteocalcin.

Bones are made up of an outer cortex and a central medulla

The outer shell of all bones, the **cortex**, is composed of strong cortical bone which supports load bearing.

The central part of the bone, the **medulla**, contains a meshwork of trabecular bone between which lies the fatty bone marrow where haematopoiesis occurs. Trabecular bone is metabolically more active than cortical bone and is therefore more prone to metabolic bone diseases such as osteoporosis.

Bones may be described according to their shape and maturity

Bones are often described according to their shape. Examples of **long bones** include the humerus and phalanx (the latter being a miniature long bone). Long bones consist of three parts: metaphysis, diaphysis, and epiphysis (Fig. 17.1). The scapula and occipital bone are examples of **flat bones**. The bones that make up the wrist and ankles are **short bones**.

Two major cell types are found in bone, osteoblasts and osteoclasts

Osteoblasts synthesize and secrete osteoid and also play a significant role in the mineralization process. The enzyme alkaline phosphatase present on the osteoblast cell surface raises local concentrations of calcium and phosphate, favouring deposition of hydroxyapatite. Osteoblasts also express receptors that bind hormones controlling bone growth such as parathyroid hormone, vitamin D, oestrogen, and glucocorticoids.

Osteoclasts resorb bone by attaching to the surface of bony tissue. Osteoclasts have a ruffled border, creating tiny spaces between the cell and the bone into which they secrete acid, which solubilizes the mineral component of bone, and enzymes that digest osteoid.

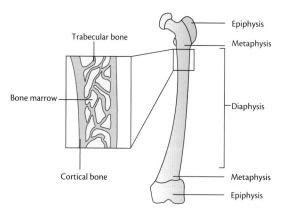

Fig. 17.1 Anatomy of a long bone.

LINK BOX

Alkaline phosphatase

Some alkaline phosphate derived from osteoblasts enters the circulation where it can be detected in blood samples. Raised serum alkaline phosphatase levels may be seen in conditions of rapid bone turnover such as Paget's disease (p. 404). Remember that alkaline phosphatase is also present on biliary epithelial cells and may also be raised in conditions causing biliary damage such as primary biliary cirrhosis (p. 189) and primary sclerosing cholangitis (p. 190).

The mature skeleton is a dynamic structure which is constantly remodelling

Bone is not an inert tissue; it is constantly undergoing renewal. **Remodelling** is the process by which old bone is removed and subsequently replaced by new bone. This cyclical process is mediated by a complex interaction between osteoclasts and osteoblasts, under the control of a large number of cytokines and growth factors.

During childhood and early adulthood, the rate of bone remodelling is high; bone formation by osteoblasts exceeds osteoclastic resorption, with a net increase in bone. At skeletal maturity, which occurs between the ages of 25 and 35, the peak bone mass is reached. From this age onwards, bone remodelling serves to repair tiny areas of stress-induced damage to the skeleton, maintaining its structure and strength.

After about 40 years of age, osteoclastic activity begins to uncouple from osteoblastic activity. The increased bone resorption compared with bone formation leads to a gradual slow loss of bone mass. In females, there is a phase of accelerated bone loss for approximately 5 years immediately after the menopause due to lack of oestrogen, before slowing down to the usual rate of loss as mentioned above.

Metabolic bone disease

Metabolic bone disease refers to a group of disorders in which there is some disturbance of bone formation and/or resorption. They include osteoporosis, Paget's disease, and osteomalacia (Table 17.1).

TABLE 17.1	Metabolic bone diseases	
Disease	**Typical presentation**	**Frequency**
Osteoporosis	Back pain	Common
	Loss of height	
	Fracture	
Paget's disease	Deformity of long bones	Common
	Pain in hips	
Osteomalacia	Generalized bone pain	Uncommon
	Muscle weakness	

Osteoporosis

Osteoporosis is the most common metabolic bone disorder

Osteoporosis is an extremely common disorder characterized by a generalized reduction in bone mass, resulting in increased bone fragility and predisposition to fracture (Fig. 17.2). Of those people surviving to the age of 80, one in three women and one in five men will go on to suffer a hip fracture due to osteoporosis. An estimated 3 million people in the UK suffer from osteoporosis, and each year more than 230 000 osteoporosis-related fractures occur, costing the NHS over £1.7 billion each year (£5 million every day!).

Bone mass in later life depends on the peak bone mass and the rate of bone loss

Bone mass in later life is a reflection of the peak bone mass attained in early adulthood and the subsequent

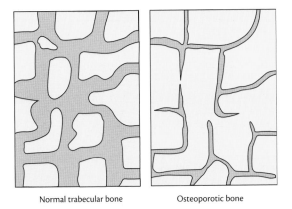

Normal trabecular bone   Osteoporotic bone

Fig. 17.2 Microarchitecture of normal and osteoporotic bone showing marked loss of trabecular bone.

JARGON BUSTER

Osteopetrosis

Be careful not to confuse osteoporosis with **osteopetrosis**. Osteopetrosis, which is much rarer than osteoporosis, is a genetic disease characterized by abnormal osteoclast function and the formation of heavy brittle bones made entirely of woven bone; these are extremely susceptible to fracture.

rate of age-related bone loss (Fig. 17.3). If peak bone mass is low, then the chance of developing osteoporosis will be higher. Genetic factors strongly influence peak bone mass, including polymorphisms of the collagen type IA1 gene. Nutrition and physical activity are also important.

Increasing age is associated with a slow but relentless loss of bone mass due to decreasing bone turnover as osteoblastic activity declines and osteoclastic activity increases. Other important factors in age-related bone loss include declining levels of physical activity and reduced calcium absorption from the gut.

In women, oestrogen deficiency markedly accelerates bone loss after the menopause. Post-menopausal bone loss is very rapid due to a marked increase in osteoclastic activity. It is thought that oestrogen deficiency reduces apoptosis of osteoclasts.

A number of other factors may also contribute to osteoporosis, most notably glucocorticoid therapy and several diseases (Table 17.2).

Glucocorticoid therapy is by far the most important exogenous factor in osteoporosis

The impact of glucocorticoids as an iatrogenic cause of osteoporosis has led to the formulation of national guidelines specifically for glucocorticoid-induced osteoporosis in the UK. Loss of bone mineral density occurs within a few months of starting therapy and is associated with a significant risk of fracture of the hip and spine. Furthermore, glucocorticoids appear to increase fracture risk beyond just the effect of lowering bone mineral density. Thus, for any given bone mineral density, the risk of fracture is higher in glucocorticoid-induced osteoporosis than in straightforward age-related osteoporosis.

Steroids exert their effects on bone in a number of ways. They decrease osteoblast activity and their active life span. Steroids also decrease calcium absorption

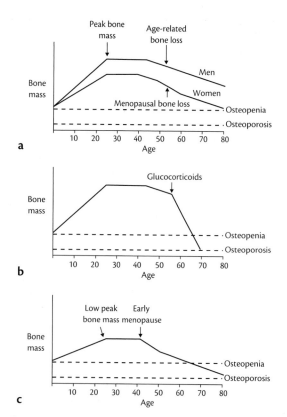

a

b

c

Fig. 17.3 Examples of pathways to osteoporosis. (a) Peak bone mass is achieved in early adulthood followed by slow age-related bone loss. In women, there is an accelerated period of bone loss during the menopause. (b) This male patient develops osteoporosis due to therapeutic administration of glucocorticoids. (c) This female patient develops osteoporosis because she failed to reach peak bone mass for genetic reasons and had an early menopause.

TABLE 17.2 Factors causing a reduction in bone mass
Glucocorticoid treatment
Cushing's syndrome
Hyperthyroidism
Hyperparathyroidism
Gluten-sensitive enteropathy
Inflammatory bowel disease

from the intestine and increase renal calcium loss. Sex hormone production is also suppressed, and the resulting hypogonadism may result in increased bone turnover and bone loss.

Osteoporotic fractures are known as fragility fractures

Osteoporosis is clinically silent until fracture occurs. Most fractures that occur in osteoporotic bones are **fragility fractures**, defined as fractures that occur spontaneously or following a fall from a standing height or less. The most common sites of osteoporotic fractures are the vertebrae, distal radius (Colles' fracture), and the neck of the femur (Fig. 17.4).

Vertebral fractures may occur spontaneously or after simple manoeuvres such as lifting or bending down. Multiple vertebral fractures lead to a loss of height and spinal deformity, typically a thoracic kyphosis.

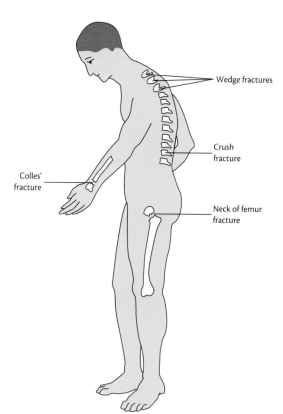

Fig. 17.4 Common fragility fractures in osteoporosis.

Colles' fractures typically occur following a fall on to the outstretched hand. Reduction of the fracture can usually be achieved in the emergency department under local anaesthetic, followed by immobilization in a plaster cast for several weeks. Although there may be problems with long-term deformities after the fracture, recovery is generally satisfactory.

Fractures of the neck of the femur are the most problematic of all the osteoporotic fractures as they necessitate hospital admission and surgical intervention. Because most patients are frail and elderly, postoperative morbidity and mortality are high.

Osteoporosis is diagnosed by dual energy X-ray absorptiometry

Standard radiographs cannot reliably assess bone mass, and blood tests are not helpful either (serum calcium, phosphorus, and alkaline phosphatase levels are all normal in osteoporosis). The best validated technique for measurement of bone density is **dual energy X-ray absorptiometry** (DEXA). Osteoporosis is defined as a bone density more than 2.5 standard deviations below the mean. This value has been chosen because a bone density below this level is associated with a high risk of fracture and is a strong indication for treatment.

At present, screening the entire population for osteoporosis with densitometry is not justified as it is not cost effective. Only patients with symptoms or signs suggestive of osteoporosis, or patients known to be at risk of osteoporosis, undergo densitometry (Table 17.3).

JARGON BUSTER

Osteopenia versus osteoporosis

Note that a bone density between 1 and 2.5 standard deviations below the mean is defined as **osteopenia**. Osteopenia is therefore also a condition of low bone mass, but is not severe enough to increase the risk of fracture significantly.

TABLE 17.3 Indications for performing bone densitometry

Fragility fracture
Loss of height or thoracic kyphosis
Glucocorticoid therapy
Disease associated with osteoporosis, e.g. hyperparathyroidism

TABLE 17.4 Drug options for osteoporosis

Bisphosphonates
Raloxifene
Teriparatide
Strontium ranelate

Management of osteoporosis

Patients with osteoporosis should be treated to strengthen their bones and prevent osteoporotic fractures. The mainstay of treatment of osteoporosis is with drugs that inhibit bone resorption and/or stimulate bone formation (Table 17.4).

First line agents in most cases of osteoporosis are **bisphosphonates** (inhibit bone resorption) and **strontium ranelate** (inhibits bone resorption and stimulates bone formation) as these reduce fractures at all three major sites (hip, spine, and wrist). Most patients are also given calcium and vitamin D supplements, although there is doubt over their benefit in osteoporosis.

Key points: Osteoporosis

- Osteoporosis is a generalized reduction in bone mass associated with a risk of fragility fracture.

- The most common fractures associated with osteoporosis are fractures of the hip, wrist, and vertebrae.

- Bone mass in later life is related to the peak bone mass achieved in early adulthood and the rate of age-related bone mass. Oestrogen deficiency in post-menopausal women causes rapid bone loss.

- A number of secondary factors increase the rate of bone loss, of which the most common is glucocorticoid treatment.

- Osteoporosis is clinically silent until a fracture occurs. Vertebral fractures lead to loss of height and thoracic kyphosis. Colles' fractures and hip fractures present acutely following a fall and require hospital admission.

- Patients known to be at risk of osteoporosis should undergo bone densitometry. Osteoporosis is defined as a bone density more than 2.5 standard deviations below the mean.

Paget's disease of bone

Paget's disease of bone is the second most common metabolic bone disease after osteoporosis, and the UK has the highest incidence in the world.

The hallmark of Paget's disease is excessive and disorganized bone turnover

Paget's disease is characterized by increased chaotic bone turnover in localized parts of the skeleton. The disease passes through a number of stages, all of which may be seen simultaneously either within the same bone or within different bones. Initially, there is intense osteoclastic bone resorption followed by frantic bone formation by osteoblasts in response to the bony destruction. The osteoblastic activity then becomes overexaggerated with the laying down of grossly thickened, weak bone prone to pathological fracture.

Quite what causes this bizarre behaviour remains unknown. A viral cause has long been suggested because viral inclusions have been seen in the osteoclasts of Pagetoid bone on electron microscopy. Subsequent work, however, has failed unequivocally to prove a viral aetiology.

Pain and bony deformity are the most common symptoms of Paget's disease

The vast majority of patients with Paget's disease are completely asymptomatic, and in many patients the diagnosis is made incidentally on a radiograph performed for some other reason (Fig. 17.5). Probably fewer than 5 per cent of patients have symptoms, which is usually bony pain related to stretching of the periosteum overlying areas of thickened bone. Clinically the affected bones are enlarged, deformed, and warm. The enlargement is particularly evident in the tibia and the skull.

Suspicion of Paget's disease may be easily confirmed on radiography of the affected bone and by measurement of serum alkaline phosphatase, which is markedly raised in Paget's disease due to the intense osteoblastic activity. Serum calcium is usually normal in Paget's disease.

Pathological fracture, deafness, and osteosarcoma are important complications of Paget's disease

Although most patients with Paget's disease do not suffer any significant problems from the disease, there are some important possible complications. Pathological fracture is a risk because Pagetoid bone is weak. Enlargement of skull bones may compress the VIIIth

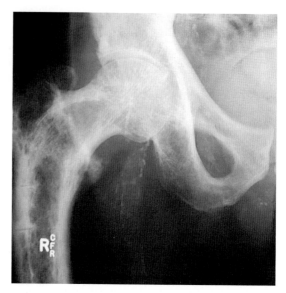

Fig. 17.5 This right femur shows a thickened cortex and bone sclerosis caused by Paget's disease. Incidentally, the hip joint also shows the features of osteoarthritis with loss of the joint space.

cranial nerve, causing profound deafness which is poorly responsive to treatment.

The most dreaded complication of Paget's disease is the development of the malignant bone neoplasm **osteosarcoma**. Although this only occurs in less than 1 per cent of all patients, it carries a very poor prognosis. Osteosarcoma should always be considered in a patient known to have Paget's disease if their pain rapidly worsens. For some reason, the humerus appears to be a particularly high risk site.

Key points: Paget's disease

- Paget's disease is a common metabolic bone disease of unknown aetiology in which there is increased bone turnover in localized areas of the skeleton.

- Only about 5 per cent of patients with Paget's disease are symptomatic, usually presenting with bone pain. The diagnosis is usually obvious on the basis of the clinical picture, supportive radiology, and a raised alkaline phosphatase level.

- The main complications of Paget's disease are pathological fracture, deafness, and osteosarcoma.

Osteomalacia

Osteomalacia is characterized by inadequate mineralization of osteoid, leading to softening of the bone. In children, the disease is called **rickets**.

Osteomalacia is usually due to vitamin D deficiency

Although in theory osteomalacia may occur if there is deficiency of calcium, phosphorus, or vitamin D, in practice virtually all cases are due to vitamin D deficiency. Osteomalacia due to low calcium or phosphate is extremely rare.

In the UK, the people most at risk of vitamin D deficiency are those who get little exposure to sunlight, as most vitamin D is produced in the skin by the action of UV light. Immigrants from Asia, particularly women and children, are at risk of osteomalacia as people with dark skin living in areas where there is less daily sunlight are less efficient at producing vitamin D, and traditional dress such as the burka stops sunlight falling on the skin.

Elderly people confined to home are also at risk of osteomalacia due to lack of sunlight, as are patients with gluten-sensitive enteropathy and Crohn's disease due to malabsorption of vitamin D.

Osteomalacia causes bony pain and muscle weakness

The main symptoms of osteomalacia are diffuse bony pain and muscle weakness. The non-specific nature of the symptoms means that the diagnosis of osteomalacia is often delayed by 2 or 3 years.

The bony pain of osteomalacia does not normally affect any one particular part of the body, and there is usually no other indication that anything is wrong. Backache is common, and sometimes a minor knock on a bone, such as the shin, is unusually painful. Sitting or lying down relieves the pain. As the disease gets worse, pain is felt everywhere, and any movement can be painful.

Some of the pain in osteomalacia is caused by slight cracks in the bone (microfractures) which are visible on radiographs as **Looser's zones**, named after the doctor who first described them. Occasionally the cracks can lead to complete breaks, but once treatment for osteomalacia begins the cracks will heal normally.

Muscle weakness in osteomalacia is thought to be related to phosphate depletion in the muscle cells resulting in disturbed glycolysis, and decreased vitamin D resulting in diminished calcium uptake by sarcoplasmic reticulum.

Alkaline phosphatase levels are raised in osteomalacia due to increased osteoblastic activity. Serum calcium is either normal or slightly low in osteomalacia; it is maintained by parathyroid hormone at the expense of the mineralization of the bone.

Key points: Osteomalacia

- Osteomalacia is bone softening due to defective mineralization of bone.

- Osteomalacia is almost always due to vitamin D deficiency as a result of lack of sun exposure. Asian immigrants and the elderly are most at risk of the disease.

- Malabsorption of vitamin D may also lead to osteomalacia in patients with gluten-sensitive enteropathy or Crohn's disease.

- The main symptoms of osteomalacia are bony pain and muscle weakness. The weakened bone is prone to microfractures and complete fractures.

- Blood tests reveal a raised alkaline phosphatase. Serum calcium is either normal or slightly low.

- Treatment involves increasing sunlight exposure and vitamin D.

Bone fractures

A **fracture** is a complete or partial interruption of a bony surface following trauma. The bones most commonly fractured are those at the wrist, ankle, and hip joints. The clinical consequence of fractures is highly variable, ranging from no symptoms to death. The outcome following a fracture depends on the site, the severity of the force causing the fracture, and the general health of the patient.

Fractures occurring in a bone weakened by a disease process are called **pathological fractures**, and typically occur due to a force that would not ordinarily fracture a healthy bone. The most common causes of pathological fracture are osteoporosis, bony metastases, myeloma, and Paget's disease.

Accurately describing a fracture is important to communicate the important information about the injury rapidly between people caring for the patient. Commonly used terms include the following:

- Incomplete or complete. Complete fractures result in two or more separated pieces of bone. A comminuted fracture is one resulting in the formation of multiple splintered fragments.

- Undisplaced or displaced. Displaced fractures refer to those where the normal contour of the bone is not maintained following fracture.

- Open or closed. If the site of the fracture is near a break in the skin, the fracture may be described as open; if the skin is intact, then it is a closed fracture.

- Stable or unstable. A stable fracture is one that is unlikely to move any further. An unstable fracture is one that will continue to move unless action is taken to secure the fracture.

Fractures heal by a sequence of procallus, bony callus, and modelling

Healing of fractures begins with the formation of **procallus** at the fracture site. Procallus is analogous to the granulation tissue of other healing sites. After a week, procallus is converted into bony callus by the action of osteoblasts. In the last phase, the new bone is modelled along the lines of mechanical force operating at that site.

Bones can only heal with correct alignment if the fractured ends of the bones are approximated and the bones immobilized. In many fractures, this can be achieved by manipulation under local anaesthesia followed by immobilization in a plaster cast. If the fracture is more complicated, adequate positioning of the bones may require general anaesthesia and the placing of nails or plates and screws by an orthopaedic surgeon.

Key points: Bone fracture

- A fracture is a partial or complete interruption of a bone surface following trauma.

- Fractures occurring in diseased bone after trivial trauma are known as pathological fractures, and may be seen in osteoporosis, Paget's disease, myeloma, and bones infiltrated by metastatic tumour.

- Fractures may be described in a number of ways including incomplete/complete, undisplaced/displaced, open/closed, and stable/unstable.

- Successful healing of fractures requires close approximation of the broken ends and immobilization. In complex fractures, this may require fixation under general anaesthesia.

Osteomyelitis

Osteomyelitis is most often due to direct implantation of bacteria in bone following injury or surgery

The term osteomyelitis literally means 'inflammation of bone and bone marrow'. However, as all cases of bone inflammation are due to infection, the term osteomyelitis has come to be defined as an infection of bone. Microorganisms may gain access to bone either by direct implantation or by haematogenous spread. The most common organism causing osteomyelitis is the bacterium *Staphylococcus aureus*.

Most cases of osteomyelitis occur due to direct implantation of bacteria, either due to open fractures or following orthopaedic surgery. Diabetics with penetrating foot ulcers are also at risk of developing osteomyelitis. Osteomyelitis following haematogenous spread is usually encountered in children, who are at particular risk because sprouting capillary loops adjacent to epiphyseal growth plates promote the localization of circulating bacteria.

Osteomyelitis presents with fever and pain in a limb, with loss of function. In young children unable to vocalize their symptoms, there may simply be a refusal to use a limb or weight bear on it. Treatment of osteomyelitis is with immobilization and antibacterials such as flucloxacillin. As well as treating the infection in the bone, the antibacterials are also important in preventing the development of septicaemia.

Early diagnosis and prompt treatment reduces the risk of bone necrosis and a chronic cycle of bone death, extension of infection, and further bone death. Antibacterials cannot work effectively in the presence of bone death, and so surgery is needed in chronic infections to clear away the dead bone and allow entry of new viable tissue, the host immune system, and the antibacterials.

Key points: Osteomyelitis

♦ Osteomyelitis is an infection of bone and bone marrow.

♦ Most cases of osteomyelitis are caused by bacteria, particularly *S. aureus*.

♦ Bacteria gain access to the bone either by direct implantation or by haematogenous spread.

♦ Osteomyelitis causes fever and pain in the affected limb. Children may present with refusal to use a limb. Treatment requires antibacterial agents effective against *S. aureus*, such as flucloxacillin.

♦ If diagnosis and treatment is delayed leading to bone necrosis, antibacterial treatment alone is often not effective and surgery is needed to clear away the dead bone.

Bone tumours

The vast majority of tumours in bone are metastatic deposits

Ninety-nine per cent of all malignant tumours found in bone are deposits of metastatic tumour. The majority of these originate from carcinomas of the lung, breast, kidney, thyroid, and prostate. With the exception of prostate carcinoma, which often stimulates new bone formation, most metastatic bony deposits are osteolytic, i.e. they destroy bone. Bone destruction by metastatic disease may be sufficient to cause elevation of serum calcium levels, and bony metastasis is one of the more common causes of hypercalcaemia.

Primary tumours of bone are rare but important

Although primary tumours of bone are rare, they are still important to know about as the malignant neoplasms typically affect children and young adults; the treatment involves mutilating surgery such as limb amputation, and the prognosis is often not good.

A few general points about primary bone tumours are worth mentioning:

♦ Individual tumours tend to show a predilection for certain sites of the skeleton.

♦ Individual tumours tend to present in characteristic age groups.

♦ Imaging plays a very important role in diagnosis, as each bone tumour tends to have characteristic radiological features.

♦ If any biopsy procedure is to be carried out, it should be performed *after* imaging studies, as the biopsy produces changes in the tissue that could be misinterpreted as representing malignancy on any subsequent imaging.

Primary bone tumours are usually classified according to their *histological type* (e.g. if they are bone forming or cartilage forming) and their *behaviour* (e.g. benign or malignant). Note, however, that there are some bone tumours intermediate between benign and malignant, in that they grow rapidly, cause local destruction, and often recur following excision, but virtually never metastasize (Table 17.5).

Benign primary bone tumours include osteochondroma, chondroma, and osteoid osteoma

Osteochondroma is a benign bone tumour which grows as a solitary exophytic nodule from the metaphysis of a long bone, close to the epiphyseal growth plate. It is a common lesion, usually found in children.

Chondroma is a benign cartilage-forming tumour. They are divided into two groups according to which part of the bone is involved. **Enchondromas** arise in the medulla of the bone, typically in the bones of the hands and feet. **Periosteal chondromas** arise on the surface of

TABLE 17.5 Primary bone tumours
Benign
Osteochondroma
Chondroma
Osteoid osteoma
Osteoma
Intermediate (locally aggressive but rarely metastasize)
Giant cell tumour
Osteoblastoma
Malignant
Osteosarcoma
Chondrosarcoma

the bone, the proximal humerus being a characteristic site. They are often discovered incidentally.

Osteoid osteoma is a benign bone-forming tumour which most commonly arises in the femur of children or young adults. It is unusual for the tumour to be palpable, but it is readily identified on plain radiographs. The tumour seldom exceeds 1 cm in maximum dimension. Despite its small size, it can cause considerable pain, particularly at night.

Giant cell tumour is a locally recurrent primary bone tumour

Giant cell tumour is a benign, locally aggressive neoplasm that arises in the ends of long bones. The tumour is composed of sheets of neoplastic ovoid mononuclear cells interspersed with large osteoclast-like giant cells. The giant cells are probably not neoplastic, but rather recruited into the tumour by the neoplastic mononuclear cells.

Giant cell tumours typically present with pain and swelling over the site of the tumour in a young adult aged 20–45. A giant cell tumour is a locally aggressive neoplasm which is notorious for its potential to recur following excision. Distant metastases are extremely rare.

Malignant primary bone tumours include osteosarcoma and chondrosarcoma

Osteosarcoma is the most common malignant primary bone tumour. Osteosarcoma is a malignant tumour defined by the production of malignant bone by the neoplastic cells. It is essentially a tumour of the immature skeleton, with most of them seen between the ages of 5 and 25. Occasional cases occur in the elderly, most as a complication of Paget's disease. Osteosarcoma is an aggressive tumour that shows rapid haematogenous dissemination, particularly to the lungs. Its precise aetiology is unknown. Whilst a history of trauma may often be elicited, it is usually felt that the trauma has drawn attention to the tumour rather than having caused it.

Chondrosarcoma accounts for about 15 per cent of primary malignant bone tumours. These tumours arise in either the marrow space or adjacent to the cortex of the bone. In contrast to enchondromas, chondrosarcoma rarely involves the distal extremities. Instead, they are particularly common in the pelvic bones. They mainly occur in adults and are rare before the age of 30.

There are a number of variants of chondrosarcoma. Some are slowly growing tumours composed of well differentiated cartilage that rarely metastasize until very late. The dedifferentiated variant, however, has a dismal prognosis, even with aggressive therapy.

> ## Key points: Bone tumours
>
> - Most bone tumours represent metastases from other sites. Primary bone tumours also occur, but are rare neoplasms.
>
> - Each primary bone tumour has characteristic features that must all be taken into account when considering a diagnosis, including the age of the patient, the site of the lesion, and the radiographic appearances.
>
> - Primary bone tumours are classified according to their histological type (e.g. if they are bone or cartilage forming) and by their behaviour.
>
> - Common begin primary bone tumours include osteochondroma, osteoid osteoma, and chondroma.
>
> - Gaint cell tumour of bone is notorious for recurring locally, but rarely metastasizes.
>
> - Common malignant primary bone tumours include osteosarcoma and chondrosarcoma.

Joint disease

Normal joints

Joints are the sites of union or articulation between bones. Three types of joint are recognized:

- **Fibrous joints** are joined by fibrous tissue and have minimal movement, e.g. the skull bones.

- **Cartilaginous joints**, in which the ends of two bones are covered by a thin layer of hyaline cartilage and are united by fibrocartilage, e.g. the pubic symphysis.

- **Synovial joints** have a joint space that allows a wide range of movement between bones, the articulating ends of which are covered by hyaline cartilage. A capsule lined by synovium encloses the joint cavity which is filled with synovial fluid for lubrication.

Most joint diseases are either degenerative or inflammatory in origin. Inflammatory joint diseases may be due to autoimmunity, crystal deposition, or infection. Tumours arising in joints, whilst recognized, are very rare.

Osteoarthritis

Osteoarthritis, or osteoarthrosis, is a very common degenerative joint disease which usually affects large weight-bearing joints such as the hip and knee, and the interphalangeal joints of the hands.

Osteoarthritis is caused by thinning and disintegration of articular cartilage

Despite its name, osteoarthritis is not an inflammatory disease; inflammatory cells are not found in increased numbers in joints affected by the disease. In the great majority of patients, osteoarthritis occurs for no apparent underlying reason and appears to be an age-related phenomenon. Obesity can accelerate the condition in weight-bearing joints due to increased loading across the joint.

Osteoarthritis therefore appears to be a 'wear and tear' disease in which articular hyaline cartilage gradually softens and disintegrates. The bone immediately underneath the cartilage, the subchondral bone, responds with highly disorganized bony remodelling, leading to loss of the normal trabecular scaffold, the development of cystic lesions, and bony outgrowths (osteophytes) at the margins of the articular surface.

Pain is the dominant symptom of osteoarthritis

Osteoarthritis causes mild to moderate joint pain which increases with joint use, and is therefore worst at the end of the day and improves with rest. The pain is probably derived from the bones of the joint, as cartilage is avascular and has no nerves. Stiffness may occur but is usually short lived, and soft tissue swelling is rare, both important distinguishing features from rheumatoid arthritis.

Surgery for osteoarthritis should be reserved for patients who have failed conservative management

Treatment for osteoarthritis should begin with simple measures such as weight loss and the use of analgesics such as paracetamol. Non-steroidal anti-inflammatory drugs (NSAIDs) are more effective as pain relievers, but their use should be balanced against their side effects, particularly peptic ulceration.

Surgical intervention is reserved for patients in whom these measures have failed to help. A number of approaches are possible, though total joint replacement remains one of the most commonly performed and most successful operations, providing immediate relief of pain and a marked improvement in joint function.

Key points: Osteoarthritis

- Osteoarthritis is a degenerative joint disease affecting large weight-bearing joints such as the hip and knee, and the interphalangeal joints of the hands.

- Osteoarthritis appears to be an age-related phenomenon in which articular cartilage softens and disintegrates.

- Exposure of the underlying bone causes pain which increases with joint use. The pain is worst at the end of the day and improves with rest.

- Increased bone remodelling leads to subchondral bone cysts and osteophyte formation, important radiological features of osteoarthritis.

Rheumatoid arthritis

Rheumatoid arthritis (RA) is a chronic systemic autoimmune inflammatory disease with the brunt of the disease falling upon synovial joints. RA is common, affecting about 1 per cent of the population worldwide. As with all autoimmune diseases, it is more common in women.

JARGON BUSTER

Rheumatoid arthritis and rheumatic fever

Take care not to confuse rheumatoid arthritis with **rheumatic fever**, the immunologically mediated disease which can lead to chronic rheumatic valvular heart disease (p. 94).

Rheumatoid arthritis causes chronic inflammation of synovium leading to destruction of joints

Joints affected by RA show chronic inflammation of the synovium. In response to the inflammation, the synovium proliferates and becomes tremendously hyperplastic; up to 100 times its original weight. The mass of hyperplastic synovial tissue, known as **pannus**, then erodes into the articular cartilage and completely destroys the joint (Fig. 17.6). RA is therefore a deforming, destructive arthropathy.

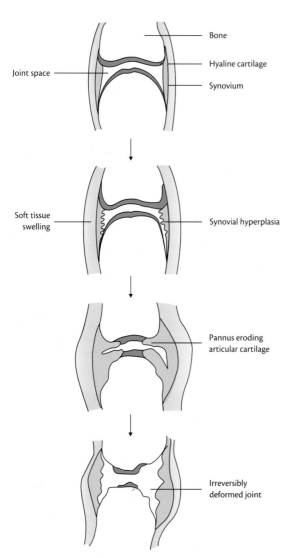

Fig. 17.6 Progression of rheumatoid arthritis. Inflammation and hyperplasia of the synovium in early rheumatoid arthritis cause swelling of the involved joints. With progression, pannus formation destroys the articular cartilage, leading to irreversible deformity of the joint.

We still know very little about the cause of rheumatoid arthritis

Despite many years of intense research, our knowledge about the aetiology and pathogenesis of RA remains at best crude. CD4+ T lymphocytes, B lymphocytes, and macrophages are all important as they are found in the inflamed synovial tissue, and certain major histocompatibility complex (MHC) class II alleles have been strongly associated with susceptibility to RA.

The classic theory for the pathogenesis of RA implicated autoreactive CD4+ T lymphocytes as the guilty cells, mediating joint damage by driving macrophages to release proinflammatory cytokines such as tumour necrosis factor-α (TNF-α) and interleukin-1 (IL-1). Antibody production was thought to be a secondary phenomenon occurring as a result of spillage of autoantigens due to the joint destruction.

Recently, however, there has been a shift in thinking. Suspicion now centres on B cells as the primary culprits, producing autoantibodies that mediate the joint damage and activate CD4+ T cells which perpetuate the inflammation.

Rheumatoid factor is an anti-IgG antibody found in most patients with RA

About 80 per cent of adults with rheumatoid arthritis are positive for **rheumatoid factor**, an autoantibody which binds the Fc portion of IgG. Although long used to aid the diagnosis of RA, rheumatoid factor is a relatively poor marker for RA. Not only can it be negative in patients with RA, it is also often positive in many other autoimmune conditions and in up to 5 per cent of healthy individuals.

Anti-CCP antibodies are highly specific for rheumatoid arthritis

More recently, antibodies against **cyclic citrullinated peptides** (anti-CCP antibodies) have been shown to be highly specific for RA. These antibodies react against proteins in which the amino acid arginine has been replaced by citrulline. Citrulline, an intermediary in the conversion of orthinine to arginine, is not normally present in proteins.

Anti-CCP antibodies, which can be easily measured using enzyme-linked immunosorbent assay (ELISA), have a similar sensitivity to rheumatoid factor but a much better specificity due to a lower-false positive rate. Measuring anti-CCP antibodies is therefore an extremely useful test in patients presenting with early synovitis to pick out those people destined to develop RA who should be treated early to prevent irreversible joint destruction.

Anti-CCP antibodies may also have a pathogenic role

Because the presence of anti-CCP antibodies may predate the onset of disease symptoms by many years, they may have a direct pathogenic role in RA. Citrullinated antigens are present in inflamed synovium, and anti-CCP-producing plasma cells have been isolated from the synovium of patients with RA.

Rheumatoid arthritis presents as a slowly progressive, symmetrical, peripheral polyarthritis

The typical presentation of RA is pain and stiffness of the small joints of the hands and feet, which evolves over a period of weeks to months. Other joints such as the wrists, elbows, ankles, and knees may also be involved. The pain and stiffness are significantly worse in the morning and tend to improve with gentle activity. On examination, the joints are swollen, warm, tender, and show limitation of movement. With increasing joint damage, the joints become irreversibly deformed (Fig. 17.7).

Rheumatoid nodules are the most common extra-articular feature of rheumatoid arthritis

Although the dominant sites of damage in RA are the joints, a number of other tissues may be involved by

TABLE 17.6 Extra-articular features of rheumatoid arthritis
Rheumatoid nodules
Vasculitis
Scleritis and episcleritis
Serositis with pleural effusion
Pulmonary fibrosis
Amyloidosis

the disease (Table 17.6). The most common extra-articular feature is the subcutaneous **rheumatoid nodule**. These are firm dermal nodules typically seen over pressure points, particularly the elbows. Microscopically, rheumatoid nodules are composed of a zone of granulomatous inflammation surrounding an area of dead collagen fibres. The reason for their formation is not clear.

More serious complications of RA include vasculitis, pulmonary fibrosis, and amyloidosis. Fortunately these are rare.

LINK BOX

Rheumatoid arthritis and secondary Sjögren's syndrome

Many patients with rheumatoid arthritis also develop secondary Sjögren's syndrome, causing dry eyes and dry mouth from immune destruction of lacrimal and salivary glands (p. 454).

Treatment of RA involves a combination of NSAIDs and DMARDs

Initial treatment of RA requires NSAIDs. These help to relieve symptoms of pain and stiffness in the joints, but do not slow the progression of the disease. NSAIDs should therefore be used in combination with **disease-modifying antirheumatic drugs** (DMARDs) such as methotrexate and sulphasalazine. There are a large number of DMARDs to choose from, and combinations of them seem to be particularly effective at preventing the irreversible joint destruction.

Newer biological DMARDs which act on specific components of the immune system are exciting new developments in the treatment of RA. Examples include

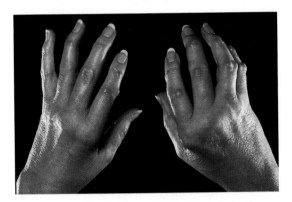

Fig. 17.7 The hands of a patient with rheumatoid arthritis showing symmetrical soft tissue swelling of the metacarpophalangeal joints and early deformity of the fingers.

anti-CD20 antibodies which deplete mature B lympho-cytes from the body (CD20 is a cell surface protein found on B lymphocytes), and CTLA4-Ig which inhibits T cell activation. Early trials with these agents have shown considerable promise. Unfortunately, many of these new therapies are enormously expensive, though the cost may be offset by savings that result from the improved long-term outcome.

Rheumatoid arthritis results in a varying degree of disability

The prognosis of RA is variable. About 25 per cent of patients will go into long-term remission. About 50 per cent will continue to have problems with mild to moderate disability. The other 25 per cent develop progressive disease with severe disability.

Key points: Rheumatoid arthritis

- Rheumatoid arthritis is a multisystem autoimmune disorder which shows a predilection for joint involvement.

- Rheumatoid arthritis is characterized by self-perpetuating synovial inflammation, leading to erosion of articular cartilage and eventually irreversible joint destruction.

- Both CD4+ T lymphocytes and B lymphocytes are important, but which one initiates the inflammation is not known.

- The typical presentation of rheumatoid arthritis is slowly progressive pain and stiffness in the small joints of the hands and feet.

- Subcutaneous rheumatoid nodules are the most common extra-articular feature of rheumatoid arthritis.

- The presence of rheumatoid factor and anti-CCP antibodies is highly suggestive of rheumatoid arthritis, and these are helpful in making the diagnosis early so that treatment can begin before joint destruction occurs.

- Treatment of rheumatoid arthritis involves NSAIDs for symptomatic relief, and combinations of DMARDs to slow the progression of the disease.

Spondyloarthropathies

The term **spondyloarthropathy** encompasses a group of inflammatory joint diseases characterized by arthritis predominantly affecting the spinal column and peripheral joints, and inflammation at the insertion site of tendons and ligaments to bone known as **enthesitis** (Table 17.7). The older term 'seronegative spondyloarthropathy', which refers to the absence of rheumatoid factor in these conditions, is largely historical and somewhat redundant now.

Once thought of as rare diseases, spondyloarthropathies are now recognized to be common diseases that, as a group, occur in 1 per cent of the population, making them the most frequent inflammatory joint diseases after RA. Although their effects can be mild, these conditions can be extremely disabling in some patients. They usually present in young people (most aged 20–40 years) and there is a slight male predominance.

Spondyloarthropathies are strongly associated with the HLA-B27 allele

Spondyloarthropathies are well recognized to cluster in families, and one of the most interesting features of the spondyloarthropathies is the strong genetic association with possession of the MHC class I allele HLA-B27. Precisely how carriage of the HLA-B27 gene leads to a spondyloarthropathy remains unknown, though numerous theories have been proposed.

The arthritogenic peptide theory is the traditional hypothesis for spondyloarthropathy

The traditional theory behind the pathogenesis of spondyloarthropathies is known as the 'arthritogenic peptide' theory. This proposes that HLA-B27 binds unique peptides and presents them to CD8+ cytotoxic T cells, leading to joint inflammation. The nature of the arthritogenic peptide, particularly whether it is of microbial or self origin, is not known.

TABLE 17.7 Spondyloarthropathies
Ankylosing spondylitis
Reactive arthropathy
Psoriatic arthropathy
Enteropathic arthropathy

Misfolding of the HLA-B27 molecule may also be important

There has been considerable interest recently in the possible importance of misfolding of the HLA-B27 protein in the pathogenesis of spondyloarthropathies. HLA-B27 is slightly unusual in that folding of the protein appears to be slower compared with other HLA alleles and so has a tendency to become misfolded. It is plausible that misfolded HLA-B27 proteins that are not broken down quickly enough accumulate in the endoplasmic reticulum of the cell, stimulating an intracellular stress response that leads to inflammation.

In addition to misfolding, HLA-B27 molecules also have a tendency to dimerize. HLA-B27 homodimers are detectable on the cell surface in patients with spondyloarthropathy, in a form which lacks the β_2-microglobulin molecule, normally an essential component of MHC class I molecules. It is possible that these abnormal HLA-B27 homodimers could function as a peptide-presenting structure to T lymphocytes.

Ankylosing spondylitis is the most common spondyloarthropathy

Ankylosing spondylitis is a common disease affecting up to 0.5 per cent of the population which usually presents in young adults between 20 and 40. The hallmark of ankylosing spondylitis is lower back pain due to spinal joint inflammation starting in the sacroiliac joints, often coupled with enthesitis. Enthesitis leads to fibrosis and the laying down of bone at the site of inflammation rather than joint destruction and instability. In the spine, enthesitis at the insertion of the annulus fibrosus (the outer part of the intervertebral disc) results in fusion of the vertebral bodies causing stiffening of the spine.

Other clinical features of ankylosing spondylitis include iritis, alveolitis, and fibrosis involving the upper lobes of the lungs, and aortic valve incompetence secondary to aortitis.

Reactive arthritis follows an infection elsewhere in the body

Reactive arthritis is a form of arthritis occurring within 1 month of an infection somewhere else in the body. In most cases, this is a genitourinary infection with *Chlamydia* or a gastrointestinal infection with *Shigella*, *Salmonella*, or *Campylobacter*. Most patients are HLA-B27 positive, though this is not obligatory. The precise cause of reactive arthritis is not known. Intact bacteria have not been isolated from affected joints, though bacterial antigens and bacterial DNA have been found, suggesting that this material may become deposited in the joints and drive the inflammatory process.

The typical picture is pain and stiffness in the lower back, knees, ankles, and feet. Enthesitis is common, often causing plantar fasciitis or inflammation of the Achilles tendon (Fig. 17.8). The majority of people with reactive arthritis have a single attack which settles completely, though some people develop a chronic relapsing and remitting arthritis.

Psoriatic arthritis affects 5 per cent of people with psoriasis

Psoriatic arthritis is a spondyloarthropathy seen in about 5 per cent of patients with psoriasis. About half of patients with psoriatic arthropathy are HLA-B27 positive. The distal interphalangeal joints are most commonly affected. The pathogenesis of psoriatic arthropathy is unknown.

Enteropathic arthritis is associated with inflammatory bowel disease

Enteropathic arthritis is a spondyloarthropathy seen in about 10 per cent of patients with inflammatory bowel disease (ulcerative colitis and Crohn's disease). The arthritis typically affects the sacroiliac joints and lower limb

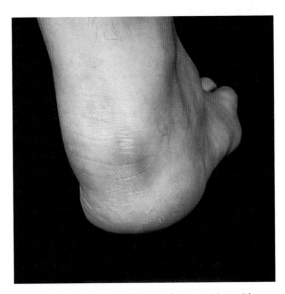

Fig. 17.8 Enthesitis of the Achilles tendon in a patient with reactive arthritis.

joints in an asymmetrical fashion. The cause of entero-pathic arthropathy is not known, though it has been proposed that ulcerated bowel becomes permeable to antigens that trigger the arthritis. The arthritis usually responds to symptomatic treatment and control of the underlying inflammatory bowel disease.

Key points: Spondyloarthropathies

- The spondyloarthropathies encompass a group of diseases characterized by inflammatory arthritis of the spine and peripheral joints, and enthesitis.

- Spondyloarthropathies include ankylosis spondylitis, reactive arthritis, psoriatic arthritis, and enteropathic arthritis.

- Spondyloarthropathies show striking familial aggregation and a strong genetic link to HLA-B27.

- Exactly how HLA-B27 leads to spondyloarthropathy remains unknown. The two main theories are the arthritogenic peptide theory and the aberrant form theory.

- Ankylosing spondylitis is the most common spondyloarthropathy. There is progressive stiffening of the spine from fusion of the vertebral joints.

- Reactive arthritis is triggered by a gastrointestinal or genitourinary infection.

- Psoriatic arthritis is a mild disease seen in 5 per cent of psoriasis sufferers.

- Enteropathic arthritis affects 10 per cent of patients with ulcerative colitis or Crohn's disease, possibly triggered by antigens leaking through the abnormally permeable gut wall.

Crystal arthropathies

The crystal arthropathies are caused by deposition of crystals in joints

Crystal arthropathies are joint diseases caused by deposition of crystals in the joint. Neutrophils ingest the crystals and degranulate, releasing enzymes that damage the joint. Two main types of crystal account for most cases of crystal arthropathy: sodium urate crystals, which cause **gout**, and calcium pyrophosphate crystals, which cause **pseudogout**.

Gout arises due to crystallization of urate in tissues

Gout is caused by inflammation in response to deposition of urate crystals in a joint. Precipitation of urate is the result of raised levels of urate in the blood (hyperuricaemia). Most cases of hyperuricaemia are due to impaired excretion of urate by the kidneys, though the underlying cause of this is not known. Although hyperuricaemia is a prerequisite for gout, it is important to note that only about 5 per cent of people with hyperuricaemia actually develop gout.

Acute gout typically presents with a red, hot, painful great toe

The classical manifestation of acute gout is a middle-aged man with the sudden onset of an agonisingly painful, swollen, red joint (Fig. 17.9). Any joint may be involved, though the first metatarsophalangeal joint is particularly characteristic. The arthritis responds well to high doses of NSAIDs.

Chronic tophaceous gout leads to tophus formation in the skin and around joints

People with very high levels of urate in the blood may develop **chronic tophaceous gout** in which large deposits of urate (**tophi**) occur in the skin and around

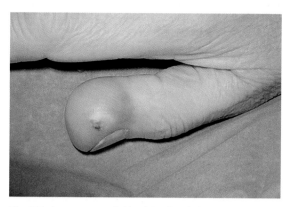

Fig. 17.9 Acute monoarthritis of the thumb due to gout.

joints (Fig. 17.10). Chronic joint pain is common, and large tophi look unsightly and may ulcerate.

LINK BOX

Gout and urate renal calculi

Large concretions of urate in the outflow tracts of the kidney can lead to renal calculi formation (p. 228).

Pseudogout is due to the deposition of calcium pyrophosphate crystals

Pyrophosphate is a byproduct of the hydrolysis of nucleotide triphosphates in chondrocytes of cartilage. Shedding of crystals into a joint precipitates an acute arthritis which mimics gout, except that it is more common in women and usually affects the knee or wrist.

Microscopic examination of crystals in joint fluid can distinguish gout from pseudogout

Although the clinical features of gout and pseudogout are often very characteristic, joint aspiration is often performed to confirm the diagnosis and, of particular importance, to rule out a septic arthritis. In a crystal arthropathy, microscopic examination of a sample of joint fluid reveals the presence of numerous crystals, both lying free and present within neutrophils. The shape of the crystals and their appearance when viewed under polarized light allow the distinction between urate and pyrophosphate crystals.

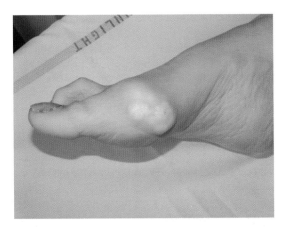

Fig. 17.10 Gouty tophus around the first metatarsophalangeal joint.

Key points: Crystal arthropathies

- Crystal arthropathies are inflammatory joint diseases caused by deposition of crystals in the joint.

- The two main crystal arthropathies are gout and pseudogout.

- Gout is caused by deposition of sodium urate crystals due to hyperuricaemia, which is usually due to impaired renal excretion of urate.

- The typical presentation of gout is an acutely painful, red, hot first metatarsophalangeal joint.

- Patients with persistently high levels of urate in the blood may develop chronic tophaceous gout in which large deposits of urate known as tophi develop in the skin and around joints.

- Pseudogout is an acute arthritis due to deposition of calcium pyrophosphate in joints.

- Pseudogout is more common in women and usually affects the knee or wrist.

Septic arthritis

Septic arthritis is usually caused by blood-borne S. aureus

Septic arthritis is infection of a joint. The infection is almost always caused by bacteria; the most common species is *S. aureus*. The bacteria usually reach the joint via the blood stream, but may occasionally enter following penetrating trauma. Once in the joint, establishment of infection is favoured by the relative inability of phagocytes to enter the joint. Pre-existing joint diseases such as rheumatoid arthritis increase the risk of septic arthritis.

Suspected septic arthritis requires urgent investigation and treatment

An infected joint is hot, red, swollen, and extremely painful. Suspected septic arthritis must be managed without delay to prevent rapid, irreversible destruction of the joint. The joint should be aspirated and the fluid sent to microbiology for urgent Gram staining and culture. Microscopic examination for crystals should also be requested to rule out an acute crystal arthropathy.

Blood cultures may also be useful as they may grow the culprit organism. Treatment is with an antibacterial agent with activity against staphylococci such as flucloxacillin.

Joint neoplasms

Neoplasms arising in joints do occur, but are extremely rare. The most important neoplasm arising in and around joints is called the **diffuse-type giant cell tumour** (also known as **pigmented villonodular synovitis**).

A diffuse-type giant cell tumour is a destructive proliferation of synovial like cells which is locally aggressive but does not metastasize. Most cases affect the knee joint or the tissue around the knee joint, typically in young adults. Patients present with a long history of pain and swelling of the joint; recurrent bleeding into the joint space is also common. Excision is the treatment of choice though local recurrence is often a problem.

Soft tissue tumours

Soft tissue tumours are neoplasms that arise from connective tissue elements of the body such as fat, smooth muscle, fibroblasts, blood vessels, and skeletal muscle.

The annual incidence of benign soft tissue tumours is in the order of 3000 per million population, whereas the annual incidence of malignant soft tissue tumours is around 30 per million population. Soft tissue sarcomas therefore account for less than 1 per cent of all malignant tumours.

Magnetic resonance imaging (MRI) is the method of choice for detecting and staging soft tissue tumours. Sometimes the MRI features of a soft tissue tumour are so characteristic that the diagnosis can be reliably predicted from the MRI alone.

Soft tissue tumours may be categorized according to their histogenesis and behaviour (Table 17.8).

Benign soft tissue tumours

Benign soft tissue tumours do not recur following excision and do not metastasize. The vast majority of soft tissue tumours behave in a benign fashion, and recurrence after surgical excision is extremely rare.

Lipoma is a benign tumour composed of mature fat cells (adipocytes). Lipomas typically occur in the subcutaneous fat, presenting as painless soft masses. Lipomas are the most common soft tissue tumour.

TABLE 17.8	Categorization of soft tissue tumours
Histogenesis	
Adipocytic tumours	
Fibroblastic/myofibroblastic tumours	
Fibrohistiocytic tumours	
Smooth muscle tumours	
Skeletal muscle tumours	
Vascular tumours	
Tumours of uncertain histogenesis	
Behaviour	
Benign	
Intermediate (locally aggressive)	
Intermediate (rarely metastasizing)	
Malignant	

Leiomyoma is a benign tumour composed of smooth muscle cells. The vast majority of leiomyomas arise from smooth muscle of the myometrium of the uterus and the smooth muscle of the arrector pili muscle in the skin.

Haemangioma is a benign soft tissue tumour composed of endothelial cells forming vascular channels of varying size. Haemangiomas most commonly arise in the skin during the first year of life and usually clear spontaneously.

Nodular fasciitis is a benign tumour composed of fibroblastic/myofibroblastic cells. Nodular fasciitis occurs mostly in young adults, rapidly appearing over 1–2 months as a tender subcutaneous mass. Although any part of the body may be involved, the trunk, head, and neck are the most frequently affected sites.

Intermediate (locally aggressive) soft tissue tumours

Intermediate (locally aggressive) soft tissue tumours are locally destructive neoplasms which often recur locally following attempted surgical excision, but do not metastasize.

Fibromatoses are fibroblastic neoplasms characterized by infiltrative growth and a tendency to local recurrence, but they do not metastasize. **Superficial fibromatoses** arise in the palmar or plantar soft tissues. Palmar fibromatosis (Dupuytren's disease) initially causes an asymptomatic firm palmar nodule adherent to the overlying skin which eventually leads to flexion contractures of the fourth and fifth fingers. Plantar fibromatosis presents as a firm nodule or thickening of the sole of the foot which is adherent to the overlying skin. Plantar fibromatosis rarely causes contractures of the toes. In troublesome cases, surgical excision may be attempted, though local recurrence is common. **Deep fibromatoses**, which arise in deep soft tissues, are rarer than their superficial counterparts. Most patients present with an asymptomatic abdominal mass, occasionally associated with mild abdominal pain. Deep fibromatoses can be extremely difficult to manage; most are large by the time they present, making complete excision impossible.

Atypical lipomatous tumour is a soft tissue neoplasm composed of mature adipocytes showing significant variation in cell size and nuclear atypia. Atypical lipomatous tumours typically present in middle-aged adults as a painless enlarging mass, most frequently located in the deep soft tissue of the thigh. The prognosis of atypical lipomatous tumours depends on their ease of surgical excision. Cure may be possible when tumours occur at a site where complete surgical excision with a wide margin can be achieved. Tumours arising in areas difficult to resect (e.g. the retroperitoneum or mediastinum) are liable to repeated local recurrence that may lead to death.

Intermediate (rarely metastasizing) soft tissue tumours

Intermediate (rarely metastasizing) soft tissue tumours are locally aggressive tumours which occasionally give rise to distant metastases.

Solitary fibrous tumour is a locally aggressive soft tissue tumour of fibroblastic/myofibroblastic type. Microscopically, the tumour contains a prominent branching vascular network which is highly characteristic. Solitary fibrous tumours have been described in many locations, though common sites include the pleura and the subcutaneous soft tissue. Although many cases of solitary fibrous tumour behave in a completely benign fashion, some behave aggressively and occasionally metastasize.

Kaposi's sarcoma is a locally aggressive soft tissue tumour composed of neoplastic endothelial cells. Kaposi's sarcoma has an infectious aetiology, being universally associated with **human herpes virus 8** (HHV-8) infection. Kaposi's sarcoma typically involves the skin, presenting with purplish red nodules and plaques. In the classical form, it occurs on the lower legs of elderly men and follows an indolent course. In patients with HIV, however, Kaposi's sarcoma follows an aggressive course with the development of multiple primary tumours in the skin, oral mucosa, lymph nodes, and internal organs. *Note that in this situation, these reflect separate primary tumours rather than metastatic deposits.*

Malignant soft tissue tumours

Malignant soft tissue tumours are locally destructive and have a high risk of metastasis.

Liposarcoma is a malignant soft tissue tumour containing a variable number of primitive adipocytic cells called lipoblasts. Most liposarcomas occur in young adults, presenting as a large painless mass within the deep soft tissue of the limbs, particularly the thigh. Local recurrence and metastases are common, making prognosis poor.

Leiomyosarcoma is a malignant soft tissue tumour composed of cells showing smooth muscle differentiation. The most common site of leiomyosarcoma is the soft tissue of the retroperitoneum. Other well recognized locations include the skin and the myometrium. Retroperitoneal leiomyosarcomas are fatal in the majority of cases as they are large (>10 cm) at presentation and impossible to excise completely, making them prone to both local recurrence and metastasis. Leiomyosarcomas at other sites tend to have a slightly better prognosis as they present earlier.

Angiosarcoma is a malignant soft tissue tumour composed of neoplastic cells showing evidence of endothelial cell differentiation. It is a rare tumour, accounting for less than 1 per cent of all sarcomas. The majority arise in the skin.

Rhabdomyosarcoma is a malignant soft tissue tumour showing skeletal muscle differentiation. Although rhabdomyosarcoma is very uncommon, it remains important as the most common soft tissue sarcoma in infants and children (p. 523).

High grade pleomorphic sarcoma refers to a sarcoma that cannot be shown to have an obvious line of differentiation. These tumours, formally known as 'malignant fibrous histiocytomas', have become much less common since the widespread introduction of immunohistochemistry has allowed many of them to be categorized to a specific line of differentiation. Genuine high grade pleomorphic sarcomas are extremely aggressive malignancies with poor survival.

Synovial sarcoma is a malignant soft tissue tumour with a specific chromosomal translocation t(X;18). Synovial sarcoma typically presents as a growing mass in the deep soft tissue of the extremities, particularly around the knee. The cell of origin of synovial sarcoma remains unknown; despite its name, synovial sarcoma has nothing to do with synovium.

> ### Key points: Soft tissue tumours
>
> - Soft tissue tumours are classified according to their behaviour and the cell type that the neoplastic cells attempt to recapitulate.
>
> - Benign soft tissue tumours include lipoma, leiomyoma, haemangioma, and nodular fasciitis.
>
> - Intermediate (locally aggressive) soft tissue tumours include fibromatoses and atypical lipomatous tumour.
>
> - Intermediate (rarely metastasizing) soft tissue tumours include solitary fibrous tumour and Kaposi's sarcoma.
>
> - Malignant soft tissue tumours include liposarcoma, leiomyosarcoma, angiosarcoma, rhabdomyosarcoma, high grade pleomorphic sarcoma, and synovial sarcoma.

Further reading

www.nos.org.uk, National Osteoporosis Society.

Nervous system and muscle disease

Introduction

The main function of the nervous system is to receive, transmit, and analyse information. Information is gathered by sensory systems, integrated by the brain, and used to generate output signals.

The nervous system has two major divisions, the **central nervous system** (CNS) and the **peripheral nervous system** (PNS). The CNS consists of the brain and spinal cord. The PNS includes all nervous tissue outside the CNS, namely the cranial and spinal nerves, and the autonomic nervous system.

Central nervous system

The brain is composed of two cerebral hemispheres and the brainstem, which is continuous with the spinal cord (Fig. 18.1). The cerebral hemispheres have a highly convoluted external cortex of grey matter, beneath which lie extensive white matter tracts and deep nuclei such as the basal ganglia and thalamus. The brainstem contains all the axonal bundles passing to and from the cerebral hemispheres and spinal cord, as well as many cranial nerve nuclei and the respiratory centres controlling breathing.

The spinal cord contains numerous ascending and descending white matter tracts which transmit information to and from the brain. The whole of the brain and spinal cord is covered by three connective tissue layers known as the **meninges**. These are, from outside in, the **dura mater**, **arachnoid mater**, and the **pia mater**.

JARGON BUSTER

Grey and white matter

The cell bodies of neurones in the central nervous system are often grouped together in layers called **grey matter** or in defined areas called **nuclei**. The axons of neurones form bundles which are grouped together to form tracts. Concentrations of tracts are called **white matter** because the axons are ensheathed in myelin which looks white.

Neurones are the functional unit of the central nervous system

The CNS contains billions of neurones, all of which are present at birth but not yet fully connected. During development and throughout adult life, new connections between neurones are established as new memories and skills are laid down.

Neurones are the functional unit of the nervous system, conveying electrical impulses throughout the CNS, and between the central and peripheral nervous systems. Neurones are made up of a cell body which contains the nucleus, elongated processes called **dendrites** that receive information from other neurones, and the **axon** which conducts impulses to other neurones, muscles, or glands.

Dendritic branching can be highly complex such that a single neurone may receive thousands of inputs. Axon branching allows several cell targets simultaneously

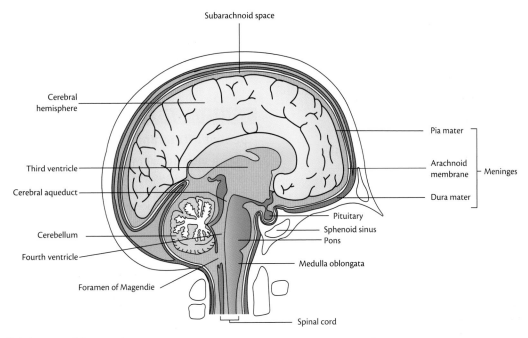

Fig. 18.1 Anatomy of the central nervous system.

to receive a signal from one neurone. Each branch of the axon terminates on another cell at a **synapse**, a specialized structure for transferring information from the axon to its target cell.

Astrocytes have a structural role and some signalling functions

Astrocytes are cells with thin delicate cytoplasmic processes extending away from the centre of the cell. These cells effectively form a scaffold for the CNS, supporting the spatial arrangement of the other cells. They may also have some signalling functions.

Another important role of astrocytes is reflected in their ability to proliferate at sites of injury (**gliosis**). Gliosis is the counterpart of scarring elsewhere in the body except, instead of laying down collagen, the astrocyte cytoplasm itself becomes the 'scar'. Gliotic 'scars' are probably the cause of many cases of epilepsy following recovery from a CNS disease.

Oligodendrocytes are the myelin producing cells of the central nervous system

Extensions of the plasma membrane of oligodendrocytes wrap around axons many times forming a myelin sheath. Gaps between myelin sheaths from neighbouring oligodendrocytes produce **nodes of Ranvier** where a small portion of the axon is exposed to the interstitial space and where voltage-dependent sodium channels are clustered in the axonal membrane. Between the nodes, myelin insulates the axon from the extracellular space, allowing action potentials to propagate rapidly by jumping from node to node in a process called salutatory conduction.

Ependymal cells line the ventricular system

Ependymal cells line the ventricular system of the CNS. A subset of ependymal cells has the capability to produce cerebrospinal fluid (CSF); these particular cells constitute the choroid plexus.

Microglia are the resident inflammatory cells of the central nervous system

Although lymphocytes and monocytes can enter and patrol the CNS from the blood, microglia are the principal immune cells of the CNS. Microglia is an unfortunate name as these cells are not glial cells at all; they are simply the resident macrophages of the CNS.

The capillaries of the brain form part of the blood–brain barrier

Although the larger blood vessels supplying the brain are identical to vessels elsewhere in the body, the capillaries of the CNS are quite different. Their endothelial cells have no fenestrations and they have a thick basement membrane making them less permeable than other capillaries in the body. Foot processes of astrocytes also surround the basement membrane of the capillary. These features allow tight control over what passes between the blood and the CNS, a property known as the **blood–brain barrier**.

Raised intracranial pressure

Any increase in volume in the cranial cavity leads to a rise in intracranial pressure

There is very little space within the rigid cranial box, so any lesion occupying volume in the cranial cavity will cause a rapid rise in intracranial pressure and deformation of the brain. Common causes of space-occupying lesions in the cranial cavity include an intracranial haematoma, a neoplasm, and a cerebral abscess.

Focal lesions in the brain are frequently accompanied by a swelling of the nearby brain parenchyma known as **cerebral oedema** which contributes further to the rise in intracranial pressure. Cerebral oedema is almost certainly the result of damage to the blood–brain barrier and accumulation of fluid in the extracellular spaces of the white matter. Clearance of fluid is poor because the brain has no lymphatics.

Symptoms and signs of raised intracranial pressure include the following:

- *Headache*, due to compression and distortion of pain and stretch receptors around intracranial blood vessels including those within the dura mater. The headache is typically worse in the morning and on movement.

- *Vomiting*, due to stimulation of vomiting centres in the pons and medulla.

- *Papilloedema*, which is swelling of the head of the optic nerve due to accumulation of axonal cytoplasm within it.

INTERESTING TO KNOW

Benign intracranial hypertension

Benign intracranial hypertension ('pseudotumour cerebri') is a rare disease in which raised intracranial pressure occurs in the absence of an intracranial mass lesion or hydrocephalus. Most patients present with a headache typical of raised intracranial pressure, and papilloedema is found on fundoscopy. No focal neurological signs are present.

The cause of benign intracranial hypertension is unknown, though the disease is more common in females and almost all patients are obese. Although rarely life threatening, benign intracranial hypertension leads to permanent visual loss in up to half of all patients due to damage to the optic nerve.

Herniation is the most important consequence of raised intracranial pressure

With increasing pressure, parts of the brain can be displaced (herniate) in relation to certain rigid structures in the cranial cavity. Herniation occurs at several characteristic sites, depending on the site of the space-occupying lesion (Fig. 18.2).

- **Subfalcine herniation** occurs when the cingulate gyrus is displaced under the falx cerebri. This may cause compression of the anterior cerebral artery and subsequent anterior cerebral infarction.

- **Transtentorial herniation** occurs when the medial aspect of the temporal lobe is displaced inferiorly over the free margin of the tentorium cerebelli. One of the first signs of transtentorial herniation is pupillary dilation and impaired ocular movements on the side of the herniation due to compression of the third cranial nerve. With progression, transtentorial herniation is frequently fatal due to haemorrhage within the midbrain from torn vessels.

- **Tonsillar herniation** occurs when the cerebellar tonsils are displaced through the foramen magnum.

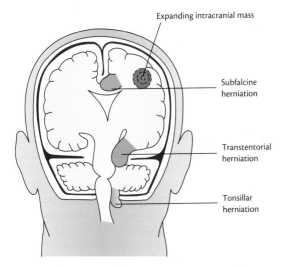

Fig. 18.2 Raised intracranial pressure due to an expanding intracranial mass may cause herniation at three typical sites: subfalcine, transtentorial, and tonsillar.

Expanding intracranial mass

Subfalcine herniation

Transtentorial herniation

Tonsillar herniation

Compression of vital respiratory and cardiac centres located in the medulla oblongata is life threatening.

Key points: Raised intracranial pressure

♦ The brain is enclosed in a rigid box with limited room for expansion.

♦ Any space-occupying lesion within the cranial cavity leads to a rise in intracranial pressure.

♦ The mass effect of a lesion within the brain is often exacerbated by cerebral oedema due to disruption of the blood–brain barrier.

♦ Symptoms of raised intracranial pressure include headache and nausea. Fundoscopy reveals a swollen optic nerve head.

♦ The main danger of raised intracranial pressure is herniation of parts of the brain from one compartment to another. The three commonest types of herniation are subfalcine, transtentorial, and tonsillar. Compression of vital structures due to herniation may lead to death.

Hydrocephalus

Hydrocephalus refers to excessive CSF within the ventricular system. In adults, most cases of hydrocephalus are due to obstruction to the normal flow of CSF (**obstructive hydrocephalus**). Expanding lesions in the posterior fossa are particularly prone to causing obstructive hydrocephalus because the narrow lumen of the aqueduct and fourth ventricle is easily blocked off.

Obstructive hydrocephalus may also result as a complication of subarachnoid haemorrhage or meningitis due to organization and fibrosis of blood or exudate blocking drainage of CSF out of the arachnoid space.

LINK BOX

Congenital hydrocephalus

Congenital hydrocephalus occurs in about 1 in 1000 births. Most are caused by congenital malformations of the CNS which obstruct flow of CSF, such as the **Arnold–Chiari malformation** and **aqueduct stenosis** (p. 508).

Coma

A **coma** is a state of unrousable unconsciousness. Normally, consciousness is maintained by communication between a region in the brainstem known as the reticular activating system and the cerebral cortex. Coma may therefore result from any of the following:

♦ A focal lesion in the brainstem affecting the reticular activating system.

♦ A focal lesion in a cerebral hemisphere raising intracranial pressure and compressing the brainstem.

♦ A diffuse problem globally affecting the function of the cerebral cortex.

Common focal lesions causing coma include intracranial bleeds, which may be spontaneous or following head injury. Common diffuse lesions causing coma include metabolic conditions such as uncontrolled diabetes, hepatic failure, toxins such as drugs and alcohol, and CNS infections such as meningitis or encephalitis.

Dementia

Dementia is a clinical syndrome characterized by the progressive decline of cognitive function without an impairment of consciousness. Dementia can be viewed conceptually as a form of 'chronic brain failure' due to any disease that causes gradual loss of cortical neurones. Dementia therefore has many possible causes (Table 18.1), though the most common are Alzheimer's disease, vascular dementia, and dementia with Lewy bodies.

Cerebrovascular disease

The CNS gains energy entirely from oxidative metabolism of glucose. The CNS cannot store glucose and so is critically dependent on a constant supply of oxygen and glucose from the blood. Cerebral blood flow, which is 800 ml/min, accounts for 15–20 per cent of the cardiac output. If the blood supply to a region of brain stops, neurones will start dying within minutes, and within a matter of hours the entire region supplied by that artery will be irreversibly damaged.

Cerebrovascular disease refers to any brain disease attributable to a vascular cause. Most cerebrovascular diseases are related to narrowing, occlusion, or rupture of a vessel supplying the brain. Cerebrovascular disease is the third leading cause of death in the Western world after ischaemic heart disease and cancer.

Stroke

Cerebrovascular accident or **stroke** is the most common manifestation of cerebrovascular disease. A stroke is a sudden neurological deficit lasting longer than 24 h that is attributable to a vascular cause. If the deficit resolves within 24 h, then the term **transient ischaemic attack** (TIA) is used. Although this clinical distinction is made, the underlying pathology is identical. Having a TIA is therefore a major risk factor for sustaining a subsequent completed stroke.

The three most common causes of stroke are:

+ **Cerebral infarction** due to blockage of a cerebral artery (80 per cent).

+ **Intracerebral haemorrhage** due to rupture of a vessel into the brain substance (15 per cent).

+ **Subarachnoid haemorrhage** due to rupture of a vessel into the subarachnoid space (5 per cent).

The most useful test to distinguish between a haemorrhage and an infarct is a computed tomography (CT) scan of the head, as haemorrhage will be immediately apparent.

Cerebral infarction is usually due to blockage of a cerebral artery by a thromboembolus

The majority of strokes are due to cerebral infarction, i.e. death of brain tissue due to insufficient blood supply (Fig. 18.3). This occurs due to sustained cerebral arterial occlusion severe enough to cause infarction of the specific territory of distribution of the compromised vessel.

Most cerebral infarctions are caused by thromboembolic occlusion of a cerebral artery. Most thromboemboli come from an internal carotid artery containing complicated atherosclerotic plaques. Emboli may also come from the left side of the heart, particularly the left atrium in patients with atrial fibrillation.

Note that only a small proportion of cerebral infarctions are due to *in situ* thrombosis complicating an advanced atherosclerotic plaque within a cerebral artery, because cerebral arteries are much less severely affected by atherosclerosis than the internal carotid arteries.

TABLE 18.1 Causes of dementia

Alzheimer's disease
Vascular dementia
Dementia with Lewy bodies
Huntington's disease
Parkinson's disease
Alcohol
Vitamin B12 deficiency
HIV infection

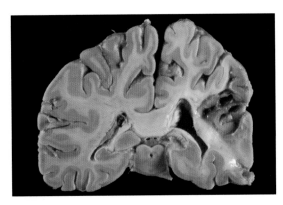

Fig. 18.3 Cerebral infarction.

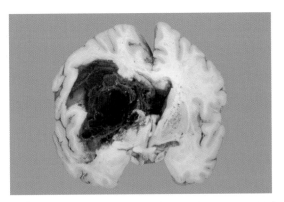

Fig. 18.4 Intracerebral haemorrhage. This is a slice of brain taken at post-mortem from a patient who suddenly collapsed and died. There is a massive intracerebral haematoma which led to a huge rise in intracranial pressure and herniation. The cause in this case was hypertension, and other changes of hypertension at post-mortem included left ventricular hypertrophy and nephrosclerosis of both kidneys.

Intracerebral haemorrhage is usually due to hypertension

An intracerebral haemorrhage produces neurological symptoms by producing a mass effect on nearby structures and from the toxic effect of blood itself (Fig. 18.4). The most common causes of spontaneous intracerebral haemorrhage are hypertension, cerebral amyloid angiopathy, and arteriovenous malformations.

- **Hypertension** is the most common cause of intracerebral haemorrhage. The haemorrhage is due to rupture of tiny aneurysms called **Charcot–Bouchard aneurysms** which form in arterioles weakened by long-standing hypertension. The basal ganglia and thalamus are common sites for rupture.

- **Cerebral amyloid angiopathy** accounts for about 10 per cent of intracerebral haemorrhages. The underlying abnormality is the deposition of amyloid in the media of small and medium sized cerebral arteries. This appears to be an age-related phenomenon and is not associated with amyloid deposition outside the brain. Haemorrhages associated with amyloid angiopathy tend to occur at the border between the grey and white matter of the cerebral hemispheres.

- **Arteriovenous malformations** are abnormal tangles of blood vessels in which arteries are directly connected to veins, without a capillary bed between them. Blood is therefore delivered at high pressure into veins, which become dilated and prone to rupture. Bleeding from an arteriovenous malformation is the most common cause of intracerebral haemorrhage in patients under 45 years of age.

JARGON BUSTER

Haemorrhagic infarct versus haemorrhagic stroke

Cerebral infarcts can bleed secondarily giving rise to a **haemorrhagic infarct**. It is thought that this happens when damaged blood vessels supplying the area of infarction are reperfused as the occlusive material dissolves. It is important to realize that this phenomenon is not the same as a **haemorrhagic stroke**, where the primary pathology is bleeding into the brain substance.

Subarachnoid haemorrhage is usually due to rupture of a berry aneurysm

Subarachnoid haemorrhage is bleeding into the subarachnoid space between the arachnoid membrane and pia mater (Fig. 18.5). A subarachnoid haemorrhage may occur following traumatic rupture of vessels at the base of the brain, but more commonly occurs spontaneously due to rupture of a **berry aneurysm**.

Most berry aneurysms arise at sites of arterial bifurcation at the base of the brain (Fig. 18.6). It is largely unknown why some people develop berry aneurysms. Although they are not present at birth, it is possible

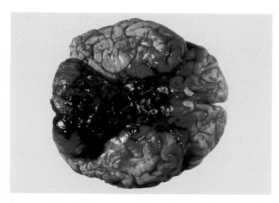

Fig. 18.5 Subarachnoid haemorrhage. This is the undersurface of the brain removed at post-mortem from a patient who suddenly cried out, collapsed, and died. Blood is seen filling the subarachnoid space. When the blood clot was cleared away, a ruptured berry aneurysm was found in the circle of Willis.

that there is a congenital defect in the tunica media of the cerebral vessels which leads to aneurysm formation later in life under the influence of atherosclerosis and hypertension. Most berry aneurysms do not rupture.

Subarachnoid haemorrhage causes a sudden severe headache; people describe it as like being struck hard on the back of the head. It is often precipitated by exertion, straining, or sexual intercourse. In about one-third of cases, massive subarachnoid haemorrhage causes instant death due to a rapid rise in intracranial pressure and fatal herniation. Another third become

unconscious and have a high risk of dying or developing permanent neurological deficit. The remaining third usually do well provided there is no rebleeding.

Key points: Stroke

- Stroke, or cerebrovascular accident, refers to the sudden onset of a neurological deficit which lasts longer than 24 h, due to a vascular event.

- The most common cause of stroke is cerebral infarction. Most cerebral infarctions are due to thromboemboli from an internal carotid artery or from the heart occluding a cerebral artery.

- Spontaneous intracerebral haemorrhage is the second most common cause of stroke. Most cases are due to rupture of a Charcot–Bouchard aneurysm caused by hypertension. In elderly people, blood vessels affected by cerebral amyloid angiopathy may rupture, causing intracerebral haemorrhage. In young people, bleeding from an arteriovenous malformation is the most common cause of intracerebral haemorrhage.

- Subarachnoid haemorrhage is bleeding into the subarachnoid space, usually due to rupture of a berry aneurysm. Berry aneurysms are thought to develop under the influence of hypertension and atherosclerosis in people with a congenital weakness in the tunica media of cerebral vessels.

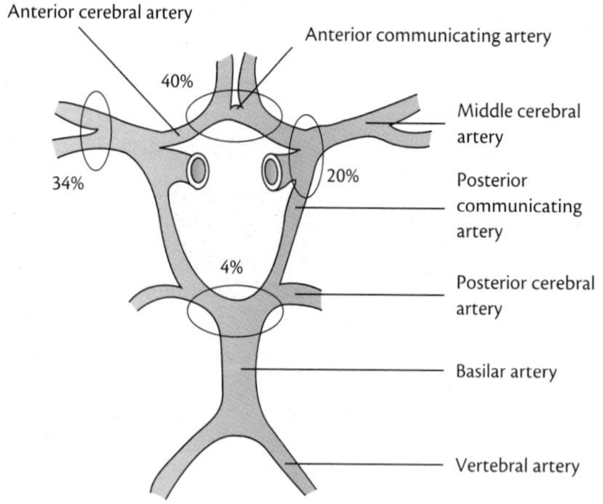

Fig. 18.6 Diagram of the circle of Willis showing common sites of berry aneurysm formation.

Vascular dementia

Vascular dementia, or **multi-infarct dementia**, is dementia resulting from cerebrovascular disease. Vascular dementia is the result of numerous small, often subclinical, infarcts and haemorrhages occurring throughout the brain due to a combination of atherosclerosis, hypertension, and cerebral amyloid angiopathy. Vascular dementia is a very common cause of dementia and probably contributes, to some degree, to virtually all cases of dementia.

Hypertensive encephalopathy

Hypertensive encephalopathy is a hypertensive emergency in which a dramatic rise in blood pressure leads to failure of cerebral autoregulation, breakdown of the blood–brain barrier, and diffuse cerebral oedema.

Hypertensive encephalopathy presents with headache, nausea, vomiting, and confusion. Left untreated, seizures occur and eventually coma ensues. A number of conditions may mimic hypertensive encephalopathy, including hypoglycaemia, Wernicke's encephalopathy, encephalitis, and tumours.

The aim of treatment is gradually to reduce diastolic blood pressure over a period of 1–2 h. The first line agent is **sodium nitroprusside**, a direct vascular smooth muscle relaxant which immediately lowers blood pressure with a short-lived effect. This enables fine control of the blood pressure to be achieved by adjusting the rate of infusion of the drug accordingly.

Trauma to the central nervous system

Trauma to the CNS is potentially very serious. Head injury is the leading cause of death in people under 45 years of age in developed countries. The number of severe head injuries in the UK each year is about 50 000, and these account for some 20 per cent of deaths in people aged 5–45, and severe disability in those who survive.

Skull fractures

If the force of a head injury is severe, the skull may fracture at the site of impact. Uncomplicated skull fractures are not in themselves a problem but, because considerable force is required to fracture the skull, they are a marker of serious head injury. A patient with a skull fracture is therefore more likely to have associated underlying intracranial disease such as contusions and haemorrhage. Skull fractures also increase the risk of developing intracranial infection.

Cerebral contusions

Cerebral contusions are bruises on the surface of the brain which occur when the brain suddenly moves within the cranial cavity and is crushed against the skull. Typically there is injury at the site of impact (the **coup** lesion) and at the site diagonally opposite this point (the **contrecoup** lesion). Oozing of blood into the brain parenchyma and the associated cerebral oedema are important contributors to raised intracranial pressure.

Intracranial haemorrhage

Bleeding in and around the brain is a common feature of head injury. Intracranial bleeds form a solid blood clot (haematoma) which increases intracranial pressure.

Extradural haematoma is due to haemorrhage between the dura and the skull. The bleeding vessel is often the middle meningeal artery which is torn following fracture of the squamous temporal bone. Accumulation of extradural blood is usually slow as the firmly adherent dura is slowly peeled away from the inner surface of the skull (Fig. 18.7). Patients with extradural haematomas may often appear well for several hours following head injury, but then quickly deteriorate as the haematoma enlarges and compresses the brain.

Subdural haematoma is due to haemorrhage between the dura and the arachnoid. The bleeding results from tearing of delicate bridging veins that traverse the subdural space to drain into the cerebral venous sinuses. Blood from these veins spreads freely through the subdural space, eventually enveloping the entire cerebral hemisphere on the side of the injury (Fig. 18.8). Subdural haematomas are often seen in elderly people following relatively minor trauma, and may present with confusion. Shrinkage of the brain due to age-related atrophy may contribute to the risk of subdural haemorrhage by placing traction on the bridging veins.

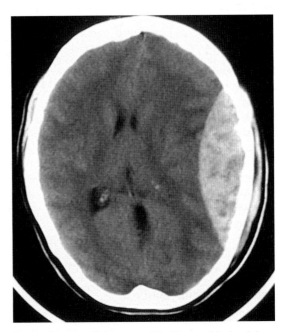

Fig. 18.7 Extradural haematoma. This CT scan of the head shows compression and shift of the left cerebral hemisphere by a biconvex high density lesion. This is an extradural haematoma caused by rupture of the middle meningeal artery following head injury.

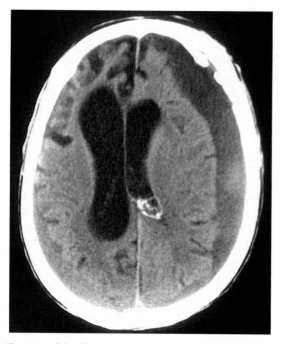

Fig. 18.8 Subdural haematoma. The lateral ventricles are shifted to the right and are enlarged. The left cerebral hemisphere is compressed by a crescent-shaped radiolucency between the left cerebral cortex and the skull. This is a subdural haematoma. The cerebral hemispheres are shrunken and atrophic which stretches the bridging veins making them easily torn by minor trauma to the head. A small subdural haematoma is also on the right side posteriorly. It is more recent as it is more dense.

Subarachnoid haemorrhage is usually seen following spontaneous rupture of a berry aneurysm (see earlier), but may also occur following trauma. Head injury may lead to subarachnoid haemorrhage if cerebral contusions bleed out into the subarachnoid space, if fractures of the skull base tear large vessels at the base of the brain, or if blood from an intraventricular haemorrhage reaches the subarachnoid space via the exit foramina of the fourth ventricle.

Intracerebral haematomas more commonly occur spontaneously due to hypertension, but may also occur in association with severe head injury.

Traumatic axonal injury

Traumatic axonal injury refers to axonal damage due to trauma, typically following sudden acceleration and deceleration of the head. Traumatic axonal injury covers a spectrum of changes ranging from involvement of a few axons to shearing of a large number of axons. The most severe form of traumatic axonal injury is known as **diffuse axonal injury**. Patients suffering diffuse axonal injury are rendered immediately unconscious from the moment of impact and usually remain unconscious until death.

Spinal cord injury

Spinal cord injury is usually the result of road traffic accidents in which a fracture or dislocation of the vertebral column crushes the spinal cord and irreversibly damages it. The level of cord injury determines the extent of disability. Lesions of the thoracic cord or below lead to loss of function of the legs (paraplegia); cervical cord lesions involve all four limbs (tetraplegia). Very high lesions paralyse the diaphragm, leading to reduced ventilation and respiratory compromise.

> ## Key points: Trauma to the central nervous system
>
> - Trauma to the central nervous system is a common cause of death and disability. Many traumas are the result of road traffic accidents.
>
> - Trauma to the head may result in skull fracture, cerebral contusions, intracranial haemorrhage, and traumatic axonal injury.
>
> - One of the main problems in patients with head injury is the development of raised intracranial pressure.
>
> - Trauma to the spinal cord is usually the result of a fracture or dislocation of the vertebral column. Depending on the level of the injury, there may be paraplegia or tetraplegia.

Infections of the central nervous system

Infection of the CNS is a difficult task for microorganisms, as the CNS is enclosed in several layers which act as good barriers to infection. The most common routes of infection to the CNS are blood-borne infection, invasion via peripheral nerves, and local invasion from nearby structures (e.g. infections in the ears or sinuses).

Meningitis

Meningitis is an infection of the subarachnoid space which leads to symptoms of fever, headache, and photophobia. The key clinical sign is **neck stiffness**, characterized by physical resistance to flexion of the neck. Focal neurological signs are usually absent, as the inflammation is restricted to the meninges with no involvement of the brain itself.

Viral meningitis is the most common type of meningitis

Viruses are the most common cause of meningitis, the most frequent culprits being members of the enterovirus family such as echoviruses and coxsackieviruses. Viral meningitis causes headache, fever, and photophobia. Neck stiffness is usually less marked than in bacterial meningitis. CSF examination typically shows a predominance of lymphocytes and a normal glucose level. Culture fails to grow a bacterial organism. If necessary, polymerase chain reaction (PCR) can be performed on CSF to identify the specific virus responsible. There is no specific treatment for viral meningitis, but fortunately the disease runs a mild course and complete recovery is the rule.

Bacterial meningitis is a very serious infection

In contrast to viral meningitis, bacterial meningitis is a potentially life-threatening infection. A number of bacteria may cause meningitis (Table 18.2), though most cases are caused by either *Neisseria meningitidis* or *Streptococcus pneumoniae*. *Haemophilus influenzae* was once responsible for many cases of meningitis, but since the introduction of the *H. influenzae* type b (Hib) vaccine, the number of cases of *H. influenzae* meningitis has fallen significantly.

Neisseria meningitidis and *S. pneumoniae* reach the CNS via the blood, in which they are able to survive because their capsule renders them resistant to phagocytosis

---

TABLE 18.2   Bacteria causing meningitis

Neisseria meningitidis
Streptococcus pneumoniae
Haemophilus influenzae
Escherichia coli
Mycobacterium tuberculosis

---

and complement. The bacteria directly infect choroid plexus cells and gain entry into the CSF. Once in the CSF, the bacteria can multiply rapidly within it because of the absence of effective host defences.

Lysis of some bacteria with release of cell wall components into the subarachnoid space stimulates an inflammatory response and the formation of a purulent exudate in the subarachnoid space. The bacteria themselves do not appear to cause significant direct tissue injury; it is the inflammatory response that causes the manifestations of the disease.

The clinical features of bacterial meningitis are similar to those of viral meningitis, with headache, fever, photophobia, and neck stiffness, though usually more severe. Any patient suspected of having bacterial meningitis should be given immediate empirical antibacterial treatment while further investigations are being performed. This action saves lives.

Laboratory identification of the responsible bacteria is absolutely essential so that the most effective antibacterial drug can be administered. The key specimens are CSF (Table 18.3) and multiple sets of blood cultures. Microscopy of CSF can be performed immediately, and typically shows large numbers of neutrophils. A Gram stain result can be ready within the hour and can help narrow down the likely causative bacteria. Definitive culture and sensitivity results on CSF or blood cultures take at least 24 h.

Meningococcal meningitis is typically seen in young children and adolescents

Neisseria meningitidis (meningococcus) is a Gram negative coccus which has a number of different serotypes. Most cases of meningococcal meningitis in the UK are now caused by type B. The number of cases caused by type C is falling since the Department of Health introduced the serotype C vaccine into the national vaccination programme.

Neisseria meningitidis is a normal commensal organism of the nasopharynx in up to 20 per cent of the population. Nasopharyngeal carriage of *N. meningitidis* can be spread from person to person by droplet infection, and transmission is therefore a problem where many people live together in close contact, such as university halls of residence.

For meningitis to occur, the bacteria must enter the blood stream and invade the meninges. How and why this occurs in some people remains unknown.

TABLE 18.3	Typical CSF changes in meningitis			
	Normal	**Viral**	**Bacterial**	**Tuberculous**
Appearance	Clear	Turbid	Purulent	Turbid
Microscopy	Few cells	Lymphocytes	Neutrophils	Lymphocytes
Glucose	1/2–2/3 blood level	Normal	Low	Low

Antibodies against antigens in the capsule of the bacterium protect against infection with *N. meningitidis*. The most susceptible people are therefore young children who have lost protection from maternal antibodies, and adolescents who have not yet encountered the organism and have no specific immunity.

As well as the typical features of meningitis, there may also be symptoms related to the associated meningococcaemia, including the well publicized 'non-blanching' skin rash due to bleeding from necrotic skin capillaries. In its most severe form, meningococcal septicaemia is a highly lethal condition causing the rapid development of septic shock, acute disseminated intravascular coagulation, and multiorgan failure.

Pneumococcal meningitis is usually seen in young children and the elderly

Streptococcus pneumoniae (pneumococcus) is a Gram positive coccus carried in the pharynx of most individuals. Invasion of the blood and meninges is rare, but may occur in those without high levels of antibody to the bacterial capsule such as young children under 2 years of age and the elderly. Pneumococcal meningitis causes the same symptoms as other forms of meningitis. The skin rash of meningococcal disease is not normally seen.

Tuberculous meningitis has a gradual onset over a few weeks

The meninges are one of the more common sites for extrapulmonary tuberculosis, though usually this occurs in people with an obvious focus of infection elsewhere. Tuberculous meningitis typically presents much more slowly than acute bacterial meningitis, starting with malaise and then proceeding slowly to photophobia and neck stiffness. Microscopy may reveal acid-fast bacilli, but definitive diagnosis requires culture of the organism from CSF. Culture takes many weeks, and PCR is increasingly being used to provide a quicker result.

Severe bacterial meningitis may cause permanent neurological complications

Death remains a very real possibility in patients with severe bacterial meningitis. Survivors of severe bacterial meningitis may be left with permanent neurological sequelae including hearing loss, learning difficulties, paralysis, and seizures.

Key points: Meningitis

- Meningitis is an infection of the subarachnoid space.

- Most cases of meningitis are caused by viruses. Viral meningitis is usually a self-limiting infection.

- Bacterial meningitis is much more serious, with more severe symptoms and a greater chance of complications such as hearing loss, learning difficulties, paralysis, and seizures.

- Patients with suspected bacterial meningitis require immediate empirical antibacterial treatment pending the results of cerebrospinal fluid and blood culture analysis.

- Meningococcal meningitis occurs when nasopharyngeal *N. meningitis* invades the blood stream and reaches the meninges. Young children and adolescents are most at risk due to lack of specific antibodies against the capsule of the organism. In its most fulminant form, meningococcal septicaemia leads to shock and multiorgan failure.

- Pneumococcal meningitis occurs if nasopharyngeal *S. pneumoniae* enter the blood stream and reach the meninges. Pneumococcal meningitis is seen mostly in young children and the elderly.

Encephalitis

Encephalitis is a destructive inflammation of the brain substance caused by direct infection of the brain. Because the substance of the brain is affected, the patient with encephalitis commonly has confusion, behavioural abnormalities, and an altered level of consciousness. Seizures may occur in severe encephalitis.

Viruses are the most common causes of encephalitis, and by far the most common culprit is herpes simplex virus (HSV). It is crucial to consider the possibility of herpes simplex encephalitis in a patient with signs of cerebral dysfunction, as prompt administration of aciclovir reduces the likelihood of death or long-term disability.

Herpes simplex encephalitis occurs following reactivation of the virus in the trigeminal ganglion, from which the virus can pass into the temporal lobe. The virus often causes a simultaneous infection around the mouth, and the presence of perioral vesicles may be a useful clue to the diagnosis. Imaging of the brain with CT or magnetic resonance imaging (MRI) is useful to highlight abnormalities in the temporal lobe. Identification of HSV can be achieved by performing PCR on a sample of CSF.

Cerebral abscess

Brain abscesses are foci of infection associated with destruction of the brain substance. Most brain abscesses arise by direct spread from an infection in a paranasal sinus, the middle ear, or a tooth. Brain abscesses may also result from haematogenous spread, usually in the form of an infected embolus from a vegetation of infective endocarditis. Fortunately, brain abscesses have become rare since the introduction of antibacterial agents.

A brain abscess typically presents with symptoms related to an infected intracranial mass, i.e. headache, nausea and vomiting, fever, epilepsy, or localizing neurological signs. A CT scan is usually diagnostic, and treatment requires surgical drainage and prolonged antibiotic treatment for at least 1 month. Brain abscesses are serious conditions; 20 per cent of patients die from the abscess, and half of survivors are left with persistent neurological deficits or epilepsy.

Demyelinating diseases of the central nervous system

Multiple sclerosis

Multiple sclerosis (MS) is a relapsing and remitting disease of the CNS in which episodes of neurological disturbance affect different parts of the CNS at different times. MS affects about 1 in 1000 people in the UK and is a major cause of disability in people of working age.

Symptoms of multiple sclerosis are caused by demyelination of axons within lesions called plaques

The neurological deficit in MS is associated with lesions called **plaques** in the white matter of the CNS. Microscopically, plaques contain inflammation with loss of oligodendrocytes and myelin. The demyelination blocks normal conduction of impulses down axons passing through the plaque.

Multiple sclerosis is thought to be an autoimmune disease

The precise aetiology and pathogenesis of MS remain unknown although an autoimmune cause is favoured. Patients with MS have autoreactive T cells against myelin basic protein and autoantibodies against myelin antigens such as myelin oligodendrocyte glycoprotein (MOG). What triggers the autoimmunity is not known, although the striking geographical link to temperate areas of the world suggests an environmental factor may be relevant.

The current prevailing theory is that the inflammation is the primary problem, and the loss of oligodendrocytes and myelin is secondary to the inflammation. However, this is only conjecture, and recent evidence has suggested that in early MS loss of oligodendrocytes may occur prior to any inflammation, suggesting that perhaps the inflammation is an appropriate response to some other primary problem causing oligodendrocyte death. This challenges the concept of a primary autoimmune pathogenesis for MS.

Initially recovery from episodes of demyelination is complete, but over time recovery becomes slower and incomplete

Episodes of demyelination lead to attacks of acute neurological deficit which develop over a period of a few days and remain for a few weeks before there is recovery of symptoms. Recovery of function may occur for a number of reasons:

◆ Remyelination occurs. Sometimes an axon may remyelinate and regain back much of its original function.

◆ Demyelinated axons continue to function despite losing their myelin, e.g. by producing more sodium channels to generate an action potential.

◆ New neuronal pathways are created to bypass the damaged neurones.

In the early stages of the disease, complete recovery is the rule. However, as the disease progresses, recovery is slower and residual deficit remains. This is presumably because the axons themselves also start to die because there are no oligodendrocytes releasing essential growth factors. Axonal death is permanent and is the chief reason for the progressive permanent neurological disability that occurs in patients with MS.

Plaques have a predilection for certain sites in the CNS

Although plaques may occur anywhere in the white matter of the CNS, they have a predilection for distinct sites, most notably the optic nerves, the periventricular region, the brainstem, and the cervical spinal cord (Fig. 18.9). Common features of MS include the following:

◆ Blurred vision and loss of colour vision due to demyelination in one of the optic nerves.

◆ Patchy numbness or tingling in a limb due to spinal cord demyelination.

◆ Vertigo and incoordination due to cerebellar demyelination.

◆ Eye movement disorders due to demyelination of brainstem white matter tracts coordinating eye movements. One highly characteristic physical sign of MS is an **internuclear ophthalmoplegia** due to demyelination of the medial longitudinal fasciculus.

With progression of the disease, the spinal cord becomes a heavy target for demyelination leading to serious disability from paraplegia, loss of sphincter control, and sexual dysfunction.

Diagnosing multiple sclerosis requires evidence of two or more attacks at different sites at different times

Making a definite diagnosis of MS requires clear evidence of at least two episodes of neurological deficit occurring at different times, and affecting different parts of the CNS. Someone who has had only one attack of demyelination does not have MS, although investigations may help establish that a diagnosis of MS is very likely.

If a brain MRI shows the typical periventricular demyelination in a patient with only one clinically apparent attack of demyelination, there is a good chance that clinically definite MS will develop within 5 years.

Visual evoked potentials measure the speed of impulse conduction along the optic nerve. Slowing of conduction may remain for many years after an attack of optic nerve demyelination, and this may provide helpful extra evidence for MS by demonstrating a second lesion.

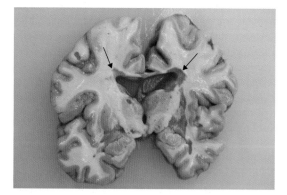

Fig. 18.9 Multiple sclerosis plaques. Brown appearance of multiple sclerosis plaques, seen here in a characteristic location around the lateral ventricles (arrows).

Key points: Multiple sclerosis

◆ Multiple sclerosis is a chronic relapsing and remitting disorder of the central nervous system characterized by episodes of neurological deficit.

◆ The neurological deficit is due to areas of white matter demyelination within lesions called plaques.

◆ Initially the plaques of multiple sclerosis show a predilection for the optic nerve, brainstem, and cerebellum. Early in the disease, episodes of demyelination often resolve, with complete recovery.

Key points: Multiple sclerosis—cont'd

- Later in the course of the disease, the spinal cord becomes a heavy target and recovery from demyelination becomes incomplete, leaving many patients wheelchair bound.

- The cause of multiple sclerosis remains unknown, though an autoimmune pathogenesis is favoured.

Neurodegenerative diseases

The term 'degenerative' as a label for a disease was much used back in the nineteenth century when there was no other apparent cause for a disease. With the advances of modern medicine, many of the degenerative diseases of old have been reclassified into their correct disease category.

Neurodegenerative diseases, however, remain a well recognized category of disease, used to describe a number of baffling diseases in which selective groups of neurones die with no appreciable inflammation (Table 18.4).

Ongoing work is slowly beginning to unravel the possible cause of these diseases. A vast amount of evidence now exists to suggest that these diseases are the result of abnormal processing and folding of proteins. Accumulation of these abnormal proteins leads to death of selective groups of neurones.

Virtually all of the neurodegenerative diseases are either inherited or have an inherited form which has an earlier age of onset than the sporadic form. The inherited forms are associated with a mutation that increases the likelihood of the relevant protein misfolding and aggregating. Precisely what makes the protein

misfold spontaneously in the sporadic forms remains unclear, but is clearly a crucial question to answer.

Alzheimer's disease

Alzheimer's disease is the most common cause of dementia. In the UK, Alzheimer's disease affects 5 per cent of people aged over 65 and as many as 20 per cent of people aged over 80. With an ever aging population, the incidence of Alzheimer's disease is likely to continue to rise.

Alzheimer's disease typically starts with memory loss. Memories of events or episodes are particularly affected, including day to day memory and new learning. As the disease progresses, there is increasing disability in managing daily activities such as finances and shopping. Loss of motor skills develops next, causing difficulty in dressing, cooking, and cleaning. Later in the disease, agitation, restlessness, wandering, and disinhibition may occur. This may cause considerable upset to family and carers. The terminal stages of the disease cause reduced speech output, immobility, and incontinence. Death occurs on average 10 years from diagnosis, often from pneumonia.

The brains of patients with Alzheimer's disease show marked atrophy of the cerebral cortex, particularly in the hippocampus (Fig. 18.10). Microscopically, there is neuronal loss associated with a number of additional lesions, namely:

- **Amyloid plaques**, composed of amyloid Aβ protein.

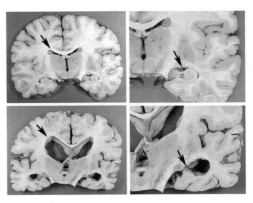

Fig. 18.10 Alzheimer's disease. The top images are from a normal patient aged 70, while the bottom images are from a patient with Alzheimer's disease. Note the ventricular dilation (left hand side) and cortical atrophy in the brain from the patient with Alzheimer's disease, particularly marked in the hippocampus (right hand side).

TABLE 18.4	Neurodegenerative disorders
Alzheimer's disease	
Dementia with Lewy bodies	
Parkinson's disease	
Huntington's disease	
Prion diseases	

◆ **Neurofibrillary tangles**, inclusions within neurones composed of *paired helical filaments*, the main constituent of which is the microtubule-binding protein tau.

◆ **Dystrophic neurites** and **neuropil threads**, distorted neuronal processes which also contain tau.

Note that none of these changes are specific for Alzheimer's disease; all of them can be found in the brains of normal elderly people, albeit in lower numbers. Alzheimer's disease is associated with a high density of these lesions throughout the cerebral cortex. Because these changes can be found in a very high proportion of normal elderly subjects, debate continues as to whether Alzheimer's disease is a distinct disease process or just the extreme end of the normal ageing process.

The pathogenesis of Alzheimer's diseases remains unclear, in particular which of the various lesions found in the brain is of primary pathogenic importance. Current evidence strongly supports the theory that the underlying pathogenic event in Alzheimer's disease is accumulation of Aβ amyloid (Fig. 18.11).

Aβ peptides are derived from a normal protein which has been called amyloid precursor protein (APP) as we do not know its normal function. APP is a transmembrane protein which is expressed on the cell surface. Aβ peptides are formed from APP by the action of two enzymes called β-secretase and γ-secretase. Genetic evidence that supports the role of Aβ peptide in Alzheimer's disease includes the early development of Alzheimer's disease in patients with trisomy 21 due to a gene dosage effect, and the discovery that two genes linked to early onset Alzheimer's disease code for components of γ-secretase.

Precisely how Aβ is related to neurofibrillary tangles, dystrophic neuritis, and neuronal loss seen in Alzheimer's disease remains unknown.

> ## Key points: Alzheimer's disease
>
> ◆ Alzheimer's disease is the most common cause of dementia.
>
> ◆ Alzheimer's disease presents initially with memory loss. With progression, there is loss of language and motor skills. Eventually patients are rendered immobile, mute, and incontinent.
>
> ◆ The cerebral cortex of patients with Alzheimer's disease shows neuronal loss and is filled with Aβ amyloid plaques, neurofibrillary tangles, dystrophic neurites, and neuropil threads.
>
> ◆ Current evidence points strongly to Aβ amyloid plaques as the underlying pathogenic lesions in Alzheimer's disease.

Dementia with Lewy bodies

Dementia with Lewy bodies (DLB) is now recognized as the second most common cause of dementia. The defining feature of DLB is the presence of **Lewy bodies** in neurones of cortical grey matter *and* subcortical nuclei. Lewy bodies are inclusions with the cytoplasm of neurones composed mainly of α-synuclein, ubiquitin, and parkin. They can only be appreciated microscopically (Fig. 18.12).

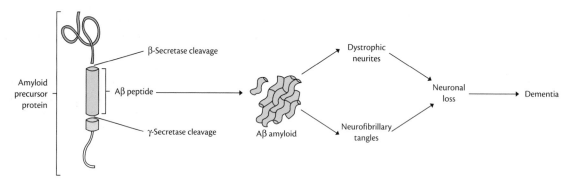

Fig. 18.11 Theory of pathogenesis of Alzheimer's disease. Accumulation of Aβ amyloid derived from amyloid precursor protein is thought to give rise to dystrophic neurites and neurofibrillary tangles, which in turn cause the neuronal loss leading to dementia.

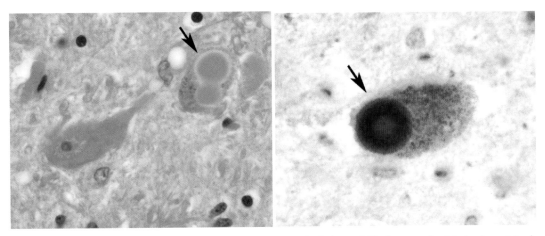

Fig. 18.12 Lewy body. Microscopic images of a neurone containing a Lewy body (arrows). The image on the right has been stained using an antibody against alpha synuclein, the main constituent of a Lewy body. Lewy bodies are seen in great number in neurones of the substantia nigra in Parkinson's disease, and in cortical neurones in dementia with Lewy bodies.

The brain of patients with DLB also often contains microscopic changes typical of Alzheimer's disease such as amyloid plaques and neurofibrillary tangles, and there is often considerable overlap between the two diseases. The key feature in distinguishing the two is the distribution of the changes; most notably, the neurofibrillary tangles in DLB spare the hippocampus, which is severely affected in Alzheimer's disease.

DLB causes a progressively worsening dementia. Features that are helpful in distinguishing it from Alzheimer's disease include *fluctuating levels of cognition*, *recurrent visual hallucinations* (often remarkably detailed), and *features of parkinsonism* (though not enough for the diagnosis of Parkinson's disease). Other features supportive of a diagnosis of DLB include recurrent falls, syncope, or transient loss of consciousness.

> ♦ Helpful clinical features to distinguish DLB from Alzheimer's disease include fluctuating cognition, recurrent visual hallucinations, and features of parkinsonism.

Parkinson's disease

Parkinson's disease is a neurodegenerative disease characterized by selective loss of dopaminergic neurones in the substantia nigra. Under normal circumstances, neurones in the substantia nigra synthesize dopamine which acts as an inhibitory neurotransmitter in the putamen and globus pallidus of the basal ganglia. Loss of control of movement generation in Parkinson's disease manifests with tremor, bradykinesia (slow movement), and rigidity typical of the disease.

Loss of the substantia nigra neurones can be appreciated macroscopically because of loss of the normal melanin pigmentation of this region (Fig. 18.13). If this region is examined microscopically, there is severe neuronal loss, and surviving neurones contain Lewy bodies (exactly the same as those seen in the cortex of patients with DLB).

The cause of the degeneration of substantia nigra neurones in Parkinson's disease is not known. There is support for an environmental cause, as there is a relative

Key points: Dementia with Lewy bodies

♦ Dementia with Lewy bodies is the second most common cause of dementia.

♦ The defining feature of DLB is the presence of Lewy bodies in cortical and subcortical neurones.

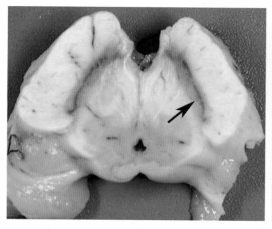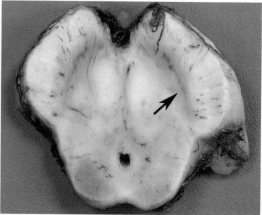

Fig. 18.13 Substantia nigra in Parkinson's disease. Slices through the midbrain of a normal person (left) and a patient with Parkinson's disease (right) showing loss of pigmentation in the substantia nigra in Parkinson's disease (arrows).

absence of identifiable genetic links, and a positive family history is unusual in Parkinson's disease. Furthermore, a synthetic heroin byproduct known as MPTP is known to cause parkinsonism; exogenous molecules that can selectively damage the dopaminergic neurones of the substantia nigra are therefore known to exist.

JARGON BUSTER

Parkinsonism

Parkinsonism refers to the combination of rigidity, bradykinesia, and resting tremor. The most common cause of parkinsonism is Parkinson's disease, but there are other causes of parkinsonism, e.g. treatment with dopamine antagonist drugs such as haloperidol and phenothiazines, and dementia with Lewy bodies.

Key points: Parkinson's disease

- Parkinson's disease is a neurodegenerative disease in which there is selective loss of dopaminergic neurones in the substantia nigra.

- Loss of dopaminergic input to the basal ganglia leads to a movement disorder characterized by tremor, rigidity, and bradykinesia.
- Microscopic examination of the substantia nigra in a patient with Parkinson's disease shows loss of neurones, with Lewy bodies present in surviving neurones.
- The cause of Parkinson's disease is not known, although an environmental agent which is selectively toxic to substantia nigra neurones has been suggested.

Huntington's disease

Huntington's disease is a slowly progressive fatal neurodegenerative disorder caused by an inherited genetic defect in a gene encoding a protein of unknown function called **huntingtin**. The normal gene contains a region with between nine and 37 continuous triplet repeats of the sequence CAG.

When the number of repeats exceeds 37, molecules of huntingtin begin to stick together, leading to malfunction of neurones. Generally speaking, the higher the number of repeats, the earlier the disease presents and the more rapid the neurological decline. The defect is inherited in an autosomal dominant fashion and the numbers of repeats within the abnormal gene tends to increase in each successive generation, a phenomenon known as **anticipation**.

The brain of a patient with Huntington's disease is reduced in weight and shows marked atrophy of the caudate nucleus, putamen, and globus pallidus. If these areas are examined microscopically, there is marked neuronal loss with astrocytic gliosis. Surviving neurons have inclusions containing massive amounts of accumulated huntingtin protein. Whether these inclusions are the cause of the neuronal damage, an incidental byproduct that serves as a marker of the disease, or even a beneficial coping response by neurones is not known for certain.

The earliest symptoms of Huntington's disease include uncontrollable muscular movements, stumbling and clumsiness, lack of concentration, short-term memory lapses, depression, and changes of mood (sometimes including aggressive or antisocial behaviour). Needless to say, this can put tremendous strain on family relationships and is a confusing and frightening time, as the patient does not understand what is happening and why. Once the diagnosis is made, there are also profound implications for the children of the affected individual.

> ## Key points: Huntington's disease
>
> ◆ Huntington's disease is an inherited neurodegenerative disorder caused by abnormally high numbers of triplet repeats in a gene encoding a protein of unknown function called huntingtin.
>
> ◆ The length of the triplet repeat inversely correlates with the age of onset of the disease, and the length of triplet repeats tends to increase through successive generations.
>
> ◆ The neuronal loss in Huntington's disease is most marked in the caudate nucleus, putamen, and globus pallidus, leading to uncontrollable muscular movements and clumsiness.

Prion diseases

Prion diseases, or **transmissible spongiform encephalopathies**, are fatal disorders of the CNS which occur in both humans and animals. Although the clinical features of each disease vary, all are linked by the accumulation of an abnormal form of a protein called **prion protein** which leads to neuronal loss and the appearance of tiny vacuoles within neuronal and astrocytic cell processes (spongiform change).

Normal prion protein (PrP) is present in neurones and is designated PrP^c. In prion diseases, the protein undergoes a conformational change into a β-pleated sheet form designated PrP^{res} (resistant) which renders it resistant to breakdown.

What has generated so much interest in prion diseases is the overwhelming evidence that PrP^{res} is itself able to stimulate the conversion of more PrP^c into PrP^{res}, and that the abnormal prion protein is itself the causal agent in prion diseases (Fig. 18.14). Needless to say, huge controversy was generated when it was suggested

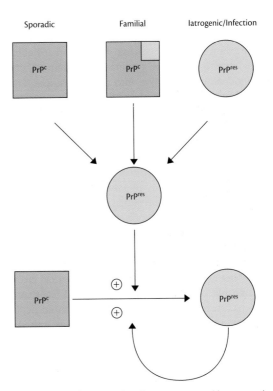

Fig. 18.14 Prion diseases. Prion diseases are caused by accumulation of PrP^{res} formed from normal PrP^c, a process which is itself stimulated by PrP^{res}. Initial acquisition of PrP^{res} may occur spontaneously in sporadic forms, due to a mutation that renders the normal PrP more susceptible to forming the abnormal form, or it may be acquired from an external source.

that a protein appeared to be able to transmit and replicate itself in the absence of any nucleic acid.

Sporadic CJD is the most common human prion disease

Sporadic Creutzfeldt–Jacob disease (CJD) is the most common human prion disease, but it is still rare, with an annual incidence of only 1 per 1 000 000 people. The cause of sporadic CJD is not known for certain, but it is thought that it arises when a normal PrP molecule spontaneously converts into the abnormal form, stimulating the conversion of more abnormal PrP molecules and eventually causing the disease. If this theory is correct, then the disease arises due to a chance event in the brain, i.e. getting sporadic CJD is simply a case of 'bad luck'.

Familial CJD is due to inherited mutations in the PRP gene

Familial cases of CJD are due to inherited mutations of the prion protein gene that produce an instability in the structure of prion protein and a higher chance of spontaneous conversion into the disease-associated form. Once the abnormal form has been produced, it then stimulates the conversion of more normal PrP into the resistant form.

Iatrogenic CJD has occurred following neurosurgery and corneal grafting

CJD has been accidentally transmitted in the course of medical treatment by neurosurgical instruments, corneal grafts, and growth hormone extracted from human pituitary glands. Subsequent measures to reduce the risk of iatrogenic transmission of prion diseases include strict selection criteria for corneal grafts and use of recombinant growth hormone. The theoretical risk of transmitting prion diseases through blood transfusion remains a concern and is the rationale behind depleting white blood cells from all donated blood in the UK.

Variant CJD is transmitted to humans by eating BSE-infected beef

In 1996, a distinct variant of CJD was recognized in the UK, known as **variant CJD** or **new variant CJD**. This form varies from sporadic CJD in a number of ways:

◆ Variant CJD affects younger individuals with an average age of onset of around 27 years, whereas sporadic CJD tends to affect middle-aged and elderly individuals.

◆ The duration of variant CJD is longer, often a year or more, whereas the duration of sporadic CJD is typically a few months or, in a few cases, a few weeks.

◆ The symptoms of sporadic and variant CJD tend to be different. In particular, sporadic CJD tends to present with an obvious neurological illness that follows a very rapidly progressive course. In variant CJD, the initial presentation is often with psychiatric or behavioural symptoms, and it may not be clear that the individual has a neurological illness until several months after the onset.

After intense study, it was discovered that the prion strain causing variant CJD is identical to the one found in bovine spongiform encephalopathy (BSE) in cattle, and the alarming possibility was raised that BSE was transmissible to humans by eating beef from cattle with BSE. As nothing was known about the natural history of this new disease in humans, there was great fear of a possible epidemic of variant CJD.

Fortunately the number of new cases of variant CJD occurring in the UK has remained very low and is not increasing. Analysis of the number of deaths from variant CJD suggests that a peak has been passed and the numbers of cases continue to decline. Only five deaths from definite or probable variant CJD occurred in the UK in 2005. However, it remains possible that the numbers of cases may rise again if genetic susceptibility affects the speed of onset.

Key points: Prion diseases

◆ Prion diseases are rare neurodegenerative diseases in which accumulation of an abnormal form of a cellular protein known as prion protein causes neuronal death and vacuolation in the brain.

◆ Prion diseases are interesting because the aetiological agent causing the conversion of normal prion protein into the abnormal form is itself the abnormal form of prion protein.

Key points: Prion diseases—cont'd

- Sporadic Creutzfeldt-Jacob disease is the most common human prion disease. It is thought to occur when a normal PrP protein spontaneously converts into the abnormal form.

- Familial Creutzfeldt-Jacob disease is caused by inherited mutations in the PRP gene which produce an unstable PrP protein that is more prone to converting into the abnormal form.

- Iatrogenic Creutzfeldt-Jacob disease has been caused by contaminated neurosurgical instruments and corneal grafts.

- Variant Creutzfeldt-Jacob disease is caused by transmission of bovine spongiform encephalopathy from cattle to humans through infected beef.

- The most common form of motor neurone disease in adults is amyotrophic lateral sclerosis.

- Loss of motor neurones in amyotrophic lateral sclerosis is thought to be related to excessive calcium influx into the cell, leading to death by apoptosis.

- Amyotrophic lateral sclerosis presents with asymmetrical limb muscle weakness. As the disease progresses, there are problems with eating, speaking, and breathing. The disease is usually fatal within a few years.

Motor neurone disease

Motor neurone disease is a degenerative disease affecting motor neurones

Motor neurone disease refers to a group of degenerative disorders of the CNS that selectively affect motor neurones. The most common form of motor neurone disease in adults is **amyotrophic lateral sclerosis**, in which there is selective degeneration of motor neurones in the motor cortex and spinal cord. There is a minimal astrocytic response and little evidence of inflammation.

The cause of amyotrophic lateral sclerosis remains unknown, although there is currently much interest in the possibility that the motor neurone loss is caused by excessive calcium influx into the cell through an abnormal type of glutamate receptor. Cellular calcium overload activates caspases, leading to neuronal death by apoptosis.

Key points: Motor neurone disease

- Motor neurone diseases are a group of neurodegenerative diseases that selectively affect motor neurones.

The initial symptom in most patients with amyotrophic lateral sclerosis is weakness of limb muscles in an asymmetrical fashion. Later there is involvement of the bulbar muscles, causing difficulty swallowing, chewing, speaking, coughing, and breathing. The disease is usually progressive, and is fatal within a few years. Death is usually the result of respiratory failure caused by pneumonia.

Metabolic disorders of the central nervous system

The high metabolic demands of the CNS render it particularly susceptible to metabolic disorders. These often present with diffuse cerebral dysfunction rather than localizing symptoms and signs.

Hepatic encephalopathy

Hepatic encephalopathy is a cardinal feature of hepatic failure

The onset of encephalopathy in a patient with severe liver disease is one of the defining features of hepatic failure. The precise underlying cause of hepatic encephalopathy is not clear, but it is likely that toxins normally cleared by the liver cross the blood–brain barrier and interfere with neurotransmission.

Wernicke's encephalopathy and Korsakoff's syndrome

Wernicke's encephalopathy and Korsakoff's syndrome are due to deficiency of thiamine

Deficiency of thiamine (vitamin B1) can lead to a neurological condition called **Wernicke's encephalopathy** characterized by the sudden onset of confusion and the presence of complex disorders of eye movement. The syndrome is particularly common in malnourished alcoholics, though it should be considered in any patient presenting with an acute confusional state, as administration of intravenous thiamine produces a striking clinical response.

Untreated Wernicke's encephalopathy may be followed by an irreversible condition known as **Korsakoff's syndrome** in which there is severe impairment of short-term memory.

Vitamin B12 deficiency

Vitamin B12 deficiency can cause myelopathy and dementia

Vitamin B12 deficiency is well recognized as a common cause of megaloblastic anaemia. Vitamin B12 deficiency can also cause CNS abnormalities. Vitamin B12 appears to be important for synthesis of CNS myelin and may also play a role in neurotransmission.

Vitamin B12 deficiency causes a spinal cord disease known as **subacute combined degeneration of the cord**, in which the posterior columns and the lateral corticospinal tracts of the spinal cord undergo degeneration. Vitamin B12 deficiency is also recognized as a cause of **dementia**, presumably due to loss of neurones in the cerebral cortex.

Mitochondrial encephalomyopathies

Mitochondrial encephalomyopathies are due to mutations in the genes of the mitochondrial respiratory chain

Mitochondrial encephalomyopathies are caused by mutations in the genes encoding the components of the mitochondrial respiratory chain. Some of these genes are encoded by nuclear DNA, but others are coded for by mitochondrial DNA. Nuclear gene defects may be inherited in an autosomal recessive or autosomal dominant manner. The mitochondrial genome is derived from the maternal line, and mutations are therefore inherited from the mother.

The mitochondrial respiratory chain is essential for aerobic metabolism, and so tissues heavily reliant on aerobic metabolism such as brain and muscle are preferentially involved in mitochondrial diseases. Common clinical features of mitochondrial diseases include ptosis, proximal myopathy and exercise intolerance, cardiomyopathy, optic neuropathy, fluctuating encephalopathy, seizures, ataxia, and stroke-like episodes.

Many affected individuals display a cluster of features that fall into discrete clinical syndromes such as **mitochondrial encephalopathy with lactic acidosis and stroke-like episodes** (MELAS), **myoclonic epilepsy with ragged red fibres** (MERRF), and **neurogenic weakness with ataxia and retinitis pigmentosa** (NARP). However, there is considerable clinical variability, and many individuals do not fit neatly into one category.

The extremely wide range of presentations means that mitochondrial diseases are almost certainly more common than we think because the diagnosis is often not considered. Based on the available data, one estimate for the prevalence of all mitochondrial diseases is as high as 1 in 8500 people.

Neoplasms of the central nervous system

Most neoplasms occurring in the CNS affect the brain rather than the spinal cord. Metastases are common in the CNS, and the incidence of metastases is roughly equal to the incidence of primary brain tumours.

Primary CNS neoplasms typically present with one or more of the following:

♦ Progressive neurological deficit

♦ Seizures

♦ Symptoms and signs of raised intracranial pressure

♦ Altered mental status.

The particular combination of clinical features varies depending on the location of the tumour and its rate of growth. Low grade tumours are more likely to present with a seizure disorder that may remain stable for many years, whereas patients with highly aggressive tumours typically develop a rapidly progressive neurological deficit and raised intracranial pressure.

Primary CNS neoplasms are classified according to their presumed cell of origin and their degree of differentiation. The distinction between benign and malignant has little meaning for primary CNS tumours as even benign tumours may have fatal consequences if they impinge on critical structures, and even very well differentiated CNS neoplasms may infiltrate into the surrounding brain with poorly defined margins, making complete excision difficult.

Astrocytic tumours

Astrocytomas are the most frequent primary intracranial neoplasm, accounting for some 60 per cent of all primary brain tumours. They usually arise in adults in the cerebral hemispheres. The cause of astrocytomas is unknown; no unequivocal specific aetiological agent has been found.

Astrocytomas show a wide range of biological behaviour, but all of them diffusely infiltrate the adjacent brain and they have an inherent tendency to progress over time and show more aggressive behaviour. While some astrocytomas remain stable for more than 10 years following diagnosis, others show a rapid transition into a highly aggressive neoplasm within 1–2 years. Astrocytomas are divided into three main tumour types.

Diffuse astrocytoma is an astrocytic neoplasm composed of well differentiated neoplastic astrocytes. The tumour slowly infiltrates the surrounding brain and eventually progresses to anaplastic astrocytoma, and then glioblastoma. The tumours tend to present with seizures, although often in retrospect subtle abnormalities of speech, sensation, or movement are recalled.

Anaplastic astrocytoma is an astrocytic neoplasm composed of a mixture of well differentiated and poorly differentiated neoplastic astrocytes. The growth of the tumour is rapid, and life expectancy is on average only 3 years.

Glioblastoma is the most aggressive astrocytic tumour, composed of poorly differentiated neoplastic astrocytes (Fig. 18.15). Glioblastoma may develop in a patient with a previous diagnosis of a diffuse astrocytoma or anaplastic astrocytoma, but often manifests *de novo* with a short clinical history of seizures and the rapid development of raised intracranial pressure. Despite its highly infiltrative growth, glioblastomas rarely metastasize outside of the CNS. Glioblastoma is one of the most aggressive neoplasms, with few patients surviving more than 1 year from diagnosis.

Oligodendroglial tumours

Oligodendroglial tumours are neoplasms in which the neoplastic cells resemble normal oligodendrocytes. Rather like astrocytomas, oligodendroglial tumours show a continuous spectrum of appearances and behaviour ranging from well differentiated neoplasms to poorly differentiated aggressive neoplasms. For ease of distinction, oligodendroglial tumours are split into two: oligodendroglioma and anaplastic oligodendroglioma.

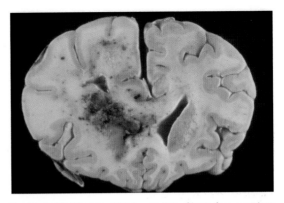

Fig. 18.15 Glioblastoma. This is a section of brain from a patient who presented with signs of raised intracranial pressure, rapidly deteriorated, and died. There is an ill defined tumour with areas of haemorrhage. Microscopy revealed this to be a glioblastoma which was much more extensive than was apparent macroscopically.

Oligodendroglioma is a well differentiated slowly growing tumour of adults composed of cells resembling oligodendrocytes. Oligodendrogliomas usually present following seizure, though there is often a long history of headaches and vague neurological symptoms. The average survival in patients with oligodendrogliomas is about 10 years.

Anaplastic oligodendroglioma is an oligodendroglial tumour containing areas of increased cellularity, marked cytological atypia, and high mitotic activity. They present in a similar way to oligodendrogliomas but with a much shorter history. The average survival is 2–3 years.

Meningioma

Meningiomas are slow growing tumours composed of neoplastic meningothelial cells (arachnoid cells). Under normal circumstances, these cells are scattered throughout the arachnoid membrane but are concentrated over the arachnoid villi.

Meningiomas are smooth well circumscribed neoplasms which are adherent to the dura mater (Fig. 18.16). Infiltration of the overlying skull bone is not uncommon, but invasion of the brain is very rare. Many small meningiomas go completely unnoticed and are often found incidentally at autopsy. Larger meningiomas present due to compression against adjacent structures, the specific nature of the symptoms depending

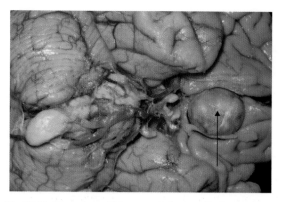

Fig. 18.16 Meningioma. This very well circumscribed tumour (arrow) has the typical macroscopic appearance of a meningioma, a suspicion which was confirmed microscopically.

on the site of the tumour. There may also be features of raised intracranial pressure.

Meningiomas are potentially curable tumours if complete surgical excision can be achieved.

Primary CNS lymphomas

Primary CNS lymphomas are lymphomas arising in the CNS *in the absence of lymphoma outside the nervous system at the time of diagnosis*. This definition therefore excludes lymphomas that have arisen outside the nervous system and then spread secondarily to the CNS. Like other intracranial neoplasms, common presentations of CNS lymphoma include focal neurological deficits, seizures, and signs of raised intracranial pressure.

The incidence of lymphomas of the CNS has continuously risen over recent decades. Much of this rise is due to increasing numbers of patients with HIV, many of whom develop a CNS lymphoma driven by Epstein–Barr virus. Virtually all CNS lymphomas are non-Hodgkin B cell lymphomas, the most common type being the **diffuse large B cell lymphoma**.

Metastases to the central nervous system

Most metastases to the CNS occur within the brain parenchyma. The most common neoplasms to metastasize to the brain are carcinomas, particularly from the breast, lung, and kidney. Malignant melanoma also has a strong propensity to metastasize to the brain.

Metastases in the brain tend to occur at the junction between the grey and white matter, presumably because the rich capillary bed at this site favours tumour deposition. Metastatic deposits in the brain are often surrounded by considerable cerebral oedema, and so may cause symptoms of raised intracranial pressure. Focal neurological deficits and seizures may also occur.

Although not strictly metastases to the CNS itself, deposits of tumour around the spinal cord or within the bones of the vertebral column may impinge on the spinal cord, leading to **spinal cord compression**. Spinal cord compression presents with numbness and loss of sensation in the legs. Patients suspected of having spinal cord compression clinically require urgent MRI scanning to visualize the spinal cord. If spinal cord compression is confirmed, radiotherapy to the site of compression is needed to prevent irreversible paraplegia.

Occasionally, metastases to the CNS may diffusely infiltrate the meninges, a condition known as **carcinomatous meningitis**. This devastating condition leads to symptoms of meningitis together with multiple cranial nerve palsies. The prognosis of patients with carcinomatous meningitis is extremely poor, with an average survival of 2–3 months.

> ## Key points: Tumours of the central nervous system
>
> ◆ Tumours of the CNS may be primary or secondary. The terms benign and malignant have less meaning in the CNS as 'benign' tumours can be life threatening if they press on critical structures.
>
> ◆ The incidences of primary CNS neoplasms and metastases are roughly equal.
>
> ◆ Primary neoplasms of the CNS may present with seizures, neurological deficits, and/or signs of raised intracranial pressure.
>
> ◆ Primary CNS neoplasms include astrocytomas, oligodendrogliomas, meningiomas, and lymphomas. Tumours arising from neurones are extremely rare.
>
> ◆ Astrocytomas are the most common primary CNS neoplasms. They show a spectrum of appearances and behaviour, but for the purposes of diagnosis and management are divided into diffuse astrocytomas, anaplastic astrocytomas, and glioblastomas in order of increasing aggression.

- Oligodendrogliomas are tumours composed of cells resembling oligodendrocytes. They show a spectrum of appearances and behaviour, but for the purposes of diagnosis and management are divided into oligodendrogliomas (low grade) and anaplastic oligodendrogliomas (high grade).

- Meningiomas are slow growing tumours composed of neoplastic cells resembling meningothelial cells. Small meningiomas may never come to clinical attention. Larger meningiomas present due to compression on nearby structures. Meningiomas are curable if complete surgical excision can be achieved.

- Primary CNS lymphomas are lymphomas arising in the CNS in the absence of lymphoma outside the nervous system at the time of diagnosis. Virtually all primary CNS lymphomas are non-Hodgkin B cell lymphomas, mostly diffuse large B cell lymphomas.

- The most common tumours metastasizing to the CNS are carcinomas, particularly breast carcinoma, lung carcinoma, and renal cell carcinoma. Malignant melanoma also frequently metastasizes to the CNS.

Epilepsy

Epilepsy is a condition in which a person has a tendency to suffer recurrent seizures. A **seizure** is a paroxysmal disorder in which sudden excess electrical discharges from cortical neurones result in intermittent attacks of altered consciousness, motor or sensory function, behaviour, or emotion. Seizures may be divided into **partial** (focal) seizures in which the seizure activity is restricted to a discrete area of the cerebral cortex, and **generalized** seizures which involve diffuse regions of the brain simultaneously.

Primarily generalized epilepsy is the most common type of epilepsy in children

Primarily generalized epilepsy is commonly seen in children. The most common type is **childhood absence epilepsy** in which the child repeatedly switches off for a moment or two, but does not convulse or fall down. When the attack finishes, the child resumes their activities and may be unaware that anything has happened.

Another type of primarily generalized epilepsy is **juvenile myoclonic epilepsy**. Children and adolescents have attacks of absence associated with sudden jerking of the limbs. Both childhood absence epilepsy and juvenile myoclonic epilepsy are genetically determined.

Secondarily generalized epilepsy is the most common type of epilepsy in adults and is usually idiopathic

Secondarily generalized epilepsy is a common problem in adults and is usually idiopathic. Presumably these patients have a lower seizure 'threshold', placing them at greater risk of seizure. The classical seizure in generalized epilepsy is known as a **tonic–clonic** or **grand mal** seizure.

The patient suddenly loses consciousness and falls to the floor. Generalized muscle stiffness (tonic phase) occurs lasting for a few seconds, followed by a clonic phase in which there are sharp repetitive muscular jerks. Tongue biting and incontinence may occur. When the jerking stops, patients usually remain unconscious for about 30 min before regaining consciousness and feeling confused and sleepy for several hours.

Partial epilepsy is much more likely to be due to an underlying structural lesion of the brain

Partial epileptic seizures are restricted to discrete areas of the brain and are more likely to arise from abnormalities such as neoplasms, infections, infarcts, or previous head injuries. It is therefore mandatory to investigate all patients with partial seizures with brain MRI to look for an underlying lesion.

The clinical features of a partial seizure depend on the site of the abnormally discharging neurones. A partial seizure in the temporal lobe may cause symptoms of déjà vu, olfactory hallucinations, and odd repetitive movements like smacking of the lips and chewing movements. A partial seizure in the motor cortex causes clonic contractions of the muscles of a hand, a foot, or one side of the face. These contractions may slowly move from one part of the body to another as the seizure focus moves along the motor cortex, a phenomenon known as **Jacksonian epilepsy**.

Key points: Epilepsy

- Epilepsy is a tendency to have recurrent seizures. Seizures may be divided into partial or generalized.

- Primarily generalized epilepsy is common in children and includes childhood absence epilepsy and juvenile myoclonic epilepsy.

- Secondarily generalized epilepsy in adults manifests with tonic–clonic (grand mal) seizures and is almost always idiopathic.

- Partial epilepsy manifests in a number of ways depending on where the seizure activity occurs.

- All adult patients newly presenting with epilepsy should have brain MRI to rule out an underlying structural brain lesion, particularly in those with partial seizures.

Peripheral nervous system

The PNS is composed of spinal nerves, cranial nerves, and the autonomic nervous system. The spinal and cranial nerves are the means by which the CNS receives information from and transmits information to the trunk and limbs, and head and neck, respectively. The autonomic nervous system is concerned with control of the internal environment through innervation of glands, the heart, blood vessels, and the gut.

Peripheral neuropathy

Diseases affecting peripheral nerves may cause varying combinations of sensory loss, weakness, and autonomic loss depending on which type of axon is involved. Peripheral neuropathy is best considered as either focal neuropathy, which affects one section of a single peripheral nerve, or polyneuropathy, which affects the entire length of all peripheral nerves.

Focal neuropathy

**Focal neuropathy affects one area
of a peripheral nerve**

Focal neuropathy is a lesion affecting one area of a peripheral nerve. The most common cause of a focal neuropathy is *trauma* (which may sever the nerve), or *compression* by surrounding tissue. Less commonly, a

focal neuropathy may result from blockage of the small blood vessels supply part of a peripheral nerve (the 'vasa nervorum').

Carpal tunnel syndrome is a good example of a focal neuropathy. It is due to compression of the median nerve as it passes under the transverse carpal ligament at the wrist. The typical symptoms are a painful tingling in the hand in the distribution of the median nerve, which is often worse at night.

LINK BOX

Carpal tunnel syndrome

Carpal tunnel syndrome may occur in patients with acromegaly due to swelling of the soft tissues in the wrist (p. 300), and in amyloidosis due to amyloid deposition in the soft tissues of the wrist (p. 483).

Polyneuropathy

**Polyneuropathies affect the entire length
of all peripheral nerves**

Polyneuropathies occur when there is injury to all peripheral nerves. Polyneuropathy affects all axons equally, but often the longest axons to the hands and feet are affected first. Polyneuropathies therefore often start with tingling or numbness of the feet and fingers, with loss of pinprick and touch sensation in a 'glove and stocking' distribution. Polyneuropathy may result from *axonal degeneration* or *demyelination*.

Polyneuropathy due to axonal degeneration affects myelinated and unmyelinated axons, so all sensory modalities are lost (joint position, vibration, pain, and temperature). Muscle wasting is marked as a result of the denervation. Axonal degeneration polyneuropathy is usually due to diabetes mellitus or a side effect of a drug (e.g. the chemotherapeutic agent vincristine). This type of polyneuropathy rarely recovers well.

Polyneuropathy due to demyelination (demyelinating polyneuropathy) only affects myelinated nerves, so whilst there is marked loss of joint position and vibration sensation, pinprick and temperature senses remain intact. There is severe muscle weakness, but the degree of muscle wasting is much less than axonal degeneration as there is no actual denervation.

Demyelinating polyneuropathy is either due to a genetic abnormality of myelination (e.g. Charcot–Marie–Tooth disease) or to an acquired abnormality of peripheral nerve myelination which is probably autoimmune in origin (e.g. Guillain–Barré syndrome, chronic inflammatory demyelinating polyneuropathy, or paraneoplastic polyneuropathy). Demyelinating polyneuropathies can recover completely over a period of months because remyelination can occur following treatment.

Guillain–Barré syndrome is an acute demyelinating polyneuropathy

Guillain-Barré syndrome is an acute demyelinating polyneuropathy which typically follows a few weeks after an upper respiratory tract or gastrointestinal infection. The most well recognized organisms which can lead to Guillain-Barré syndrome are *Campylobacter jejuni*, *Mycoplasma pneumoniae*, and Epstein–Barr virus.

The precise pathogenesis remains unknown, but the widely held theory is that in some individuals the immune response to the organism cross-reacts with peripheral nerve myelin leading to immune-mediated demyelination of peripheral nerves.

Guillain-Barré syndrome presents with the sudden onset of tingling and numbness of the fingers and toes. Over a period of weeks, the weakness then spreads proximally to involve the legs and arms. The danger in Guillain-Barré syndrome is involvement of the muscles required for ventilation. Patients with Guillain-Barré syndrome must be very carefully monitored, with ventilatory support close at hand.

Chronic inflammatory demyelinating polyneuropathy has a slower onset

Chronic inflammatory demyelinating polyneuropathy is similar to Guillain-Barré syndrome except that the symptoms come on more slowly, peaking over about 8 weeks. Chronic inflammatory demyelinating polyneuropathy rarely causes significant respiratory muscle weakness, but is a lifelong disease that does not often resolve.

Malignancies can also cause a polyneuropathy

A symmetrical polyneuropathy often occurs in patients with underlying malignancies, as a paraneoplastic effect. This is most commonly seen with small cell carcinoma of the lung, and appears to be due to a circulating antibody which causes inflammation in dorsal root ganglia.

Tumours of peripheral nerves

The major tumours of peripheral nerves to be aware of are schwannoma, neurofibroma, and malignant peripheral nerve sheath tumour.

Schwannoma

Schwannomas are encapsulated benign tumours composed of neoplastic Schwann cells. Schwannomas may arise anywhere in the PNS, in nerves of any size. Schwannomas are particularly common in the head and neck region, most notably in the vestibular division of the eighth cranial nerve (p. 465).

Schwannomas present in a number of ways depending on their location. Schwannomas arising in skin present as a subcutaneous lump. Paravertebral schwannomas are often picked up incidentally on imaging. Vestibular schwannomas present with unilateral tinnitus or deafness.

Schwannomas are slowly growing tumours that only rarely undergo malignant transformation. If excised completely, cure is the norm.

Neurofibroma

Neurofibromas are tumours composed of a mixture of cell types including Schwann cells, perineurial cells, and fibroblasts. Neurofibromas are common, and most occur as sporadic solitary tumours in the skin (localized cutaneous neurofibromas).

Multiple neurofibromas are typical of the condition **neurofibromatosis type 1** (von Recklinghausen's disease), due to an inherited mutation of the NF1 gene. Large rope-like neurofibromas arising from major nerve trunks, known as plexiform neurofibromas, are virtually pathognomic of neurofibromatosis. Extraneural manifestations of neurofibromatosis include freckling, café au lait spots, and Lisch nodules, all of which involve alterations of melanocytes. Café au lait spots are flat light brown lesions predominantly found on unexposed body surfaces. Lisch nodules are small elevated pigmented hamartomas on the surface of the iris.

Malignant peripheral nerve sheath tumour

Malignant peripheral nerve sheath tumour is a malignant soft tissue tumour showing evidence of nerve sheath differentiation. Malignant peripheral nerve sheath tumours are uncommon neoplasms; about half of them occur in patients with neurofibromatosis 1. The tumours tend to arise from large peripheral nerves, particularly in the buttock, thigh, and upper arm. The most common presentation is with an enlarging mass related to one of these sites. Malignant peripheral nerve sheath tumours are highly aggressive neoplasms with a poor prognosis.

Skeletal muscle

Normal skeletal muscle is made up of numerous muscle fibres, or myocytes, which form a syncytial network. The connective tissue elements of skeletal muscle includes the **endomysium**, which surrounds individual muscle fibres, the **perimysium**, which groups muscle fibres into bundles, and the **epimysium**, which groups whole muscle bundles.

The cardinal sign of muscle disease is *weakness*, particularly of proximal limb muscles. Proximal myopathy is usually noticed by the patient when trying to get out of a chair, climbing stairs, or lifting their arm above their head to comb their hair or hang washing on a line. The most important primary diseases of muscle are polymyositis, muscular dystrophy, and myasthenia gravis.

LINK BOX

Proximal myopathy

Proximal muscle weakness may also be a feature of Cushing's syndrome (p. 303), thyrotoxicosis (p. 312), and osteomalacia (p. 405).

Polymyositis

Polymyositis is an inflammatory myopathy in which muscle fibres are destroyed by T lymphocytes

Polymyositis is an inflammatory muscle disease in which muscle fibres are gradually destroyed by an inflammatory infiltrate. The cause of the inflammation remains unclear, but there is evidence that the muscle fibre injury may be due to an autoimmune process involving predominantly T lymphocytes.

The inflammatory infiltrate in polymyositis contains a high proportion of activated CD8+ cytotoxic T lymphocytes and no B lymphocytes. Electron microscopic studies looking closely at the interaction between T lymphocytes and muscle fibres in polymyositis have shown that the T lymphocytes invade, replace, and

eventually destroy muscle fibres. The T lymphocytes express perforin granules orientated towards the muscle fibre, indicating that this mechanism is responsible for much of the muscle fibre destruction.

Polymyositis typically presents with muscle weakness developing gradually over the course of a few weeks or months in large proximal muscles. By the time a person develops symptoms, over half their muscle fibres have been lost.

Interstitial lung disease is a frequent manifestation of polymyositis

Interstitial lung disease is a group of disorders characterized by inflammation and fibrosis in the interstitial compartment of the lung parenchyma (p. 126). Interstitial lung disease is frequently seen in patients with polymyositis, although the pathogenesis is not clear. The severity of the lung disease varies markedly, ranging from asymptomatic to rapidly progressive disease with respiratory failure and death.

The strongest predictive factor for interstitial lung disease in polymyositis is the presence of positive anti-aminoacyl tRNA synthetase antibodies, of which the anti-histidyl tRNA synthetase antibody (anti-Jo1) is the most frequently found. More than 70 per cent of patients with anti-Jo1 antibodies will have interstitial lung disease.

Glucocorticoids are the mainstay of treatment for polymyositis

Most patients with polymyositis respond to glucocorticoids. Recall, however, that a proximal myopathy is a common side effect of glucocorticoids; patients whose symptoms are worsened by glucocorticoid treatment may require alternative immunosuppressants. Patients with polymyositis should also have regular investigations to check for the presence of interstitial lung disease, such as chest radiograph, high resolution CT scanning of the lungs, pulmonary function tests, and measurement of anti-Jo1 antibodies.

Muscular dystrophy

The **muscular dystrophies** are a group of inherited diseases of muscle which lead to progressive muscle destruction and weakness. The molecular genetics of the muscular dystrophies are now being unravelled. Mutations in a number of different genes may lead to a muscular dystrophy, including genes coding for contractile proteins, proteins that anchor the contractile proteins in the muscle cell membrane, or proteins involved in energy generation in the muscle cells.

Muscular dystrophies range in severity from a severe disease presenting in childhood (e.g. **Duchenne muscular dystrophy**) to a mild weakness presenting in middle age (e.g. limb girdle dystrophies). Some muscular dystrophies can be diagnosed with confidence purely on clinical grounds because the pattern of muscular involvement is so distinctive (e.g. fascioscapulohumeral dystrophy).

Myasthenia gravis

Myasthenia gravis is a rare autoimmune disease caused by the production of antibodies to the nicotinic acetylcholine receptor at the neuromuscular junction. The autoantibodies bind to the acetylcholine receptors, blocking the action of acetylcholine. Muscles become weak after prolonged use, a phenomenon known as fatiguability. Most patients have mild symptoms, particularly intermittent drooping of the eyelids, or difficulty on long walks and prolonged exercise.

The cause of the generation of the autoantibodies is not known, though interestingly over half of all patients have an abnormality of the thymus gland, either an enlarged hyperplastic gland or a neoplasm of the thymus known as a thymoma. It is thought that the autoantibodies are generated in the thymus, and removal of the thymus often helps recovery.

> ### Key points: Muscle disease
>
> ◆ Muscle disease typically presents with proximal myopathy.

> ### Key points: Muscle disease—cont'd
>
> ◆ The most common primary muscle diseases are polymyositis, muscular dystrophy, and myasthenia gravis.
> ◆ Other important causes of proximal myopathy include glucocorticoid therapy, Cushing's syndrome, thyrotoxicosis, and osteomalacia.
> ◆ Polymyositis is an idiopathic inflammatory myopathy in which cytotoxic T lymphocytes destroy muscle fibres, causing muscle weakness in middle life. The cause is unknown.
> ◆ Muscular dystrophies are inherited disorders of muscle proteins which lead to progressive loss of muscle fibres. They range in severity from severe forms that present in childhood to mild diseases of adult life.
> ◆ Myasthenia gravis is an autoimmune disease in which antibodies to the nicotinic acetylcholine receptor at the neuromuscular junction cause muscle weakness. Intermittent drooping of the eyelids is a typical feature of the disease.

Further reading

www.cjd.ed.ac.uk, National Creutzfeldt-Jacob Disease Surveillance Unit.

Head and neck disease

Introduction

Head and neck disease traditionally covers diseases of the oral cavity, ears, nose, and throat (Fig. 19.1). Trivial conditions affecting these sites are a common cause of consultation to general practitioners and dentists. More complex problems involving these sites are the realm of ear, nose, and throat (ENT) surgeons and maxillofacial surgeons.

Oral cavity

The oral cavity comprises the lips, teeth, gums, tongue, buccal mucosa, soft and hard palates, and uvula. The major and minor salivary glands also open into the mouth.

The inner surface of the mouth is covered by oral mucosa, composed of stratified squamous epithelium overlying a layer of loose connective tissue called the corium. These layers equate to the epidermis and dermis of the skin. The main differences between skin and oral mucosa are that the squamous epithelium of oral mucosa is not keratinized, and there are no skin adnexal structures such as hair follicles, sebaceous glands, or sweat glands in the oral mucosa.

The similarity of the oral mucosa to skin means that it may be affected by inflammatory dermatological conditions including lichen planus, pemphigus vulgaris, and erythema multiforme.

Infections of the oral cavity

The main defences against infection in the oral cavity are the competition for colonization by low virulence organisms of the normal commensal flora, and saliva, which contains IgA antibodies and antibacterial substances such as lysozyme. Salivary flow itself is also important in mechanically flushing the mouth; the reduction in salivary flow in unwell dehydrated patients is an important cause of microbial overgrowth and oral cavity infections in hospitalized patients.

Infections of the oral cavity may result from the activity of the normal oral commensal flora, e.g. dental caries, chronic periodontal disease, and oral candidiasis. Infections may also be caused by acquired oral pathogens, e.g. herpetic gingivostomatitis.

Dental caries is a common cause of oral pain and discomfort

Dental decay or caries is a very common chronic disease which causes much pain and discomfort. Dental caries are caused by the bacterium *Streptococcus mutans*. The bacteria attach to salivary glycoproteins covering the teeth and multiply, synthesizing a sticky polysaccharide which forms a film called **dental plaque** in which numerous bacteria become embedded. The bacteria in plaque convert dietary sugar into lactic acid which slowly erodes the enamel layer of the tooth. Erosion into the pulp cavity causes acute pulpitis that manifests with a persistent throbbing pain, often keeping the patient awake at night (Fig. 19.2a).

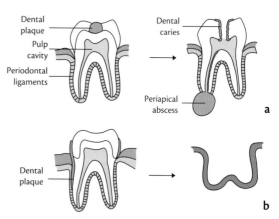

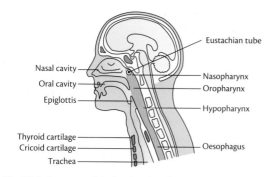

Fig. 19.1 Anatomy of the head and neck.

Fig. 19.2 (a) Dental caries. Dental plaque erodes through tooth enamel. If the pulp cavity is entered, acute pulpitis leads to throbbing pain related to the tooth and risks the development of a deep periapical abscess. (b) Chronic periodontal disease. Dental plaque eroding down the sides of a tooth destroys the periodontal ligaments that hold the tooth in the socket. Over many years, the tooth becomes gradually loosened and is eventually lost.

Chronic periodontal disease leads to tooth loosening and loss

Chronic inflammation of the gingiva and periodontal tissue caused by dental plaque is referred to as chronic periodontal disease (Fig. 19.2b). Some degree of chronic periodontal disease affects everyone, starting in early adult life. Its severity varies widely between individuals, and in some people the disease is progressive, eventually leading to tooth loss in old age.

Candidal infection of the mouth is common

Candida is a commensal fungus of the mouth carried by about 40 per cent of the population, the dorsum of the tongue being the main reservoir for the organism. *Candida* are notorious opportunistic pathogens which readily cause infection if the balance between the host and the organism is disturbed. The infection typically manifests with cream-coloured soft material coating the palate.

Oral candidiasis is commonly seen in hospitalized patients and in immunosuppressed people (it is the most frequent oral manifestation of HIV). Oral candidiasis may also be seen in patients taking inhaled steroids, particularly if their technique is poor and much of the steroid is deposited orally rather than in the respiratory tract (Fig. 19.3).

Herpes simplex causes recurrent crops of vesicles around the mouth

The herpes simplex viruses are the most frequent cause of a viral infection in the mouth. HSV is transmitted by droplet spread or contact with active lesions. Most people acquire the virus in childhood, and in many people the infection remains subclinical. Some people however develop numerous small painful vesicles on the gums and lips, known as herpetic gingivostomatitis.

During the primary infection, HSV gains access to sensory neurones, and viral DNA is transported to the sensory ganglion where the virus establishes latent infection. Later in life, about 1 in 3 infected people develop recurrent HSV infections; transcription of HSV DNA resumes, viral particles travel down the axons to gain access to the epithelium of the gums and lips, and a new crop of vesicles develops.

> ## Key points: Infections of the oral cavity
>
> ◆ Dental caries are caused by erosion of tooth enamel by acid generated by *Streptococcus mutans* bacteria from dietary sugar. Erosion into the pulp cavity causes severe throbbing toothache due to acute pulpitis.
>
> ◆ Chronic periodontal disease is the result of chronic inflammation around the edges of the tooth socket, leading to loosening and eventual loss of the tooth.
>
> ◆ Candidal infection of the mouth manifests with a cream-coloured material coating the soft palate and is common in immunosuppressed people and hospitalized patients.
>
> ◆ Herpes simplex virus is a common cause of recurrent ulceration of the mouth and gums.

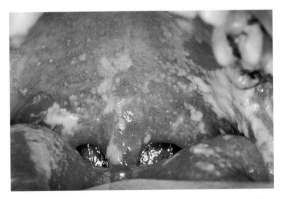

Fig. 19.3 Oral candidiasis. This infection was due to oral deposition of steroid in an asthmatic patient with a poor inhaler technique.

Squamous cell carcinoma of the oral cavity

Squamous cell carcinoma is the most common malignancy of the oral cavity

More than 90 per cent of all malignant tumours of the oral cavity are squamous cell carcinomas arising from the lining mucosa. Squamous cell carcinomas of the oral cavity have a particular propensity for early and extensive spread to lymph nodes of the neck, and occur predominantly in heavy smokers and alcohol drinkers. Infection with high risk human papillomavirus (HPV) type 16 is also an important causative agent; more than half of all oral cavity squamous cell carcinomas

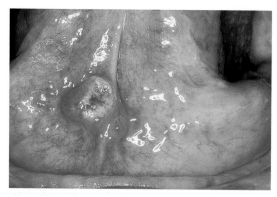

Fig. 19.4 Early squamous cell carcinoma of the oral cavity presenting as a persistent ulcerated lesion on the undersurface of the tongue.

harbour HPV DNA integrated into the genome of the neoplastic cells.

Squamous cell carcinomas may arise in any part of the oral cavity, but the lower lip and tongue base are the most common sites. Whilst some patients present with small tumours (Fig. 19.4), many do not present until they have a large ulcerated tumour mass causing pain and difficulty with speaking and eating. Sometimes patients present with enlarged lymph nodes in the neck without any symptoms from the oral lesion.

The mainstays of treatment for oral squamous cell carcinomas are surgery and radiotherapy, which may be used alone or in combination depending on the site and stage of the tumour.

Squamous cell carcinomas arise from areas of epithelial dysplasia

Squamous cell carcinomas of the oral cavity develop from areas of epithelial dysplasia. Most, but not all, areas of dysplasia give rise to a clinically visible lesion, typically a white patch (leukoplakia) or a red patch (erythroplakia) which cannot be scraped off the mucosal surface. Note that identical lesions can occur from other, non-dysplastic, epithelial changes, and so biopsy is mandatory to identify the underlying cause of the lesion.

When examined microscopically, the majority of plakias show simple hyperplasia of the squamous epithelium with no dysplasia. If dysplasia is present, the pathologist will grade it into mild, moderate, or severe. Higher degrees of dysplasia are associated with a greater likelihood of progression to malignancy. It is important to note, however, that most areas of dysplasia do not undergo malignant change and may even regress if aetiological factors such as smoking and alcohol are removed.

> ## Key points: Squamous cell carcinoma of the oral cavity
>
> - Squamous cell carcinomas account for virtually all malignant tumours of the oral cavity.
> - As with other squamous cell carcinomas of the upper aerodigestive tract, there is a strong association with smoking and alcohol abuse.
> - The lip and tongue base are the most common sites for oral squamous cell carcinomas.
> - Oral squamous cell carcinomas show a propensity for early and extensive spread to lymph nodes of the neck.
> - Oral squamous cell carcinomas present either with an ulcerated mass in the mouth, or due to rapidly enlarging cervical lymph nodes.
> - Oral squamous cell carcinomas arise from areas of epithelial dysplasia which may give rise to patches of leukoplakia or erythroplakia. Biopsy of such lesions is important to determine if there is dysplasia, and how severe it is.

Miscellaneous lesions of the oral cavity

Fibroepithelial polyps, which also occur on the skin (skin tags), are the most common type of nodule in the oral cavity (Fig. 19.5). Their aetiology is unknown but they may be related to chronic low grade trauma from teeth or dentures.

Lobular capillary haemangiomas (pyogenic granulomas), again similar to their cutaneous counterparts, may arise in the mouth (Fig. 19.6).

Mucoceles are small cystic nodules with a blue tinge, usually on the lower lip, which arise due to obstruction of a minor salivary gland duct.

Odontogenic cysts are lined by epithelial residues of the tooth-forming organ. Some of them are seen in the mouth; others are discovered on radiographs taken to investigate the cause of toothache. They are fairly common in oral medicine practice. Examples of

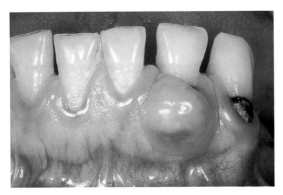

Fig. 19.5 This firm lesion on the lower gum was excised and shown to be a fibroepithelial polyp on microscopic examination.

odontogenic cysts include radicular cysts, dentigerous cysts, and odontogenic keratocysts.

JARGON BUSTER

Epulis

An **epulis** (plural epulides) is a non-specific term which literally means 'on the gum' and refers to any localized lump on the gum. It does not imply any specific underlying diagnosis, although in some circles the terms 'fibrous epulis' and 'vascular epulis' have come to be used synonymously for fibroepithelial polyp and lobular capillary haemangioma respectively.

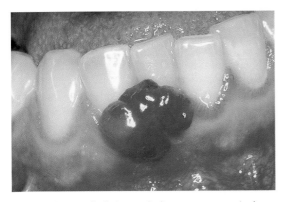

Fig. 19.6 This vascular lesion on the lower gum was excised and shown to be a lobular capillary haemangioma (pyogenic granuloma) on microscopic examination.

Salivary glands

Salivary glands are exocrine organs responsible for the production and secretion of saliva. There are three pairs of **major salivary glands**: the parotid, submandibular, and the sublingual glands. In addition, there are many **minor salivary glands** widely distributed throughout the mouth and oropharynx.

Salivary gland calculi

Salivary calculi usually arise in the submandibular gland

Most salivary calculi are composed of calcium phosphate. It is thought that they develop during periods of secretory activity due to deposition of calcium salts around a stagnant organic nidus made up of detached epithelial cells and microorganisms.

Salivary calculi are most common in middle-aged adults and may form in the main excretory ducts or in smaller ducts within the substance of the gland. The submandibular gland is most commonly affected, followed by the parotid gland. Sialolithiasis in sublingual glands or the minor glands is very uncommon.

Salivary calculi cause pain and enlargement of the salivary gland at mealtimes

The typical presentation of a salivary calculus is pain and sudden enlargement of the affected salivary gland when salivary excretion is stimulated at mealtimes. If there is partial obstruction of the gland or duct, the swelling lasts for a few minutes to a few hours. Complete obstruction leaves the gland enlarged for several days and predisposes to infection of the gland.

The management of salivary calculi depends on their location. A palpable and visible calculus near the opening of the salivary gland duct in the mouth can often be removed easily under local anaesthetic. Calculi further back in the duct usually require removal under general anaesthetic. Stones within the submandibular gland itself are usually an indication for removing the whole gland.

Key points: Salivary calculi

- Salivary calculi are composed of calcium phosphate and are thought to arise due to accumulation of calcium salts on stagnant debris in the salivary ducts.

Continued

> ## Key points: Salivary calculi— cont'd
>
> ♦ Salivary calculi most commonly affect the submandibular gland, followed by the parotid gland.
>
> ♦ Salivary calculi present with pain and sudden enlargement of the affected salivary gland when salivary flow is stimulated. Complete obstruction of the gland predisposes it to infection.

Sjögren's syndrome

Sjögren's syndrome is an autoimmune condition which causes progressive destruction of salivary and lacrimal glands. About half a million people are affected in the UK and, like all autoimmune diseases, it is much more common in women.

Many patients with Sjögren's syndrome also have a multisystem autoimmune disorder such as rheumatoid arthritis, systemic lupus erythematosus, or primary biliary cirrhosis. In this setting, the Sjögren's syndrome is called *secondary* Sjögren's syndrome to distinguish it from *primary* Sjögren's syndrome in which there is no associated disease.

Although the processes that underlie the autoimmunity are not known, B and T lymphocytes and ductal epithelial cells of the salivary gland are all involved. Of note, antigen-presenting cells have not been found in significant numbers within the inflammatory cell infiltrate in Sjögren's syndrome. Recent studies suggest that ductal epithelial cells may directly present antigens to T lymphocytes, stimulating inflammation.

Sjögren's syndrome presents with symptoms related to dry eyes and dry mouth

Most patients with Sjögren's syndrome present with symptoms related to dryness and soreness of the eyes and mouth. The dry mouth may be associated with difficulty in swallowing and speaking, and disturbance of taste. The lack of saliva predisposes to oral candidiasis and dental caries. Lack of tear production by lacrimal glands causes a gritty burning sensation in the eye and predisposes to conjunctivitis.

It is important to note that symptoms of dry eyes and dry mouth are common, especially in the elderly, and most patients with these symptoms do not have Sjögren's syndrome.

> ### JARGON BUSTER
>
> #### Keratoconjunctivitis sicca
>
> Sicca means 'dryness', and the term keratoconjunctivitis sicca simply describes the combination of dry eyes and mouth. It does not imply the underlying cause.

Lip biopsy is an important investigation in establishing a diagnosis of Sjögren's syndrome

Histological examination of salivary gland tissue is a helpful diagnostic test in patients suspected of having Sjögren's syndrome. As all salivary glands are affected, the minor salivary glands of the lip are usually the easiest to sample. The typical microscopic feature is focal collections of lymphocytes within the salivary tissue associated with destruction of the glands. Quantification of the degree of inflammation in the biopsy forms one part of the diagnostic criteria for Sjögren's syndrome.

> ### LINK BOX
>
> #### Sarcoidosis versus Sjögren's syndrome
>
> Sarcoidosis is an important differential diagnosis with Sjögren's syndrome as this can also involve the salivary glands and lacrimal glands, causing dry eyes and mouth. The lip biopsy is a useful way to distinguish the two conditions, as in sarcoidosis there will be numerous non-caseating granulomas (p. 482).

Serology is also helpful in the investigation of possible Sjögren's syndrome

Hypergammaglobulinaemia (raised levels of circulating immunoglobulins) is the most common serological finding in Sjögren's syndrome. A number of different autoantibodies are present, including rheumatoid factor, antinuclear antibodies, and antibodies against other cellular antigens. Antibodies directed against two ribonucleoproteins known as **Ro** (SSA) and **La** (SSB) are often found in patients with Sjögren's syndrome. Whilst these two autoantibodies are useful in conjunction with other supportive evidence of Sjögren's syndrome, they are *not* specific for the syndrome and may be found in other autoimmune diseases, particularly systemic lupus erythematosus.

Both primary and secondary Sjögren's syndrome are associated with a risk of lymphoma

Treatment of Sjögren's syndrome is symptomatic, though patients must be carefully monitored for the development of lymphoma. Patients with Sjögren's syndrome have a greater than 40 times higher relative risk of developing lymphoma, most of which are marginal zone B cell lymphomas (a type of non-Hodgkin lymphoma). The lymphoma usually arises in the salivary glands and tends to remain localized for many years.

LINK BOX

Chronic inflammation and marginal zone lymphomas

Other sites where chronic inflammation is known to increase the risk of developing a marginal zone lymphoma include the stomach due to *Helicobacter pylori* chronic gastritis (p. 149) and the thyroid due to autoimmune thyroiditis (p. 317).

Key points: Sjögren's syndrome

- Sjögren's syndrome is an autoimmune disease in which there is destruction of the lacrimal and salivary glands resulting in dry eyes and dry mouth.

- Both B lymphocytes and T lymphocytes are present in tissues involved by Sjögren's syndrome, though we do not know which cell is the dominant cause for the immune destruction.

- Primary Sjögren's syndrome must be distinguished from Sjögren's syndrome secondary to other diseases such as rheumatoid arthritis and systemic lupus erythematosus, and from other causes of dry eyes and dry mouth such as drugs and sarcoidosis.

- Helpful tests to diagnose Sjögren's syndrome include a lip biopsy, and measurement of a panel of autoantibodies including anti-Ro and anti-La.

- Both primary and secondary Sjögren's syndrome are associated with a risk of the development of lymphoma, normally a marginal zone B cell lymphoma.

Salivary gland tumours

The salivary glands can give rise to a remarkable number of different tumours, though only some are commonly seen (Table 19.1). Most salivary gland neoplasms are benign, with the ratio of benign to malignant being around 2:1. Most of them arise in major salivary glands, with the parotid being most commonly affected. The vast majority of salivary gland neoplasms are of epithelial origin. The most notable exception to this is non-Hodgkin's lymphoma.

Pleomorphic adenoma is the most common salivary gland tumour

By far the most common type of salivary tumour is the **pleomorphic adenoma**. Pleomorphic adenoma is a benign tumour which shows a complex intermingling of epithelial components and mesenchymal areas (Fig. 19.7). It is this diversity of different cell types within the tumour that gives rise to the name 'pleomorphic'; the term does not imply pleomorphism of the cells themselves, which are usually bland and benign looking. The relative amount of epithelial and mesenchymal cells varies widely between each tumour.

Pleomorphic adenomas usually present as slowly growing, painless, rubbery swellings. Most occur in the parotid gland. Although pleomorphic adenomas are benign tumours, local recurrence of the tumour is common unless they are excised with a margin of

TABLE 19.1 Common salivary gland tumours

Pleomorphic adenoma
Warthin's tumour
Mucoepidermoid carcinoma
Adenoid cystic carcinoma

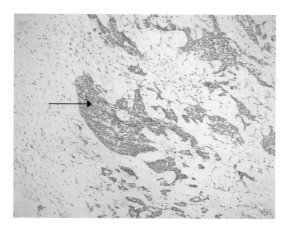

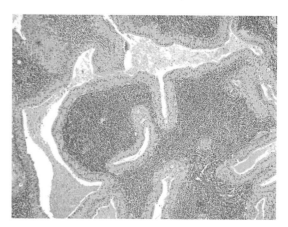

Fig. 19.7 Pleomorphic adenoma. Typical microscopic appearance of a pleomorphic adenoma with an intermingling of epithelial elements (arrow) set within a mesenchymal component.

Fig. 19.8 Warthin's tumour. Classical microscopic appearance of a Warthin's tumour with a double layer of eosinophilic epithelial cells (bright pink cells) overlying a dense lymphoid stroma (dark blue area).

normal salivary gland tissue. This is because the tumour often contains outgrowths from the main tumour mass which may be left behind if simple enucleation is performed.

Warthin's tumour has a highly characteristic microscopic appearance

Warthin's tumour, the second most common salivary gland tumour, is an interesting tumour which occurs almost exclusively in the parotid gland. The microscopic appearance of the tumour is highly characteristic, comprising a double layer of epithelial cells with markedly eosinophilic (pink) cytoplasm intermingled with dense lymphoid tissue which often includes numerous germinal centres (Fig. 19.8).

Quite how the tumour arises is uncertain, though it is thought that it develops from islands of epithelium entrapped within intraparotid lymph nodes. Warthin's tumours are benign, with a very low rate of recurrence following surgical excision.

Mucoepidermoid carcinoma is the most common salivary gland malignancy

Mucoepidermoid carcinoma is a malignant neoplasm characterized by a mixture of mucus-producing cells, squamoid (epidermoid) cells, and epithelial cells of intermediate type. The proportion of each of these cell types varies within and between tumours.

Mucoepidermoid carcinomas present as firm, fixed, painless swellings. Whilst most mucoepidermoid

carcinomas occur in the parotids, they account for a large proportion of tumours in other glands, particularly the minor salivary glands. The prognosis of the tumour is related to its pattern of infiltration of the surrounding tissues. Those that invade with an irregular front behave more aggressively than those with a broad front.

Adenoid cystic carcinoma commonly invades nerves and has a poor prognosis

Adenoid cystic carcinoma is a malignant tumour composed of epithelial and myoepithelial cells arranged in solid sheets with large punched out spaces. Adenoid cystic carcinoma has a particular propensity to invade nerves, and the tumour typically causes a painful slowly growing salivary gland mass. The neoplasm has a relentless course, and the outcome is usually fatal.

> ## Key points: Salivary gland tumours
>
> ♦ Salivary gland neoplasms may be benign or malignant. Most arise in the parotid gland.
>
> ♦ Pleomorphic adenoma is the most common benign salivary gland tumour. Surgical removal is curative provided a wide excision is achieved.

Key points: Salivary gland tumours—cont'd

- Warthin's tumour is a benign salivary gland tumour with a characteristic microscopic appearance.

- Mucoepidermoid carcinoma is the most common salivary gland malignancy made up of a mixture of mucin-producing, squamoid, and intermediate epithelial cells.

- Adenoid cystic carcinoma has a propensity to invade nerves and has a poor prognosis.

Nose and paranasal sinuses

The **nose** serves to warm and humidify inspired air, as well as removing large airborne particles. It also acts as the outflow tract for expired air, and is the organ of olfaction. The external nose is made up of skin-covered cartilage plates attached to the two nasal bones of the skull. The nasal cavities are separated by a midline septum composed of bone and cartilage, and are lined by respiratory type epithelium (pseudostratified ciliated columnar epithelium).

The **paranasal sinuses** are hollow cavities also lined by respiratory epithelium which communicate with the nasal cavity. They include the paired frontal sinuses, ethmoid sinuses, and maxillary sinuses, and the single midline sphenoid sinus. Their purpose is not known for certain though they do add resonance to the voice and give shape to the face.

Epistaxis

Most nose bleeds are trivial events, but in some situations the haemorrhage can be life threatening. In children and young people, nose bleeds usually follow nose picking or insertion of foreign bodies into the nose. The bleeding site is usually the anterior septum.

In older people, nose bleeds are usually from the posterior part of the nose, often from arterioles affected by hypertension or age-related arteriolosclerosis. Epistaxis is common in elderly patients on aspirin or warfarin.

Allergic rhinitis

Allergic rhinitis is an allergic reaction to inhaled allergens leading to sneezing attacks, watery nasal discharge, and nasal itch. The reaction is a typical immediate (type I) hypersensitivity reaction in which allergen binds to IgE antibodies on the surface of mast cells. Degranulation of mast cells leads to stimulation of afferent nerve endings causing sneezing, and inflammation of the nasal passages with symptoms of itchy nose and watery discharge.

Allergic rhinitis is divided into seasonal rhinitis and perennial rhinitis

Allergic rhinitis can be divided into seasonal rhinitis (hayfever) present for a limited period of the year, and perennial rhinitis which occurs throughout the year.

Seasonal rhinitis, due to an allergic reaction to pollen, is the most common allergic disease; up to 30 per cent of people suffer symptoms in the summer months. In addition to sneezing, discharge, and nasal irritation, there is often itching of the eyes and soft palate as well. Most patients' symptoms are worse during June and July when grass pollen grain numbers are at their highest.

Perennial rhinitis is usually due to household allergens, particularly house dust mite and allergens from domestic pets. The house dust mite survives by absorbing moisture and oxygen directly from the atmosphere, and thrives in areas which are warm, dark, and damp. Modern beds are particularly good breeding grounds for house dust mites where they can gain nourishment from desquamated skin cells.

Both forms of allergic rhinitis may lead to the formation of inflammatory polyps in the nose

The persistent oedema associated with chronic allergic rhinitis can lead to the formation of inflammatory polyps, which bulge into the nasal cavity and contribute to symptoms of nasal obstruction. In troublesome cases, the polyps can be removed surgically, though they often recur.

Sinusitis

Sinusitis is an inflammation of the mucosa of a paranasal sinus. Sinusitis is usually caused by bacterial infection of the sinuses following impaired drainage of secretions from the sinus caused by a preceding viral infection of the nasopharynx (common cold). Bacterial infection of the maxillary sinusitis may also be caused by direct spread from an infection around an upper first or second molar tooth.

Sinusitis causes the sinus to fill up with purulent exudate, leading to facial pain and altered vocal resonance. Decongestant treatment may help to improve drainage from the sinus. Antibacterial agents are not normally given in uncomplicated cases.

Tumours of the nasal cavity and paranasal sinuses

A large number of different tumours can occur in the nasal cavity and paranasal sinuses, but all are rare, together accounting for less than 1 per cent of all malignant neoplasms. The two most common tumour types are squamous cell carcinoma and non-Hodgkin lymphoma, of which the most common in the nasal cavity is **extranodal NK/T cell lymphoma** and in the paranasal sinuses **diffuse large B cell lymphoma**. Extranodal NK/T cell lymphoma is a highly aggressive, destructive malignancy which exhibits a mixture of natural killer (NK) and T cell markers. It used to be known as 'lethal midline granuloma'.

Key points: Nose and paranasal sinuses

- Epistaxis is usually due to trauma in the young but spontaneous in the elderly. Most nose bleeds are trivial, but occasionally can be life threatening.

- Allergic rhinitis is a type I hypersensitivity reaction to inhaled environmental allergens leading to sneezing, nasal discharge, and nasal itch.

- Seasonal allergic rhinitis (hayfever) is worse in the summer months when grass pollen levels are at their highest.

- Perennial allergic rhinitis occurs all year round. Household allergens, particularly the house dust mite, are the culprit allergens.

- Chronic allergic rhinitis can lead to the formation of inflammatory nasal polyps.

- Sinusitis is an infection of the paranasal sinuses, which typically complicates a common cold.

- Tumours of the nose and paranasal sinuses are rare. The most common are squamous cell carcinoma and non-Hodgkin lymphoma.

Nasopharynx

The **nasopharynx** lies above the soft palate and behind the posterior nares. It is lined by respiratory type epithelium and contains the adenoid tonsil which forms part of **Waldeyer's ring**. Waldeyer's ring is a circumferential mass of lymphoid tissue situated right underneath the surface epithelium which surrounds and protects the openings to the respiratory and digestive tracts.

Common cold

The common cold is caused by viral infection of the nasopharynx

A number of viruses may infect the nasopharynx and cause the common cold (Table 19.2). Most of these viruses have surface molecules enabling them to bind firmly to epithelial cells of the upper respiratory tract, protecting them from the flushing effect of cilia. Infection of the nasopharynx causes the production of a secretion rich in viral particles which streams out of the nose and triggers the sneezing reflex, discharging large numbers of viral particles into the air. There is no specific treatment for the common cold, and thus no need to perform laboratory tests to identify the culprit virus.

Nasopharyngeal carcinoma

Nasopharyngeal carcinoma is common in the Far East and linked to EBV infection

Nasopharyngeal carcinoma is a squamous cell carcinoma arising in the nasopharyngeal mucosa. Whilst rare in most parts of the world, there are certain populations with a high incidence, notably those in South East Asia (particularly Hong Kong, China, Thailand, and the Philippines).

Epstein–Barr Virus (EBV) infection is known to be important, and EBV genetic material can be found in all tumour cells. Diet is also thought to be important;

TABLE 19.2   Viruses causing the common cold

Rhinoviruses
Coronaviruses
Coxsackie A virus
Parainfluenza virus
Adenovirus

preserved foods such as salted fish eaten in higher quantities in South East Asia may be relevant.

The most common symptoms of nasopharyngeal carcinoma are persistent nasal and/or aural symptoms such as nasal discharge and obstruction, tinnitus, ear ache, and deafness. Nasopharyngeal carcinoma should therefore be considered in any patient presenting with new persistent unilateral ear or nose symptoms. Lymph node metastases in cervical lymph nodes are common at presentation, and many patients present because they notice a rapidly enlarging neck mass.

Nasopharyngeal carcinoma is notorious for its highly malignant behaviour, with extensive local spread and early involvement of cervical lymph nodes, and haematogenous spread to distant organs such as bone, lung, and liver. The mainstay of treatment for nasopharyngeal carcinoma is radiotherapy, which can achieve 5 year survival rates of up to 80 per cent in patients without distant metastases.

Key points: Nasopharynx

- The common cold is a viral infection of the nasopharynx. The infection stimulates production of a watery discharge rich in viral particles which is disseminated into the environment by triggering of the sneeze reflex.

- Nasopharyngeal carcinoma is associated with EBV infection and typically presents with persistent unilateral nasal or aural symptoms. Nasopharyngeal carcinoma has an aggressive behaviour with extensive local spread and early involvement of cervical lymph nodes.

Oropharynx

The **oropharynx** lies between the soft palate and the epiglottis. Each lateral wall of the oropharynx contains a palatine tonsil, another part of Waldeyer's ring.

Pharyngitis

The term 'pharyngitis' tends to be used to refer to infection of the oropharynx. The main symptom of pharyngitis is a sore throat. Most cases of pharyngitis occur as an extension of a common cold and are therefore caused by viruses, particularly adenoviruses.

Bacteria may also cause pharyngitis, but much less commonly. The most common bacterium is *Streptococcus pyogenes* (also known as group A β-haemolytic streptococci). The vast majority of streptococcal sore throats are self-limiting; however, a small proportion of cases may be associated with certain complications:

- **Otitis media** and **sinusitis**, due to local spread of the infection.

- **Rheumatic fever**. This is an immunological disorder in which antibodies formed to streptococcal antigens cross-react with various tissues of the body, including the heart and joints. Although in most tissues the initial inflammation resolves, scarring can develop over years in the endocardium of the heart valves, leading to chronic rheumatic disease. Rheumatic fever is now uncommon, though it remains the most common cause of mitral stenosis in elderly people who had the disease as a child.

- **Post-streptococcal glomerulonephritis**. This is also an immune-mediated disease in which immune complexes of streptococcal antigens and antibodies become deposited in the glomeruli, fix complement, and cause inflammation in the glomeruli. The typical presentation is an episode of the nephritic syndrome with haematuria, proteinuria, hypertension, and oedema developing 1–2 weeks after the sore throat.

Because of these possible complications, it is usually recommended to treat cases of pharyngitis thought to be bacterial in origin with penicillin. A laboratory diagnosis can be made by taking a throat swab for culture, though the decision whether to give penicillin is often made based on the clinical picture.

Infectious mononucleosis is an important cause of pharyngitis

Infectious mononucleosis (glandular fever) is a common and important cause of pharyngitis. The disease is caused by infection with EBV and is transmitted by exchange of saliva, particularly during kissing. Most people acquire the virus during close contact in childhood, with no significant effects. Those that do not acquire the infection until adolescence tend to develop an acute illness (infectious mononucleosis).

EBV has a surface receptor that binds to the C3d receptor on the surface of B lymphocytes and epithelial cells. T lymphocytes respond to the infected B cells and appear in blood films as odd-looking cells called 'atypical lymphocytes'.

The manifestations of infectious mononucleosis appear to be due to the T cell response, accounting for the absence of disease in children who mount a weaker T cell response. Older people, however, develop infectious mononucleosis about 5–6 weeks after the initial infection, characterized by fever, sore throat, and lethargy. Lymphadenopathy and splenomegaly may be found on physical examination.

The initial investigations for infectious mononucleosis include visualizing atypical lymphocytes in a peripheral blood film and performing the **Monospot test**. The Monospot test looks for the presence of heterophil antibodies released by EBV-infected B lymphocytes that agglutinate horse red blood cells (after removal of non-specific heterophil antibodies in the serum using guinea pig kidney). Not all patients with infectious mononucleosis have a positive Monospot test. Monospot-negative patients suspected of having infectious mononucleosis should have measurement of anti-EBV antibodies or polymerase chain reaction (PCR) testing for EBV DNA.

There is no specific treatment for infectious mononucleosis and thus treatment is symptomatic. In most patients, the virus establishes a latent infection in a small number of B lymphocytes.

LINK BOX

EBV as an oncogenic virus

EBV has been linked to certain malignancies, particularly B cell lymphomas in immunosuppressed patients (p. 50) and nasopharyngeal carcinoma (p. 458).

Acute tonsillitis

Acute tonsillitis refers to a pharyngitis associated with enlargement of the palatine tonsils. About half of all cases of acute tonsillitis are due to bacteria, particularly the group A β-haemolytic streptococcus. Viruses account for the other cases; infectious mononucleosis in particular may frequently be mistaken for a bacterial tonsillitis.

Acute tonsillitis is seen mostly in children, with fever, sore throat, enlarged cervical lymph nodes, and often referred pain in the ears. In cases of acute tonsillitis, a throat swab should be taken and sent for culture. Treatment should be given with oral penicillin pending the result of the throat swab.

Key points: Oropharynx

- Infection of the oropharynx is known as pharyngitis and is usually caused by viruses as an extension of a common cold.

- Bacterial pharyngitis is less common but is important, as streptococcal infections may rarely be complicated by acute rheumatic fever and post-streptococcal glomerulonephritis.

- Infectious mononucleosis is caused by Epstein–Barr virus and typically presents in adolescents with fever, pharyngitis, cervical lymphadenopathy, and splenomegaly. Atypical lymphocytes are seen on the blood film, and the Monospot test is usually positive.

Hypopharynx

The hypopharynx (also known as the laryngopharynx) lies behind the larynx and extends between the epiglottis and inferior border of the cricoid cartilage, where it becomes continuous with the oesophagus.

Hypopharyngeal carcinoma

The most important disorder of the hypopharynx is squamous cell carcinoma. The diagnosis of **hypopharyngeal carcinoma** should always be considered in any patient presenting with dysphagia or hoarseness, particularly if they are heavy smokers and drinkers. Generally speaking, these tumours present late; hoarseness implies that the tumour has already spread anteriorly into the larynx. The prognosis is poor.

Larynx

The larynx extends from the tip of the epiglottis to the inferior border of the cricoid cartilage and is divided into three compartments: supraglottis, glottis, and subglottis. The supraglottis comprises the epiglottis, aryepiglottic folds, false vocal cords, ventricles, and saccules. The glottis consists of the true vocal cords and the anterior and posterior commissures. The subglottis extends from below the vocal cords to the top of the trachea.

The larynx is mostly covered with respiratory type epithelium, with the exception of the epiglottis and the true vocal cords, which are covered by squamous epithelium.

Acute epiglottitis

Acute epiglottitis is an important cause of upper airway obstruction

Acute epiglottitis is an inflammation of the epiglottis typically caused by *Haemophilus influenzae* infection. Initially there is a severe pharyngitis at the junction of the oropharynx and hypopharynx, which then progresses to involve the whole of the laryngeal inlet, with severe oedema of the aryepiglottic folds and epiglottis.

Acute epiglottitis can occur in adults but is much more important in children, who can rapidly develop upper airway obstruction with stridor and drooling of saliva. There is often bacteraemia, and the diagnosis can be confirmed by growing the bacteria from blood cultures.

Children with acute epiglottis require careful and expert airway management whilst being treated with antibiotics to combat *H. influenzae* (e.g. cefotaxime, chloramphenicol). Fortunately, cases of acute epiglottitis are becoming rarer due to the *H. influenzae* type b (Hib) vaccine.

Acute laryngitis

Acute laryngitis often occurs as an extension from a common cold, particularly those caused by parainfluenza viruses. The development of laryngitis causes hoarseness and loss of voice. The infection is self-limiting and settles quickly if the patient rests the voice.

Laryngeal carcinoma

The most common malignancy of the larynx is squamous cell carcinoma, which originates either from the native squamous epithelium of the true vocal cords or following squamous metaplasia of the respiratory epithelium. Like other head and neck squamous cell carcinomas, cigarette smoking and alcohol abuse are major risk factors.

Carcinomas of the larynx are divided into supraglottic, glottic, and subglottic

Laryngeal carcinomas are subdivided according to their site of origin into supraglottic, glottic, and subglottic carcinomas. The glottis is the most common site, followed by the supraglottis. Subglottic tumours are uncommon.

The most common early symptom of glottic carcinoma is persistent hoarseness. Supraglottic carcinomas tend to cause a change in the quality of the voice and a sensation of a foreign body in the throat. Subglottic tumours are more likely to present with breathlessness and stridor.

Glottic carcinomas tend to remain localized for quite long periods, usually spreading to the opposite vocal cord in the late stages of the disease. Supraglottic carcinomas spread into the pyriform sinus and the tongue base. Subglottic carcinomas may spread anteriorly into the thyroid gland, posteriorly into the hypopharynx and oesophagus, and inferiorly into the trachea.

All laryngeal carcinomas are likely to spread to regional cervical lymph nodes. Haematogenous spread to distant organs is less frequent, but can be seen in advanced disease.

The two most important determinates of prognosis are the stage of the disease, and the presence or absence of lymph node metastases. Glottic carcinomas have the best prognosis, with a 5 year survival rate of up to 85 per cent, probably because they present early with hoarseness and tend to remain localized for longer.

Miscellaneous lesions of the larynx

Vocal nodules (singer's nodules) are benign thickenings of both vocal folds which occur in people who use their voice at a loud volume, e.g. singers and teachers. The nodules arise bilaterally at the junction of the middle and anterior third of the vocal cords, the point which receives the most contact during speech. They start out as soft swellings, but become more fibrous and thickened with time. Vocal nodules usually present with a change in vocal quality, variously described as 'rough', 'harsh', and 'scratchy'. The nodules often resolve spontaneously with vocal rest and speech therapy, though they can be removed surgically.

Vocal cord polyps are unilateral lesions which may be associated with cigarette smoking or vocal abuse. Vocal polyps are large fleshy lesions that hang off the vocal cord and usually require surgical removal. They cause symptoms similar to vocal nodules.

Laryngeal papillomas occur mainly in children and are caused by papillomaviruses. The infection is probably acquired at birth when the baby passes through a genital tract infected with human papillomavirus. Because the papillomas grow quickly, young children may find it difficult to breathe when sleeping. The papillomas are removed by laser surgery to maintain the voice and airway.

Key points: Larynx

◆ Acute epiglottitis is an important infection in children as it may cause acute upper airway obstruction. The incidence of the disease is falling since the introduction of the *H. influenzae* type b vaccination.

◆ Acute laryngitis is a self-limiting viral infection of the larynx which causes hoarseness and loss of voice.

◆ Laryngeal carcinomas may be divided into supraglottic, glottic, and subglottic. The diagnosis should be considered in any patient with persistent hoarseness or change in quality of the voice.

◆ Vocal nodules are benign thickenings of both vocal folds seen in people who use their voice at a loud volume.

◆ Vocal cord polyps are unilateral fleshy lesions associated with smoking.

◆ Laryngeal papillomas are benign neoplasms seen in children caused by infection with papillomaviruses.

External ear

The external ear consists of the **pinna** and the **ear canal**. The pinna is made of cartilage covered by tightly adherent skin. The ear canal is about 3 cm in length and lined by skin, with underlying cartilage in the outer two-thirds and underlying bone in the inner one-third. The skin covering the bony part of the ear canal is specialized; it does not shed like normal skin but rather migrates outwards along the ear canal, such that the ear canal is self-cleaning.

The pinna is a common site of minor congenital malformations

There are a variety of congenital malformations of the pinna, though they are usually of no clinical consequence (however, as with any external malformation, they may be a source for teasing). The most common malformations are bat ears and accessory lobules.

Trauma often affects the external ear

The external ear often bears the brunt of blunt trauma, which can lead to haematoma formation between the skin and the cartilage of the pinna. As the cartilage of the pinna has no other blood supply other than that derived from the overlying skin, if the haematoma is not evacuated the cartilage will die and will be replaced by scar tissue, leading to a deformed 'cauliflower ear' seen mostly in rugby players and boxers.

Chondrodermatitis nodularis helicis is a painful nodule occurring on the helix of the ear

The rather elaborate name **chondrodermatitis nodularis helicis** describes a small, solitary, crusted nodule which is typically seen on the helix of elderly men. The lesion may be exquisitely painful and may be severe enough to keep the patient awake at night if the affected area touches the pillow. The cause of chondrodermatitis nodularis helicis is not known, though persistent trauma is thought to be important as the site of the lesion is typically on the most protuberant part of the helix.

Chondrodermatitis nodularis helicis is often mistaken for a cutaneous malignancy such as squamous cell carcinoma or basal cell carcinoma, though the history of pain is unusual for these malignancies. Nevertheless, excision and microscopic examination is usually performed to confirm the diagnosis and exclude a malignancy.

The pinna is a common site for cutaneous malignancies

Because of its position, the uppermost part of the pinna is particularly vulnerable to sun damage and is a very common location for malignant cutaneous tumours related to sun exposure, such as basal cell carcinoma and squamous cell carcinoma.

Otitis externa

Otitis externa is a common inflammatory disorder of the external ear

Otitis externa refers to inflammation of the skin of the ear canal. This may be caused by involvement of the ear canal by a number of conditions including psoriasis, atopic dermatitis, seborrhoeic dermatitis, contact dermatitis due to ear drops, and infection by bacteria or fungi. The inflammation halts the normal skin migration process and debris begins to collect in the canal, promoting infection. Otitis externa causes severe pain worsened by movement of the pinna.

Ear wax

Wax in the external ear canal is the most common cause of conductive hearing loss

Ear wax, or **cerumen**, is produced by **ceruminous glands** which are modified apocrine glands located in the skin of the cartilaginous part of the external ear canal. Ear wax prevents maceration of the skin of the ear canal by soaking up water. Blockage of the ear canal by ear wax is the most common cause of conductive hearing loss.

Key point: External ear

◆ The pinna is a common site for congenital malformations, trauma, and cutaneous malignancies.

◆ Chondrodermatitis nodularis helicis is a painful lesion of the helix seen in elderly men. It is thought to be related to persistent trauma.

◆ Otitis externa is inflammation of the external ear which may be caused by inflammatory skin conditions or infections.

Middle ear

The middle ear is a space in the temporal bone which is lined by respiratory type epithelium. The lateral wall of the middle ear is the **tympanic membrane** (ear drum). Anteriorly, the Eustachian tube connects the middle ear to the nasopharynx. The medial wall of the middle ear contains the **oval window** where sound is conducted into the inner ear. The tympanic membrane and the oval window are connected by a chain of small bones that traverse the middle ear, the **malleus**, **incus**, and **stapes**.

Acute otitis media

Acute otitis media is a common inflammatory condition of the middle ear

Acute otitis media is a very common infection in infants and young children. The infecting organisms access the middle ear via the Eustachian tube which has a wide opening at this age. At least half of all cases of acute otitis media are caused by viruses, particularly respiratory syncytial virus. Bacterial invaders are normal nasopharyngeal commensals such as *Streptococcus pneumoniae*, *H. influenzae*, and *Moraxhella catarrhalis*.

Acute otitis media typically causes earache which makes the infection easy to localize. However, in children unable to vocalize their symptoms, it should be considered in any child with unexplained fever, diarrhoea, or vomiting. The diagnosis is made by visualizing the ear drum, which bulges outwards due to the underlying inflammation.

Treatment is with amoxicillin which has activity against all the common bacterial causes. Perforation of the ear drum is a frequent complication of otitis media. Most perforations heal with no serious consequences.

Glue ear

Glue ear is an important cause of deafness in children

Glue ear (secretory otitis media, otitis media with effusion) is a very common condition in which the middle ear becomes filled with thick fluid, causing conductive hearing loss. The precise cause of glue ear is still not known, but is probably related to poor function of the Eustachian tube preventing adequate drainage of middle ear fluid. Whilst glue ear may follow a middle ear infection, in many cases there is no obvious preceding infection.

Fortunately most cases of glue ear spontaneously resolve within 6 weeks of onset. If, however, the problem persists at a time when the infant is learning to speak, the hearing impairment can lead to delayed speech, behavioural problems, and reading and learning difficulties at school. The only effective way of treating glue ear is insertion of ventilation tubes (grommets) through the tympanic membrane to drain the fluid, often combined with removal of the adenoid tonsils near the opening of the Eustachian tube in the nasopharynx.

LINK BOX

Middle ear effusions in adults

Middle ear effusions in adults are rare but may be seen associated with an upper respiratory tract infection. A persistent unilateral middle ear effusion in an adult should always be viewed with suspicion, as it may be caused by a nasopharyngeal carcinoma blocking the opening of the Eustachian tube (p. 458).

Cholesteatoma

Cholesteatoma is a destructive lesion of the middle ear with potentially fatal complications

A **cholesteatoma** is an abnormal mass of keratin-producing squamous epithelium in the middle ear (recall the middle ear is normally lined by respiratory type epithelium). The name cholesteatoma is a complete misnomer as it does not contain cholesterol and it is not a neoplasm. Although it is not a neoplasm, it may act like one in that it has a propensity for local destruction and recurrence after excision.

The normal middle ear does not contain squamous epithelium and precisely how the squamous epithelium of a cholesteatoma arises in the middle ear remains controversial. The most likely explanation is that it grows into the middle ear from the external ear canal through a perforation in the tympanic membrane caused by acute otitis media.

The importance of cholesteatoma lies in its potential to expand and erode through surrounding structures. Problems that can arise include conductive deafness from erosion of the middle ear bones, and facial paralysis from involvement of the geniculate ganglion of the facial nerve. Erosion through the skull base may lead to life-threatening complications such as meningitis and a cerebral abscess.

Fortunately most patients with a cholesteatoma present before complications have occurred, with a foul-smelling ear discharge and conductive hearing loss. The treatment of cholesteatoma is complete surgical excision.

Otosclerosis

Otosclerosis of the stapes is a common cause of conductive hearing loss in young adults

Otosclerosis is a condition in which excess amounts of new bone are laid down in the middle ear. Although any part of the middle ear may be affected, the most common site is immediately anterior to the oval window. If the new bone extends and infiltrates around the footplate of the stapes, the stapes becomes increasingly immobilized, leading to conductive hearing loss.

Although otosclerosis affects as many as 10 per cent of the population, only 10 per cent of patients with otosclerosis (i.e. 1 per cent of the population) have involvement of the stapes and develop significant hearing loss. Otosclerosis affects women twice as often as men, and often rapidly worsens during pregnancy. The cause of otosclerosis remains obscure, though the condition often runs in families.

Otosclerosis usually presents in young adults with a very gradual hearing loss. The hearing loss occurs so slowly that many people only become aware of it when friends or relatives call attention to it. Many compensate by inadvertently learning to lip read. The hearing loss can be easily shown with a hearing test, but the otosclerosis can only be diagnosed by exploring the middle ear at surgery.

> ## Key points: Middle ear
>
> ◆ Acute otitis media is a very common infection in young children and should always be considered in any child who is unwell.
>
> ◆ Glue ear (otitis media with effusion) is a condition in which the middle ear becomes filled with thick fluid due to malfunction of the Eustachian tube. Cases that do not resolve spontaneously and cause problems with hearing loss can be treated by grommet insertion.
>
> ◆ Cholesteatoma is a non-neoplastic destructive condition of the middle ear which presents with a foul-smelling ear discharge. Surgical excision of the abnormal squamous epithelium is required to prevent erosion into adjacent structures.
>
> ◆ Otosclerosis is a condition in which excess amounts of bone are laid down in the middle ear. If this immobilizes the footplate of the stapes, conductive hearing loss may occur.

Inner ear

The inner ear is made up of a series of fluid-filled spaces running through the petrous temporal bone of the skull. The bony tubes (the bony labyrinth) are filled with a fluid called **perilymph** within which lies a series of interconnected membranous sacs (the membranous labyrinth) filled with a fluid called **endolymph**. Together, the bony and membranous labyrinths make up the organ of hearing, the **cochlear**, and the organs of balance, the **utricle**, **saccule**, and **semicircular canals**.

Perilymph is a typical extracellular fluid with an ionic composition similar to plasma, the main cation being sodium. Endolymph is a totally unique extracellular fluid, with an ion composition unlike that anywhere else found in the body. The major cation in endolymph is potassium, and there is virtually no sodium.

Disorders of the inner ear typically present with sensorineural deafness, tinnitus (high pitched ringing in the ear), and/or vertigo.

Presbyacusis

Presbyacusis is a term used to describe the hearing loss related to old age

Presbyacusis (or presbycusis) is a disorder of old age caused by degenerative loss of cochlear hair cells and/or loss of the neurones with which hair cells synapse. Presbyacusis leads to sensorineural hearing loss which usually starts at the high frequency range. Because the consonants of speech lie within this range, speech discrimination becomes difficult.

Vestibular schwannoma

Vestibular schwannoma is an important cause of unilateral deafness and/or tinnitus

Vestibular schwannoma (previously known as acoustic neuroma) is a slow growing benign tumour composed of neoplastic Schwann cells which arises from the vestibular division of the eighth cranial nerve. Although the tumour involves the vestibular nerve, the early symptoms of unilateral sensorineural deafness and tinnitus are related to stretching of the adjacent cochlear nerve over the tumour. Continued growth eventually leads to compression of adjacent cranial nerves and raised intracranial pressure. Ideally patients with any unilateral ear symptom should have brain magnetic resonance imaging (MRI) to rule out a vestibular schwannoma.

Ménière's disease

Ménière's disease causes episodic inner ear symptoms due to increased endolymphatic pressure

Ménière's disease is a disorder in which there is increased pressure in the endolymphatic system of the inner ear. The reason for the increase in endolymphatic pressure is not clear. The disease manifests with four symptoms: *fluctuating hearing loss, episodic vertigo, tinnitus, and a sensation of aural fullness*. Although the disease is not lethal, the symptoms can be extremely distressing and disabling to the sufferer.

Physical distension within the inner ear caused by increased endolymphatic pressure causes distortion of the basilar membrane and inner and outer hair cells of the cochlear, leading to hearing loss and tinnitus. Low frequency hearing loss probably occurs preferentially because the apex of the cochlear, which is wound more tightly than the base, is more sensitive to pressure changes.

The vertigo in Ménière's disease is thought to be due to the result of small breaks in the membrane separating endolymph from perilymph caused by the increased endolymphatic pressure. Mixing of potassium-rich endolymph with potassium-poor perilymph causes sudden changes in the firing of the vestibular nerve, leading to symptoms of vertigo.

> ### Key points: Inner ear
>
> - Presbyacusis is a sensorineural hearing loss seen in old age due to degeneration of cochlear hair cells and/or the neurones with which they synapse.
>
> - Vestibular schwannoma is a benign neoplasm composed of Schwann cells arising in the vestibular division of the vestibulocochlear nerve. The diagnosis should be ruled out in any patient with unilateral sensorineural hearing loss or tinnitus by brain MRI.
>
> - Ménière's disease is a disorder in which increased endolymphatic pressure causes fluctuating hearing loss, episodic vertigo, tinnitus, and a sensation of aural fullness.

Neck

The neck contains a number of structures lying in close proximity. Most neck problems present with a lump in the neck and may be related to cervical lymph nodes, the thyroid gland, or developmental remnants (Fig. 19.9).

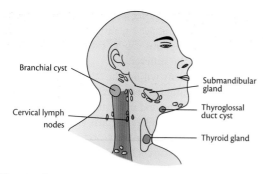

Fig. 19.9 Common origins of lumps in the neck.

TABLE 19.3	Causes of cervical lymphadenopathy
Infections of oral cavity or pharynx	
Infectious mononucleosis	
Tuberculosis	
Lymphoma	
Metastatic carcinoma	

Cervical lymphadenopathy

Enlargement of the cervical lymph nodes (cervical lymphadenopathy) may be due to a number of causes (Table 19.3). Most cases of cervical lymphadenopathy are mild and transient, in association with an infection of the tonsils, teeth, pharynx, or sinuses. Other important infections to remember that may cause cervical lymphadenopathy include infectious mononucleosis and tuberculosis.

The possibility of a malignant cause for cervical lymphadenopathy must never be forgotten. A lymphoma often presents with enlargement of cervical lymph nodes, and metastatic carcinoma from the oral cavity, pharynx, larynx, and thyroid often spreads to cervical lymph nodes. Involvement of supraclavicular lymph nodes may occur in metastatic breast, lung, and gastric carcinoma.

Fine needle aspiration cytology is a very useful investigation for enlarged cervical lymph nodes as it can usually readily distinguish between a reactive lymph node and a lymph node involved by malignancy.

Thyroid swellings

A solitary nodule related to the thyroid gland is an important clinical problem which is discussed further on p. 318. As a reminder, the most common causes are a dominant nodule in a multinodular goitre, a benign follicular adenoma, or a thyroid carcinoma.

Again, fine needle aspiration cytology is the investigation of choice.

Developmental remnants

Remnants of embryonic development can sometimes present as a lump in the neck. Because they are often cystic, their fluctuance to palpation and their location are often good clues to the underlying cause.

Thyroglossal duct cyst is a remnant left from incomplete involution of the thyroglossal duct down which the developing thyroid gland migrates from the back of the tongue to the neck. A thyroglossal duct cyst typically presents as a fluctuant lump in the midline anterior neck either in a child or in a young adult.

Branchial cysts are derived from remnants of the branchial clefts. They typically present as a fluctuant lump in the lateral aspect of the neck.

Key points: Neck lumps

- Neck lumps may be due to cervical lymphadenopathy, thyroid swelling, or developmental remnants.

- Careful clinical examination can often narrow down the possible causes according to the character of the lump and its site.

- Fine needle aspiration cytology is a quick, simple investigation of neck lumps.

CHAPTER 20

Eye disease

Chapter contents

Introduction

The eye is the organ of vision, converting light waves into electrical impulses that are transmitted via the optic nerves to the optic cortex for analysis (Fig. 20.1). Many common eye diseases are intrinsic to the eye, though the eye may also be often involved in systemic diseases such as diabetes mellitus, hypertension, and Graves' disease.

Though many eye diseases are trivial, some are sight threatening and can lead to blindness. A person can be registered blind if their visual acuity is 3/60 or worse, i.e. they can see at 3 m (or less) what a person with normal vision can see from 60 m.

Eyelid

The eyelid is a flap of tissue comprising skin covering part of the orbicularis oculi muscle. Blinking of the eyelids serves to distribute the tear film over the exposed parts of the cornea and sclera and to act as 'windscreen wipers' when foreign bodies come into contact with the eye.

Blepharitis

Blepharitis is inflammation of the eyelid. It is a chronic condition that typically affects both eyes and is usually due to infection by staphylococci or is seen in seborrhoeic dermatitis.

Staphylococcal blepharitis affects the anterior eyelid margin and tends to cause matted, hard scales around the eyelids, often with eyelash misdirection and loss.

Seborrhoeic blepharitis also affects the anterior eyelid margin and is associated with seborrhoeic dermatitis involving other areas of the body. Blepharitis due to seborrhoeic dermatitis causes an oily, greasy eyelid deposit. Loss or misdirection of the eyelashes is rare.

Chalazion and stye

A **chalazion** is a firm painless swelling of the eyelid caused by blockage of one of the sebaceous glands in the eyelid (also called Meibomian glands). A chalazion is different from a **stye** which is a painful swelling of the eyelid due to *infection* of a Meibomian gland.

Neoplasms of the eyelid

The eyelid is covered by skin and so may be affected by cutaneous neoplasms. The most common neoplasm affecting the eyelid is **basal cell carcinoma**, which usually starts as a small papule that then ulcerates and does not heal.

The eyelid may also be affected by neoplasms arising from the cutaneous appendages. The **syringoma** is a benign neoplasm derived from the sweat gland duct often seen on the lower eyelid. The eyelids may also be the site of a malignant neoplasm derived from the sebaceous (Meibomian) glands called a **sebaceous carcinoma**.

> ### Key points: Eyelid
>
> - Blepharitis is inflammation of the eyelid which may be caused by staphylococcal infection or as part of the inflammatory skin condition seborrhoeic dermatitis.
>
> - A chalazion is a firm painless swelling of the eyelid due to blockage of a Meibomian gland.
>
> - A stye is a painful swelling of the eyelid due to infection of a Meibomian gland.
>
> - The most common neoplasm of the eyelid is basal cell carcinoma.
>
> - Cutaneous appendage neoplasms such as syringoma may also arise in the eyelid.

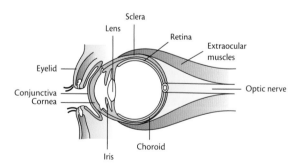

Fig. 20.1 Anatomy of the eye.

Conjunctiva

The **conjunctiva** is a thin membrane that lines the inner surface of the eyelid (the palpebral conjunctiva) and is then reflected over the sclera (the bulbar conjunctiva) where its epithelium becomes continuous with that of the cornea. The palpebral conjunctiva is lined by pseudostratified columnar epithelium, whereas the bulbar conjunctiva is lined by non-keratinizing stratified squamous epithelium.

Conjunctivitis

Conjunctivitis is inflammation of the conjunctiva, which is usually due to infection or allergy.

Viral conjunctivitis, usually due to adenovirus, causes a red eye with watery discharge which is typically unilateral. Although viral conjunctivitis is self-limiting in most cases, the disease is highly contagious and patients must undertake strict hygiene measures to prevent spreading infection to close contacts or reinfecting themselves. Bacterial conjunctivitis, usually due to *Staphylococcus aureus* or *Streptococcus pneumoniae*, causes a red eye with sticky purulent discharge and is typically bilateral. Treatment is with topical antibacterial eye drops.

Allergic conjunctivitis is due to an immediate (type I) hypersensitivity reaction to environmental allergens in the conjunctiva. The inflammation leads to a red, itchy eye. Often there is an associated allergic rhinitis too, with watery nasal discharge, nasal itch, and sneezing.

Pinguecula and pterygium

Pinguecula and **pterygium** are abnormal deposits of collagen underneath the conjunctival epithelium. They are thought to be caused by UV radiation and are most common in people who spend a lot of time outdoors. A pinguecula appears as a small yellow raised area on the bulbar conjunctiva. A pinguecula that extends out on to the cornea is called a pterygium.

Key points: Conjunctiva

- Conjunctivitis may be caused by infection or allergy.
- Viral conjunctivitis is usually caused by adenovirus and results in a unilateral red eye with watery discharge. It is highly contagious.
- Bacterial conjunctivitis is usually due to *S. aureus* or *S. pneumoniae*, and causes bilateral red eyes with purulent discharge.

- Allergic conjunctivitis is due to an immediate hypersensitivity reaction to allergens on the conjunctiva, causing a red itchy eye.
- Pinguecula is a thickening under the bulbar conjunctival epithelium caused by deposition of collagen in response to prolonged exposure to sunlight. A pinguecula that extends out over the cornea is called a pterygium.

Cornea

The **cornea** is a dome-shaped structure covering the front of the eye which forms the main refractive surface of the eye. The cornea is completely avascular to make it as transparent as possible, and so relies on the aqueous humour for nourishment.

Refractive errors

Refractive errors occur when the curve of the cornea or the shape of the eye results in light failing to be focused on the retina. If the cornea is curved too much or the eye is too long, then faraway objects will appear blurry because they are focused in front of the retina (short sightedness, or myopia). Hypermetropia, or long sightedness, is the opposite problem; the eye is too short, resulting in the image being focused behind the retina.

Corneal abrasion

A **corneal abrasion** is an area of loss of the corneal epithelium due to superficial trauma. Common culprits include fingers, finger nails, twigs, dust, sand, and prolonged wearing of contact lenses. A corneal abrasion causes pain and the sensation of a foreign body in the eye. Visual acuity is not impaired.

Corneal abrasions can be easily visualized by instilling a drop of flourescein dye on to the eye and illuminating the eye with a blue light. Fluorescein binds to exposed corneal stroma but not to intact corneal epithelium, thus highlighting corneal abrasions.

Keratitis

Keratitis is inflammation of the cornea, usually due to infection. Corneal infections can be extremely serious with significant risk of losing vision in the affected eye.

The most common cause of keratitis is herpes simplex virus (HSV). Primary orogingival infection with HSV is almost universal in childhood, following which the virus remains latent in the nerve cell bodies of the trigeminal ganglion. If the virus reactivates later in life and passes down the ophthalmic nerve, it can reach the cornea. Infection of corneal epithelial cells by HSV causes cell lysis and the formation of a branching ('dendritic') corneal ulcer.

> # Key points: Cornea
>
> ◆ Refractive errors are extremely common and are caused by an abnormal curve in the cornea resulting in light failing to be focused correctly on the retina.
>
> ◆ A corneal abrasion is a defect in the corneal epithelium caused by trauma to the eye. The defect can be readily highlighted using fluorescein drops and a blue light.
>
> ◆ Keratitis is a serious corneal disorder which may lead to loss of sight in the affected eye. The most common cause is infection with herpes simplex virus.

Anterior chamber

The **anterior chamber** is the space between the cornea and the iris. It contains **aqueous humour**, a fluid that maintains the metabolism of avascular structures (such as the cornea and lens) and regulates intraocular pressure, keeping the dimensions of the eyeball constant. Aqueous humour is secreted by the ciliary processes into the posterior chamber. It then passes into the anterior chamber through the pupil and drains out through the canal of Schlemm at the iridocorneal angle.

Glaucoma

Glaucoma is a group of diseases in which the pressure within the eye is raised sufficiently to cause damage to the optic nerve (optic neuropathy) and visual impairment. Glaucoma is a common cause of blindness in the UK.

Glaucoma is described in a number of ways:

◆ *Acute* or *chronic*. Acute glaucoma is due to a rapid rise in intraocular pressure, leading to a severely painful red eye and a rapid deterioration in vision. Chronic glaucoma is due to a gradual rise in intraocular pressure, leading to a slow deterioration in vision if untreated.

◆ *Primary* or *secondary*. Secondary glaucoma occurs as a complication of other eye diseases which obstruct the drainage of aqueous humour out of the eyeball. In primary glaucoma, the blockage to drainage of aqueous humour occurs in the absence of another underlying eye disease.

◆ *Open angle* or *closed angle*. This refers to the drainage angle where the iris joins the cornea (Fig. 20.2). If this is normal, it is termed open angle. If it is abnormal, it is termed closed angle.

Primary open angle glaucoma is the most common form of glaucoma. The raised intraocular pressure results from reduced drainage of aqueous humour through the trabecular meshwork for reasons that are not clear. Primary open angle glaucoma is a form of chronic glaucoma, causing a gradual, painless loss of vision beginning with the peripheral visual field. Central vision remains good until the late stages of the disease.

Primary closed angle glaucoma occurs due to reduced drainage of aqueous humour as a result of an ageing lens pushing the iris forward against the trabecular meshwork. Hypermetropes are at particular risk of developing closed angle glaucoma as the shape of their eyes gives them shallow anterior chambers. Primary closed angle glaucoma typically presents acutely, with the sudden onset of a severely painful red eye and blurred vision. The patient feels unwell with nausea and vomiting. Acute closed angle glaucoma is a medical emergency, requiring prompt treatment to lower intraocular pressure and preserve sight.

Secondary open angle glaucoma is caused by eye conditions which lead to clogging of the trabecular meshwork by particulate matter, e.g. proteins seeping out from a lens affected by a cataract, or blood cells following trauma to the eye.

Secondary closed angle glaucoma is caused by eye conditions that result in closure of the iridocorneal angle, such as uveitis or trauma to the eye.

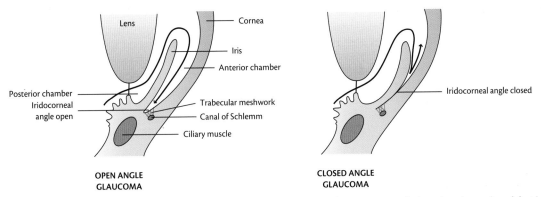

Fig. 20.2 Open angle and closed angle glaucoma. In open angle glaucoma, aqueous humour can reach the trabecular meshwork but is unable to drain through it. In closed angle glaucoma, the iris becomes pushed up against the cornea, preventing aqueous humour from reaching the trabecular meshwork.

Key points: Glaucoma

- Glaucoma occurs when intraocular pressure rises too high, risking damage to the optic nerve and blindness.

- Primary open angle glaucoma is the most common form of glaucoma. It is caused by poor drainage of aqueous humour through the trabecular meshwork for reasons that are unclear. Primary open angle glaucoma usually causes progressive loss of the peripheral visual field. Central vision remains good until the disease is advanced.

- Primary closed angle glaucoma occurs due to an ageing lens pushing the iris against the cornea, blocking flow of aqueous humour to the trabecular meshwork. Primary closed angle glaucoma usually presents acutely with a severely painful red eye and blurred vision.

- Secondary forms of glaucoma are caused by eye conditions which clog the trabecular meshwork or cause closure of the iridocorneal angle.

Lens

The **lens** is a transparent structure composed almost entirely of stiff epithelial cells tightly packed in a highly organized manner. Most of the cytoplasm of the epithelial cells of the lens is occupied by proteins called **crystallins** which are responsible for the refractile properties and transparency of the lens. Alterations in the shape of the lens by the action of the ciliary muscles allows the refractive power of the lens to be varied, enabling adjustment for close or distance vision.

Presbyopia

Presbyopia is a progressive loss of the focusing power of the lens that occurs with age. It is caused by loss of the inherent elasticity of the lens, which is no longer able to assume the near spherical shape required for near vision. People usually start to notice the condition at about age 45, when they find themselves holding reading material further away in order to focus on it.

Cataract

Cataract refers to opacification of the lens, and is one of the most common causes of visual impairment (Fig. 20.3). Most cataracts are age related ('senile cataracts') and arise due to degeneration of the crystallins in the lens. Cataracts may also occur in association with diabetes mellitus, as a side effect of glucocorticoid treatment, and following trauma to the eye.

Decreased visual acuity is the most common presenting symptom in patients with cataract. Many patients also complain of increased glare, which may be noticed in brightly lit rooms or when facing oncoming car headlights when driving at night.

Removal of an opacified lens and replacement by a synthetic lens is one of the most common procedures performed by ophthalmic surgeons.

> ## Key points: Lens
>
> ◆ Presbyopia is a progressive loss of the focusing power of the lens that occurs with ageing.
>
> ◆ Cataract is an opacification of the lens which causes clouding of vision. Most cataracts are age related due to crystallin degeneration. Cataracts are also associated with diabetes mellitus, glucocorticoid treatment, and eye trauma.

Uvea

The **uvea**, or **uveal tract**, comprises the iris, ciliary body, and choroid. The **iris** is a smooth muscle diaphragm with a central aperture (the pupil) that controls the amount of light entering the eye. The **ciliary body** is the source of aqueous humour and also contains the ciliary muscles which control the shape of the lens. The **choroid** is the richly vascular connective tissue on which the retina sits. It contains pigment cells which absorb any light traversing beyond the retina, preventing internal reflection within the vitreous humour.

Uveitis

Uveitis refers to inflammation in the uveal tract and may be divided into anterior uveitis affecting the iris and/or ciliary body, and posterior uveitis involving the choroid.

Anterior uveitis presents with a red, painful eye and photophobia. In severe cases, there may also be blurring of vision due to accumulation of inflammatory cells in the anterior chamber. Anterior uveitis may be seen in association with a number of systemic disorders including ankylosing spondylitis, sarcoidosis, and inflammatory bowel disease. In about half of cases, however, no underlying cause is found.

Posterior uveitis causes blurring of vision and floaters, due to inflammatory cells in the vitreous. Pain and photophobia are unusual. Posterior uveitis is uncommon, but may be seen in sarcoidosis and infections, e.g. toxoplasmosis.

Uveal melanocytic neoplasms

The choroid contains resident melanocytes from which neoplasms may develop. Benign melanocytic nevi may occur in the uvea, as can malignant melanoma. Malignant melanoma is the most common primary malignant neoplasm of the eye. The prognosis of melanoma of the choroid is generally poor.

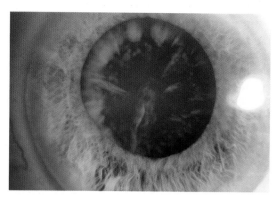

Fig. 20.3 Cataract.

> ## Key points: Uvea
>
> ◆ Anterior uveitis is inflammation in the iris and ciliary body which presents with a red painful eye and photophobia.
>
> ◆ Anterior uveitis is often idiopathic but is associated with a number of underlying disorders such as ankylosing spondylitis, sarcoidosis, and inflammatory bowel disease.
>
> ◆ Posterior uveitis is inflammation in the choroid which presents with blurring of vision and floaters.
>
> ◆ Posterior uveitis is less common than anterior uveitis but may be seen in sarcoidosis and infections such as toxoplasmosis.
>
> ◆ Benign melanocytic nevi can occur in the choroid, as can malignant melanoma.

Retina

The **retina** is the sensory layer of the eye. Near the centre of the retina is an elliptical yellow area, the **macula**, which contains a central depression known as the **fovea** where visual resolution is highest.

The retina consists of a neurosensory layer sitting on the retinal pigment epithelium (Fig. 20.4). The neurosensory layer contains the specialized photoreceptors, the rods and cones, and the neurones with which they synapse. The retinal pigment epithelium provides metabolic support to the neurosensory layer and acts as an antireflective layer.

Retinal detachment

Retinal detachment refers to separation of the layers of the retina

Retinal detachment occurs when the neurosensory layer of the retina separates from the underlying retinal pigment epithelium. Left untreated, the detached part of the retina degenerates due to loss of metabolic support, with devastating damage to vision.

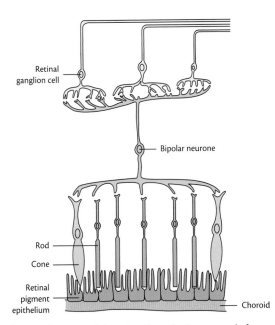

Retinal ganglion cell

Bipolar neurone

Rod

Cone

Retinal pigment epithelium

Choroid

Fig. 20.4 Structure of the retina. The retina is composed of a neurosensory layer comprising rods, cones, and neurones, which sits on the retinal pigment epithelium.

Retinal detachment is therefore considered an ocular emergency that requires immediate medical attention.

There are three types of retinal detachment

- *Break within the retina.* The most common type of retinal detachment occurs when there is a break within the neural layer of the retina, allowing vitreous fluid to seep underneath and separate the retinal layers. Those who are very short sighted, have undergone eye surgery, or have experienced a serious eye injury are at greater risk for this type of detachment. High myopes are more susceptible because their eyes are longer than average from front to back, causing the retina to be thinner and more fragile.

- *Traction of the surface of the retina.* The second most common type occurs when strands of vitreous or scar tissue create traction on the retina, pulling it loose. Patients with diabetes are more likely to experience this type.

- *Exudation of fluid beneath the retina.* The third type happens when fluid collects underneath the layers of the retina, causing it to separate from the back wall of the eye. This type usually occurs in conjunction with another disease affecting the eye that causes swelling or bleeding.

Initial symptoms commonly include the sensation of a flashing light accompanied by a shower of floaters. Over time, the patient may report a shadow in the peripheral visual field, which, if ignored, may spread rapidly to involve the entire visual field in a matter of days.

Age-related macular degeneration

Age-related macular degeneration is the most common cause of blindness in the UK

Age-related macular degeneration (ARMD) is a disease in which there is selective loss of central vision, leaving only peripheral vision intact. ARMD may be divided into dry (atrophic) and wet (exudative) ARMD.

Dry ARMD is characterized by extracellular deposits called **drusen** in the basement membrane of the retinal pigment epithelium associated with atrophy of the retinal pigment epithelium. Drusen are thought to be derived from shed fragments of retinal pigment epithelial cells that have become filled with ingested photoreceptor segments.

Wet ARMD is associated with growth of new vessels from the capillaries of the choroid into the retinal pigment epithelium for reasons that are not well understood. Organization of blood leaking from the new vessels leads to macular scars and loss of vision.

In the early stages of ARMD, central vision may be blurred or distorted. Objects may take an unusual size or shape. This process can happen quickly or develop over several months. People with the condition may become very sensitive to light or actually see lights that are not there.

Central retinal vessel occlusion

Occlusion of the central retinal vessels leads to sudden painless loss of vision

The retina is supplied with blood from the central retinal artery which is a branch of the ophthalmic artery. Blood drains from the retina into the central retinal vein which drains into the cavernous sinus. The central retinal vessels lie side by side within the centre of the optic nerve.

Central retinal artery occlusion is usually due to thrombosis overlying a complicated atherosclerotic plaque within the retinal artery, though embolism from the carotid arteries is also a recognized cause. Retinal arterial occlusion causes infarction of most of the retina, resulting in sudden painless loss of vision.

Central retinal vein occlusion is due to thrombosis causing obstruction to the outflow of blood from the retina. The retinal veins dilate, leading to retinal haemorrhage and oedema, causing a sudden painless loss of vision. The pathogenesis of central retinal vein occlusion is not clear, although patients with hypercoaguable states are at increased risk, and anything compressing on the retinal vein increases the chance of thrombosis, e.g. glaucomatous swelling of the optic nerve or atherosclerotic disease stiffening the neighbouring central retinal artery.

Hypertensive retinopathy

The arterioles of the retina are affected by hypertension much like arterioles elsewhere in the body. Long-standing hypertension thickens the arterioles, and these may be seen as irregular, tortuous vessels on fundoscopy. Severe hypertension (usually a diastolic pressure 120 mmHg or higher) may damage retinal vessels, leading to leakage or closure of the vessels. Leakage of blood from fine capillary branches causes flame haemorrhages. Closure of capillaries supplying the retina leads to small infarcts in the retina known as cotton wool spots. Swelling of the optic nerve head (papilloedema) in severe hypertension implies hypertensive damage to the capillaries supplying the optic disc, or cerebral oedema due to hypertensive encephalopathy.

Diabetic retinopathy

The retina is a common site for microvascular disease in diabetes mellitus. Diabetes leads to thickening of the basement membrane of retinal capillaries due to binding of plasma proteins (such as albumin) to glycated basement membrane proteins. Although the basement membrane is thickened, the capillaries become weaker and leakier.

The earliest changes that can be seen are the formation of capillary microaneurysms and areas of leakage of blood and lipid-rich fluids into the retina. These features constitute the clinical term **background retinopathy**, which is not sight threatening.

If progressive disease leads to occlusion of thickened retinal capillaries, then retinal ischaemia results. Oedema from small infarcts can be seen as cotton wool spots on fundoscopy (the same as may be seen in hypertensive retinopathy). These changes are termed **pre-proliferative retinopathy** and are an indication for routine ophthalmological referral.

Ongoing retinal ischaemia leads to the release of a vasoproliferative substance which stimulates the growth of new vessels in the retina. The presence of new vessels is known as **proliferative retinopathy** and is an indication for urgent referral to an ophthalmologist as it is potentially sight threatening. The new vessels are prone to bleeding because they branch repeatedly and are very fragile as they lack the supportive tissue of normal vessels. Small bleeds incite a fibrotic reaction which can lead to retinal detachment, while larger bleeds cause haemorrhage into the vitreous, both of which are sight threatening,

Key points: Retina

- Retinal detachment refers to separation of the neurosensory layer from the underlying retinal pigment epithelium. Loss of metabolic support leads to rapid death of the detached portion of the retina if prompt treatment is not instituted.

Key points: Retina—cont'd

- Age-related macular degeneration is a common cause of blindness in the UK. Selective loss of central vision occurs due to macular disease. Dry ARMD is caused by drusen deposits in the macula. Wet ARMD is caused by organization of haemorrhage into the macula from new blood vessels.

- Occlusion of the central retinal vessels causes sudden painful loss of vision.

- Hypertensive retinopathy refers to changes in retinal blood vessels as a result of hypertension. Changes in the retinal vessels at fundoscopy are useful in assessing the severity of hypertension.

- Diabetic retinopathy is the result of thickening of the basement membrane of retinal capillaries. The changes are divided into background retinopathy, pre-proliferative retinopathy, and proliferative retinopathy. Proliferative retinopathy is potentially sight threatening.

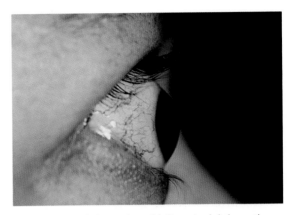

Fig. 20.5 Proptosis in a patient with Graves' ophthalmopathy.

Orbit

The **orbit** is the bony cavity which houses the eyeball, as well as the extraocular muscles controlling eye movement, and parts of the optic, oculomotor, trochlear, and abducent nerves, the ophthalmic and maxillary divisions of the trigeminal nerve, and the ophthalmic vessels.

Because the orbit is enclosed on all sides except anteriorly, diseases of the orbit often present with forward displacement of the eyeball known as **proptosis** or **exophthalmos** (Fig. 20.5). Exposure of the cornea is dangerous as the tear film cannot be distributed evenly and the eyelids can no longer completely shield the cornea, leading to pain and risk of keratitis.

Graves' ophthalmopathy

Graves' ophthalmopathy is an orbital disease seen in patients with Graves' disease. Graves' disease is due to circulating thyroid-stimulating hormone (TSH) receptor-stimulating antibodies which bind to thyroid follicular epithelial cells and cause hyperthyroidism. As well as causing thyrotoxicosis, Graves' disease also leads to orbital disease because the TSH receptor-stimulating antibodies also bind to antigens on cells within the orbit and trigger inflammation and swelling. The precise antigen in the orbit which binds the TSH receptor-stimulating antibody remains unidentified.

The most common symptoms of Graves' ophthalmopathy are soreness and watering of the eyes. The patient themselves, or others around them, may notice a staring appearance due to proptosis. A minority of patients have more severe disease associated with limitation of eye movement and pain. In its most severe form, Graves' ophthalmopathy leads to compression of the optic nerve and visual impairment. Fortunately this only occurs in about 5 per cent of patients with Graves' disease.

LINK BOX

Thyrotoxicosis and eye signs

Note that thyrotoxicosis of any cause may produce lid retraction and lid lag due to overactivity of the sympathetic nervous system, but only Graves' disease causes orbital disease and thus proptosis (p. 314).

Orbital neoplasms

Neoplasms arising in the orbit may also be a cause of proptosis. The most common benign neoplasms of the orbit are vascular neoplasms such as haemangiomas. The most common malignant tumour of the orbit is a low grade lymphoma. Malignant tumours from elsewhere in the body may also metastasize to the orbit.

> ## Key points: Orbit
>
> - Orbital disease typically presents with protrusion of the orbit, a clinical sign known as proptosis or exophthalmos.
>
> - The most common orbital disease is Graves' ophthalmopathy. This is seen in patients with Graves' disease because the TSH receptor-stimulating antibody binds to retro-orbital tissues and causes swelling behind the eye.
>
> - Neoplasms may also arise within the orbit. The most common primary orbital neoplasms are haemangiomas and low grade lymphomas.

Multisystem disease

Introduction

There are a group of diseases whose effects cannot easily be assigned to any one particular organ system. Many of these so-called 'multisystem' diseases are immunologically mediated and often produce prolonged non-specific symptoms such as fatigue, weight loss, and fever, together with symptoms related to a variety of different organ systems. Multisystem diseases may therefore present to a number of specialties including rheumatology, dermatology, nephrology, and haematology.

Systemic lupus erythematosus

Systemic lupus erythematosus (SLE) is the classic example of a multisystem disease, in which there is inflammatory damage to multiple organ systems. The incidence of SLE in the UK is about 4 per 100 000 people each year and, like most autoimmune conditions, most cases occur in women of childbearing age.

SLE has an episodic course, characterized by flares and remissions. It is highly variable in severity between individual patients, ranging from a mild condition to a life-threatening disease. Tissues frequently involved in SLE include the skin, joints, kidneys, blood, and brain.

A critical defect in SLE appears to be impaired clearance of apoptotic cells

The precise pathogenesis of SLE is not known; however, one interesting observation is that clearance of apoptotic bodies appears to be impaired in patients with SLE. Normally, apoptotic bodies are rapidly ingested by adjacent cells to prevent an immune response to cellular material. If this mechanism is slow, normal cellular material could be taken up by antigen-presenting cells, initiating an immune response to self-antigens with formation of autoantibodies (Fig. 21.1).

Patients with SLE have a host of autoantibodies

One of the cardinal features of SLE is the presence of a number of autoantibodies directed against a range of nuclear and cytoplasmic antigens. Virtually all patients with SLE have antinuclear antibodies (ANAs) against nuclear constituents. In particular, the presence of antibodies to double-stranded DNA (dsDNA) and antibodies to the so-called Smith antigen is virtually diagnostic of SLE.

Patients with SLE also often have antibodies directed against red blood cells and platelets, leading to autoimmune haemolytic anaemia and autoimmune thrombocytopenia.

Antibodies to proteins complexed to phospholipids are also well recognized. Because these antiphospholipid antibodies interfere with laboratory clotting tests, giving rise to a spuriously prolonged prothrombin time, they are sometimes referred to as **lupus anticoagulant**. Rather confusingly, despite *in vitro* prolongation of clotting, these patients actually have a *hyper*coagulable state, being at risk from arterial and venous thromboses.

LINK BOX

Antiphospholipid syndrome

Patients with antiphospholipid antibodies and disease related to them (such as thromboses and recurrent miscarriages) but without associated SLE are said to have the antiphospholipid syndrome (p. 354).

Deposition of immune complexes underlies several of the clinical features of SLE

The most frequent mechanism by which autoantibodies cause disease in SLE is through the generation of large

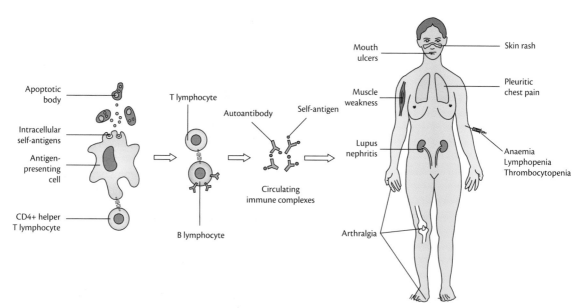

Fig. 21.1 Postulated pathogenesis of systemic lupus erythematosus. Defective phagocytosis of apoptotic bodies leads to priming of the immune system to intracellular antigens and activation of autoreactive B and T lymphocytes. Circulating immune complexes formed between autoantibodies and self-antigens then become deposited in various tissues around the body (skin, joints, kidneys), stimulating inflammation and tissue damage.

numbers of immune complexes which circulate in the blood and become deposited in certain tissues where they cause inflammation and damage. This mechanism is particularly important in the kidneys, joints, and skin.

Autoantibodies may also bind directly to a target molecule and activate inflammation. This mechanism is important in the haematological abnormalities seen in SLE.

The clinical presentation of SLE is extremely variable

True to its nature as a multisystem disease, patients with SLE can present in numerous different ways. Often the disease presents in a subtle and confusing fashion, with apparently non-specific features that makes the diagnosis difficult to reach.

At presentation, SLE may be clearly multisystemic or may involve just one organ system, with other manifestations appearing at a later date. In some patients, the clinical diagnosis is preceded for months or years by insidious symptoms. In others, the presentation is dramatic, with severe, life-threatening manifestations such as renal failure. Features seen in SLE include the following:

- *Constitutional symptoms.* Fatigue is a particularly troublesome symptom and is difficult to treat. Weight loss and a persistent low grade fever are also common.

- *Joints.* Arthralgia is the most common symptom in SLE, reported by almost all patients with SLE. The joints are painful, but appear outwardly normal (an important distinction from the swollen joints seen in rheumatoid arthritis).

- *Mouth.* Mouth ulcers are common. They are usually painless and therefore not troublesome to the patient, but nonetheless are common enough to be a useful diagnostic feature and should always be enquired about.

- *Skin.* Cutaneous lesions are common in SLE, particularly on sun-exposed areas. The lesions are extremely variable and may mimic many other skin disorders. The most characteristic manifestation is the well described 'butterfly rash' which is a scaly, erythematous rash located on the bridge of the nose and on the cheeks.

- *Lungs.* The most common pulmonary feature of SLE is inflammation of the pleura, which may cause pleuritic chest pain or breathlessness due to a pleural effusion. A pneumonitis is less common, but important as parenchymal lung disease can lead to irreversible pulmonary fibrosis.

- *Kidneys.* The kidneys are often affected in SLE because the circulating immune complexes become stuck in the glomeruli causing glomerular damage (**lupus nephritis**). The precise nature of the response varies between individuals, but may involve a proliferative response leading to haematuria and proteinuria, or a mainly structural response with thickening of the glomerular basement membrane leading to predominantly proteinuria. Persistence of glomerular injury and subsequent loss of nephrons is more likely in those patients found to have widespread proliferative changes in their glomeruli on a renal biopsy, and this is an indication for immunosuppressive therapy. Although renal involvement is often not present at diagnosis, many patients will develop it at some point in their lives.

- *Blood.* The most common haematological abnormality in SLE is anaemia, which is usually a mild anaemia of chronic disease. Anaemia may also be due to an autoimmune haemolytic anaemia, and this may pre-date the appearance of other features of SLE. The most consistent finding in the white cell count in SLE is lymphopenia, seen in about half of all SLE patients at some stage. A mild thrombocytopenia is also common in SLE and may be the presenting feature. More severe thrombocytopenia leading to petechiae may produce a picture virtually indistinguishable from idiopathic thrombocytopenic purpura. *SLE should always be carefully excluded before diagnosing ITP* (p. 348). Serum complement levels are reduced during active disease due to consumption of complement components in areas of inflammation.

Because the clinical features are so variable, the American College of Rheumatology (ACR) has published a list of criteria that can be applied to SLE to distinguish it from other closely related conditions. The most recent classification takes into account 11 criteria, with a diagnosis of SLE made if four or more are present at any point in time (Table 21.1).

Treatment of SLE depends on the activity of the disease

The treatment of SLE must be tailored to the individual patient according to the activity of the disease. The three most reliable tests of disease activity are the

TABLE 21.1 American College of Rheumatology criteria for the diagnosis of SLE

1.	Malar rash
2.	Discoid rash
3.	Photosensitivity
4.	Oral ulcers
5.	Arthritis
6.	Serositis
7.	Renal disorder
8.	Neurological disorder
9.	Haematological disorder
10.	Immunological disorder
11.	Antinuclear antibody in raised titre

- Common presenting features of SLE include joint pain, skin rash, and a haematological abnormality such as anaemia, thrombocytopenia, or lymphopenia.

- Diagnosis is made using the ACR criteria together with the presence of ANAs, particularly anti-dsDNA and anti-Sm.

- Although renal involvement is unusual at presentation, most patients will develop lupus nephritis which can lead to chronic renal failure.

- Treatment with steroids and immunosuppressants has improved life expectancy, but SLE remains a serious and potentially fatal disorder.

erythrocyte sedimentation rate (ESR), degree of complement depletion, and high anti-dsDNA antibody levels.

Patients with mild disease confined to arthralgia, tiredness, and a mild rash, with a low ESR and low titres of anti-dsDNA antibodies, can be treated symptomatically with analgesics as needed. If these symptoms are more severe, then the antimalarial drug hydroxychloroquine may be useful.

Patients with severe flares of arthritis, pleuritis, pericarditis, or autoimmune haemolytic anaemia require oral steroids such as prednisolone until symptoms improve, followed by a slow reduction in the dosage. Renal flares of SLE require the most aggressive immunosuppressive

treatment, generally with both steroids and cyclophosphamide, to prevent irreversible renal damage.

Systemic sclerosis

Systemic sclerosis is a chronic disease in which fibrous tissue accumulates in multiple organs. The skin is most commonly affected, but other organs such as the gastrointestinal tract and lungs are also frequently involved.

The aetiology and pathogenesis of systemic sclerosis are not fully understood. The likely sequence of events is an abnormal immune response to some trigger which results in the production of cytokines and growth factors that act on fibroblasts and stimulate collagen production.

The disease has been classified into two categories: limited systemic sclerosis and diffuse systemic sclerosis (Table 21.2).

Limited systemic sclerosis runs a benign course

Limited systemic sclerosis is the more common form of systemic sclerosis. Patients are usually young women with long-standing Raynaud's phenomenon who gradually notice the development of worsening tightening and thickening of the skin of the fingers, face, and neck. Calcium deposition is common, particularly in the finger pads. Evidence of structural blood vessel damage can be seen as telangiectasia on the fingers and face.

Key points: Systemic lupus erythematosus

- SLE is an autoimmune disorder involving many different organs.

- Disordered apoptosis leading to an immune response to cellular material appears to be pivotal in the pathogenesis of SLE.

- Deposition of immune complexes in the kidneys, joints, and skin appears to be important in causing disease at these sites in SLE. Autoantibodies may also form against red blood cells and platelets.

TABLE 21.2 Features of limited and diffuse systemic sclerosis

Limited systemic sclerosis
Raynaud's phenomenon for years
Skin involvement limited to face, hands, and feet
Late incidence of pulmonary hypertension, skin calcification, telangiectasia
Anticentromere antibodies in 80 per cent
Diffuse systemic sclerosis
Raynaud's phenomenon for <1 year
Skin involvement truncal and acral
Early incidence of lung disease, acute renal failure, gastrointestinal disease
Antitopoisomerase-1 (Scl-70) antibodies in 30 per cent

Often the patient is otherwise well and remains healthy for many years. The two major complications that may arise after 10–15 years are small bowel involvement and pulmonary hypertension. Small bowel involvement leads to malabsorption with anaemia, weight loss, and bulky stools.

Isolated pulmonary hypertension, occurring without other lung disease, is characteristic of limited systemic sclerosis. It is due to obliterative lesions in small pulmonary vessels which resemble those seen in primary pulmonary hypertension. The prognosis is extremely poor due to the rapid development of severe right heart failure.

JARGON BUSTER

Raynaud's phenomenon

Raynaud's phenomenon refers to episodic pallor of the digits of the hands or feet. There is a typical sequence in change of colour from white, through blue, to red. Most cases of Raynaud's phenomenon are primary, due to exaggerated vasomotor responses. There is no structural abnormality in the arterial wall.

In contrast, secondary Raynaud's phenomenon occurs due to arterial insufficiency caused by conditions such as systemic sclerosis or SLE. Raynaud's phenomenon is often the first manifestation of such diseases; all patients with Raynaud's phenomenon should be investigated to rule out a secondary cause, especially when the age of onset is over 30 years.

JARGON BUSTER

CREST syndrome

The CREST syndrome is an old term which refers to a constellation of features seen in advanced limited systemic sclerosis, namely calcinosis, Raynaud's phenomenon, oesophageal dysmotility, scleroderma, and telangiectasia.

Diffuse systemic sclerosis runs a more aggressive course

Diffuse systemic sclerosis presents much more abruptly. There is widespread thickening of the skin which becomes bound to underlying structures leading to impaired mobility in tendons and joints. Contractures and stretching of the skin over bony points often lead to painful ulcers which are slow to heal.

In diffuse systemic sclerosis, visceral involvement occurs early in the course of the disease. Lung involvement occurs in most patients, particularly those with the anti-topoisomerase I (Scl-70) autoantibody, leading to pulmonary fibrosis. Systemic sclerosis should always be considered in the differential diagnosis of a patient with lung fibrosis.

Key points: Systemic sclerosis

- Systemic sclerosis is an autoimmune disease characterized by fibrosis in multiple organs.

- There are two main forms: limited systemic sclerosis and diffuse systemic sclerosis.

- Limited systemic sclerosis begins with Raynaud's phenomenon, followed by the gradual onset of skin tightening and telangiectasia. After a period of 10–15 years, malabsorption and pulmonary hypertension occur.

- Diffuse systemic sclerosis causes the abrupt development of widespread skin thickening, lung fibrosis, and severe hypertension. Acute renal failure due to severe hypertension is the most life-threatening complication of systemic sclerosis.

An important complication of diffuse systemic sclerosis is the development of severe hypertension due to obliterative changes in blood vessels. About 20 per cent of patients with diffuse disease develop severe hypertension with hypertensive encephalopathy and a rapid deterioration in renal function ('scleroderma renal crisis').

Sarcoidosis

Sarcoidosis is a curious disease in which many tissues and organs become filled with non-caseating granulomas. The typical sarcoid granuloma is a well circumscribed collection of epithelioid macrophages with only a few surrounding lymphocytes. Caseous necrosis is not seen in the core of the granulomas, one important distinction for excluding the possibility of tuberculosis.

The cause of sarcoidosis remains an utter mystery. The current theory is that sarcoidosis is an inflammatory response to some unidentified environmental agent in a susceptible host. An infective cause has long been sought, in particular a mycobacterium due to the granulomatous response. However, no study has unequivocally proven an infectious aetiology for sarcoidosis.

Sarcoidosis can involve virtually any organ of the body, but some are involved more than others:

* *Lymph nodes.* Virtually all cases of sarcoidosis involve lymph nodes. Any lymph node may be involved, but the most common are the hilar and mediastinal lymph nodes. Enlargement of these nodes are usually picked up on a chest radiograph.

* *Lungs.* The lungs are frequently involved by sarcoidosis, with the non-caseating granulomas typically surrounding lymphatics in the interstitial compartment. Healing of the granulomas may lead to varying degrees of lung fibrosis. Severe sarcoidal lung disease may lead to right heart failure and respiratory failure.

* *Skin.* Skin lesions due to non-caseating granulomas often manifest with an asymptomatic maculopapular rash seen on the face and the trunk. One characteristic pattern is the appearance of purple shiny rubbery plaques on the nose, known as **lupus pernio**. Erythema nodosum may also be associated with sarcoidosis. *This is not due to non-caseating granulomas but appears to be a response to immune complexes trapped in the subcutaneous fat.*

* *Eyes.* Sarcoidosis involving the eye typically causes **uveitis**, meaning inflammation in the uveal tract. Anterior uveitis, which causes a red, painful eye with photophobia, is often self-limiting. Posterior uveitis, which causes floaters due to inflammatory cells appearing in the vitreous with some blurring of vision, is a more chronic form of the disease.

* *Lacrimal and salivary glands.* Involvement of the lacrimal and salivary glands may lead to dry eyes and dry mouth. Sarcoidosis is an important differential diagnosis of Sjögren's syndrome.

* *Nervous system.* Sarcoidosis can affect both the central and peripheral nervous systems. A seventh cranial nerve palsy is a common complaint in sarcoidosis. Hypothalamic involvement is also common, resulting in diabetes insipidus due to destruction of antidiuretic hormone-producing neurones.

Simple haematological and biochemical parameters can support a diagnosis of sarcoidosis

Simple haematological and biochemical blood tests can be helpful in supporting a suspected diagnosis of sarcoidosis, though they are not specific. The ESR is often raised, and hypercalcaemia is seen in about 10 per cent of cases due to conversion of vitamin D into active 1,25-dihydroxycholecalciferol within the granulomas. Serum levels of angiotensin-converting enzyme (ACE) are raised in most patients with active sarcoidosis.

In typical cases of sarcoidosis, the clinical picture and other simple investigations can be sufficient to make an accurate diagnosis of sarcoidosis. In less clear-cut cases, biopsy of an affected organ may be necessary to demonstrate the presence of non-caseating granulomas and exclude other differential diagnoses.

Sarcoidosis may be divided into an acute form and a chronic form

One useful way of considering sarcoidosis is by dividing it into acute and chronic forms. Most patients have the acute form, associated with manifestations that include erythema nodosum, bilateral hilar lymphadenopathy, anterior uveitis, and a seventh cranial nerve palsy. These patients do well, with spontaneous resolution within 1–2 years from diagnosis.

About 5 per cent of patients with sarcoidosis develop the chronic form of the disease, which is associated with lupus pernio, pulmonary fibrosis, and posterior uveitis. These patients are at higher risk of developing organ failures as a result of the disease. End-stage lung fibrosis is the most common problem for patients with severe chronic sarcoidosis, leading to respiratory failure and right heart failure.

Key points: Sarcoidosis

- Sarcoidosis is a multisystem disease of unknown aetiology characterized by the presence of non-caseating granulomas in tissues.

- The common organs to be affected are the hilar lymph nodes, lungs, skin, eyes, lacrimal and salivary glands, and nervous system.

- Supportive biochemical evidence of sarcoidosis include a raised ESR, hypercalcaemia, and a raised serum ACE. Definitive diagnosis requires histological demonstration of non-caseating granulomas on a biopsy, though often this is not required if the clinical picture is distinctive.

- Most patients with sarcoidosis have an acute form of the disease which typically resolves within 2 years from diagnosis with no long-lasting consequences.

- A minority of patients with sarcoidosis have a chronic form of the disease which tends to persist and lead to permanent organ damage. End-stage lung fibrosis is the most serious consequence, leading to respiratory failure and right heart failure.

Amyloidosis

Amyloidosis describes a *group* of conditions (not a single disorder) in which there is excess deposition of **amyloid** in tissues. Amyloid is a term for any protein which has assembled abnormally into β-pleated sheets, a feature which renders the protein exceptionally insoluble. The body cannot easily break down these proteins, so they slowly build up in extracellular spaces, leading to cell strangulation and death.

TABLE 21.3   Examples of amyloid proteins

Amyloid protein	Precursor protein
Amyloid AA	Serum amyloid A
Amyloid Aβ	Amyloid precursor protein
Amyloid AL	Immunoglobulin light chain
Amyloid ATTR	Transthyretin

Interestingly the body does not seem to react to amyloid; there is no inflammatory response to it. Amyloid proteins are designated 'A' followed by an abbreviation to designate the protein of origin (Table 21.3).

Amyloid may be deposited locally within a single organ

Localized amyloid deposits may be found in a number of clinical disorders. For instance, amyloid deposits are found in the brain of patients with cerebral amyloid angiopathy and Alzheimer's disease, in the islets of the pancreas in patients with type 2 diabetes mellitus, and in the thyroid in patients with medullary carcinoma of the thyroid.

Amyloid may also be deposited in multiple organs

When amyloid deposits affect multiple organs, the condition is known as generalized, or systemic, amyloidosis. This form of amyloidosis is much more significant than the localized form as it leads to gradual failure of multiple organs. Because of the variable manifestations of the disease, most patients with systemic amyloidosis often go undiagnosed until they are gravely ill due to the effects of failure of many organs. Although systemic amyloidosis may affect any organ, the most important and common are the kidneys, heart, and gastrointestinal tract.

Renal amyloidosis is the most common and serious site of amyloidosis. Amyloid becomes stuck in the glomeruli, disrupting the filtration system and causing the glomeruli to become abnormally leaky to protein. Amyloidosis should be considered in the differential diagnosis in any patient presenting with heavy proteinuria or the nephrotic syndrome.

Cardiac amyloidosis leads to stiffening of the chambers of the heart, preventing adequate filling of the chambers during the cardiac cycle. Amyloidosis is an

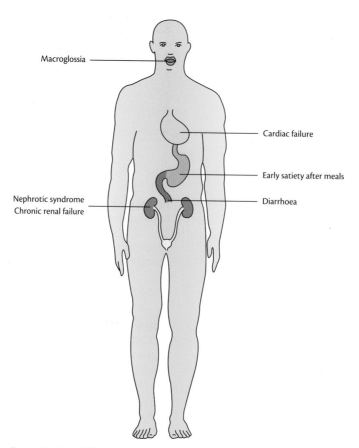

Fig. 21.2 Clinical features of generalized amyloidosis.

important cause of chronic heart failure in patients with no other clear cause to explain it. Rhythm disturbances may also occur if amyloid deposition affects the conducting system of the heart.

Gastrointestinal tract amyloidosis may lead to diarrhoea due to small bowel disease or a feeling of early satiety after a meal due to poor motility of the stomach. Enlargement of the tongue (macroglossia) is also a well recognized feature and can be massive, interfering with eating and drinking.

The two most common types of systemic amyloidosis are **AA amyloidosis** and **AL amyloidosis**.

AA amyloidosis is a complication of chronic inflammatory conditions

The AA protein is a fragment of the circulating acute phase protein **serum amyloid A**. Serum amyloid A is made in hepatocytes in response to cytokines released by activated inflammatory cells. Its function is not yet known.

AA amyloidosis occurs in conditions associated with long-term persistent inflammatory activity. AA amyloidosis is relatively rare in developed countries. Most cases are due to a chronic inflammatory rheumatological condition such as rheumatoid arthritis, ankylosing spondylitis, or juvenile chronic arthritis. Note that amyloidosis is rare in SLE and systemic sclerosis because the inflammatory activity does not induce production of serum amyloid A.

Chronic infections such as tuberculosis, leprosy, and osteomyelitis are common causes of AA amyloidosis in the developing world.

AL amyloidosis is a plasma cell disorder with a poor prognosis

AL amyloidosis is a rare and aggressive disease which affects only about 600 people in the UK each year. AL amyloidosis is a plasma cell disorder in which the amyloid is derived from large amounts of free immunoglobulin light chain secreted from an abnormal clone of plasma cells in the bone marrow. In most cases, the plasma cell disorder is subtle and does not in itself give rise to any problems, i.e. *these patients do not have myeloma, but rather a low grade version of it.*

The prognosis of AL amyloidosis is poor, with relentless amyloid deposition leading to cardiac and renal failure within 1 year.

Diagnosis of amyloidosis requires histological demonstration of the amyloid deposits

The diagnosis of amyloidosis is histological, i.e. proof of amyloid deposition in biopsy material. The biopsy may be directed at an organ giving rise to disease manifestations, e.g. a renal biopsy in someone with proteinuria, or directed at a site likely to show amyloid even if there are no symptoms related to it but is easy to access e.g. a rectal biopsy (positive in 80 per cent of amyloid patients) or a subcutaneous fat aspirate (positive in 60 per cent of amyloid patients).

Key points: Amyloidosis

- Amyloidosis describes a group of conditions in which amyloid is deposited in tissues.

- Amyloid is a term for an abnormally folded protein which is poorly broken down by the body.

- Extracellular accumulation of amyloid protein leads to cell death.

- Amyloid proteins are named according to the protein they are derived from.

- The two most common examples of generalized amyloidosis are AA and AL amyloidosis.

- AA amyloidosis is caused by deposition of serum amyloid A protein in the setting of chronic inflammation. In developed countries, the most common causes of AA amyloidosis are chronic inflammatory rheumatological conditions such as rheumatoid arthritis.

- AL amyloidosis is caused by deposition of light chain immunoglobulin molecules produced in large quantities by an abnormal clone of plasma cells. AL amyloid has a poor prognosis, with death from cardiac and renal failure occurring within 1 year.

Vasculitis

Vasculitis is a pathological process defined by *inflammation and damage to blood vessels*. Inflammatory cell infiltration of the blood vessel causes swelling, necrosis, and disruption of the vessel wall. Subsequent remodelling of the damaged tissue causes fibrosis and thickening of the vessel wall. The inflammatory changes and their sequelae can lead to a number of problems including tissue ischaemia, bleeding, and aneurysmal dilation. Blood vessels of any size may be affected.

Vasculitis may be primary or secondary

It is important to realize that vasculitis may be a primary disease process or, alternatively, a secondary manifestation of another underlying disease. The blood vessel damage in the secondary forms of vasculitis is due to *deposition of circulating immune complexes in blood vessel walls* which activate complement and stimulate acute inflammation. Secondary vasculitis may therefore be seen in a number of disorders associated with immune complex formation, including infections, drug reactions, and multisystem autoimmune diseases such as rheumatoid arthritis and SLE.

The blood vessel damage in primary forms of vasculitis is quite different. Immune complexes are rarely demonstrable in the vessel wall in primary vasculitis, and so do not appear to be important. Instead, the pathogenesis of primary vasculitis appears to be *direct autoimmune attack against endothelial cells lining the blood vessel.*

Primary vasculitis is best classified according to the size of the vessels involved

There have been many different attempts to classify the various types of primary vasculitis. The most useful one is based on the size of the blood vessels that are inflamed, i.e. large, medium, or small (Table 21.4). The autoimmune mechanisms leading to each type of vasculitis appear to be different.

In a large or medium sized vessel vasculitis, T lymphocytes appear to be the main mediators of damage; autoantibodies are not consistently found. Autoantibodies may, however, be relevant in small vessel vasculitis as most patients have antibodies against neutrophil cytoplasmic antigens (**ANCA**), the levels of which correlate well with disease activity.

Giant cell arteritis

Giant cell arteritis is the most common cause of large vessel vasculitis

Giant cell arteritis typically causes vasculitis of the branches of the external carotid artery and ophthalmic arteries. Giant cell arteritis is most common in older people, being rare before 50 years of age. Patients present with severe throbbing headache and jaw claudication (ischaemic pain in the muscles of mastication after prolonged chewing) due to involvement of the superficial temporal artery. Examination reveals scalp tenderness, and the temporal artery may feel nodular with reduced pulsation.

Involvement of the ophthalmic artery can lead to ocular symptoms including diplopia and transient or complete loss of vision. The latter is the most dreaded complication of giant cell arteritis. Giant cell arteritis may also involve the aorta, causing a thoracic aortitis which may be complicated by aneurysm formation, dissection, and rupture.

In almost all patients with giant cell arteritis, a syndrome of systemic inflammation accompanies the vascular manifestations. These non-specific symptoms include malaise, anorexia, weight loss, fever, and night sweats.

A useful clue to the diagnosis is the presence of a markedly raised ESR. Clinching the diagnosis requires microscopic proof of inflammation in a large blood vessel (usually a temporal artery biopsy). Note that, despite the name, giant cells do not have to be part of the inflammatory cell infiltrate to make the diagnosis. Unfortunately, the disease affects the artery in a focal manner, so a negative biopsy does not exclude the diagnosis. Given the potential consequences of delayed or no treatment, it is therefore often necessary to treat some patients with steroids without biopsy confirmation.

Polyarteritis nodosa

Polyarteritis nodosa affects medium sized muscular arteries

Polyarteritis nodosa is a primary vasculitis in which medium sized arteries become inflamed, leading to areas of aneurysm formation and narrowing of the involved vessel. Strict application of the criteria for the diagnosis of polyarteritis nodosa makes it a rare disease, as the co-existence of small vessel disease leads to a diagnosis of microscopic polyarteritis instead.

The clinical manifestations of the disease are related to organ dysfunction as a result of tissue ischaemia. The main organs affected by polyarteritis nodosa are the gastrointestinal tract, nervous system, and muscles. Lesions in the gut often lead to abdominal pain and the passage of altered blood. Nervous system involvement is typically in the form of palsies of multiple peripheral nerves ('mononeuritis multiplex'). Tiredness is often very prominent in polyarteritis nodosa, due to a combination of persistent generalized inflammation and damage to muscles.

A diagnosis of polyarteritis nodosa may be confirmed by a number of tests. Arteriography of renal or

TABLE 21.4 Types of primary vasculitis
Large vessel vasculitis (aorta and its major branches)
Giant cell arteritis
Medium vessel vasculitis (larger muscularized arteries)
Polyarteritis nodosa
Kawasaki disease
Small vessel vasculitis (small arteries, arterioles, capillaries, venules)
Wegener's granulomatosis
Microscopic polyarteritis

mesenteric arteries showing areas of vessel narrowing and irregularity with aneurysm formation is highly suggestive. A muscle biopsy showing a necrotizing vasculitis of medium sized vessels is also helpful. Patients with true polyarteritis nodosa should be ANCA negative.

Small vessel vasculitis

Small vessel vasculitis is defined by the presence of necrotizing vasculitis involving small arteries, arterioles, capillaries, and venules. ANCAs are found in virtually all patients with a small vessel vasculitis and are a very useful diagnostic tool. It is not clear if ANCAs directly cause the vasculitis or are merely a marker for it, but they are useful for helping to diagnose the vasculitis and in monitoring its response to treatment.

Wegener's granulomatosis and microscopic polyarteritis are the most common small vessel vasculitides

Wegener's granulomatosis is characterized by a necrotizing small vessel vasculitis, together with granulomatous inflammation involving the upper respiratory tract. **Microscopic polyarteritis** is characterized by a necrotizing small vessel vasculitis but without granulomatous inflammation elsewhere. The two diseases therefore share many clinical features related to the small vessel vasculitis, though Wegener's granulomatosis may have a number of additional manifestations related to the granulomatous inflammation in the upper respiratory tract (e.g. persistent nasal discharge and ear blockage).

The kidneys and lungs bear the brunt of a small vessel vasculitis

The kidneys and lungs are common targets in small vessel vasculitis as these organs rely particularly on the integrity of the fine capillaries for ultrafiltration and gas exchange, respectively. In the kidneys, the small vessel vasculitis hits the glomeruli hard, typically causing a necrotizing glomerulonephritis which in severe cases may stimulate crescent formation and present with acute renal failure.

In the lungs, the small vessel vasculitis manifests as an alveolar capillaritis with bleeding into the alveolar spaces. Alveolar haemorrhage presents with haemoptysis and breathlessness. Investigations reveal hypoxia and diffuse alveolar shadowing on the chest radiograph.

JARGON BUSTER

Goodpasture's syndrome

Goodpasture's syndrome is the combination of a rapidly progressive glomerulonephritis and alveolar haemorrhage. It is most commonly due to Wegener's granulomatosis, microscopic polyarteritis, or antiglomerular basement membrane disease.

Diagnosis of a small vessel vasculitis is based on the clinical picture, ANCA results, and histology

A diagnosis of small vessel vasculitis is usually based on a combination of the clinical history, the presence of ANCA, and histological proof of a small vessel vasculitis, almost invariably from a renal biopsy showing a necrotizing glomerulonephritis.

Demonstrating granulomatous inflammation in biopsies from the upper respiratory tract is also required for a diagnosis of Wegener's granulomatosis.

Key points: Vasculitis

◆ Vasculitis is a pathological process characterized by inflammation and destruction of blood vessel walls.

◆ Secondary vasculitis may be seen as part of a systemic disease due to immune complex deposition in blood vessel walls.

◆ Primary vasculitis is due to direct autoimmune attack on blood vessels, and is classified according to the size of the blood vessels involved.

◆ Giant cell arteritis is the most common large vessel primary vasculitis. Inflammation affecting the superficial temporal artery leads to headache and jaw claudication. Urgent treatment with steroids is needed to prevent the potential complication of blindness due to involvement of the ophthalmic artery.

Continued

Key points: Vasculitis—cont'd

◆ Polyarteritis nodosa is a primary vasculitis affecting medium sized arteries. Symptoms usually relate to the gastrointestinal tract, nervous system, and muscles. Arteriography showing areas of vessel narrowing and irregularity is highly suggestive of the diagnosis.

◆ Wegener's granulomatosis and microscopic polyarteritis are the most common small vessel vasculitides. The kidneys and lungs bear the brunt of the disease, causing necrotizing glomerulonephritis and alveolar haemorrhage. ANCA positivity is a useful diagnostic feature.

Paediatric disease

Introduction

Paediatrics is a distinct speciality related to the care of children in the age span that begins with the fetus and extends through adolescence (Table 22.1). During this period, there are dynamic changes, not only in the child's growth and development, but also in its immediate environment. So, diseases in children must be understood against the background of these changes.

Although there is an overlap between the diseases of childhood and those of adults, there are several important differences:

- Specific disorders, such as prematurity, are unique to children. At the same time, some diseases, such as breast and lung cancers, which are common in adults, are not reported in children.

- Susceptibility to injury varies considerably between adults and children. For example, the rapidly growing and maturing central nervous system (CNS) is particularly susceptible to injury during the first 2 years of life.

- Diagnosis of diseases in childhood requires knowledge of each stage of development, with regard to the anatomical, biochemical, physiological, intellectual, and psychological functions. Appropriate reference

TABLE 22.1 Periods of early childhood

Fetus	10 weeks–birth
Neonate	Birth–1 month
Infant	Birth–1 year

values, for example growth charts, are available for each stage of development.

- Treatment in relation to drugs, such as dose and toxicity, is also considered in comparison with various stages of growth and development. For instance, treatment with chemotherapy or radiotherapy increases the risk of developing a second malignancy many years later; this problem is of little consequence to an elderly person, but is of great concern to a child.

- The outlook for recovery from the same disease varies between children and adults. Bone fractures heal with complete structural restoration in a child as the bone remodels and reshapes with general growth. In an adult, a similar fracture may result in permanent deformity.

Because of the special knowledge, skills, and experience required to care for children, there is subspecialization within paediatrics, such that there are dedicated paediatric surgeons, gastroenterologists, cardiologists, nephrologists, radiologists, and pathologists. Together, they form multidisciplinary teams to share their expertise in caring for children. Often children present with diseases that pose a challenge even to the most experienced specialist. It makes the job all the more interesting!

Fetus

The fetus enjoys a well protected environment within the uterus, with a dedicated blood supply from the placenta. The main problems faced by the developing fetus are infections crossing the placenta or an inadequate placental blood supply.

Intrauterine infection

The main route of infection of a fetus is transplacental spread, by which infection passes from the maternal circulation to the fetal circulation across the placenta. The mother may not necessarily be symptomatic or show signs of infection. Note that infection in the mother is not inevitably followed by infection of the fetus. Transplacental spread of infection is characteristic of the so-called 'TORCH' group of pathogens: *Toxoplasma*, Others (parvovirus B19, *Listeria*), Rubella, Cytomegalovirus, and Herpes simplex virus.

Congenital infections cause fetal injury by various mechanisms

Microorganisms cause fetal damage by their ability to inhibit cell division and migration, to stimulate (or suppress) a host immune response, and to cause ischaemic necrosis of cells and tissues. Many of the TORCH group of organisms also act as teratogens (agents that cause congenital defects).

Intrauterine infection can manifest in a variety of ways at different periods of gestation

Depending on the organism and the severity and timing of the infection, intrauterine infection may result in a wide spectrum of effects. The fetus may not survive infection, leading to intrauterine death. If the fetus does survive, it may be born prematurely, show intrauterine growth restriction, or have congenital anomalies.

Cytomegalovirus and rubella virus infection are the most well characterized congenital infections

Cytomegalovirus (CMV) is the most common congenital infection, with an incidence of 1 per cent of all births. Early gestational infections are the most devastating. Severely affected infants have intrauterine growth restriction, microcephaly (an abnormally small head), hydrocephalus, and hepatitis. The majority of infected newborns, however, are asymptomatic at birth, but are at risk of deafness due to damage to the inner ear.

Rubella virus can reach the fetus in emboli of necrotic placental tissue. The greatest risk to the fetus arises if the mother has a primary infection during the first trimester. Congenital heart defects occur during this period. Neurological deficits, deafness, and cataracts are the other major manifestations of intrauterine rubella infection. Rubella infection arising in the last trimester is unlikely to produce malformations.

Intrauterine growth restriction

Intrauterine growth restriction (IUGR) refers to a fetus that fails to reach its own intrinsic full growth potential. There are three broad categories of causes of IUGR:

- *Uteroplacental insufficiency*, which may be due to an umbilical vascular anomaly, maternal hypertension, or pre-eclampsia. Compromised blood flow to the fetus results in diminished fetal growth. When there is continued hypoperfusion, the brain is initially spared, but if perfusion continues to be decreased other tissues such as the kidneys and the myocardium are affected, resulting in oligohydramnios and fetal heart decelerations. The ultimate consequence of uteroplacental insufficiency is fetal distress and death (Fig. 22.1).

- *Maternal causes*, such as illicit narcotic intake, heavy cigarette smoking, and alcohol abuse during the second and third trimesters. Other important causes are infections such as rubella, and medications such as phenytoin (an antiepileptic), steroids, warfarin, and chemotherapy. Fifty per cent of cases of IUGR involve a maternal risk factor. Worldwide, the single greatest cause of IUGR is malaria.

- *Fetal causes*, which arise from fetal chromosomal abnormalities, structural abnormalities, or multiple gestations.

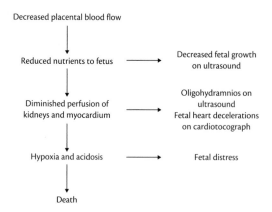

Fig. 22.1 Effects of placental insufficiency on the fetus and correlation with diagnostic features.

IUGR infants have an increased number of complications and a high perinatal mortality rate

Approximately half of IUGR infants suffer from conditions such as perinatal asphyxia and hypoglycaemia (poor fat and glycogen stores). A twofold increase in cerebral dysfunction is seen in the long term, ranging from minor learning disabilities to cerebral palsy. The perinatal mortality rate is also higher for any given gestational age in these infants. The prognosis for normal post-natal growth and development varies by the degree and cause of the IUGR.

Infants

Infants are children in the first year of life. The term neonate is also used specifically for a baby within the first 4 weeks of life. Most diseases of infancy are related to being born too early, too late, too small, too large, or with congenital anomalies.

Prematurity

Prematurity may result from spontaneous pre-term labour, multiple pregnancy, polyhydramnios, or premature rupture of membranes. A baby may also be forced to be delivered early if the risks of continuing the pregnancy outweigh the risks of prematurity.

Immaturity of the organs is the main reason for the major problems seen in premature neonates. Such problems include respiratory distress syndrome, germinal matrix haemorrhage, necrotizing enterocolitis, and infection. The earlier the gestation, the higher the risk of these complications.

Respiratory distress syndrome

Respiratory distress syndrome is due to surfactant deficiency

Respiratory distress syndrome (RDS) is a disease principally associated with prematurity as a result of inadequate production of surfactant by the immature lungs. Surfactant is a lipoprotein that lowers the surface tension in the alveoli, resulting in less pressure being required to keep the alveoli patent, and preventing collapse of the alveoli during expiration.

Production of surfactant does not begin in significant amounts until 30 weeks gestation. Premature babies born before 30 weeks lack surfactant; the high surface tension in the alveoli leads to collapse of the alveoli and hence impaired gas exchange.

Hyaline membrane disease is the pathological hallmark of RDS

If the lungs of a neonate with RDS are examined microscopically the terminal airways and alveoli are seen to be lined by structureless membranes called hyaline membranes. These are composed of necrotic pneumocytes, fibrin, and other proteins that have leaked out of damaged capillaries.

> # Key points: Intrauterine infection and IUGR
>
> - Some maternal infections can pass to the fetus via the placenta. These may be mild or subclinical in the mother.
>
> - Once infected, the fetus may die, but if it survives it may be born with the infection or show characteristic malformations.
>
> - Intrauterine growth restriction refers to a fetus that fails to reach its full growth potential.
>
> - IUGR may be due to problems with the placenta, maternal factors, or fetal factors.
>
> - Fetuses with IUGR who survive to birth are at increased risk of neonatal morbidity and mortality.

RDS, ARDS, HMD, and DAD

Respiratory distress syndrome and hyaline membrane disease are the clinical and pathological counterparts, respectively, of acute respiratory distress syndrome and diffuse alveolar damage seen in adults (p. 108).

RDS presents with clinical features of respiratory distress

RDS presents within 4 h of birth with tachypnoea (respiratory rate >60 breaths/min), sternal and intercostal recession, and expiratory grunting. Chest radiography shows a diffuse, finely granular appearance to both lungs (Fig. 22.2).

Infants with RDS are at risk of chronic lung disease of prematurity

Without effective treatment, infants with RDS are at risk of developing permanent lung disease known as **chronic lung disease of prematurity**. The lungs of these infants show poor blood vessel development, scarring, and cyst formation.

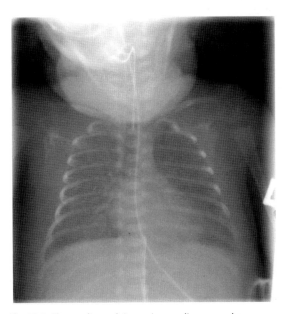

Fig. 22.2 Chest radiograph in respiratory distress syndrome showing diffuse fine shadowing throughout both lungs.

Chronic lung disease of prematurity is not only a result of scarring caused by RDS but is also due to iatrogenic damage caused by oxygen therapy (oxygen concentrations >40 per cent are toxic to the neonatal lung), and mechanical trauma caused by artificial ventilation. The incidence of this form of severe lung disease is increasing, as survival of premature infants improves. Infants with chronic lung disease of prematurity are at increased risk of respiratory infections, particularly with respiratory syncytial virus, and pulmonary hypertension.

Germinal matrix–intraventricular haemorrhage and periventricular leukomalacia

Germinal matrix–intraventricular haemorrhage and periventricular leukomalacia are two distinct forms of CNS injury seen in the pre-term infant.

Germinal matrix–intraventricular haemorrhage is due to rupture of capillaries in the germinal matrix

Germinal matrix-intraventricular haemorrhage (GMH-IVH) is characterized by bleeding within the germinal matrix, a bilateral structure located in the periventricular zone composed of proliferating immature neurones that eventually migrate peripherally to form the cerebral cortex. The germinal matrix involutes early in third trimester, and so GMH-IVH is rare in infants born over 32 weeks' gestation.

The germinal matrix is vulnerable to bleeding because its intrinsically fragile capillaries are easily ruptured. Bleeding from these capillaries is considered to be the result of alterations in cerebral flow. Such alteration is caused by fluctuations in the systemic blood pressure because of poor autoregulatory mechanisms of the premature neonate. Hypoxic injury to the capillaries also makes them more prone to damage, and so RDS also contributes to GMH-IVH.

The long-term sequelae of GMH-IVH are hydrocephalus and cerebral palsy. It is not possible to predict which infants will develop such sequelae.

Periventricular leukomalacia is an ischaemic lesion in the white matter around the cerebral ventricles

Periventricular leukomalacia (PVL) is a form of hypoxic–ischaemic brain injury in the pre-term infant. The most widely held theory is that PVL is caused by impaired perfusion of watershed zones of the periventricular white matter. Infection and septicaemia appears to be associated with PVL. An important consequence in surviving infants is cerebral palsy.

Necrotizing enterocolitis

Necrotizing enterocolitis (NEC) occurs almost exclusively in premature infants. NEC is the clinical end-point of three interacting factors:

- *Mucosal damage*, due to causes such as artificial hyperosmolar milk feeds which cause gut flora to proliferate.

- *Ischaemia*, related to hypoxia and hypotension.

- *Infection*, particularly with gas-forming organisms such as *Clostridium perfringens*.

The most common sites of involvement in NEC are the terminal ileum and the colon, but any part of the large or small intestine may be affected. In the early stages, there is erosion and sloughing of the mucosa with blood in the lumen of the intestine. With persisting injury, the necrosis extends from involvement of the superficial portions of the wall to full thickness infarction.

Submucosal or subserosal gas-filled cysts are seen in severely affected areas. In the more advanced cases, there is bowel perforation and peritonitis. NEC has a mortality of approximately 20–30 per cent in those who perforate.

Treatment requires surgical resection of the affected bowel. Microscopic examination of the resected bowel is crucial to exclude other causes of enterocolitis, such as Hirschsprung's disease. Another important reason for examining the surgical specimen is to see if the resection margins are viable, because an ischaemic bowel may heal by fibrosis, resulting in stricture formation. An important long-term complication is short bowel syndrome, which is due to severe malabsorption that follows extensive resection of the small intestine. It is likely to occur if less than 40 cm of small bowel is left behind.

Infection in the premature infant

Premature infants are susceptible to infections because of immature physical defences and poorly developed immunity. Humoral immunity is deficient as infants born before the third trimester have not received maternal IgG antibodies, which are transferred to the fetus during the last 3 months of pregnancy.

The thin skin of the pre-term infant is easily damaged and infected. The necrotic umbilical stump, and various tubes and catheters that are invariably present in these babies, allow pathogenic organisms to enter the body. The lower the gestational age and birth weight, the higher the risk of any infection and the greater the severity of the illness.

Key points: Prematurity

- Premature neonates suffer problems related to immaturity of their organ systems.

- Respiratory distress syndrome is due to surfactant deficiency making the work of breathing extremely difficult.

- Germinal matrix–intraventricular haemorrhage is bleeding within the germinal matrix due to poor autoregulation of blood flow. Severe cases may cause permanent neurological sequelae.

- Necrotizing enterocolitis causes death of the bowel due to a combination of mucosal damage from hyperosmolar feeds, ischaemia, and infection.

- Infections are common in premature neonates due to their immature immune system and the presence of multiple tubes and lines.

Perinatal asphyxia

Perinatal asphyxia (birth asphyxia) is the failure of oxygen delivery to tissues and organs occurring around the time of birth. Some degree of hypoxia is a normal event during labour; the fetus can adapt to periods of hypoxic stress by redistributing blood flow to important organs and switching to anaerobic glycolysis.

There are many causes of perinatal asphyxia, including placental abruption, cord compression, anaesthetic or opiate administration to the mother (causing fetal respiratory depression), congenital cardiac or pulmonary anomalies, an obstructed airway, birth trauma, and congenital sepsis. Some of these may have already led to IUGR.

Post-term infants and infants of diabetic mothers are most at risk of perinatal asphyxia

Post-term infants are more susceptible to asphyxia for two main reasons. First, the declining placental function that accompanies post-maturity results in decreased maternal blood flow to the baby. The baby utilizes its fat and glycogen stores to compensate for the relative lack of nutrients from the mother. This leaves it with no reserve of glucose to meet metabolic demands during episodes of hypoxia. Secondly, these infants are large, and so are at risk of difficult labour and birth trauma.

Diabetic mothers with hyperglycaemia cause fetal hyperglycaemia because glucose crosses the placenta. As maternal insulin does not cross the placenta, the fetus responds by producing insulin. This leads to increased growth of the fetus by increasing cell numbers and size. These large babies are at increased risk of birth trauma and perinatal asphyxia.

There are two typical manifestations of perinatal asphyxia: hypoxic–ischaemic encephalopathy and meconium aspiration syndrome.

Hypoxic–ischaemic encephalopathy is due to neuronal necrosis

Hypoxic–ischaemic encephalopathy (HIE) is the clinical manifestation of brain injury occurring immediately or up to 48 h after asphyxia. Hypoxic–ischaemic brain injury selectively damages *grey* matter neurones. The neurones in the deep grey matter (hippocampus, basal ganglia, and thalamus) are more severely affected in the premature infant. The vulnerable areas of the term infant are the cerebral and cerebellar cortices. In severe hypoxia, all susceptible areas are affected.

In severe HIE, the mortality rate is as high as 50 per cent. Twenty per cent of the survivors of HIE have neurological impairment, particularly cerebral palsy. Infants with mild HIE, and those who are neurologically normal by 10 days of age, have an excellent long-term prognosis.

INTERESTING TO KNOW

TOBY trial

At present there is no specific treatment for asphyxia other than stabilization with treatment aimed at reducing seizures. Recent studies have suggested that cooling may help the neonate with moderate or severe perinatal asphyxia.

The TOBY trial aims to determine if the use of whole body cooling at 6 h of age will improve survival and reduce neurological impairment. The neonate is cooled to 33.5°C and kept at this temperature for 3 days followed by gradual warming to normal temperature. The neurological and neurodevelopmental assessment of survivors takes place at 18 months of age.

Meconium aspiration syndrome is due to inhalation of meconium into the lungs

Meconium is the first faeces of the newborn. It is a sticky, thick, green/black substance composed of intestinal contents and amniotic fluid debris. During anoxia, the fetus relaxes its anal sphincter and expels meconium into the amniotic fluid. Normally a fetus takes shallow breaths of amniotic fluid *in utero*. If meconium is present in the amniotic fluid or upper airway before, during, or immediately after delivery, it can be inhaled further into the airways and down into the lungs. This is more likely to happen in severe anoxia, when the fetus begins to take deep gasps.

It is important to remember that meconium staining of the amniotic fluid is seen in up to 10 per cent of normal births and so other signs of asphyxia, such as a low arterial pH and a low Apgar score at birth, must be identified before a meconium-stained placenta is accepted as being of any significance. Meconium aspiration syndrome is confined to mature infants, since pre-term infants rarely pass meconium *in utero*.

JARGON BUSTER

Apgar score

The **Apgar score**, named after its deviser, is a method used for assessing and quantifying the physiological state and responsiveness of a newborn infant. Five signs are evaluated: heart rate, respiratory effort, muscle tone, response to a catheter in the nostril, and colour of the skin (pink or blue). A score of 0, 1, or 2 is given for each parameter. Apgar scores therefore range from 0 to 10, with 10 representing an infant in the best possible condition.

Meconium aspiration has three major effects:

- Collapse of areas of lung due to airway obstruction by meconium plugs.
- Pneumonitis caused by the irritant effect of meconium constituents such as enzymes and bile salts.
- Surfactant deficiency as meconium strips surfactant from the alveolar surface.

Most infants recover within 4–10 days with respiratory support and surfactant replacement. A few develop pneumothorax and chronic lung disease following mechanical ventilation, and infections.

Key points: Perinatal asphyxia

- Perinatal asphyxia is failure of oxygen delivery to the various tissues and organs.

- It is due to failure of physiological adaptive responses to asphyxia.

- Multiple organ systems are affected by acute perinatal asphyxia.

- Asphyxia is due to either maternal or fetal causes.

- Hypoxic–ischaemic encephalopathy and meconium aspiration syndrome are two important clinical manifestations of asphyxia.

- Asphyxia is a major contributor to childhood morbidity and mortality.

Neonatal infection

Infection in the newborn remains an important cause of morbidity and mortality at all birth weights and gestations. Most neonatal infections are acquired from the mother during transit through an infected birth canal, e.g. herpes simplex virus, *Chlamydia trachomatis*, group B streptococci, *Escherichia coli*, and *Neisseria gonorrhoeae*.

Infection may also be acquired in the first week after birth via contact with infected adults or other neonates. *Escherichia coli*, group B streptococcus, and *Staphylococcus epidermidis* are responsible for 80–85 per cent of severe neonatal infections

LINK BOX

Vertical transmission of HBV and HIV

Contact between the neonate and maternal blood during delivery facilitates transmission of hepatitis B virus (p. 183) and HIV (p. 49) to the baby.

Escherichia coli and group B streptococci may cause pneumonia and meningitis

Neonates exposed to *E. coli* or group B streptococci in the maternal genital tract may go on to develop pneumonia and meningitis. Pneumonia usually develops in the first week of life; meningitis may be seen either during or after the first week of life. Bacterial meningitis is a very serious condition with a mortality of up to 50 per cent. Neonates surviving meningitis may develop neurological complications such as cerebral palsy, or hearing impairment in later life.

Ophthalmia neonatorum is an infection of the eye of the neonate

Ophthalmia neonatorum presents with a red eye with purulent discharge. It is caused by infection with *N. gonorrhoea*, *C. trachomatis*, or staphylococci. Swabs should be taken to identify the causative organism. As both *N. gonorrhoea* and *C. trachomatis* are sexually transmitted infections, the mother should be counselled and treated appropriately, as should her sexual contacts.

The umbilical stump can become infected

Omphalitis refers to inflammation of the umbilicus. It is usually caused by *Staphylococcus aureus* and can be treated presumptively with flucloxacillin. The only major potential complication of omphalitis is spread of the infection via the umbilical vessels causing septicaemia.

Key points: Neonatal infection

- Neonatal infection and sepsis remain an important cause of morbidity and mortality at all birth weights and gestations.

- Most neonatal infections are acquired following passage through the mother's genital tract. Others may be picked up after birth following contact with infected adults.

- *Escherichia coli* and group B streptococci are important causes of pneumonia and meningitis.

- Ophthalmia neonatorum is an infection of the eye caused by *N. gonorrhoeae*, *C. trachomatis*, or staphylococci.

- Omphalitis is an infection of the umbilical stump caused by *S. aureus*.

Neonatal screening

All neonates in the UK are screened for phenylketonuria and congenital hypothyroidism on a blood sample taken from the heel within the first 2 weeks of life (the Guthrie test). Although these disorders are rare, early recognition and treatment can prevent permanent brain damage.

Phenylketonuria is caused by deficiency of the enzyme phenylalanine hydroxylase

Phenylketonuria is an autosomal recessive disorder with an incidence of 1 per 10000 births in the UK. In phenylketonuria, there is decreased activity of the liver enzyme phenylalanine hydroxylase which converts the dietary amino acid phenylalanine to tyrosine.

Normally tyrosine is converted to neurotransmitters (dopamine, noradrenaline, and adrenaline) and also to melanin. Upon ingestion of phenylalanine, affected patients develop hyperphenylalanaemia and produce a variety of phenylalanine metabolites such as phenylpyruvic acid, which is the ketone that gives the disease its name. The block also results in tyrosine deficiency.

Through mechanisms that are not entirely understood, phenylalanine accumulation in the brain results in defective synthesis of myelin and inadequate development of neurones. Cerebrospinal fluid (CSF) shows decreased levels of the neurotransmitters due to inhibition of their synthesis.

Patients with untreated phenylketonuria develop severe mental retardation, and 25 per cent have seizures. The melanin deficiency in the iris and hair is manifest clinically as blue eyes and blond hair. Early restriction of phenylalanine in the diet prevents mental retardation.

Congenital hypothyroidism causes irreversible brain damage

Congenital hypothyroidism is a developmental abnormality of the thyroid gland that results in low thyroxine levels. It occurs in 1 in 4000 live births in the UK. Some infants develop irreversible brain damage because the development of the CNS is intrinsically reliant on thyroxine from early fetal life. Thyroxine therapy within 2 weeks of birth enables many infants to achieve normal intellectual development. Screening for congenital hypothyroidism involves looking for high concentrations of thyroid-stimulating hormone in neonatal blood.

> ### Key points: Neonatal screening
>
> ◆ All neonates born in the UK are screened for phenylketonuria and congenital hypothyroidism.
>
> ◆ Phenylketonuria is due to severe deficiency of the enzyme phenylalanine hydroxylase. Early dietary restriction of phenylalanine can prevent severe mental retardation.
>
> ◆ Congenital hypothyroidism causes irreversible brain damage as the central nervous system requires thyroxine for normal development. Infants in whom hypothyroidism is detected early respond well to treatment with thyroxine.

Sudden infant death syndrome

Sudden infant death syndrome (SIDS) is the diagnosis given for the sudden death of an infant where the cause of death remains unexplained after a review of the clinical history, death scene investigation, and a thorough post-mortem examination. The manner of death is presumed to be natural, although the cause is unknown.

SIDS accounts for about 5 per cent of deaths in infancy, and 90 per cent of SIDS deaths occur in infants younger than 6 months. The pathophysiological mechanisms responsible for SIDS remain unknown, although there are a number of associated risk factors (Table 22.2).

A SIDS diagnosis results from a multiprofessional investigation

The recommended procedure in the event of a sudden infant death is for the paediatrician, police, and social services to interview the parents and investigate the scene of the death. This should be done as soon as possible, preferably on the same day as the death. As soon as the child is brought into hospital, a senior paediatrician examines the child and orders appropriate investigations, including radiology and laboratory tests.

The Coroner must be informed, and within 48 h of death a paediatric pathologist performs a detailed post-mortem examination. The preliminary findings of the investigations are communicated to the parents.

The final results of the post-mortem are not available until 2–3 months after death. It takes this long for the

TABLE 22.2 Risk factors for sudden infant death syndrome

Sleeping prone (on the abdomen)
Premature birth
Low socio-economic status
Overheating due to excess clothing or bedding
Maternal drug abuse or smoking during pregnancy
Smoking in the household

large number of investigations and tests to be available for complete assimilation. These are considered with the findings of the police and social services to establish the cause of death. A diagnosis of SIDS is reached by excluding all other natural or unnatural causes.

> ## Key points: Sudden infant death syndrome
>
> - Sudden infant death syndrome is a cause of death given after exclusion of all other causes of death
>
> - A thorough laboratory investigation includes toxicological, microbiological, and biochemical tests, and a full post-mortem examination.
>
> - The main objective of the professional team is to identify a cause of death, if possible, and to provide help and support to the bereaved family.

Congenital anomalies

Congenital anomalies are structural defects present at birth. Two per cent of neonates have a major abnormality which is either incompatible with life or requires major surgery. Congenital anomalies may be caused by the following:

- *Single gene disorders*. These are due to mutation of a single gene and follow a Mendelian pattern of inheritance (autosomal dominant, autosomal recessive, X-linked recessive).

- *Chromosomal disorders*. These arise from chromosomal aneuploidy, which is reduplication or deletion of whole chromosomes or parts of chromosomes.

These disorders affect autosomal or sex chromosomes. Trisomy 21 (Down's syndrome) and Turner's syndrome (45,X) are two important examples of chromosomal disorders.

- *Teratogens*. Recognized teratogenic agents include intrauterine infections (e.g. rubella), maternal alcohol abuse, nutritional deficiencies (e.g. folic acid), and certain drugs (e.g. warfarin).

- *Multifactorial*. Both genetic and environmental factors are involved in causing a birth defect, e.g. facial clefting.

In up to 60 per cent of cases of congenital anomaly, no clear underlying cause can be found.

Congenital heart disease

Congenital heart disease (CHD) is the most common group of structural disorders in children, with an incidence of approximately 8 per 1000 live births. With advances in medical and surgical care, the majority of children with CHD are now surviving into adulthood.

Congenital heart diseases can be described in a number of ways

CHD may be described according to the anatomical defect, the haemodynamic alteration, and the status of tissue oxygenation (Fig. 22.3).

- *Anatomical defects* describe the actual structural abnormality, e.g. a ventricular septal defect, atrial septal defect, or patent ductus arteriosus.

- *Haemodynamic alterations* describe the presence of any shunting and/or obstruction to blood flow as a result of the anatomical defect. Shunting refers to the flow between the normally separate systemic and

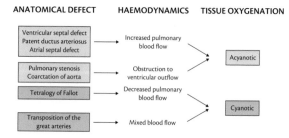

Fig. 22.3 Congenital heart disease. Summary of pathophysiological and clinical features of the common congenital heart diseases.

pulmonary circulations due to the anatomical defect. The direction of the blood flow depends upon the relative pressures of the two circulations, flowing from areas of high pressure to areas of low pressure. Obstructive lesions can occur anywhere in either circulation. In general, right-sided obstruction produces decreased pulmonary blood flow and cyanosis, while left-sided obstruction results in decreased systemic blood flow. If obstruction is severe, the flow through the obstructed circulation depends on the ductus arteriosus. These are known as duct-dependent lesions, and the symptoms in these types of CHD appear soon after birth when the duct begins to close.

- *Tissue oxygenation status* is assessed by the presence or absence of cyanosis in the child. Acyanotic defects usually involve left-to-right shunts. When the blood is directed away from the lungs before having reached them (right-to-left shunt), there is hypoxia sufficient to cause cyanosis.

Complications of CHD include cardiac failure, infective endocarditis, and pulmonary hypertension

The following are the important complications of CHD:

- **Cardiac failure.** Cardiac failure commonly occurs in CHD due either to volume overload in shunting defects, or pressure overload in obstructive defects. The principal symptoms of cardiac failure are breathlessness and fatigue. In infants, this typically presents with rapid tiring during feeding (the most strenuous activity for the majority of infants!).

- **Infective endocarditis.** Turbulent flow across shunts results in haemodynamic injury to the endocardium, predisposing to infective endocarditis.

- **Pulmonary hypertension.** Excessive pulmonary blood flow through a large left-to-right shunt leads to raised pulmonary artery pressure. If these shunts are not repaired, the pulmonary hypertension may become irreversible. The child will then become cyanotic due to reversal of the shunt (i.e. the shunt becomes right-to-left). This is known as Eisenmenger's syndrome.

Ventricular septal defect is the most common type of CHD

Ventricular septal defect (VSD) comprises one or more holes in the interventricular septum. They can occur

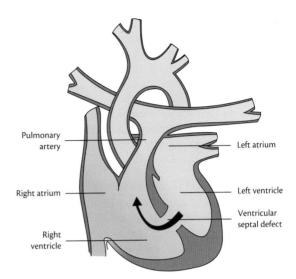

Fig. 22.4 Ventricular septal defect. In the presence of a ventricular septal defect, blood flows from the higher pressure left ventricle into the right ventricle, resulting in a left-to-right shunt.

anywhere in the ventricular septum; three-quarters of them occur in the upper part of the septum (Fig. 22.4).

A small VSD may have little functional significance and may close spontaneously as the child matures. There remains, however, a risk of infective endocarditis at the site of the defect and so children with a VSD should be given prophylactic antibiotics before any invasive procedure.

A larger VSD causes flow of blood from the left ventricle to the right ventricle (i.e. a left-to-right shunt). Increased volume load is placed on both sides of the heart (the right side receives blood through the VSD and the left heat receives more venous return), leading to symptoms of cardiac failure. Large VSDs are repaired surgically in infancy.

Patent ductus arteriosus allows post-natal left-to-right shunting

Patent ductus arteriosus (PDA) is persistence of the ductus arteriosus after 10 days of life. In the fetal circulation, the ductus arteriosus connects the pulmonary artery to the descending aorta, allowing blood exiting the right ventricle to bypass the lungs. As pulmonary vascular resistance falls after birth, and systemic vascular resistance rises, the duct closes, first functionally, by constriction, and then anatomically, ending up as a ligament (ligamentum arteriosum).

In the presence of a PDA, systemic blood flows from the higher pressure aorta to the lower pressure pulmonary artery through the patent duct, causing a left-to-right shunt. As a result, blood flow to the lungs is increased twofold. Twice the volume returns from the lungs to the left atrium, which therefore expands in response to this volume overload. The left ventricle also enlarges and its myocardium becomes hypertrophied. Infective endocarditis in the region of the ductus arteriosus is a frequent complication.

Atrial septal defect is due to a hole in the atrial septum

Atrial septal defect (ASD) is an abnormal opening in the septum between the two atria. The most common site of an ASD is in the middle of the septum away from the atrioventricular valves. This allows blood to flow from the left atrium to the right atrium, resulting in an increase in the amount of blood flowing through the lungs. Many children with an ASD are asymptomatic, but some may notice easy fatiguability. ASDs typically manifest in early adulthood due to atrial arrhythmias.

Atrioventricular septal defect is the most common CHD seen in Down's syndrome

The atrioventricular septum is the partition that separates the atria and the ventricles from each other. In a complete atrioventricular septal defect (AVSD), the defect comprises a low ASD that is continuous with a high VSD. Essentially it is a hole in the centre of the heart. A complete AVSD with a large ventricular component will function similarly to a VSD, with volume overload to the right ventricle. Approximately half of children with Down's syndrome have some form of AVSD.

Tetralogy of Fallot is the most common cyanotic CHD

The most frequently seen congenital cardiac anomaly to cause a right-to-left shunt is **tetralogy of Fallot**. Tetralogy of Fallot comprises four defects (Fig. 22.5):

♦ *Stenosis of the outflow tract of the right ventricle.* This is the fundamental abnormality, and is usually due to thickening of the muscular tissue immediately below the pulmonary valve. The severity of the obstruction influences the haemodynamics and the resulting clinical picture.

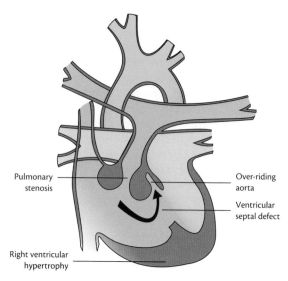

Fig. 22.5 Tetralogy of Fallot. Tetralogy of Fallot comprises pulmonary stenosis, a ventricular septal defect, an over-riding aorta, and right ventricular hypertrophy.

♦ A *ventricular septal defect*, which is usually large, allowing for equalization of pressure between the ventricles.

♦ An *over-riding aorta* which receives blood from both the ventricles.

♦ *Right ventricular hypertrophy*, which is secondary to the pulmonary obstruction and the increased right ventricular pressure.

The pulmonary stenosis decreases the blood flow to the lungs, and consequently the amount of oxygenated blood returning to the left side of the heart. As the pulmonary outflow obstruction increases, the right ventricular pressure increases above the systemic pressure, and deoxygenated blood flows from the right ventricle to the left ventricle across the VSD. The net effect is that deoxygenated blood from the right-sided circulation enters the systemic circulation, and so there is cyanosis.

Transposition of the great arteries results in two parallel circulations

Transposition of the great arteries (the aorta and the pulmonary artery) is the second most common cyanotic CHD. In this condition, the main arteries arise from the wrong ventricle: the aorta exits from the right ventricle and the pulmonary artery exits from the left ventricle. If there is no communication between the pulmonary and systemic circulations, the abnormality is incompatible with life. For survival, 'mixing' of blood from both circulations must occur. This is usually achieved through a VSD or a PDA.

Coarctation of the aorta is localized narrowing of the aortic arch

Coarctation of the aorta is a congenital developmental abnormality in which there is a localized area of narrowing (stenosis) of the lumen of the aortic arch, distal to the origin of the left subclavian artery. There are two forms of aortic coarctation, distinguished by the age at which they usually present (Fig. 22.6).

In the 'infantile' form, there is a PDA distal to the coarctation. This allows adequate cardiac output to the whole body, but much of the cardiac output is deoxygenated blood coming from the right side of the heart via the pulmonary artery and PDA, and so there is cyanosis of the lower half of the body. Many infants with this type of coarctation do not survive early life without some form of surgical or catheter intervention.

In the 'adult' form, there is no PDA and the stenosis is located in the region of the attachment of the closed ductus arteriosus. Blood flow to the upper part of the body is increased, and eventually most patients develop upper extremity systolic hypertension. The stenosis, however, restricts the amount of blood flowing to the lower part of the body, so the blood pressure in the lower limbs is low and the strength of the femoral pulse is decreased. There is also radiofemoral delay (delayed pulses in the legs). Most children with this type of coarctation are asymptomatic, and the condition may not be recognized until later in adult life.

> ### Key points: Congenital heart disease
>
> - Congenital heart disease is the most common group of structural abnormalities.
> - Congenital heart disease can be considered at three levels: anatomical, haemodynamic, and oxygenation status.
> - Cardiac failure, infective endocarditis, and pulmonary hypertension are the main complications of CHD.

> - VSD is the most common acyanotic CHD and tetralogy of Fallot is the most common cyanotic CHD.

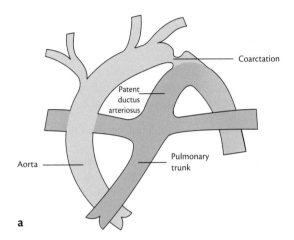

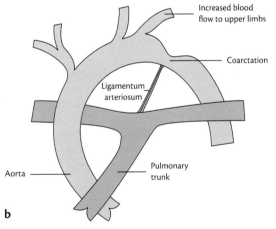

Fig. 22.6 Coarctation of the aorta. (a) In the infantile form, a patent ductus arteriosus allows an adequate cardiac output to the systemic circulation, but much of this is deoxygenated blood and so there is cyanosis. (b) In the adult form, there is no patent ductus arteriosus. There is no cyanosis, but blood flow to the upper limbs is increased, resulting in upper limb hypertension. Decreased blood flow to the lower limbs causes radiofemoral delay.

Respiratory tract malformations

Congenital diaphragmatic hernia is a defect in development of the diaphragm

Congenital diaphragmatic hernia is a hole in diaphragm caused by failure of the pleuroperitoneal canals to close during 8–10 weeks of gestation. Other anomalies are also present in 40 per cent of cases.

The main problem with congenital diaphragmatic hernia is that bowel loops and the liver pass through the hole into the thorax and squash the developing lungs. The lung on the same side as the hernia becomes hypoplastic and shows structural abnormalities in the form of reduced numbers of airways, alveoli, and pulmonary artery branches, as well as maturation arrest of pneumocytes. The infant presents with respiratory failure, and 50 per cent die within 24 h of birth.

Congenital adenomatoid malformation is a mass of abnormal lung tissue

Congenital adenomatoid malformation is a lung mass composed of terminal bronchioles. There are no normal alveoli. Usually a single lobe is involved. Many cases are diagnosed by antenatal ultrasound at 20 weeks gestation. Most congenital adenomatoid malformations cause a degree of respiratory distress and so are surgically removed.

Sequestration is a mass of non-functional embryonic lung that does not communicate with the airways

Pulmonary sequestration is a discrete mass of lung tissue that has no normal connection with the respiratory tract. Sequestrations have a systemic blood supply. The majority are intrapulmonary and found in the left lower lobe. Up to half of the extrapulmonary sequestrations may be associated with other anomalies. Pulmonary sequestrations may become infected or cause massive haemoptysis.

Laryngomalacia is the most common anomaly of the upper respiratory tract

Laryngomalacia is a relatively common condition in which the epiglottis and arytenoid cartilages collapse during inspiration. The infant presents within the first few weeks of life with inspiratory stridor. The stridor may worsen until about 6 months of age, and then gradually improves. Most children are symptom free by 24 months.

> ## Key points: Respiratory tract malformations
>
> - Congenital diaphragmatic hernia is a hole in the diaphragm which allows abdominal contents to enter the thorax and squash the developing lungs.
> - Congenital adenomatoid malformation is a lung mass composed of terminal bronchioles. Most are surgically removed as they cause respiratory distress.
> - Pulmonary sequestration is an abnormal mass of embryonic lung found within the substance of the lung. Complications include infection and haemorrhage.
> - Laryngomalacia causes collapse of the upper airways and inspiratory stridor. After 6 months of age the condition spontaneously improves.

Gastrointestinal and hepatobiliary malformations

Cleft lip and palate are due to failure of complete fusion of the developing facial structures

Cleft lip is an opening in the upper lip between the mouth and the nose. Infants with a cleft lip do not normally have feeding difficulties and usually develop normal speech.

Cleft palate is a failure of the palate to join in the midline, and its appearance ranges from a trivial bifid uvula to complete midline separation of both the soft and the hard palates. Infants with cleft palates may have feeding difficulties as it makes forming a vacuum in the mouth difficult. Special bottles and teats can usually overcome this problem. Following surgical repair of a cleft palate, most children develop good speech, although the repaired palate can make it difficult to pronounce some sounds clearly.

Exomphalos and gastroschisis are congenital anterior wall defects

Exomphalos is a ventral wall defect at the umbilicus that causes the abdominal contents to protrude through the umbilicus. This protrusion is covered by a delicate transparent sac made up of amniotic membrane and peritoneum. The abnormality arises due to failure of the midgut to return to the abdomen from the umbilical coelom during embryogenesis.

Gastroschisis literally means 'split stomach'. It refers to an abdominal wall defect that lies to the side of the umbilicus, through which loops of bowel protrude, but, unlike exomphalos, there is no protective covering sac.

Both defects can be detected antenatally as early as 10 weeks of gestation. With adequate supportive and surgical management in specialized centres, the prognosis is generally good.

Atresia is a congenital failure of the development of a lumen

Atresia is a term that can be applied to any situation where part of an epithelial-lined tube fails to develop its lumen. In the gastrointestinal tract, the most common sites for atresia are the oesophagus and the small intestine. The gut proximal to the atretic segment ends in a blind pouch, causing obstruction.

Bearing in mind that during the fourth month of gestation one-third of the amniotic fluid is normally swallowed by the fetus and then resorbed in the proximal jejunum, one can appreciate that oesophageal and duodenal atresia will cause polyhydramnios, due to the inability of swallowed material to pass through the gut.

Oesophageal atresia occurs in 1 in 3500 live births. It results from faulty division of the foregut into the tracheal and oesophageal channels during the first month of embryonic life. In the majority of cases, there is a communication between the distal oesophagus and the trachea, known as a tracheo-oesophageal fistula (Fig. 22.7). The affected neonate will present with coughing and choking during feeding. Oesophageal atresia is usually diagnosed when attempts to pass a catheter into the stomach fail. At least half of affected infants have other congenital abnormalities, and cardiac defects account for the majority of deaths in infants with oesophageal atresia.

Duodenal atresia is less common. Failure of epithelial apoptosis results in incomplete canalization of the duodenal lumen by 8 weeks of gestation. The obstruction is usually distal to the ampulla of Vater. Duodenal atresia is associated with Down's syndrome in 30 per cent of cases. A pre-natal ultrasound scan showing a dilated proximal duodenum and stomach, and polyhydramnios is highly suggestive of duodenal atresia.

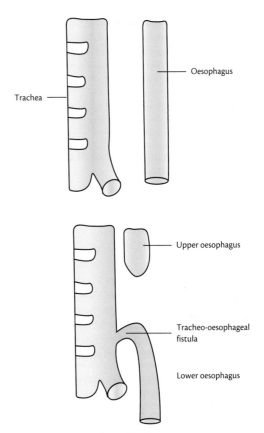

Fig. 22.7 Tracheo-oesophageal fistula.

Atresias elsewhere in the small bowel are usually isolated abnormalities; however, as 15 per cent of them are associated with meconium ileus, affected infants must be tested for cystic fibrosis.

Biliary atresia is an important cause of jaundice in infants

Biliary atresia is a rare, but serious disease of infancy in which there is inflammatory destruction of the extrahepatic biliary tract, resulting in obstruction to bile flow. Typically the gallbladder is also absent or poorly formed. Although it has been considered to be a congenital anomaly, there is now some evidence emerging to suggest that it may well be an acquired disease.

Biliary atresia presents with jaundice at around 4–8 weeks of age, often with other features of biliary obstruction such as pale stools and dark urine. Some infants develop pruritus which can be very distressing.

The main differential diagnoses to consider are neonatal hepatitis and α_1-antitrypsin deficiency.

Although biliary atresia is rare (incidence of 1 in 10 000), it is nonetheless extremely important to make the diagnosis as soon as possible, as prompt surgery is essential to prevent irreversible liver cirrhosis. The earlier surgery is performed, the better the chance of success.

Malrotation is an important cause of bowel obstruction and infarction

Malrotation refers to malpositioning of the intestine and mesentery due to a failure of rotation of the developing gut as it returns from the umbilical coelom to the abdomen during development.

A malrotated bowel is likely to have a narrow mesenteric base, predisposing to volvulus around the superior mesenteric artery. Compromised arterial blood supply leads to ischaemic necrosis of the entire midgut, extending from the duodenum to the transverse colon. The injured bowel wall leads to bleeding into the lumen, and a high risk of perforation. Without prompt surgical intervention, the condition can be fatal.

Meckel's diverticulum is the most common congenital gastrointestinal anomaly

Meckel's diverticulum represents a remnant of the vitellointestinal duct, the structure that connects the primitive gut to the yolk sac. The anomaly is estimated to be present in 2 per cent of the normal population. Within the mucosa of the diverticulum there may be areas of acid secreting-type mucosa, as found in the stomach, or pancreatic tissue (gastric or pancreatic 'heterotopia').

Most children with a Meckel's diverticulum are asymptomatic. The most common symptom is painless rectal bleeding, caused by ulceration within a diverticulum containing gastric-type mucosa. Small bowel obstruction may also occur, related to intussusception or incarceration.

Hirschsprung's disease is the congenital absence of ganglion cells in the wall of the intestine

Congenital absence of ganglion cells in the digestive tract results from the failure of neuroblasts to migrate all the way from the oesophagus to the anal canal during weeks 5–12 of gestation. These neuroblasts form the ganglion cells that comprise the submucosal and intramuscular nerve plexuses of the bowel wall.

Ganglion cells play an important role in peristalsis, the rhythmic process propelling intestinal contents distally.

In Hirschsprung's disease, a variable length of the distal bowel is aganglionic. The absence of ganglion cells results in loss of the fine control of muscle tone in the bowel, and the net result is spasm of the circular muscle coat in the aganglionic part of the bowel. The spasm causes intestinal obstruction and failure to pass meconium after 24 h following birth. Twenty per cent of cases of intestinal obstruction in neonates is due to Hirschsprung's disease.

Rectal biopsy is the gold standard for the diagnosis of Hirschsprung's disease (Fig. 22.8). The submucosa shows an absence of ganglion cells on routine staining. A special laboratory technique (acetylcholinesterase staining) is utilized to identify the increased number of nerve fibres in the abnormal bowel segment, which is another histological feature of Hirschsprung's disease. This test can only be performed on fresh tissue (i.e. not formalin fixed), and so it is important that such a biopsy is transported to the laboratory immediately after it has been taken.

Imperforate anus reflects a malformation in the region of the anorectum

Conditions encompassing atresia or agenesis of the rectum and anus are often grouped together under the umbrella heading 'imperforate anus'. Such lesions can range in severity from a stenosed anal canal through to anorectal agenesis.

From a surgical point of view, they are best considered as being either high or low abnormalities, depending on the level of the termination of the bowel with respect to the level of the pelvic floor. Low defects are relatively easy to correct, and postoperative function is good. With higher defects, the opposite holds true, the reason being that such defects are more likely to be associated with fistulae between the rectum and the genitourinary tract, as well as a deficient pelvic floor.

Key points: Gastrointestinal tract malformations

- Cleft lip and palate disorders are the most common congenital anomalies of the orofacial structures.

Key points: Gastrointestinal tract malformations—cont'd

♦ Exomphalos and gastroschisis are due to congenital anterior wall defects.

♦ Atresia may occur in the oesophagus, duodenum, and small bowel.

♦ Malrotation with midgut volvulus is an important cause of bowel ischaemia.

♦ Meckel's diverticulum is the most common congenital gastrointestinal anomaly.

♦ Hirschsprung's disease is the congenital absence of ganglion cells in the distal large bowel, causing intestinal obstruction.

♦ Rectal biopsy is the gold standard for the diagnosis of Hirschsprung's disease.

♦ Anorectal anomalies can be relatively easy to correct if they occur below the pelvic floor. Those above the pelvic floor often involve a fistula to other pelvic structures.

Genitourinary tract malformations

Malformation of the urinary tract is among the most common of all congenital malformations: more than one-third of all malformations diagnosed on antenatal ultrasound affect the urinary tract. Approximately 10 per cent of the population have some congenital anomaly of the genitourinary tract.

Renal agenesis refers to congenital absence of the kidney. Unilateral renal agenesis is not rare and is easily diagnosed on ultrasound. Bilateral renal agenesis is very rare and always fatal.

Renal hypoplasia is a rare condition in which the kidney is simply small, but otherwise normal. The prognosis is good provided that the other kidney undergoes compensatory hypertrophy.

Horseshoe kidney refers to a single kidney formed by fusion of the two developing kidneys, producing a horseshoe-shaped organ that crosses the midline. Overall renal function is not significantly affected (though there is an increased risk of nephrolithiasis).

Ureteral duplication is a common anomaly in which two separate pelves in the kidney are accompanied by

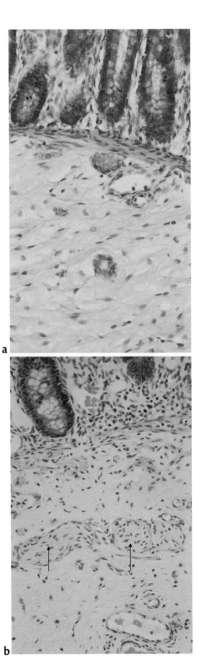

Fig. 22.8 Hirschsprung's disease. (a) A microscopic image from a normal rectal biopsy. At the top you can see the base of the rectal crypts. Beneath the muscularis mucosae is the rectal submucosa, within which ganglion cells are present. (b) A microscopic image from a rectal biopsy taken from an infant with Hirschsprung's disease. No ganglion cells are present in the submucosa; instead abnormally large nerve trunks are seen (arrows).

partial or complete reduplication of the ureter. When there is complete reduplication, the upper ureter typically enters the bladder posteriorly at the normal site of the ureteric orifice on the trigone of the bladder. The lower ureter usually enters the bladder laterally and has a short intramural course. Because of this site of implantation, there is often vesicoureteric reflux up this ureter.

Multicystic dysplastic kidney describes a dysplastic, non-functioning kidney replaced by many large cysts. It is the most common cystic lesion identified antenatally and the most common cause of an abdominal mass in the perinatal period. There is little or no intervening normal renal parenchymal. The condition is usually unilateral and almost always associated with atresia of the ureter.

Renal dysplasia is recognized microscopically by the presence of immature tubules, usually accompanied by islands of cartilage, neither of which are features of a normal kidney. *Note that in this context, the term dysplasia refers to the abnormal organization and differentiation of the kidney and does not imply a pre-neoplastic lesion as in adults.* The outcome in children with a normal contralateral kidney is excellent.

Obstruction in the urinary tract leads to hydronephrosis

Congenital disorders causing obstruction in the urinary tract are important because they are potentially treatable causes of chronic renal failure. The characteristic consequence of congenital obstructive uropathy is dilation of the renal pelvis and calyces (hydronephrosis), which can be detected on antenatal ultrasound. Hydronephrosis is in fact the most common urinary tract abnormality detected antenatally, but bear in mind that it is not the primary abnormality; rather it is a reflection of some other problem (Fig. 22.9).

Pelviureteric junction (PUJ) obstruction is one of the most common causes of congenital obstructive uropathy. It is due to an intrinsic malformation of the smooth muscle of the wall in that particular region of the drainage system.

Posterior urethral valves are mucosal folds in the posterior prostatic urethra. They cause distension of the bladder, bladder wall hypertrophy, and bilateral hydroureter and hydronephrosis. Bilateral hydronephrosis due to posterior urethral valves is usually detected by routine antenatal ultrasound. Endoscopic resection

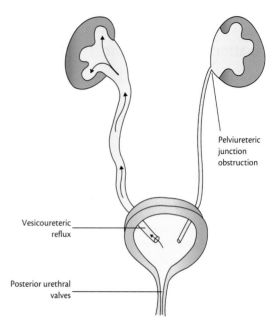

Pelviureteric junction obstruction

Vesicoureteric reflux

Posterior urethral valves

Fig. 22.9 Structural anomalies of the urinary tract causing hydronephrosis.

of the valve(s) should be performed as soon as possible after birth.

Vesicoureteric reflux may also lead to hydronephrosis

Antenatal hydronephrosis can also be the result of a non-obstructive process such as severe vesicoureteric reflux. Abnormal reflux of urine from the bladder back up into the urinary tract causes dilation of the ureter and the kidney which may be picked up on antenatal ultrasound scanning.

Severe vesicoureteric reflux is extremely important as it is associated with the development of permanent renal scarring which can lead to chronic renal failure in later life (see later).

Undescended testis is the most common congenital genitourinary anomaly in males

Cryptorchidism (incomplete descent of the testis) is said to occur when the testis has not descended into its normal intrascrotal position. It is not clear why some testes fail to descend. Orchidopexy (mobilization of testis and spermatic cord, followed by fixation of the testis in the scrotal sac) should be performed by 2 years of age as the potential for fertility becomes compromised after then.

LINK BOX

Cryptorchidism and testicular malignancy

Cryptorchidism is one of the few well recognized risk factors for the development of testicular tumours (p. 241).

Hypospadias is the most common congenital anomaly of the penis

In hypospadias, the urethral meatus opens out on to the undersurface of the penis. It is usually an isolated problem, though the incidence of cryptorchidism in those with hypospadias is higher than that in the general population.

Key points: Genitourinary tract malformations

- Renal agenesis is congenital absence of a kidney.

- Renal hypoplasia is a congenitally shrunken kidney.

- Multicystic dysplastic kidney is a cystic disorganized kidney with no normal renal parenchyma.

- Pelviureteric junction obstruction and posterior urethral valves are common causes of urinary tract obstruction which may be picked up as antenatal hydronephrosis.

- Severe vesicoureteric reflux may also present with antenatal hydronephrosis.

- Cryptorchid testes should be surgically implanted in the scrotum to preserve fertility. Cryptorchid testes are at increased risk of developing a testicular tumour.

- Hypospadias is a malformation in which the urethra opens out onto the ventral surface of the penis.

Bone and joint malformations

Developmental dysplasia of the hip (DDH) and talipes equinovarus (club foot) are the most common osteoarticular anomalies.

DDH should be diagnosed and treated promptly to ensure the best outcome

Developmental dysplasia of the hip is an imperfect development of the hip joint which predisposes the joint to dislocation. The anomaly may affect the femoral head, the acetabulum, or both. DDH affects 1–2 per 1000 live births and should be screened for during the routine clinical examination performed on all newborn babies.

The typical form of DDH occurs in a neurologically normal child, commonly affecting the left hip, and is four times as common in girls than it is in boys. A positive family history, being first born, breech delivery, and oligohydramnios all predispose children to DDH. DDH should be treated promptly to prevent the development of osteoarthritis of the hip.

Talipes equinovarus, or clubfoot, is a deformity of the foot and ankle involving several joints

Talipes equinovarus, or clubfoot, describes a deformity in which the forefoot is adducted (toward the midline of the body) and supinated (upturned), and the hindfoot points downwards (equinus deformity). It affects about 1 in 1000 live births. It is usually an isolated, idiopathic abnormality, but may be associated with spina bifida or compression *in utero* secondary to oligohydramnios. The severity of the deformity is variable. If conservative treatment is ineffective, surgical treatment can be considered.

Key points: Bone and joint malformations

- Developmental dysplasia of the hip can cause dislocation of the hip. Hip instability should always be looked for at birth so that subsequent joint malformation can be avoided.

- Talipes equinovarus (club foot) is a deformity of the foot and ankle, of variable severity, which in most cases is idiopathic.

Central nervous system malformations

Malformations of the CNS are common (5 to 10 per 1000 live births). Their causes may be genetic (gene mutation or chromosomal anomaly) or environmental (viruses, chemicals, and drugs).

Neural tube defects result from failure of the fusion of the neural tube

The neural tube is formed between days 20 and 28 of embryogenesis when the neural groove closes off. Failure of this process, or subsequent reopening of a region of the tube, may result in a variety of problems.

- **Anencephaly** is due to defective closure of the rostral end of the neural tube. Neonates have no cerebral cortex or cranium. This is a fatal condition.

- **Meningoencephalocele** is protrusion of the brain and meninges through a midline skull defect, usually in the occipital region. It is often associated with other cerebral malformations.

- **Spina bifida** is due to defective closure of the neural tube, usually towards the caudal end of the tube (Fig. 22.10). **Meningocele** is a posterior outpouching of the meninges through the defect in the vertebral arch. **Meningomyelocele** is similar, except that the meningeal-lined protrusion also contains a loop of spinal cord. This may lead to problems such as urinary incontinence, constipation, and variable degrees of motor and sensory impairment of the legs.

The incidence of neural tube defects has declined because of maternal folic acid supplementation around the time of conception, and termination of pregnancy following their detection on antenatal ultrasound scans.

Congenital hydrocephalus may be due to aqueduct stenosis or the Arnold–Chiari malformation

Hydrocephalus reflects excessive expansion of the ventricles due to excess CSF, and results from abnormal production, flow, or absorption of CSF. The most common cause of congenital hydrocephalus is aqueduct stenosis, in which an abnormally narrowed cerebral aqueduct obstructs the normal flow of CSF from the third to the fourth ventricle.

The Arnold–Chiari malformation is a malformation of the base of the skull associated with inferior displacement of the cerebellum and medulla oblongata

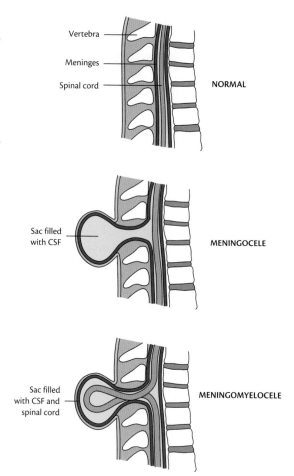

Fig. 22.10 Types of spina bifida.

into the upper spinal canal. The foramina of Magendie and Luschka, by which CSF normally exits the fourth ventricle, are compressed by the bony ridge of the foramen magnum, and so CSF flow is obstructed.

Key points: Central nervous system malformations

- Neural tube defects result from failure of the fusion of the neural tube before 28 days of gestation.

- Such defects include anencephaly, meningocele, and meningomyelocele.

> ## Key points: Central nervous system malformations—cont'd
>
> ◆ Congenital hydrocephalus is usually the result of impaired flow of CSF caused by either cerebral aqueduct stenosis or Arnold–Chiari malformation.

The older child

Beyond 1 year of life, most childhood diseases are related to infection. In the western world, most deaths in children older than 1 year are due to accidents, malignant neoplasms, or the effects of congenital anomalies.

Cardiovascular disease

The most common cardiac diseases affecting older children are the effects of CHDs. Acquired cardiovascular disease is uncommon in children compared with adults because children have not yet developed atherosclerosis. The most common acquired cardiac condition affecting children in the developed world is Kawasaki disease.

Kawasaki disease

Kawasaki disease is an acute vasculitis of childhood which was first described in Japan but has now been described in children of all races and ethnicities. The majority of affected children are under the age of 5 years. The precise cause remains unknown, though an infectious cause is suspected.

Kawasaki disease causes the sudden onset of fever that lasts for 5 days or longer. On examination, there is an inflamed throat, an erythematous tongue, and dry, red, cracked lips. Cervical lymphadenopathy is often prominent. There may be erythema and pain of the hands and feet.

The importance of Kawasaki disease is related to the effect that the vasculitis has on the coronary arteries. During the healing process, the coronary arteries are prone to developing aneurysms. Although in most cases these coronary artery aneurysms cause no symptoms and regress over time, thrombosis within an aneurysm may occur, causing myocardial infarction in the child.

Aneurysm formation can be prevented by the prompt administration of intravenous immunoglobulin.

> ## Key points: Kawasaki disease
>
> ◆ Kawasaki disease is a vasculitis of childhood which presents with fever, oral changes, and cervical lymphadenopathy.
>
> ◆ Kawasaki disease is important because, untreated, coronary artery aneurysms may develop.
>
> ◆ Thrombosis in a coronary artery aneurysm can cause myocardial infarction in a child.
>
> ◆ Prompt recognition and treatment of Kawasaki disease is important to prevent coronary artery aneurysm formation.

Respiratory disease

Respiratory disorders are responsible for up to one-third of acute paediatric admissions to hospital. Many of these are due to infections, and indeed respiratory infections are the most common infections in childhood.

The risk factors for respiratory tract infections include premature birth, congenital heart disease, chronic lung disease, and immunocompromise. Parental smoking is also a major factor, so much so that it has been estimated that 10–15 per cent of all acute paediatric beds could be closed if parental smoking could be eliminated, or at least significantly reduced.

Most respiratory pathogens can cause any one of the respiratory infections, ranging from mild rhinitis to potentially life-threatening bronchiolitis and pneumonia. Viruses cause 80–90 per cent of childhood respiratory infections. Dual infections with a viral and a bacterial pathogen, or two viruses, are also common.

> ### LINK BOX
>
> ### Recurrent respiratory tract infections
>
> If a child has persistent or recurrent symptoms of respiratory infections, consider the possibility of an underlying disorder such as a primary immunodeficiency (p. 48) or cystic fibrosis (p. 518).

Croup

Croup is an infection of the larynx, trachea, and bronchi ('laryngotracheobronchitis') caused by viruses such as parainfluenza. Croup is characterized by the sudden onset of hoarseness with a barking cough. The child may be breathless and also have stridor. The infection is usually self-limiting.

Epiglottitis

Epiglottitis is an infection of the upper respiratory tract by the bacterium *Haemophilus influenzae* which causes acute inflammation and swelling of the epiglottis. In severe cases, the markedly swollen epiglottis may suddenly obstruct the upper airway. Thankfully, epiglottitis is a rapidly disappearing disease due to immunization against *H. influenzae*.

Bronchiolitis

Bronchiolitis is a viral infection of the bronchioles which commonly occurs in infancy, particularly during the winter months. Respiratory syncytial virus (RSV) accounts for 70 per cent of cases. Parainfluenza, adenovirus, and influenza virus are responsible for many of the other cases. The peak incidence of bronchiolitis is between 2 and 4 months of age.

RSV replicates in the epithelium lining the nasopharynx and the bronchus, and in the lung alveolar macrophages. It causes necrosis of the epithelial cells and proliferation of the goblet cells, stimulating mucus production. Luminal debris and mucus, combined with submucosal oedema and host inflammatory cells in the wall of the airway, cause airway obstruction, which is manifested clinically as expiratory wheezing.

As the airways of infants have a smaller luminal diameter relative to the wall thickness compared with older children, as well as higher airway resistance, the bronchiolitis is more severe in infants. The bronchiolar obstruction causes increased airway resistance, with patchy atelectasis (collapse of lung tissue) and, due to the added effect of coughing, alveolar tearing leading to interstitial emphysema.

In infants under 6 months, bronchodilators are usually ineffective, as the airflow obstruction is mainly due to mucus plugging and mucosal oedema. Resolution of bronchiolitis begins within 3 or 4 days as the epithelial cells start to regenerate. By 2 weeks, most infants will have recovered clinically, though approximately half of them will continue to have wheezing episodes over the next few years. In some of these children, the wheezing may in fact be an early manifestation of asthma. This is more likely if the child has a family history of atopic disease or is exposed to parental smoking.

Pneumonia

In older children, bacterial pneumonia is usually more common than viral pneumonia. As in adults, the vast majority of these are caused by *Streptococcus pneumoniae*. In school age children, *Mycoplasma pneumoniae* is also a common cause of pneumonia.

Resolution of pneumonia follows in most cases within 3 weeks. However, complications such as pleural effusion, empyema, lung abscess, and septicaemia may develop in a small proportion of cases. These are more common in children with underlying chronic lung disease, congenital heart disease, or neurological disease.

Asthma

Asthma is a chronic airways disease in which bronchial hyper-reactivity causes episodic symptoms of cough, breathlessness, and wheeze due to airway narrowing.

Asthma is the most common chronic disease in childhood, affecting up to 10 per cent of all children. It is responsible for 10–20 per cent of all acute medical admissions to paediatric wards. The incidence of asthma is increasing, alongside an increase in atopic disease generally. The reason for this rise is not clear, although there are theories that this could be related to a fall in common childhood infections altering the way the immune system develops.

Key points: Respiratory disease

- Respiratory infections are the most common infections in childhood.

- Croup is an infection of the larger airways caused by parainfluenza virus leading to hoarseness and a barking cough.

- Epiglottitis is an infection of the upper airways caused by *H. influenzae* which can result in marked swelling of the epiglottis and sudden upper airway obstruction.

Key points: Respiratory disease—cont'd

- Bronchiolitis is a common infection of infants caused by respiratory syncytial virus.

- Pneumonia in older children is usually caused by *S. pneumoniae*.

- Asthma is a very common cause of chronic illness in childhood and its incidence is increasing.

Gastrointestinal disease

Gastro-oesophageal reflux disease

Gastro-oesophageal reflux disease (GORD) refers to symptoms attributable to reflux of gastric contents into the lower oesophagus. In children, it is most common in infancy due to their supine position and a liquid diet. Other conditions that predispose to GORD include cerebral palsy and Down's syndrome.

Symptoms in infants are usually vomiting, crying, and irritability. Older children with GORD usually vocalize their symptoms and complain of a burning retrosternal pain (heartburn) as in adults. In 80 per cent of patients, the symptoms resolve by 18 months. The sequelae of GORD in children include aspiration, erosive oesophagitis, leading to stricture, and failure to thrive. Barrett's oesophagus is an uncommon complication in children.

In children, 24 h monitoring of oesophageal pH, and upper gastrointestinal tract endoscopy are useful to establish the diagnosis and to grade the severity of GORD.

Pyloric stenosis

Pyloric stenosis is an obstruction at the level of pylorus of the stomach due to marked hypertrophy of the muscularis propria of the pyloric wall. It presents between 2 to 4 weeks of age with recurrent projectile, nonbilious vomiting within 30 minutes of a feed.

Pyloric stenosis occurs in approximately 1 out of 300 live births, and is most prevalent in Caucasians. After inguinal hernia, it is the second most common condition requiring surgery during the first two months of life.

Gastroenteritis

Gastroenteritis is a common reason for hospital admission as very young children can rapidly become dehydrated. Rotavirus and adenovirus are the most common causes of gastroenteritis in children under 2 years of age. Rotavirus accounts for 60 per cent of cases in outbreaks, particularly during winter months.

Bacterial gastroenteritis is accompanied by blood in the stools, with or without mucus, and is most likely to occur in the summer months. *Salmonella*, *Shigella*, and *Campylobacter* species are the three most common causes of bacterial infection in children worldwide.

The majority of children recover from an episode of acute gastroenteritis, but a few lapse into a malabsorptive state lasting for weeks or months (post-enteritis enteropathy).

Gluten-sensitive enteropathy

Gluten-sensitive enteropathy is a dietary intolerance to gluten leading to inflammation in the small bowel and malabsorption (p. 153). In children, it is an important cause of failure to thrive and delayed puberty.

As in adults, measurement of serum endomysial antibodies is useful as a screening test for gluten-sensitive enteropathy, though in children under 2 years antigliadin levels may be of more value. Histopathological examination of a duodenal biopsy remains the gold standard for the diagnosis.

Acute appendicitis

Acute appendicitis is the most common cause of an acute abdomen in children. It may occur at any age, but is most common after 5 years of age and is rare in children less than 2 years old. Acute appendicitis is caused by obstruction of the lumen of the appendix, and in children this is usually due to either a faecolith, enlarged lymphoid follicles in the appendiceal mucosa, or *Enterobius vermicularis* worms filling the lumen.

Mesenteric adenitis

Mesenteric adenitis is infection and enlargement of mesenteric lymph nodes which may be seen in association with an upper respiratory tract infection. It is thought to occur due to swallowing of infected sputum. Mesenteric adenitis presents as a systemic illness with abdominal symptoms and is an important differential diagnosis for acute appendicitis.

Intussusception

Intussusception occurs when a segment of bowel 'telescopes' in on itself, causing obstruction. Intussusception is the most frequent cause of intestinal obstruction between 3 months and 2 years of age. The cause is unknown in the majority of cases though it may follow adenoviral infection of the lymphoid tissue of the gastrointestinal tract. A lead point, such as an inverted Meckel's diverticulum, is discovered in fewer than 10 per cent of cases. Intussusception is also seen in cystic fibrosis (possibly related to faecal overloading with a bolus of sticky thick faeces acting as a lead point) and Henoch Schönlein purpura (with a haematoma acting as a lead point).

Inflammatory bowel disease

Crohn's disease (p. 155) and ulcerative colitis (p. 163) are chronic relapsing intestinal disorders believed to be caused by an inappropriate immune response to commensal gut bacteria. Approximately 25 per cent of patients with chronic inflammatory bowel disease present before the age of 20.

Crohn's disease occurring in childhood is an important cause of growth failure. In addition to the usual characteristic gastrointestinal manifestations of Crohn's disease (diarrhoea, abdominal pain, and weight loss), children and adolescents may also exhibit prominent extraintestinal manifestations, such as joint symptoms, delayed puberty, and growth failure.

INTERESTING TO KNOW

Infliximab for Crohn's disease in children

Infliximab is a monoclonal antibody against TNF-α, which is used for treatment of Crohn's disease that is resistant to standard treatment. Evidence so far indicates that it may be more potent in children than in adults because some children who have received it early in the development of the disease have shown sustained remission for several years. If this response is seen consistently in further studies, infliximab could be used as the first line therapy at the onset of the disease.

Ulcerative colitis diagnosed in patients before the age of 20 is more likely to be associated with a positive family history of the disease. In contrast to adults, rectal biopsies from children with ulcerative colitis may be normal or show only minimal architectural abnormalities and inflammation. Regular colonoscopic screening of patients for colonic dysplasia should begin 10 years after the onset of symptoms even if the patient is still young.

Infectious colitis

Children infected with invasive bacteria such as *Salmonella*, *Shigella*, or *E. coli* may develop bloody diarrhoea as in adults. One important complication of infection with *E. coli* O157 is the development of haemolytic-uraemic syndrome (HUS) which is the most common cause of acute renal failure in children.

Key points: Gastrointestinal disease

- Gastro-oesophageal reflux disease is common in infants due to their supine position and liquid feeds. It usually causes vomiting, crying, and irritability. Older children may vocalize symptoms of heartburn.

- Pyloric stenosis is gastric outflow obstruction caused by marked hypertrophy of the muscularis propria of the pyloric wall. It causes projectile vomiting after feeds and requires surgery.

- Gastroenteritis in children should be taken seriously as young children can become rapidly dehydrated.

- Gluten-sensitive enteropathy is an important cause of failure to thrive or delayed puberty in children.

- Acute appendicitis is the most common cause of the acute abdomen in children. It is commonly caused by obstruction of the appendix by a faecolith, enlarged lymphoid tissue, or *Enterobius* worms.

- Mesenteric adenitis is an inflammation and enlargement of mesenteric lymph nodes which may present similarly to acute appendicitis.

Liver disease

Liver diseases are generally uncommon in childhood, but they are an important cause of morbidity and mortality. As in adults, liver diseases may come to light either following a clinically apparent episode of acute liver injury with jaundice and deranged liver function tests, or more insidiously with features of chronic liver disease.

Hepatitis A infection is the most common viral hepatitis seen in children. It is acquired through contaminated food or water and typically causes an episode of acute icteric hepatitis which resolves completely over a period of weeks with no lasting complications. Hepatitis B and C are not often newly acquired by children as these are transmitted sexually or by blood.

Non-alcoholic liver disease refers to a range of liver disorders with identical features to alcoholic liver disease but which occur in association with obesity and diabetes rather than alcohol (p. 187). The rising epidemic of obesity in children and adolescents has resulted in increasing cases of non-alcoholic fatty liver disease and non-alcoholic steatohepatitis (NASH). NASH is important as there is a danger of progressive fibrosis culminating in cirrhosis.

Autoimmune hepatitis is primarily a disease of adults (p. 188) but may appear at any age. It may present as an acute liver disease or as a chronic liver disease. The clinical features in children are similar to those in adults.

Primary sclerosing cholangitis is a biliary disease in which large bile ducts are destroyed by an inflammatory attack (p. 189). Although seen mostly in adults, it is being increasingly recognized in children. The clinical and histological features of childhood PSC are often different from those of the adult form, raising some doubt as to whether PSC occurring in childhood is in fact a different disease process.

α_1-Antitrypsin deficiency is an inherited disorder in which liver disease is caused by the accumulation of α_1-antitrypsin in the liver. The progress of the liver disease is extremely unpredictable. It may produce jaundice and liver disease early in the neonatal period within days of birth, or present during childhood, or in adult life.

Wilson's disease is an inherited disorder that results in accumulation of copper, particularly in the liver, brain, and eyes (p. 191). Wilson's disease may present as an episode of acute liver disease or with chronic liver disease. Any child with liver disease must have the diagnosis considered, as missing this treatable form of liver disease is a disaster.

Liver transplantation is the definitive and life-saving treatment for children who have acute fulminant liver failure or end-stage chronic liver disease. Chronic liver disease accounts for three-quarters of liver transplants in children, most of which are due to biliary disorders and α_1-antitrypsin deficiency.

Continued

> ## Key points: Liver disease—cont'd
>
> ◆ α_1-Antitrypsin deficiency and Wilson's disease are important inherited causes of liver disease in children.
>
> ◆ Liver transplantation may be performed for children with acute liver failure or end-stage chronic liver disease.

Renal disease

Acute renal failure

Acute renal failure is a potentially reversible sudden decline in renal function over a period of days or weeks. As in adults, the causes of acute renal failure can be divided into pre-renal, renal, and post-renal. Unlike adults, however, pre-renal causes are much less common in developed countries because of improved resuscitation of children with conditions such as diarrhoea, trauma, and burns.

Haemolytic–uraemic syndrome is the most common cause of childhood acute renal failure

In the UK, the most frequent cause of acute renal failure in children is HUS. HUS is a serious complication of infectious colitis caused by verocytotoxin-producing *E. coli* (VTEC), usually of the serotype O157. The toxin enters the blood stream where it damages the endothelial cells of the microcirculation.

HUS is one of the **thrombotic microangiopathies**, in which microthrombi develop in capillaries, shearing up red blood cells as they pass through. HUS therefore presents with the sudden onset of haemolytic anaemia, thrombocytopenia, and acute renal failure following an attack of bloody diarrhoea.

Glomerulonephritis is the other major cause of childhood acute renal failure

About 20 per cent of childhood acute renal failure is due to a severe glomerulonephritis. The most common form is post-streptococcal glomerulonephritis. Severe renal involvement in Henoch Schönlein purpura (see later) may also cause acute renal failure.

Chronic renal failure

Chronic renal failure is a slowly progressive decline in renal function. The causes of chronic renal failure in children are closely related to the age of the child. Before age 10, congenital anomalies and obstructive uropathy are the most common causes. After age 10, glomerular diseases and reflux nephropathy are the important causes.

One of the main complications of chronic renal failure in children is failure of growth as a result of medication, endocrine abnormalities, and renal bone disease.

Glomerular disease

By far the most common glomerular disease in children is **minimal change disease**, which typically presents with the nephrotic syndrome. Because most children with the nephrotic syndrome have minimal change disease, a renal biopsy is not normally performed. The child is started on steroid therapy, and steroid responsiveness is a good indicator of the diagnosis. Renal biopsy is therefore only performed if the clinical picture is atypical or if there is a poor response to steroid treatment.

> ## Key points: Renal disease
>
> ◆ The most common cause of acute renal failure in childhood is haemolytic–uraemic syndrome, a thrombotic microangiopathy that follows an attack of bloody diarrhoea caused by *E. coli* O157.
>
> ◆ The most frequent causes of chronic renal failure in children are congenital anomalies of the urinary tract and reflux nephropathy.
>
> ◆ Minimal change disease is the most common glomerular disease in children, presenting with the nephrotic syndrome.

Urological disease

Urinary tract infection

Urinary tract infections (UTIs) are among the most common bacterial infections of children and are responsible for many acute febrile illnesses in childhood. Like adults, the most common organism is *E. coli*.

UTIs in children are often a marker of an underlying abnormality in the urinary tract. About 40 per cent of children with UTIs have an associated urinary tract abnormality. Half of these are due to vesicoureteric reflux; the remainder have malformations such as duplications or an obstruction.

The danger of UTI in children is the risk of *renal scarring*, which if severe may lead to chronic renal failure many years later. The risk of permanent renal damage is greatest in infants with severe vesicoureteric reflux (VUR) and so a priority is to investigate whether VUR is present and if so how severe it is. This is usually achieved using a technique known as a **micturating cystourethrogram**.

Children found to have VUR are usually given prophylactic antibiotics until 4 years of age, after which time new renal scars do not seem to occur. Surgical reimplantation of the ureters is also an option in severe cases.

Testicular torsion

Testicular torsion occurs when a freely mobile testis twists completely on the spermatic cord and cuts off its own blood supply. An ischaemic testis presents with a unilateral red swollen painful testis.

Although other disorders may cause similar features (e.g. a torsion of the hydatid of Morgagni or epididymo-orchitis), if there is any suspicion of testicular torsion then surgical exploration of the scrotum is mandatory. Provided surgical intervention takes place within 6 h, the testis should still be viable and it can be untwisted and fixed to the scrotum. Any further delay risks irreversible infarction of the testis which will appear black at operation and must be excised.

Key points: Urological disease

- Urinary tract infections are extremely common bacterial infections of childhood.

- A UTI in a child may be a marker of an underlying structural anomaly of the urinary tract and should be investigated.

- The danger of recurrent urinary tract infections in children is the development of permanent renal scarring which if severe may lead to chronic renal failure in later life.

- Renal scarring is most likely to occur in infants with severe vesicoureteric reflux and this should always be investigated in a child with UTI aged under 5 years.

- Testicular torsion occurs when the testis twists on the spermatic cord and cuts off its own blood supply.

- Testicular torsion is a paediatric surgical emergency requiring immediate exploration of the scrotum and fixation of the testis before it irreversibly infarcts.

Bone and joint disease

Septic arthritis

Septic arthritis is a bacterial infection of the joint space which requires prompt diagnosis and treatment to prevent subsequent joint destruction.

The main portals of entry into the joint space for bacteria are haematogenous spread and direct spread from the surrounding soft tissues. Bacteria may also gain entry through the epiphysis of a bone or joint affected by osteomyelitis.

A single joint is commonly affected, usually the hip, shoulder, or elbow. It generally occurs either in the first 2 years of life or in adolescence. *Staphylococcus aureus* is generally the most common bacteria, and in children this is followed by *H. influenzae* (children under 2), salmonella, streptococci, and gonococci (late adolescence).

Juvenile chronic arthritis

Juvenile chronic arthritis (JCA) is a chronic inflammatory joint disease affecting 1 in 1000 children. The peak age of onset is 1–3 years, with a second peak occurring during adolescence.

JCA is defined by the presence of joint swelling, or two of the following features: joint tenderness, decreased range of motion, pain on range of motion, or joint warmth. To make the diagnosis, these features must have been present for 6 weeks, and the affected individual must be younger than 16 years of age.

The exact events which trigger and perpetuate the joint inflammation in JCA have yet to be defined. Although the weight of evidence favours the hypothesis that joint inflammation is antigen driven, it is still unclear whether such antigens are derived from infectious agents or are true autoantigens.

Juvenile chronic arthritis differs from rheumatoid arthritis in four ways

Features distinguishing JCA from rheumatoid arthritis (p. 409) are as follows:

- Oligoarthritis is more common in JCA, rather than polyarthritis.

- Large joints are commonly affected in JCA.

- Systemic disease is more common in JCA (spiking fevers, skin rash, hepatosplenomegaly, serositis).

- Fewer than 10 per cent of JCA patients are positive for rheumatoid factor.

The management of JCA is, however, similar to that of rheumatoid arthritis. Complications of the disease are joint destruction, impaired growth, and infections secondary to immunosuppressive therapy. A significant proportion of patients will still have the disease 10 years following diagnosis.

Key points: Bone and joint disease

- Septic arthritis is a bacterial infection of the joint, usually caused by *S. aureus*. Urgent diagnosis and treatment are needed to prevent joint destruction.

- Juvenile chronic arthritis is a chronic inflammatory joint disease of children which may manifest with or without systemic symptoms.

- Treatment of juvenile chronic arthritis is similar to that of rheumatoid arthritis.

Nervous system and muscle disease

Meningitis

Meningitis is an infection of the arachnoid space (p. 429). We have already seen how in neonates, *E. coli* and group B streptococcus are common causes. In older children, *N. meningitidis* and *S. pneumoniae* are the main pathogens. *Haemophilus influenzae* has become less common since the introduction of a vaccine against the organism. Bacterial meningitis is a serious disease; mortality is 5–10 per cent and permanent neurological sequelae occur in 10–20 per cent of survivors.

Cerebral palsy

Cerebral palsy is an umbrella term covering a group of non-progressive disorders of movement, tone, and posture due to a defect of the immature brain. The severity of cerebral palsy varies considerably from extremely mild to extremely severe. It is the most common cause of physical disability in the UK, with an incidence of 2 in every 1000 live births. Pre-term and low birth weight infants are at particular risk of cerebral palsy.

As well as motor problems, there may also be epilepsy, learning difficulties, and impairment of vision, hearing, and speech. Important complications are gastro-oesophageal reflux disease and aspiration pneumonia. Therefore, a multidisciplinary approach is essential for management of children with cerebral palsy.

Although complications during birth leading to cerebral hypoxia have been implicated in cerebral palsy, these cases account for a minority (~10%). Most cases appear to be due to antenatal insults to the developing brain, including intrauterine infections.

Muscular dystrophy

Muscular dystrophy encompasses a number of diseases characterized by progressive muscle wasting. **Duchenne muscular dystrophy** (DMD) is the most common form of muscular dystrophy and is also the most severe, with symptoms presenting in infancy, and most affected individuals are wheelchair bound by the age of 11. **Becker muscular dystrophy** (BMD) is a similar but much less aggressive form of the disease with a later age of onset and milder symptoms.

DMD and BMD are both caused by mutations in the DMD gene

Both DMD and BMD are single gene disorders caused by a malfunctioning gene on the X chromosome. They are both recessive diseases, and therefore occur much more commonly in males than in females. The occurrence of DMD is about 1 in 3500 males, while BMD is much less common, with an occurrence of 1 in 20 000 males.

The disease gene is named DMD and is the largest known gene in the human genome (2.2 million base pairs of DNA). The protein is called dystrophin, and is located under the membranes of muscle cells. The function of the protein is to join the muscle cell's cytoskeleton to the extracellular matrix.

In DMD, very little dystrophin is produced and the muscle cells become more permeable, causing them to swell and burst. In BMD, near normal amounts of dystrophin are produced, but there are subtle differences in the structure of the protein which adversely affects its function.

Muscular dystrophy causes progressive muscle weakness

DMD affects boys from about 3 years of age, with gradually worsening muscle weakness. The first symptoms include difficulties with walking normally and getting up off the floor. Progressive deterioration leaves the patient relying on a wheelchair by age 11 and the disease is generally fatal by age 18 due to a combination of respiratory failure and cardiac failure.

Although the disease is characterized by loss of muscle cells, the overall size of certain muscles, such as those of the calves, appears to increase as the muscle fibres are replaced by fat and connective tissue ('pseudohypertrophy').

The symptoms of BMD are very similar, but they usually do not appear until the patient is in his teens, and may present much later in life. The progression of the disease is much slower than DMD, and BMD patients can expect a near normal lifespan.

Treatment of muscular dystrophy is supportive

The diagnosis of DMD and BMD is now confirmed by analysis of the DMD gene for mutations. Although regular physiotherapy can help to prolong mobility, no curative treatment is available for DMD or BMD. However, these diseases are prime targets for gene therapy because they represent defects in a single gene affecting an easily accessible tissue.

Key points: Nervous system and muscle disease

- Meningitis in older children is usually caused by *N. meningitidis* and *S. pneumoniae*. Bacterial meningitis in children is a serious disease, with a significant risk of permanent neurological sequelae.

- Cerebral palsy is a non-progressive neuromuscular disorder due to damage to the immature brain. In most cases, the damage appears to occur before birth.

- Muscular dystrophies are a group of inherited disorders which cause progressive muscle wasting.

- Duchenne muscular dystrophy is the most common form. It is also the most severe, with most children wheelchair bound by age 11.

- Becker muscular dystrophy is a much less aggressive form with a later age of onset and milder symptoms.

- Both Duchenne and Becker muscular dystrophy are caused by mutations in the DMD gene on the X chromosome.

Multisystem disease

In adults, multisystem diseases are mostly immunologically mediated diseases. In children, immune diseases may also cause multisystem disease, e.g. Henoch Schönlein purpura, though genetic diseases are also important, e.g. cystic fibrosis and Down's syndrome.

Down's syndrome

Down's syndrome is a chromosomal disorder due to the presence of an extra chromosome 21 (trisomy 21). The presence of an extra autosome is usually incompatible with full-term development, and results in spontaneous abortion. Trisomy 21 is the only autosomal trisomy compatible with a normal lifespan; this is probably because chromosome 21 contains only about 240 genes.

The incidence of Down's syndrome is strongly related to maternal age. Down's syndrome has an incidence of 1 in 1500 in mothers in their early 20s, but rises sharply to as much as 1 in 30 by the time the mother is 45.

Down's syndrome is usually caused by non-disjunction of chromosome 21 during meiosis

The most common mechanism leading to trisomy 21 is **non-disjunction** during meiosis. The paired chromosomes fail to separate as the cell divides, leaving one cell with two copies and the other with none. If this gamete fertilizes with a normal egg or sperm, it will produce an embryo with three copies of the chromosome.

Down's syndrome is associated with a number of abnormalities

Features of Down's syndrome include mild to moderate mental retardation, limited growth, characteristic facial features (slanting eyes sometimes with a squint, small ears, open mouth with protruding tongue, small nose), and a single palmar crease.

Other problems associated with Down's syndrome include structural congenital anomalies of the heart (mostly AVSD and VSD) and duodenal atresia (Fig. 22.11). Hypothyroidism and acute leukaemia are also more common.

The life expectancy of Down's individuals is lower than normal because of these associated disorders. However, life expectancy can be as high as 40–50 years, and there is no effect on fertility.

LINK BOX

Down's syndrome and Alzheimer's disease

Older Down's patients are at increased risk of developing Alzheimer's disease, presumably because they inherit an extra copy of the APP protein which becomes the Aβ amyloid in amyloid plaques (p. 434).

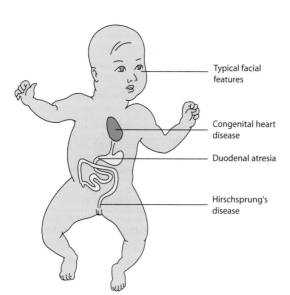

Fig. 22.11 Features of Down's syndrome.

Typical facial features

Congenital heart disease

Duodenal atresia

Hirschsprung's disease

Antenatal screening picks up most cases of Down's syndrome

Many cases of Down's syndrome are diagnosed pre-natally, and pre-natal testing is recommended for older mothers. If the diagnosis is not picked up antenatally, Down's syndrome can be diagnosed at birth by the facial appearance of affected babies and the characteristic hypotonia (poor muscle tone) resulting in floppiness. Blood tests are then carried out to confirm the diagnosis by looking for the extra copy of chromosome 21 or other abnormalities involving this chromosome.

Key points: Down's syndrome

♦ Down's syndrome is one of the most common chromosomal disorders.

♦ Down's syndrome is associated with trisomy 21.

♦ The incidence of Down's syndrome is strongly linked to maternal age.

♦ Individuals with Down's syndrome have a typical facial appearance. There is a strong association with a number of underlying structural anomalies including congenital heart disease and duodenal atresia.

♦ Most cases of Down's syndrome are diagnosed on antenatal screening.

Cystic fibrosis

Cystic fibrosis (CF) is the most common lethal genetic disease, with an incidence of 1 in 2500 in Caucasians. It is a multisystem disease affecting many organs including the lung, pancreas, and gastrointestinal tract. The spectrum of the disease is extremely wide, ranging from mild disease to patients with severe disease who die early from respiratory failure.

Cystic fibrosis is caused by mutation in the CFTR gene

Cystic fibrosis is caused by a mutation in the **cystic fibrosis transmembrane conductance regulator** (CFTR) gene. CFTR is a chloride channel present in the apical surface of epithelial cells lining the luminal passages of the sweat ducts, intestines, bile ducts, pancreatic ducts, airways, and vas deferens.

More than 1000 disease-associated mutations have been described in the CFTR gene, though 70 per cent of CF patients have a deletion of the codon for phenylalanine at position 508 (the ΔF508 mutation).

Defective CFTR leads to impaction of thick secretions in secretory organs

Defects in CFTR function result in chloride impermeability. As a consequence, the epithelial cells lining luminal passages reabsorb excess sodium and water, and the luminal secretions become extremely thick and tenacious, blocking the lumen (Fig. 22.12).

Meconium ileus is the first presentation of cystic fibrosis in 15 per cent of cases

Cystic fibrosis may present in the newborn with a type of bowel obstruction called **meconium ileus**, which is caused by thick inspissated meconium. Typically, the distal one-third of the ileum contains meconium concretions, while the middle third of ileum is dilated by greenish black, thick meconium. Fifty per cent of cases are complicated by volvulus or perforation.

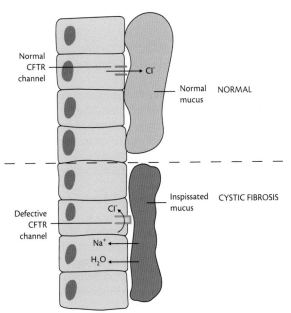

Fig. 22.12 Cystic fibrosis. Dysfunction of CFTR leads to excess sodium and water reabsorption by luminal epithelial cells, resulting in thick viscid secretions on epithelial surfaces.

Pancreatic insufficiency occurs in over 90 per cent of cases

Dehydrated pancreatic secretions plug the pancreatic ducts, and stasis eventually leads to autodigestion of the pancreas. The majority of the patients with cystic fibrosis have pancreatic enzyme insufficiency early in life. Pancreatic insufficiency typically leads to florid steatorrhoea due to fat malabsorption. Some children develop diabetes.

Biliary cirrhosis and gallstones may occur in cystic fibrosis

In cystic fibrosis, the viscosity of bile is increased and the biliary channels may become plugged with inspissated secretions, leading to chronic liver disease and cirrhosis. Abnormal mucin in the gallbladder and malabsorption of bile acids results in gallstones in many patients.

Progressive pulmonary disease is the major cause of morbidity and mortality in cystic fibrosis

Blockage of airways in the lungs by thick secretions provides a fertile ground for colonization of the lung by microbes. *Pseudomonas aeruginosa* is often a dominant infection, causing repetitive resistant infections. Recurrent lung infections often lead to bronchiectasis. The majority of the deaths associated with cystic fibrosis result from progressive lung disease.

> ## Key points: Cystic fibrosis
>
> - Cystic fibrosis is caused by an inherited mutation in the CFTR gene.
>
> - CFTR codes for a chloride channel found in the apical membrane of epithelial cells lining secretory passages.
>
> - Defective activity of the chloride channel results in sodium and water reabsorption and the creation of thick viscid secretion in the lumens of affected organs.
>
> - Blockage of the small bowel by thick meconium in cystic fibrosis may cause meconium ileus in the neonatal period.

Continued

> ### Key points: Cystic fibrosis—cont'd
>
> - Blockage of pancreatic ducts causes chronic pancreatitis and pancreatic insufficiency.
>
> - Blockage of airways leads to recurrent pulmonary infections and bronchiectasis.
>
> - The majority of deaths in cystic fibrosis are related to progressive pulmonary disease.

Henoch Schönlein purpura

Henoch Schönlein purpura (HSP) is a systemic vasculitis of children. It typically involves the skin, gastrointestinal tract, joints, and kidneys. The cause of the vasculitis is not known for certain, though about half of all cases appear to be triggered by a streptococcal upper respiratory tract infection.

The typical presentation of HSP is with a purpuric rash over the backs of the legs and buttocks, with abdominal pain, vomiting, and painful knees and ankles. In about half of cases, there is also a glomerulonephritis leading to haematuria and proteinuria. Acute renal failure only occurs in a minority of cases.

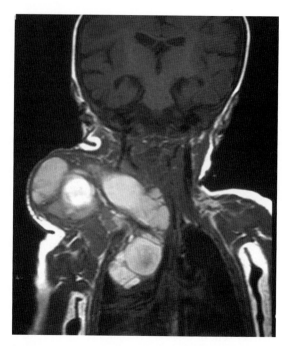

Fig. 22.13 MRI scan showing a huge lymphangioma arising in the neck. You can see how even a benign tumour can be extremely difficult to remove completely if it grows in a critical location.

> **LINK BOX**
>
> ### HSP and IgA nephropathy
>
> HSP and IgA nephropathy (p. 215) are related disorders in that the renal involvement is identical in both, with mesangial IgA deposition. IgA nephropathy affects young adults and only affects the kidneys, whereas HSP occurs mostly in children and also affects the skin, gastrointestinal tract, and joints.

Paediatric tumours

As in adults, paediatric tumours are classified into benign or malignant categories.

Lymphangiomas and haemangiomas are common benign childhood neoplasms

Lymphangiomas are benign neoplasms composed of dilated lymph channels which can attain large sizes (Fig. 22.13). Although benign, large lymphangiomas may be extremely difficult to excise completely if the lymphatic channels creep into the surrounding tissues.

Haemangiomas are benign neoplasms composed of dilated blood vessels of various sizes. They are the most common skin and soft tissue tumours of infancy. They proliferate rapidly over the first year, then involute over the next 5–7 years. A small number may cause permanent disfigurement and functional compromise.

Cancer is an important cause of death and morbidity in childhood

Cancer is one of the leading causes of death in childhood, accounting for over 20 per cent of deaths in children between 1 and 14 years of age. In the UK, approximately 1500 new cases of childhood cancer are diagnosed every year and approximately 300 children die from cancer every year.

In adults, environmental factors are of major importance in the development of malignancy, e.g. smoking in lung carcinoma and diet in colorectal carcinoma.

In contrast, the aetiology of many childhood cancers remains uncertain. Important causative factors of childhood cancers include the following:

- Genetic predisposition. Children with Down's syndrome have 10–20 times greater risk of developing leukaemia than healthy children.

- Ionizing radiation. Exposure to radiation in the third trimester increases the risk of childhood cancer.

Children suffer from different types of cancer than adults

The spectrum of cancers in childhood is very different from that in adults. Many childhood tumours arise from embryonal tissue and such embryonal tumours rarely occur in adults. On the other hand, the common adult tumours, such as carcinomas of the lung, stomach, and bowel, are extremely rare in children.

The overall cure rate is high in childhood cancers

In contrast to the very small improvements in survival rates for the common adult cancers, the outcome for most types of childhood cancers has improved dramatically over the last 20 years. The survival rate for all malignant cancers rose from 50 per cent in 1977 to 77 per cent in 2002. This is due to improvements in combined modality therapy (chemotherapy, surgery, and radiation) as well as better supportive care. Children with cancers are now treated in specialist centres where appropriate expertise is available. Children in a similar diagnostic group are entered into national and international trials that are leading to improved treatment.

INTERESTING TO KNOW

Childhood cancer

By the year 2010, it is estimated that 1 in every 250 adults will be a survivor of childhood cancer.

There may be significant long-term consequences of treatment

The most important long-term side effects of therapy for malignant tumours are growth failure, reduced fertility, major organ damage, and a 10- to 20-fold increase in the risk of secondary cancer in adulthood. With that in mind, increasing attention is now being focused on minimizing the toxic effects of chemotherapy.

Extensive pathological work-up is necessary to provide an accurate diagnosis

It is imperative to have an accurate diagnosis before embarking on therapy for a childhood malignancy as the treatment varies considerably according to the specific tumour type. It is therefore extremely important that the sample of tumour is taken from the best possible site and that it is transported immediately to the pathology laboratory.

Depending on the amount of tissue available, the biopsy is divided into several smaller portions for specific studies. The majority of the sample is put into formalin to be made into haematoxylin and eosin stained sections for morphological analysis. The remaining tissue is divided up for genetic tests such as fluorescence in situ hybridisation (FISH) studies and cytogenetics. These tests may be extremely helpful in making a diagnosis if a highly characteristic genetic change is present in the neoplastic cells.

Small round cell tumours of childhood all have a very similar appearance

Small round cell tumours are a number of different childhood tumours which all have a very similar appearance down the light microscope (Fig. 22.14). Unsurprisingly, they are all made up of similar looking small round cells!

Tumours which can give this appearance include acute lymphoblastic lymphoma, neuroblastoma,

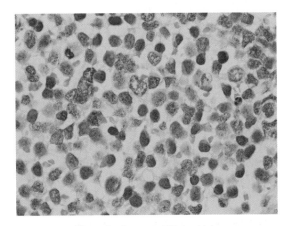

Fig. 22.14 Small round cell tumour. This is a high power microscopic image of a small round cell tumour. On the basis of this appearance alone, the tumour could be any one of a number of possibilities including neuroblastoma, lymphoma, rhabdomyosarcoma, or primitive neuroectodermal tumour.

rhabdomyosarcoma, and primitive neuroectodermal tumour. In these cases, additional tools such as immuno-histochemistry and genetic studies are necessary to identify the precise tumour.

Acute leukaemia

Acute leukaemia is the most common malignancy in childhood

Acute leukaemia is a haematological malignancy derived from haematopoietic stem cells in the bone marrow. The neoplastic cells differentiate into primitive lymphoid or myeloid cells ('blasts') which have a huge proliferative capacity. The bone marrow becomes rapidly overwhelmed by the malignant blasts, leading to the sudden onset pancytopenia due to bone marrow failure. Malignant blasts also spill into the peripheral blood and infiltrate organs such as lymph nodes, liver, spleen, and bones.

Eighty per cent of childhood leukaemia is acute lymphoblastic leukaemia (ALL) in which the neoplastic cells differentiate into lymphoid blasts. The remainder are acute myeloid leukaemia (AML) in which the neoplastic cells differentiate into myeloid blasts.

The diagnosis of acute leukaemia is usually established by examination of a bone marrow aspirate which shows large numbers of primitive blasts.

Central nervous system neoplasms

Brain and spinal cord tumours are the second most common form of childhood cancer. In contrast to adults where most primary brain neoplasms arise in the cerebral hemispheres ('supratentorial'), most paediatric brain neoplasms arise in the brainstem or cerebellum ('infratentorial').

Pilocytic astrocytoma is a slow growing type of astrocytoma which commonly occurs in the cerebellum of children. The typical age group is 5–10 years of age, and 90 per cent of cases can be cured.

Medulloblastoma is a solid primitive neuroectodermal tumour that arises from the cerebellar vermis and extends to fill the cavity of the fourth ventricle. They typically present with features of raised intracranial pressure, and signs of cerebellar dysfunction. One highly characteristic feature of medulloblastoma is its tendency to spread along the CSF pathways.

Ependymoma is a slow growing neoplasm derived from the ependymal lining of the cerebral ventricles. They cause clinical symptoms by blocking CSF pathways.

Lymphomas

Lymphomas are malignancies derived from mature lymphocytes that have left the bone marrow and taken up residence in lymphoid tissue such as lymph nodes. As in adults, lymphomas in children can be divided into non-Hodgkin's lymphoma and Hodgkin's lymphoma.

Non-Hodgkin's lymphoma is the more common form in younger children. The most common subtypes in childhood are Burkitt's lymphoma, lymphoblastic lymphoma, diffuse large B cell lymphoma, and anaplastic large cell lymphoma. All are high grade lymphomas.

Hodgkin's lymphoma presents in adolescence or young adulthood. Hodgkin's lymphoma is characterized by the presence of the Hodgkin–Reed–Sternberg cell and has different histological subtypes. The treatment depends on the histological type and stage of the disease.

Neuroblastoma

Neuroblastoma is a malignant tumour derived from neural crest cells that mature into the ganglion cells of the sympathetic nervous system. They may occur in the adrenal medulla or the sympathetic ganglia located in the neck, thorax, abdomen, and pelvis. The tumour cells secrete high amounts of catecholamines and associated metabolites, which can be detected in the urine and are an important diagnostic test.

For the purposes of treatment, children with malignant tumours are stratified into risk groups depending on various clinical, biochemical, histological, and biological factors. The most powerful biological factor is the status of the MYCN gene, which is available from FISH and molecular genetic studies. MYCN gene amplification, which is identified in approximately 25 per cent of tumours, is associated with aggressive and advanced disease.

Wilms' tumour

Wilms' tumour (nephroblastoma) is a malignant renal tumour of childhood which typically affects children aged 2–4 years old.

These tumours replace part or whole of the kidney (Fig. 22.15). With progressive growth, they invade the renal capsule and extrarenal structures. They may spread into the renal vein and inferior cava and metastasize to the lymph nodes and distant organs such as the liver and lungs.

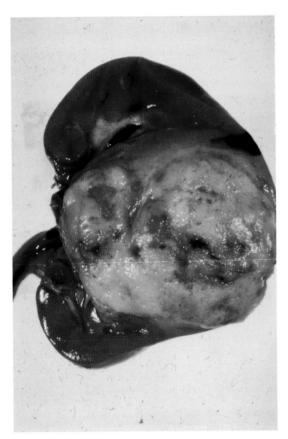

Fig. 22.15 Wilms' tumour of the kidney.

The diagnosis is made by examination of a needle biopsy or resection of the renal mass. Histologically, Wilms' tumour mimics normal renal development and shows three components. The blastema cells represent the parent or precursor cells. These show variable differentiation into two other components, the epithelial (glomeruli and tubules) and the mesenchymal component.

Osteosarcoma

Osteosarcoma is a malignant tumour of bone that produces osteoid. The peak incidence is in the second decade of life, a period characterized by rapid bone growth. It commonly affects the metaphyseal growth plates of long bones. The bones commonly affected are distal femur, proximal tibia, and proximal humerus.

While the imaging may be very suggestive, a biopsy is necessary for definitive diagnosis.

Ewing's sarcoma

Ewing's sarcoma is a group of neoplasms that arise in soft tissue and bone which share similar histological and molecular features. Histologically they are small round cell tumours with varying degrees of neural differentiation. Both show a characteristic chromosomal translocation t(11;22), which is detected by FISH or molecular studies.

Rhabdomyosarcoma

Rhabdomyosarcoma is the most common soft tissue sarcoma in children. The most common areas of the body to be affected in children are the head and neck, urinary bladder, or testes. They are more common in boys.

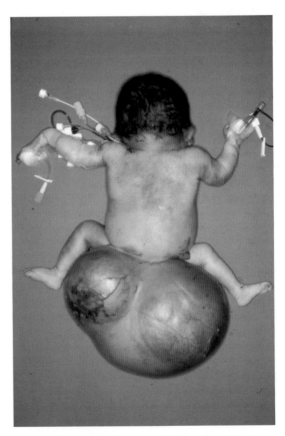

Fig. 22.16 Sacrococcygeal teratoma. This baby was born with this large sacrococcygeal teratoma.

Children with certain rare genetic disorders (such as Li Fraumeni syndrome) have a higher risk of developing rhabdomyosarcoma.

Retinoblastoma

Retinoblastoma is a rare malignant embryonal tumour of the retina. Sixty per cent of retinoblastomas are sporadic with no relevant family history, while in the inherited form there is often family history.

Teratoma

Teratomas are germ cell tumours composed of tissue differentiating down all three germinal layers. They may occur in the gonads or in extragonadal locations such as the sacrococcygeal region (Fig. 22.16), mediastinum, and neck. Teratomas may present as a congenital tumour present at birth.

Key points: Paediatric tumours

- The majority of tumours in children are benign, although even these may be problematic if they are large and arise in critical locations.

- Childhood cancers have a good cure rate, although adverse long-term effects of treatment remains a concern.

- Extensive pathological work-up is necessary to provide an accurate diagnosis of a childhood tumour, especially in cases where the histological appearance is non-specific, e.g. a small round cell tumour.

- Acute leukaemia is the most common malignancy in childhood. Children with acute leukaemia become rapidly unwell due to bone marrow failure.

- Primary central nervous system tumours are the second most common form of childhood cancer. Examples include pilocytic astrocytoma, medulloblastoma, and ependymoma.

- Lymphomas are malignant solid tumours of lymphoid cells.

- Neuroblastoma is a malignant solid tumour of the adrenal medulla and sympathetic nervous system.

- Wilms' tumour is a malignant solid tumour of the kidney.

- Osteosarcoma is the most common primary malignant bone tumour in childhood and adolescence.

- Ewing's sarcoma is a family of soft tissue and bone tumours that all show the same chromosomal translocation t(11;22).

- Teratoma is the most common germ cell tumour, and may present as a congenital tumour.

PART III

Pathology in real life

CHAPTER 23

Pathology as a clinical discipline

Chapter contents

Introduction

So far in this book we have talked about pathology as a scientific subject. Pathology also exists as a clinical speciality, being one of the core diagnostic services in the hospital. As a junior hospital doctor, you will be sending samples to the pathology laboratory many times every single day, so it is useful to have a basic understanding of what actually happens in that somewhat mythical place 'the lab'.

Pathology laboratories are split into different specialist departments which will usually include haematology, clinical biochemistry, microbiology, and cellular pathology. Some of your patients who die either in hospital or in the community will require a post-mortem examination, and as these are performed by pathologists the mortuary should also be included in a list of pathology departments.

Haematology

Full blood count

The **full blood count** is the most common test requested from the haematology laboratory. A busy haematology laboratory may receive over 1000 requests for a full blood count every day. Fortunately these are performed by automated cell counters, which are extremely accurate provided they are carefully calibrated. When blood results are abnormal, the instruments are designed to flag the result for review. The full blood count typically includes a cell count of red cells, platelets, and white cells, together with a number of other parameters (Table 23.1).

TABLE 23.1 Parameters measured in a full blood count
Haemoglobin concentration
Red cell count
Mean corpuscular volume
Packed cell volume
Mean corpuscular haemoglobin concentration
Red cell distribution width
Platelet count
White blood count

Haemoglobin is measured using the haemoglobin-cyanide (HiCN) method, in which a sample of blood is diluted in a solution containing potassium cyanide and potassium ferricyanide. Haemoglobin is converted into HiCN and the absorbance of the solution is then measured in a spectrometer at a wavelength of 540 nm, allowing calculation of the haemoglobin concentration.

Red blood cell count is measured by passing a suspension of the sample through the aperture of an impedance counter or through the beam of a light of a light-scattering instrument. The electrical impulse that is generated by each red cell allows the red blood cell count to be measured.

The height of the electrical impulse generated allows the **mean cell volume** (MCV) or the **packed cell volume** to be determined. The MCV is used to categorize anaemia into microcytic, macrocytic, or normocytic. Note that the MCV is an average across many cells, and so whilst a value in the normal range may represent a single population of normal sized red blood cells, it may also occur if there are similar numbers of microcytic and macrocytic red blood cells.

The **mean corpuscular haemoglobin concentration** (MCHC) measures the concentration of haemoglobin within the red blood cell. If there is a reduction in cell volume that is not matched by a reduction in red cell haemoglobin, then the MCHC rises. This is most often due to spherocytosis.

The **red cell distribution width** (RDW) estimates the variation in size of the red blood cells. A raised RDW should prompt examination of a blood film to help elucidate the underlying cause.

Platelet count is measured using the same techniques as are employed for counting red cells, except the thresholds are altered to account for the smaller size of platelets.

White cell counts are performed on diluted blood in which the red cells have been either lysed or rendered transparent so they do not interfere with leukocyte counting. Modern automated counters are now able to count different types of leukocyte differentially and even detect the presence of immature neutrophils. Cells which the machine does not recognize may be reported as 'large atypical cells'. These may be the result of cells such as the atypical lymphocytes seen in infectious mononucleosis.

Reticulocytes can also be counted automatically by combining various dyes and fluorochromes with the

RNA in reticulocytes and enumerating them using a flow cytometer.

Blood film

A **blood film** is made by spreading a drop of blood across a glass slide. Films may be spread by hand, but nowadays this is usually done by automated blood counters. Examination of the blood film is an essential part of haematological examination in order to assess the morphology of the cellular elements of the blood, so it is useful to be familiar with some of the more common terms used on blood film reports.

Red cell morphology

Anisocytosis refers to increased variation in red cell size. Anisocytosis may be due to red blood cells that are large (macrocytes) or small (microcytes), or a combination of the two. Macrocytes are commonly seen in megaloblastic anaemias, myelodysplastic syndromes, and alcohol excess. Microcytes are seen if there is defective haemoglobin synthesis, e.g. iron deficiency anaemia and thalassaemia.

Poikilocytosis refers to increased variation in red cell shape. This is seen in association with abnormal erythropoiesis, e.g. megaloblastic anaemia, iron deficiency anaemia, thalassaemia, myelodysplastic syndromes, and myelofibrosis.

Hypochromic red cells stain palely. This usually is due to a lowered haemoglobin concentration, of which the most common cause is iron deficiency. In iron deficiency, the red cells are also microcytic. Hypochromic red cells are also seen in thalassaemia; the presence of target cells favours a diagnosis of thalassaemia rather than iron deficiency.

Spherocytes are red cells which are more spherical than normal red cells, i.e. their diameter is less than normal and their thickness is greater than normal. Spherocytes may result from inherited defects in the red cell membrane such as hereditary spherocytosis, or result from loss of chunks of red cell membrane in haemolytic anaemias.

Schistocytes are red cell fragments which are smaller than normal red cells and have varying shapes, often with sharp angles. Schistocytes are found in many blood disorders, including thalassaemias, megaloblastic anaemia, myelodysplastic syndromes, and in microangiopathic haemolytic anaemias.

Target cells are red cells with a central stained area and a peripheral stained area separated by poorly staining cytoplasm, creating a 'target' appearance. Target cells may be conspicuous in chronic liver disease and thalassaemia.

Leukocyte morphology

Examination of the neutrophil lineage may show hypersegmented neutrophils (neutrophils with >5 nuclear lobes) in megaloblastic anaemia, large numbers of the whole range of neutrophil precursors in chronic myeloid leukaemia, or numerous myeloid blasts in acute myeloid leukaemia.

Examination of lymphoid cells may show atypical lymphocytes in infectious mononucleosis, numerous small lymphoid cells and smear cells in chronic lymphocytic leukaemia, and numerous lymphoid blasts in acute lymphoblastic leukaemia.

Clotting screen

A clotting screen should be taken into a citrate tube as the citrate chelates calcium, preventing the blood from clotting. In the laboratory, calcium and other clotting stimulators are added to the plasma and the time taken for a clot to generate is measured. Depending on which clotting stimulators are added, different clotting factors can be assessed.

In the **prothrombin time** (PT), thromboplastin is used to stimulate clot formation. The test is known to depend on factors V, VII, X, and fibrinogen. The **international normalized ratio** (INR) is a way of expressing the PT by adjusting for local variations in the thromboplastin used in that particular laboratory.

In the **activated partial thromboplastin time** (APTT), the plasma is incubated with kaolin to activate clotting. Phospholipid is then added to generate a clot. The APTT depends on factors XII, XI, X, IX, V, prothrombin, and fibrinogen.

Abnormalities in clotting tests may be seen in a number of disorders, and the PT and APTT results often help to distinguish between the causes (Table 23.2).

Erythrocyte sedimentation rate

The **erythrocyte sedimentation rate** (ESR) is taken into a 100 mm long tube which is stood vertically. At the end of 1 h, the fall of the red cell level compared with the original plasma meniscus at the top of the tube is the ESR. A very high ESR is seen in myeloma,

TABLE 23.2 Causes of abnormal clotting tests

Prolonged prothrombin time
    Warfarin treatment
    Liver disease
    DIC

Prolonged activated partial thromboplastin time
    DIC
    Liver disease
    Heparin treatment
    Haemophilia
    von Willebrand's disease

DIC, disseminated intravascular coagulation.

malignancy, and chronic inflammatory conditions due to proteins around red cells reducing their negative charge and causing repulsion.

Blood products

Red cell concentrates

Red cell concentrates are the most commonly administered form of blood product. They are given to anaemic patients to increase the circulating red cell mass rapidly and improve the oxygen supply to the tissues.

A red cell transfusion is indicated for patients with a haemoglobin concentration below 7 g/dl, or patients with symptoms related to anaemia. Many red cell transfusions are given inappropriately, and with that in mind the following points should be noted:

- A haemoglobin of 8–10 g/dl is safe, even in patients with significant cardiovascular disease.

- In acute blood loss, studies have shown that up to a 30 per cent blood loss can be treated with crystalloid or colloid solutions only. Even in an elderly population, there is no increase in mortality provided the haemoglobin is kept above 8 g/dl.

- Postoperative patients, who are limited in their activity, are unlikely to have oxygen demands that exceed supply. Wound healing is not affected unless oxygen tension decreases below 6.5 kPa, or the haematocrit is <18%.

Stringent pre-transfusion testing is required before issuing red cell concentrates

When a red cell transfusion is needed, stringent pre-transfusion testing must be performed before donated red cells are issued. Pre-transfusion testing includes the following:

- **Group and screen**, involving ABO and D grouping of the recipient, and an antibody screen.

- **Donor red cell selection and cross-matching**, which may involve serological testing between the recipient's serum and donor red cells, or electronic selection.

ABO grouping is the single most important serological test performed on pre-transfusion samples, and the accuracy of testing systems must not be compromised. ABO grouping is performed by testing the patient's red cells against monoclonal anti-A and anti-B antibodies. In addition, a reverse ABO grouping is performed in which the patient's serum is tested against known group A red cells and group B red cells. D status is detected using monoclonal IgM anti-D antibody. The ABO and D group must, where possible, be verified against previous results for the patient.

Antibody screening is used to detect any antibodies to red cell antigens other than ABO or D. Most patients develop alloantibodies due to previous blood transfusions or during pregnancy when the mother is exposed to fetal red cell antigens inherited from the father and not shared by the mother. Antibody screening is performed using an **indirect antiglobulin test**, in which the recipient's serum is mixed with a set of screening red cells suspended in low ionic strength solution. Agglutination of the red cells indicates the presence of an alloantibody. If an alloantibody is detected in the screening process, it must be identified and its likely clinical significance assessed.

Antibody screening tests are now very reliable at picking up relevant red cell antibodies, such that in recent years the traditional approach of performing a further indirect antiglobulin test between the actual donor red cells and the recipient's serum is being replaced by abbreviated serological techniques such as the immediate spin cross-match.

In the immediate spin cross-match, the recipient's serum is briefly incubated with the donor red cells followed by centrifugation and examination for agglutination; this rapid cross-match is an acceptable way of excluding major ABO incompatibility in patients with a negative antibody screen. Many hospitals have gone one step further and eliminated all serological cross-matching for certain categories of patient and rely entirely on electronic issuing of red cells based on the group and screen alone.

Patients found to have antibodies on the antibody screen must have a full indirect antiglobulin test cross-match performed between the recipient's serum and the donor red cells before issuing the blood.

Immediate haemolytic transfusion reaction is the most serious complication of blood transfusion

An immediate haemolytic transfusion reaction is usually due to ABO incompatibility. Recipient IgM antibodies bind to the donor red cells and activate complement, leading to fever, breathlessness, hypotension, and renal failure. Haemoglobin liberated from the lysed red cells is filtered at the glomerulus and may lead to toxic acute tubular necrosis and acute renal failure. The development of acute disseminated intravascular coagulation is a poor prognostic sign.

ABO incompatibility usually results from errors outside the haematology laboratory such as failure to check the identity of the patient when taking the sample for pre-transfusion testing, mislabelling the sample with the wrong patient's details, collecting and delivering the wrong blood, and failure to identify the patient correctly before starting the transfusion.

Delayed haemolytic transfusion reactions are due to IgG alloantibodies

Delayed haemolytic transfusion reactions occur in patients with alloantibodies to donor red cells at a level too low to be detected by the pre-tranfusion testing. When the blood is transfused, the immune response is amplified and the transfused red cells are destroyed by IgG antibodies.

Many episodes of delayed haemolytic transfusion reaction are clinically silent. Overt episodes typically present with anaemia and jaundice about a week after the transfusion. A blood film shows spherocytosis.

Non-haemolytic febrile transfusion reactions are due to antibodies to leukocytes

Transfusion reactions may occur due to alloantibodies to antigens on leukocytes in the packed red cell transfusion, leading to fever, flushing, and tachycardia. Non-haemolytic transfusion reactions were commonly seen in patients alloimmunized by previous transfusions or pregnancies, but are now less common following the introduction of leukocyte-depleted blood in the UK over worries about transmission of variant Creutzfeldt–Jacob disease.

There is a small risk of transmitting infections through donated blood

All donated blood in the UK is screened for hepatitis B virus, hepatitis C virus, human immunodeficiency virus (HIV), and human T cell lymphotrophic virus type 1 (HTLV-1). Whilst stringent measures are taken to ensure transfused blood is safe, this can never be guaranteed. The incidence of transmission of HBV is 1 in 900 000 units transfused, less than 1 in 30 million units for HCV, and under 1 in 8 million units for HIV. Concerns of the theoretical risk of transmitting variant Creutzfeldt–Jacob disease led to leukocyte depletion from all donated blood in the UK in 1999.

Platelet concentrates

Platelet concentrates are prepared by centrifugation of whole blood. They are stored at 22°C for up to 5 days. They are used to treat bleeding in patients with severe thrombocytopenia. ABO antigens are present on platelets and so ABO-compatible platelets should be given where possible to patients. Rhesus antigens are not present on platelets and so transfusing rhesus-incompatible platelets does not affect platelet survival. However, some rhesus-negative patients may be immunized against Rhesus D from residual red cells present in the concentrate.

Current recommendations suggest that Rhesus D-negative platelets should where possible be given to Rhesus D-negative patients, especially to females who have not yet reached the menopause.

Fresh frozen plasma

Fresh frozen plasma is prepared by removing plasma from a single unit of blood by centrifugation within 8 h of donation. The plasma is then snap frozen at –80°C and maintained deep frozen until use. The product is ABO and Rhesus D grouped.

Fresh frozen plasma should only be used in patients who have severe bleeding due to multiple clotting factor deficiencies, such as acute disseminated intravascular coagulation or overanticoagulation with warfarin.

Clinical biochemistry

Most commonly performed clinical biochemistry tests are carried out by automated instruments capable of processing large numbers of samples. The machines must, however, be carefully calibrated by laboratory staff to ensure accurate results.

Electrolytes

Serum electrolyte concentrations are measured using **ion-selective electrodes**, which are coated with a membrane that only allows passage of the ion of interest. A sample of the test serum enters the testing chamber and the ion in question equilibrates across the membrane, generating a voltage difference between the measuring electrode and the reference electrode. Sensitive potentiometers measure the voltage difference and the microprocessor in the machine calculates the electrolyte concentrations. Ion-selective electrodes are now available for measurement of most ions, though the most commonly used are those for sodium, potassium, and calcium.

Renal function tests

Urea may be measured in a number of different ways. One popular method is an enzymatic method in which the enzyme urease (the main source of which is the jack bean) is used to hydrolyse urea to ammonia and water. The ammonium ion is quantified and used to calculate the original urea concentration.

Creatinine may be measured in a number of different ways, but most employ the *Jaffe reaction* in which creatinine reacts with picrate in an alkaline medium to yield an orange–red complex that can be quantified by photometry. Despite being first described way back in 1886, the precise reaction mechanism and the structure of the product still remain unclear today!

Liver function tests

Liver transaminases are measured by coupling a transaminase reaction to a dehydrogenase reaction. Oxaloacetate formed from aspartate by aspartate transaminase (AST) is reduced to malate in the presence of malate dehydrogenase, whilst pyruvate formed by alanine transaminase (ALT) is reduced to lactate in the presence of lactate dehydrogenase. As the reactions proceed, NADH is oxidized to NAD. The disappearance of NADH can be followed by spectrophotometry and used to calculate the original concentrations of AST and ALT.

The most popular method for measuring alkaline phosphatase (ALP) is addition of 4-nitrophenyl phosphate which, under alkaline conditions, is converted to 4-nitrophenoxide (4-NP) which is an intense yellow colour. The rate of formation of 4-NP by the action of the enzyme can be monitored with a recording spectrophotometer.

γ-Glutamyltransferase (GGT) activity is measured using the substrate L-γ-glutamyl-3-carboxy-4-nitroanilide which is split by GGT, yielding a yellow nitroaniline product which can be measured by spectrophotometry.

C-reactive protein

C-reactive protein (CRP) is one of the acute phase proteins synthesized in the liver during an inflammatory response. CRP binds to foreign microbes and activates the complement cascade via the classical pathway (p. 35). CRP is the most sensitive acute phase protein as a marker of inflammation, increasing within 6–12 h and exhibiting a huge range of elevation (up to 2000 times normal).

CRP is normally measured by immunochemical methods. A specific antibody to the protein is added to the sample and, after a timed interval, the number of immune complexes that have formed can be measured by the light-scattering properties of the immune complexes.

Arterial blood gases

Arterial blood gas measurements are an important part of the work-up of many patients, particularly those with severe respiratory and metabolic conditions. Although modern blood gas analysers may measure a number of parameters, the main three are the pH, pO_2, and pCO_2.

These three measurements are all made using ion-selective electrodes. The pH is calculated as the negative logarithm of the hydrogen ion concentration which is measured via an ion-selective glass electrode. The pO_2 and pCO_2 are measured using gas electrodes which are separated from the test solution by a thin membrane permeable to gas but not solutions.

The carbon dioxide electrode works by measuring the change in pH in a bicarbonate solution surrounding the electrode produced by CO_2 in the sample, and then calculating pCO_2 using the Henderson–Hasselbalch equation.

The oxygen electrode works in a slightly different way. It measures the current which flows when oxygen from the test solution diffuses through the gas membrane and on to the electrode where it is reduced. The pO_2, which is directly proportional to the flowing current, can then be calculated.

Microbiology

The main aims of a diagnostic microbiology laboratory are to identify microorganisms responsible for infections and to provide guidance on appropriate antimicrobial therapy. Identification of infectious organisms can be achieved by a number of methods which range from simple tests performed in minutes to prolonged cultures taking weeks to complete (Table 23.3).

Specimen collection is the single most important determinant of accurate results in microbiology

The accuracy of a microbiological report can only be as good as the quality of the specimen on which it is based. The specimen should be taken from the site of suspected infection and if possible be collected before antimicrobial therapy is given. The best specimen is one taken from a normally sterile site, such as blood. The limitations of other sites with their own indigenous flora need to be taken into account during laboratory processing.

Specimens should be transported as quickly as possible to the laboratory because in some specimens, such as urine, bacterial and fungal contaminants may rapidly multiply, giving falsely high counts on culture and masking true pathogenic organisms. Unlike histopathological specimens, microbiological specimens should never be placed into formalin as this will kill any organisms present!

Infectious agents may be identified by detecting the organism itself or the patient's response to it

Tests performed in a microbiology laboratory to identify infectious agents fall into four main categories:

◆ *Direct visualization by microscopy.* Detection of organisms may be achieved at its simplest by visualizing the organism in the specimen by either light microscopy or electron microscopy.

◆ *Culture.* Most microorganisms can be grown in the laboratory either on artificial media (bacteria and yeasts) or in tissue culture (viruses). Culturing organisms is the slowest method of identification; results cannot be achieved in less than 18 h, and may take much longer. Culture does, however, allow antimicrobial sensitivity testing to be performed.

◆ *Identification of a specific microbial product.* These include structural components of the microbe (e.g. cell wall antigens), toxins, or genetic material.

◆ *Antibody detection.* This is particularly helpful when the organism in question cannot be cultured or culture may be hazardous to laboratory staff.

Microscopy

Light microscopy is a fundamental part of microbiological specimen examination which is quick and easy to perform. Specimens for light microscopy may either be placed directly on to a glass slide for examination or dried, fixed with heat or alcohol, and then stained.

Direct preparations are made by placing the specimen on a glass slide

Direct preparations are easily made by placing a drop of the specimen in the centre of a glass slide and gently lowering a clean coverslip on to the specimen so it spreads out to the edge of the coverslip. Some specimens are seen more clearly if a drop of water is added to the slide before the coverslip is lowered ('wet preparation' or 'wet mount'). Common examples

TABLE 23.3   Common microbiological techniques

Time	Method	Examples
Minutes/hours	Light microscopy	Bacteria, fungi, cysts/ova of parasites
	Electron microscopy	Viruses
	Antigen detection	Hepatitis B surface antigen
	Antibody detection	Anti-HIV, anti-hepatitis C virus
	Molecular techniques	*Chlamydia*
Days	Solid and liquid culture	Bacteria and yeasts
	Tissue culture	Viruses
	Toxin detection	*Clostridium difficile* cytotoxin
Weeks	Lowenstein–Jensen agar	*Mycobacteria*

of specimens examined with direct preparations include the following:

- Urine to quantify neutrophil and red cell numbers.
- Faeces to look for cysts, eggs, and parasites.
- Skin scrapings for fungi.
- Vaginal discharge for *Trichomonas* or fungi.

Stained preparations are dried, fixed, and then stained

Organisms which are better visualized and categorized with special stains are examined with a stained preparation. A sample of the specimen is placed on the microscope slide, dried, and then fixed on to the slide with either heat or alcohol before staining. The most commonly used stain in microbiology is the **Gram stain** which allows the division of bacteria into Gram positive (violet) and Gram negative (red).

Electron microscopy is needed to visualize viruses

Viruses cannot be seen by light microscopy because they are too small. Electron microscopy is therefore a useful tool to identify viruses which are difficult or impossible to culture, e.g. rotaviruses. The problem with electron microscopy is that a large number of viral particles must be present to be detectable, so the sensitivity of the test is not brilliant.

Culture

Most bacteria and fungi can be cultured on solid nutrient media

The vast majority of bacteria and fungi can be cultured on solid, agar-based nutrient media. Most media are **selective media**, designed to support the growth of possible pathogens and inhibit the growth of likely commensal organisms, thus increasing the chances of growing a pure culture of the offending organism.

A sample of the specimen is spread on to a plate containing the media and, after incubation, the organisms grow as visible colonies on the surface of the media. For blood cultures, the individual taking the sample directly inoculates the sample into paired liquid media bottles for aerobic and anaerobic incubation.

Possible pathogens are then examined using simple tests to identify them. Sometimes the appearance of the colony is quite characteristic and can be used as a

preliminary clue to the likely identity of the organism, which is confirmed by performing further tests such as Gram staining, growth requirements, and enzyme production.

Sometimes it is important to go beyond the identification of a specific species to give further information. As an example, in the investigation of an outbreak of food poisoning caused by *Escherichia coli*, identification of the *E. coli* serotype O157 would predict a higher risk of haemolytic–uraemic syndrome, a major cause of acute renal failure in children suffering from diarrhoea due to this organism.

Viruses and intracellular bacteria must be grown in cell or tissue culture

Obligate intracellular organisms such as viruses and bacteria like *Mycoplasma* and *Chlamydia* must be grown in a cell or tissue culture as they are incapable of growth outside of cells. The specimen is inoculated into the cell culture medium and the presence of the organism is detected by observing for a cytopathic effect. Intracellular organisms that do not produce a cytopathic effect or which grow poorly in cell culture must be detected in other ways, e.g. serology or polymerase chain reaction (PCR).

Susceptibility tests are a valuable aid to the antibacterial treatment of an infection

Once an organism has been identified that is likely to be the cause of the presumed infection, its antibiotic sensitivities can be tested. There are two main types of tests:

- *Diffusion tests*. The organism is inoculated onto an agar plate, and filter paper discs containing relevant antibacterials are applied to the surface. After incubation, the plate is examined for zones of inhibition around each antibacterial disc and the organism is classified as sensitive, intermediate (meaning the organism may respond to high doses), or resistant.

- *Dilution tests*. These allow a more quantitative assessment of susceptibility by determining the **minimum inhibitory concentration** (MIC) and the **minimum bactericidal concentration** (MBC) of the antibacterial. The MIC is the lowest concentration that inhibits visible growth of the bacteria. The MBC is the lowest concentration of antibacterial required to kill the organism.

LINK BOX

Infective endocarditis

Determining the MBC and measuring serum levels of antibacterials is important in the management of patients with infective endocarditis to ensure that a therapeutic concentration of drug is maintained during treatment (p. 99).

Antigen detection

Detection of specific microbial antigens relies on the use of specific monoclonal antibodies raised in mice against the antigen of interest to test for the presence of the antigen of interest.

Agglutination techniques are qualitative tests for antigens

Antigen detection using antibodies involves mixing the specimen with a specific antibody to the antigen of interest, and testing for the presence of antibody bound to antigen. The simplest technique involves coating latex particles with the antibody, such that in the presence of antigen the latex beads agglutinate, forming a clump which is visible to the naked eye. This merely tells you if the antigen is present or not, e.g. the *Streptococcus pneumoniae* capsule.

ELISAs and fluorescent techniques are quantitative tests for antigens

Extensions of this technique have been developed that allow actual measurement of the level of antigen according to the level of binding to a standard amount of added antibody. This is achieved by binding an enzyme (enzyme-linked immunosorbent assay) or a fluorescent probe to the antibody which generates a visual signal, the strength of which is used to measure the antigen concentration. Examples include measurement of levels of hepatitis B surface antigen.

Nucleic acid detection

PCR uses specific nucleic acid primers to probe microbial genetic material

PCR is currently available for the detection of a number of infectious agents including *Chlamydia* *trachomatis*, *Mycobacterium tuberculosis*, HIV, hepatitis C, and cytomegalovirus.

PCR tests are often used qualitatively for diagnostic purposes but may also be useful quantitatively for management purposes. A good example would be the measurement of HIV viral load in the blood of an HIV-infected person.

Antibody detection

Infections can also be identified by detecting the presence of antibodies reactive to a particular infectious agent. Such antibodies are usually detected by ELISA on the patient's serum. Examples of infections commonly diagnosed through antibody detection include HIV, hepatitis C, and rubella.

Cellular pathology

Most diseases are associated with structural changes in cells which can be identified microscopically. Cellular pathology is concerned with the examination of cells and is divided into two distinct disciplines: histopathology and cytopathology.

Histopathology

Histopathology refers to the microscopic examination of intact tissues

The majority of the workload of a histopathology department involves receiving and examining intact tissue specimens for diagnosis. Material for histopathology may be sent in two main forms: tissue biopsies and surgical resections.

Biopsies are small samples of tissue which are sent for the purposes of establishing a diagnosis. Common examples include a core biopsy from a lump in the breast or transrectal ultrasound-guided biopsies of the prostate. Once the diagnosis is established, further treatment can be performed depending on the findings.

Surgical resections are usually larger specimens which are performed as a part of the patient's treatment. Although the diagnosis is usually known before the surgery, the pathologist still performs a vital role in sampling the organ to establish the extent of the disease.

Processing of tissue samples and making slides takes time

Tissue sent for histopathology undergoes a complex journey before arriving on a glass slide for examination by a histopathologist. Before anything can be done, the tissue must be fixed in formalin for 24 h to prevent the immediate autolysis (decay) that occurs as soon as any tissue is removed from the body.

After fixation, the histopathologist provides a macroscopic description of the specimen and then samples small postage stamp-sized pieces for examination. These pieces are placed in plastic cassettes which then undergo a further round of overnight processing in which the water content of the tissue is gradually removed and replaced with wax. The tissue is then embedded in melted paraffin wax blocks which set and harden around the tissue. Extremely thin slices through the tissue can then be cut, mounted on to glass slides, and stained with haematoxylin and eosin for examination.

Immunohistochemistry allows the identification of cell type by staining for cell proteins

Immunohistochemistry is a technique which has become an extremely useful tool for histopathologists. Before immunohistochemistry, histopathologists had to rely entirely on the appearances of the tissue on haematoxylin and eosin stained slides to make a diagnosis. Before immunohistochemistry, it was impossible to distinguish between some conditions which looked identical on simple morphology.

Immunohistochemistry has improved diagnosis by allowing further characterization of cell type by staining for proteins which the cells are expressing. Identification of cell type using this method has become enormously helpful in diagnosis, particularly of tumours. As an example, a poorly differentiated carcinoma may appear exactly the same as a high grade lymphoma on morphology alone. Simple immunohistochemical stains can help distinguish the two, as the carcinoma will stain positively for **cytokeratin** whereas the lymphoma will stain positively for **leukocyte common antigen**.

One of the main reasons for delay in the issuing of histopathology reports is the use of immunohistochemistry which takes an extra 1–2 days to perform.

Frozen sections are requested when an immediate answer is needed during an operation

A **frozen section** is a technique by which tissue can be prepared for immediate histopathological diagnosis.

Rather than fixing the tissue in formalin for 24 h, the specimen is snap frozen in liquid nitrogen to make it hard enough to cut thin sections for staining.

The problem with frozen sections is that the freezing severely damages the tissue, making the slides much more difficult to interpret than those prepared in the normal manner. For this reason, frozen sections should only be used in situations where the answer critically determines what will happen to the patient on the operating table.

Examples of appropriate frozen section requests include the following:

◆ Determining tissue identity in parathyroid surgery. Often during parathyroid surgery, the parathyroid glands may look identical to other structures such as lymph nodes or pieces of fat. Frozen sections may therefore be requested to confirm that the tissue removed is indeed parathyroid tissue.

◆ Checking excision margins following removal of a tumour. When a tumour is being excised from a location where only a minimal amount of surrounding tissue wants to be removed, the surgeon may send samples of the excision margin to check they are clear of tumour before finishing the operation. This is often done in head and neck surgery for squamous cell carcinomas.

◆ To exclude secondary deposits of a malignancy before curative surgery is attempted. When curative surgery is attempted for a malignant neoplasm, the presence of distant metastases is a contraindication to surgery as cure becomes impossible by local resection of the primary tumour. Sometimes at operation, small nodules may be seen which are suspicious for metastases that were not picked up on imaging before the operation. These may be sent for frozen section to confirm or exclude the presence of malignancy.

Please remember that requesting frozen sections when the result does not *immediately* affect patient management is both a waste of resources and potentially dangerous for the patient.

Cytopathology

Cytopathology, or **cytology**, refers to the microscopic examination of *individual* cells smeared directly on to a glass slide. There are three main ways in which cells may be sampled for cytology:

◆ *Spontaneously shed cells in body fluids*. Common examples include sputum, urine, pleural effusions, and ascitic fluid. As the number of cells in these specimens is often low, the cytology laboratory will usually concentrate the cells by centrifuging the fluid when preparing the specimens.

◆ *Cells scraped off body surfaces*. Common examples include cervical smears (p. 260), brushings from the oesophagus at endoscopy, or brushings from the bronchi at bronchoscopy.

◆ *Fine needle aspiration*. Cells from virtually any organ or tissue can also be sampled by aspirating cells out through a fine needle. Tissues such as lymph nodes, salivary glands, breast, and thyroid can be easily aspirated in an outpatient clinic. Deeper organs such as lung, mediastinum, and liver can also be aspirated but require imaging guidance such as ultrasound or computed tomography (CT) (Fig. 23.1). These aspirates are therefore usually performed by radiologists.

The advantage of cytology over histopathology is that the specimens can be obtained much more easily and with less trauma than by a needle biopsy. The results

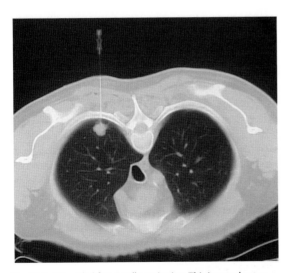

Fig. 23.1 CT-guided fine needle aspiration. This image shows a thin needle being introduced into a peripheral lung tumour under CT guidance to obtain material for cytological examination.

are also quicker as the cells are smeared immediately on to a slide and stained; there is no need for 24 h formalin fixation.

The main downside of cytology is that determination of tissue architecture is not possible as all of the cells have been dissociated from one another. For this reason, cytology is generally used as a quick assessment to decide if a lesion is benign or malignant, and then histopathology is used to elucidate the precise nature of a malignancy.

Mortuary

The **mortuary** is a storage facility for the bodies of patients who have died in the hospital, or for patients who have died in the community but require a post-mortem examination.

Death certification

The doctor has a number of duties to fulfil when a patient dies, including making the diagnosis of death, deciding whether the death should be referred to the Coroner, and if not, correctly completing a death certificate.

The diagnosis of death is usually made by confirming fixed dilated pupils and the absence of a carotid pulse, heart sounds, and breath sounds. This should be documented in the medical notes, recording the time and date clearly.

A death certificate must be issued before the body can be disposed of. A death certificate should only be filled in if the cause of death is known and there are no reasons to refer the death to the Coroner. The death certificate is completed with the disease or condition directly leading to death in the 1A slot. Conditions that led to the condition stated in 1A may be listed in 1B and 1C, though these must be ordered logically such that 1A is due to 1B that is due to 1C. Other conditions contributing to the death but not directly related to the disease in 1A can be listed in part 2. For example:

1A Acute myocardial infarction

1B Coronary artery atherosclerosis

2 Diabetes mellitus

Post-mortems

Post-mortems or **autopsies** are an important means of establishing the cause of death. The data from post-mortem studies are widely used in national statistics which in turn dictate health spending needs in the future.

Coroner's post-mortems are performed to determine if death was by natural causes

The vast majority of post-mortems performed in the UK are Coroner's post-mortems. The Coroner is an independent officer with statutory responsibility for the legal investigation of certain categories of death such as the following:

- Sudden and unexpected deaths
- Deaths where the cause is unknown and the doctor cannot issue a certificate
- Where the cause of death may be due to accident or industrial disease.

In these circumstances, a death certificate is not completed and the death is referred to the Coroner. If the Coroner decides that a post-mortem is necessary, an autopsy must be performed by law and consent of the relatives is not required. The pathologist performing the post-mortem acts for the Coroner and not for the hospital. The main aim of the Coroner's post-mortem is to decide if the death was natural or unnatural. In cases of unnatural deaths, e.g. industrial-related diseases such as mesothelioma, the Coroner may then hold a formal inquest into the death.

Note that in any death where there is a suspicion of criminal involvement (i.e. murder or manslaughter), the autopsy is performed by specially trained forensic pathologists who work for the Home Office.

Hospital post-mortems are performed for medical interest

Hospital, or medical interest, post-mortems are done at the request of doctors with the relatives' agreement. For hospital post-mortems, the cause of death is known and a death certificate is issued, but a post-mortem is requested to find out more information such as the extent of the disease or the effect of treatment.

Hospital post-mortems are important in education, audit, and research. Despite advances in imaging and other diagnostic tests, studies have shown that the presumed cause of death is often wrong. Nevertheless, the number of hospital post-mortem examinations performed in the UK has continued to fall and is now at its lowest level ever. The reasons for this fall are probably related to a combination of lack of interest from clinicians and pathologists, and increasing difficulties in getting consent from the next of kin.

Ideally, the consultant who looked after the deceased patient should be the one to ask the relatives for consent to the post-mortem. Often, however, this task falls to junior members of the medical team, so it is important that all doctors understand what happens during a post-mortem so they are able to explain it to the relatives.

Post-mortems are carried out as soon as possible after death

A post-mortem is usually performed within 2–3 days of death. This is to minimize the effects of tissue autolysis on the macroscopic features of the organs. A typical post-mortem takes about 1–2 h and begins with a thorough review of the clinical history and an external examination of the body. The internal organs are then completely removed (eviscerated), often in three blocks or 'plucks' from the body (Fig. 23.2), via a single longitudinal incision down the front of the body. The brain is removed by reflecting the scalp through an incision concealed in the hair at the back of the head and then removing the skull vault using an electric saw.

After removal, the organs are weighed, sliced, and examined for pathology. At the end of the examination, the organs, including the brain, are replaced in a bag in the body cavity and the incision is sutured up. The cranial cavity is packed and the skull vault replaced before resuturing the scalp. Reconstruction of the body is performed with great skill, and in most cases the incisions cannot be seen when the body is dressed for the funeral.

The pathologist then writes a complete report on the findings in each organ and constructs a clinicopathological summary. In Coroner's post-mortems, where a death certificate has not yet been issued, the pathologist will give the cause of death in the usual format (1A, 1B, etc.). In hospital post-mortems, the death certificate has already been issued and the pathologist instead compiles a list of relevant findings. If the cause of death found at autopsy differs significantly from the stated cause of death, then the death certificate may be amended accordingly.

Retention of organs and tissue from post-mortems is a controversial issue in pathology

In the past, small pieces of tissue from relevant organs and even whole organs were retained by the pathologist

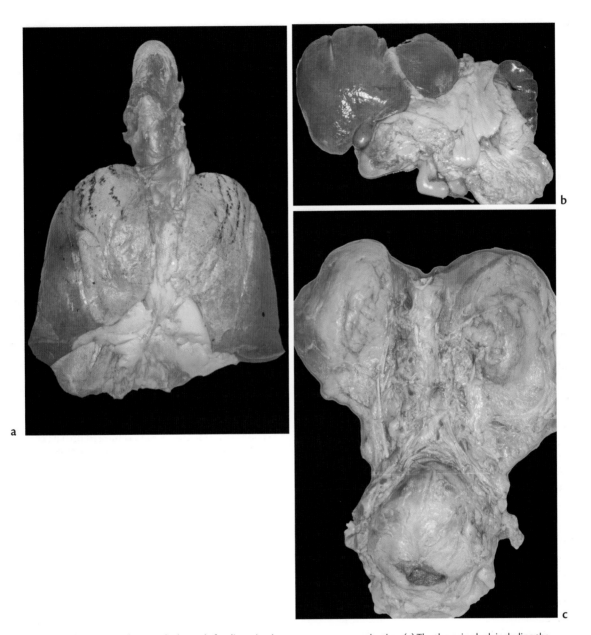

Fig. 23.2 Freshly eviscerated organ plucks ready for dissection in a post-mortem examination. (a) The thoracic pluck including the heart, lungs, and neck structures. (b) Upper gastrointestinal pluck including the stomach, duodenum, liver, gallbladder, pancreas, and spleen. (c) The retroperitoneal pluck viewed from behind including the abdominal aorta, adrenal glands, kidneys, ureters, and bladder. In a female, this pluck also includes the uterus, fallopian tubes, and ovaries.

to examine histologically to further the information gained from the post-mortem. Recently, the retention of such tissue has became extremely controversial when the parents of children who underwent Coroner's post-mortem examinations discovered that tissues and whole organs had been retained without their knowledge.

The public outcry led to formal inquiries which culminated in a new Human Tissue Act which came into force in April 2006. This has set strict limits on the retention of human tissue from post-mortems; contravening the legislation is a criminal offence punishable with a prison sentence, so pathologists need to be extremely careful to document precisely what material they are retaining, why they need the tissue, and how long they intend to keep it for.

Further reading

www.dh.gov.uk/PolicyAndGuidance/HealthAndSocial CareTopics/Tissue/fs/en, information about use of human tissue from the Department of Health.

CHAPTER 24

Case studies

Case 1

A 48-year-old woman is referred to her local hospital. She discovered a breast lump whilst showering which her GP was concerned about. The breast clinic at the hospital operates a 'one-stop' breast clinic where the triple approach to breast lumps is used.

Q What is meant by the term 'triple approach'?

A The triple approach refers to the combination of clinical, pathological, and radiological assessment of a breast lump. Together, these three modalities are very good at accurately diagnosing or excluding breast cancer.

Q Why is the clinic 'one stop'?

A Most breast lumps can be assessed with the triple approach in a single visit to the outpatient clinic, meaning that most women will have an answer as to the nature of the lump the same day.

You are working in the clinic and the consultant asks you to see the patient first. After taking a history, you consent the lady for a breast examination. Clinically you are concerned that this lump is malignant.

Q What features of a breast lump would make you suspicious that it might be malignant?

A Breast carcinomas are usually hard and poorly mobile because of the fibrosis that forms around them. They may be fixed to the chest wall or overlying skin if they have invaded into them. Traction on the ducts connected to the nipple may cause the nipple to invert.

As part of the investigation of the lump, you perform a fine needle aspiration for cytological examination.

Q What is fine needle aspiration cytology and why is it a useful test?

A Fine needle aspiration cytology is a technique by which a fine needle is passed into the lump, and cells are aspirated into the hub of the needle. The cells are then spread on to a glass slide, dried, and stained for immediate microscopic examination. This is a very useful test for distinguishing benign from malignant breast lumps; it can be performed easily in the outpatient clinic and the result can be available very quickly.

The cytologist in the clinic examines the slides you made and the report comes back 10 min later. It says: 'This is a cellular aspirate containing numerous discohesive groups of malignant cells with pleomorphic nuclei. Myoepithelial cell nuclei are inconspicuous. Summary: C5, malignant cells seen.'

Q What does 'pleomorphic' mean? Why do you think there is a lack of myoepithelial cell nuclei in the preparation? What does C5 mean?

A Pleomorphic means a variable size and shape. The presence of cells with pleomorphic nuclei is one important feature suggestive of malignancy. Myoepithelial cells are features of normal breast ducts and lobules. Breast carcinomas are composed of a proliferation of neoplastic epithelial cells that destroy the normal breast tissue and so do not contain myoepithelial cells. All breast lump aspirates are given a cytology code from 1 to 5 to indicate the findings. C1 is a non-diagnostic aspirate, C2 is benign, C3 is atypical probably benign, C4 is atypical probably malignant, and C5 is an unequivocally malignant aspirate.

While the cytology is being performed, the patient goes to radiology for imaging of the lesion. The radiologist concurs with the clinical and cytological findings of malignancy. The patient is informed of the diagnosis, and undergoes a wide local excision and axillary clearance 2 weeks later.

One week after her surgery you are at the breast multi-disciplinary meeting where the patient has been listed for discussion. The pathologist shows a series of slides from the specimen and summarizes her findings as 'a grade 3 invasive ductal carcinoma with areas of admixed high grade DCIS, which appears completely excised. ER and PR negative, Her2 positive. None of the six lymph nodes retrieved from the axillary sampling contain metastatic carcinoma.'

Q   Explain the terms 'grade 3', 'high grade DCIS', and 'Her2'.

A   All breast carcinomas are graded by the pathologist examining the specimen according to how well differentiated the tumour appears microscopically. Using set criteria, the tumours are graded from 1 to 3, with grade 3 representing the least degree of differentiation.

DCIS means ductal carcinoma in situ. DCIS is a precursor lesion of breast carcinoma in which malignant cells are present but still confined to the duct system. Once the malignant cells break out of the duct and into the breast tissue, it has become an invasive breast carcinoma. The grade of the DCIS is determined by how atypical the nuclei of the cells appear. Usually grade 3 invasive carcinomas are accompanied by high grade DCIS.

Her2 is a growth receptor which is overexpressed by some breast carcinomas due to an amplification in the number of copies of the gene. Her2-positive breast carcinomas are generally more poorly differentiated and have a worse prognosis.

Knowing the Her2 status is important not only as a prognostic marker but also because it predicts response to the Her2 receptor antagonist trastuzumab.

Cross-reference: breast carcinoma (p. 291).

Case 2

You are the F1 medical house officer on call for the day. A 59-year-old overweight banker presents to your team with severe central chest pain. He looks pale and grey and is sweating.

Q   What common and important conditions present with central chest pain?

A   Common causes of central chest pain are acute myocardial infarction, acute coronary syndrome, oesophagitis, and musculoskeletal chest pain. Less common, but very important to consider is the possibility of aortic dissection.

The nursing staff perform an electrocardiogram whilst you are taking a history from the patient. The ECG shows ST elevation in leads V1–V4. You diagnose an anterior ST elevation myocardial infarction (STEMI) and treat him with aspirin and streptokinase.

Q   What is a STEMI and what is the underlying pathology causing it? How is this different from an acute coronary syndrome?

A   STEMI is infarction of the full thickness of a region of myocardium. It is caused by thrombosis over a complicated atherosclerotic plaque occluding a coronary artery and starving the supplied area of myocardium of oxygen. Acute coronary syndromes are a spectrum of conditions of myocardial ischaemia in which there is no ST elevation on the ECG, and include unstable angina and non-ST elevation myocardial infarction.

Q   Does it surprise you that this man never suffered from attacks of angina?

A   No. This man's myocardial infarction was probably caused by an unstable plaque that ruptured, but was too small to cause symptoms of reversible ischaemia.

Q Why are aspirin and streptokinase effective in treating an STEMI?

A The occlusive thrombus is composed of platelets and fibrin. Aspirin is an antiplatelet agent that stops platelet aggregation, and streptokinase is a fibrinolytic agent that breaks down fibrin. Together these agents dissolve the thrombus blocking the coronary artery.

He is admitted to the coronary care unit where you are working the following day. His blood troponin result is back from the biochemistry laboratories, and is raised at 13.

Q What is troponin and why is it a useful test in people with chest pain?

A Troponins are molecules that regulate the interaction of actin and myosin in muscle. Troponins are released into the blood from damaged muscle. Because cardiac troponins are distinct from skeletal muscle troponins, cardiac troponins are highly sensitive and specific markers of myocardial necrosis, and the level of the rise correlates with the amount of myocyte damage. The troponin level allows risk stratification in patients with acute coronary syndromes as the more myocardial necrosis there has been, the higher the risk to the patient. The main drawback of troponins are that they may not rise until 12 h after the myocardial damage, meaning that the test cannot be used as an immediate test to rule out a significant cardiac cause of chest pain in A&E.

Later that morning, you are fast bleeped to the unit because he has become drowsy with a systolic blood pressure of 60 mmHg.

Q What possible causes of this turn of events run through your mind?

A This is most likely to be an early complication of the acute myocardial infarction such as an arrhythmia, acute left ventricular failure (LVF), or an acquired ventricular septal defect.

The cardiac monitor shows ventricular tachycardia, and he is successfully shocked out of the rhythm.

He then makes an uneventful recovery and is discharged from hospital the following week.

Ten years later, the man presents to his GP complaining of worsening shortness of breath. On examination, his apex beat is displaced, there is a pansystolic murmur, and he has bilateral basal crepitations in his lungs. The GP suspects chronic LVF due to a combination of ischaemic heart disease and mitral regurgitation.

Q What is chronic LVF? Why do you think he may have mitral regurgitation?

A Chronic LVF is a syndrome in which a variety of symptoms and signs occur due to an inadequate cardiac output. Chronic LVF has a number of possible causes, the most common being ischaemic heart disease, hypertension, and valvular disease. We know this gentleman has ischaemic heart disease (he has had an acute myocardial infarction), but he also appears to have valvular heart disease in the form of mitral regurgitation. The mitral regurgitation is almost certainly also ischaemic in origin—the previous myocardial infarction may have affected the function of the papillary muscles of the mitral valve. Also, dilation of the heart as a result of the LVF pulls the valve leaflets apart, predisposing to regurgitation.

Q What further tests could you do to confirm a suspicion of chronic LVF?

A An echocardiogram should be performed. This can measure left ventricular function by calculating the ejection fraction (the percentage of blood the left ventricle pumps out in systole) and also confirm the presence and severity of mitral regurgitation. A chest radiograph will also show an enlarged heart and pulmonary venous congestion. Measurement of circulating B-type natriuretic peptide (BNP) levels is also becoming a useful screening test for chronic LVF as this is released when the left ventricle is stretched.

Q What is the prognosis of chronic LVF?

A Not good. In fact, many people diagnosed with chronic LVF die within only a few years of diagnosis. Although symptoms can be controlled and prognosis can be improved with drugs, the natural course of chronic LVF is of progressively worsening cardiac function and death.

Cross-references: atherosclerosis (p. 75), ischaemic heart disease (p. 87), mitral regurgitation (p. 95).

Case 3

A healthy 25-year-old female is invited for her first cervical smear test.

Q What is a cervical smear and how is the test performed?

A A cervical smear is a screening test for cervical neoplasia. Cells of the transformation zone of the cervix are scraped away using a spatula and examined microscopically.

The smear is sent to the local pathology laboratory. Two weeks later, the report comes back saying: 'Mild dyskaryosis seen. Please repeat smear in 6 months.'

Q What is dyskaryosis?

A Dyskaryosis is a cytological term for abnormalities in the nucleus of a cell. In cervical screening, dyskaryosis is divided into mild, moderate, or severe.

The patient returns for the repeat smear test. The result comes back as: 'Moderate dyskaryosis seen. Refer to colposcopy.'

Q What is colposcopy?

A Colposcopy is a close examination of the cervix using a special binocular microscope and a bright light source. Special stains can be painted on to the cervix to highlight any abnormalities.

At colposcopy, a biopsy is taken from an area of abnormality. The histology report reads: 'A biopsy from the transformation zone showing evidence of CIN 2 and wart virus change.' At the follow-up colposcopy appointment, a diathermy loop excision of the transformation zone is performed.

Q What is CIN? What is the relevance (if any) of the wart virus change?

A CIN stands for cervical intraepithelial neoplasia. CIN is the precursor lesion of cervical squamous cell carcinoma. Microscopically it is defined by dysplasia of the squamous epithelium but without invasion through the basement membrane. The wart virus change refers to microscopic features suggestive of infection of the transformation zone epithelium by human papilloma virus (HPV). This is often seen in association with CIN as HPV is the underlying cause of cervical neoplasia.

Q Why was her transformation zone excised?

A Patients with high grade CIN (grade 2 or 3) are advised to have their entire transformation zone excised. Although only a minority of patients with CIN develop invasive squamous cell carcinoma, there is no way of predicting who will progress and who will not, so excision of the transformation zone is recommended for CIN 2 or 3.

Cross-reference: cervical squamous neoplasia (p. 257).

Case 4

A mother brings her 1-year-old daughter to the GP surgery because of poor appetite, irritability, and increased crying for the past 2 days. The infant had *Haemophilus influenzae* b and meningococcal group C vaccine at 2, 3, and 5 months of age. Both the parents smoke cigarettes.

On examination, the child is active and not in distress. She has a temperature of 38°C. The pulse and blood pressure are normal. ENT examination reveals a bulging congested left tympanic membrane. The right tympanic membrane is clear. The throat does not look inflamed. The lungs are clear to auscultation. The rest of the examination is normal. In particular, there is no neck stiffness, bulging fontanelle, or skin rash.

Q What is the most likely diagnosis?

A The history suggests an upper respiratory tract infection. The appearance of the left tympanic membrane confirms a diagnosis of acute otitis media.

Q What is the peak age of presentation of acute otitis media?

A The peak age is 6–18 months of age, though 20 per cent of children aged under 4 are affected at least once a year.

Q What are some risk factors for acute otitis media?

A Cigarette smoke exposure, craniofacial abnormalities, Down's syndrome, and attendance in nurseries.

Q What are the three most common bacteria that cause acute otitis media?

A *Streptococcus pneumoniae*, *H. influenzae*, and *Moraxella catarrhalis*.

Q How is acute otitis media different from otitis media with effusion (secretory otitis media, 'glue ear')?

A Acute otitis media is a bacterial infection of the middle ear. Otitis media with effusion refers to a middle ear filled with thick fluid which is a common cause of conductive hearing loss in children. Otitis media with effusion is thought to be related to dysfunction of the Eustachian tube.

Q What are the indications for treating otitis media with effusion?

A Fortunately most cases of otitis media with effusion resolve spontaneously within 6 weeks. Insertion of ventilation tubes into the tympanic membrane to drain the effusion should be considered in children with persistent disease with significant conductive hearing loss or associated problems with speech or difficulties at school.

Cross-reference: otitis media (p. 463).

Case 5

You are working in A&E when a 16-year-old girl is rushed in by ambulance. The paramedics briefly tell you that she had been feeling unwell for the past few weeks, with tiredness and marked weight loss. She was due to see her GP that day, but felt too ill to get out of bed. She then started vomiting and was becoming drowsy. Her mother phoned the general practice and was told to phone immediately for an ambulance. As the girl is rushed into the resuscitation room, the paramedics tell you her blood pressure is 85/50 mmHg and her pulse rate is 110 beats per min. Her oxygen saturations are 95 per cent. She looks pale and dehydrated, and feels cold and clammy.

Q What are your initial priorities for managing this girl?

A This young lady is extremely unwell and requires immediate active management. She is in shock, with a low blood pressure and tachycardia. The cause of the underlying shock can be determined once she is stabilized. Large bore intravenous access should be secured and rapid fluid replacement given. Blood should also be taken for a battery of tests. Although she is not pyrexial and the features do not fit precisely with septic shock (normally warm peripheries), blood cultures should also be taken as overwhelming sepsis is a common cause of severe shock in young people (particularly meningococcal).

Q What is shock and what are the possible underlying causes?

A Shock is a clinical term for a global reduction in tissue perfusion. Left untreated, shock is lethal due to multiorgan failure. There are four broad categories of shock: hypovolaemic shock, cardiogenic shock, distributive shock, and obstructive shock. In this young lady, cardiogenic shock and obstructive shock are less likely. Hypovolaemic shock and distributive shock are more likely. Particular causes at the top of one's differential in this case would include septic shock, anaphylactic shock, and hypovolaemic shock. In the absence of clear fluid loss (she is not bleeding all over the floor), other possibilities include loss through the kidneys such as uncontrolled diabetes, an acute presentation of Addison's disease, or intra-abdominal losses such as a ruptured ectopic pregnancy.

The laboratory phones the results through as soon as they are available:

Sodium	130 mmol/l
Potassium	5.7 mmol/l
Urea	21 mmol/l
Creatinine	79 μmol/l
Glucose	36 mmol/l

An arterial blood gas sample performed in A&E shows:

pH	7.26
pCO_2	2.1 kPa
pO_2	11.0 kPa

On the basis of the history and blood results, your team diagnose diabetic ketoacidosis.

Q What is diabetic ketoacidosis? Which of the above results are needed to confirm a diagnosis?

A Hyperglycaemia (usually >25 mmol/l) together with systemic acidosis on an arterial blood gas diagnoses diabetic ketoacidosis. There will also be large amounts of ketones in the urine, although this is not a diagnostic criteria as small amounts of urinary ketones can be normal, especially in fasting individuals. Note that isolated high blood glucose in a poorly controlled diabetic may be 'hyperglycaemia secondary to insulin lack' but is not diabetic ketoacidosis unless there is also acidosis. Equally, hyperglycaemia together with a large amount of ketones in the urine is not sufficient to diagnose ketoacidosis, unless there is a systemic acidosis.

Q Outline the treatment concepts for diabetic ketoacidosis.

A Fluid resuscitation is the treatment priority in the management of diabetic ketoacidosis. The combination of renal fluid loss due to the osmotic diuresis and vomiting leads to profound volume depletion. Patients commonly require several litres of fluid within the first 24 h. Once fluid replacement has started, insulin should be given intravenously in the form of a sliding scale at a rate which is regularly adjusted according to the blood glucose level. All patients with diabetic ketoacidosis should be kept nil by mouth. This is because there is commonly an associated gastroparesis and patients may vomit profusely if fed, with risk of potentially fatal aspiration. If there is any sign of an underlying infection causing the disturbance leading to ketoacidosis, this must also be treated with appropriate antibiotics.

The following day you are asked by the nurses on the ward to prescribe more fluids for the patient. You write up two bags of normal saline with potassium.

Q A medical student asks you why you are adding potassium to her fluids, pointing out the electrolyte tests showing the potassium concentration at the high end of normal. What is your answer?

A At the outset, plasma potassium levels are usually raised in diabetic ketoacidosis, although total body potassium has in reality been profoundly depleted. Once treatment has started, potassium levels begin to fall dramatically as insulin treatment drives potassium out of the extracellular fluid and into cells. Once plasma levels are within the upper limit of normal, replacement should begin in subsequent fluid bags. Patients should have electrolyte measurements every few hours to guide fluid replacement.

Cross-references: shock (p. 68), diabetes mellitus (p. 323).

Case 6

A 44-year-old man presents to A&E with a severely painful red hot first metatarsophalangeal joint. There is no history of trauma to the joint. You suspect a diagnosis of acute gout but want to exclude a septic arthritis.

Q What is gout and why does it cause joint inflammation?

A Gout is a crystal arthropathy in which crystals of urate become deposited in joints. Neutrophils phagocytose the crystals and degranulate in the joint, causing acute inflammation.

Q Why is it important urgently to rule out a septic arthritis?

A Infection in the enclosed space of a joint can rapidly, and irreversibly, destroy it.

Q What other causes of acute monoarthritis might you consider lower down your list of differential diagnoses?

A Other joint diseases more commonly associated with a polyarthritis may present with a monoarthritis, including rheumatoid arthritis or a spondyloarthropathy.

You perform an aspirate of the joint and the fluid is slightly cloudy. You send some of the fluid to microbiology for a white cell count, Gram stain, and culture. The rest of the fluid you send to histopathology to look for crystals.

Q What results would you expect from these tests for acute gout and for a septic arthritis?

A In gout, one would expect small numbers of white cells in the fluid, the presence of urate crystals, and no organisms seen on Gram stain or grown on culture. In septic arthritis, one would expect large numbers of white cells in the fluid, no crystals, and organisms to be seen on Gram staining, with a positive culture.

Cross-references: gout (p. 414), septic arthritis (p. 415).

Case 7

A 72-year-old man presents to you with a history of breathlessness on exertion. On examination, he has a harsh ejection systolic murmur and a slow rising carotid pulse. An echocardiogram shows aortic stenosis with a normal ejection fraction.

Q What are the two most common causes of aortic stenosis?

A The most common cause of aortic stenosis is calcific aortic stenosis which occurs due to calcification of the valve limiting opening of the valve cusps during systole. This is the result of longstanding haemodynamic stress on the valve over many years. Some cases of aortic stenosis are due to chronic rheumatic valvular disease. This is due to fibrosis and fusion of the valve cusps as a consequence of acute rheumatic heart disease occurring earlier in life.

Q Why is he breathless?

A The breathlessness is a symptom related to heart failure as a result of the aortic stenosis.

Q What other symptoms of aortic stenosis would you ask him about?

A The other two main symptoms of aortic stenosis are angina and episodes of syncope.

Q If the systolic function is normal, why is he getting symptoms of breathlessness due to heart failure?

A LVF may be systolic or diastolic. Systolic failure is the more common form (typically due to ischaemic heart disease). Diastolic heart failure occurs due to inadequate filling of the left ventricle and is often seen in left ventricular hypertrophy due to hypertension or aortic stenosis even in the presence of normal systolic function.

His wife tells you that she too was diagnosed with aortic stenosis last year when someone picked up a heart murmur, but she was not told she needed an operation.

Q Why is his wife not having aortic valve replacement?

A Aortic valve replacement is indicated for *symptomatic* aortic stenosis as the risk of sudden death is much higher in people with symptoms. People with asymptomatic aortic stenosis are generally just kept under close follow-up.

Cross-reference: aortic stenosis (p. 96).

Case 8

A 50-year-old housewife presents to A&E with severe right-sided loin pain which comes in waves and radiates down towards her groin. Microscopic haematuria is present on a dipstick. She is not febrile. A plain radiograph shows a 4 mm ureteric calculus at the vesicoureteric junction. Routine blood tests are sent off.

Q What are most renal calculi composed of?

A Calcium oxalate or a mixture of calcium oxalate and calcium phosphate.

She is given pain relief and she settles down. When the blood results come back, the calcium level is raised at 2.80 mmol/l. All her other blood tests are normal.

Q What are the common causes of hypercalcaemia? What is the most likely diagnosis in this lady?

A The most common causes of hypercalcaemia are primary hyperparathyroidism and malignancy. Malignancy may cause hypercalcaemia either by releasing parathyroid hormone-related peptide or through bony metastases. Rarer causes include thyrotoxicosis and sarcoidosis. The most likely cause in this lady is primary hyperparathyroidism.

Q What further blood test could be done to confirm primary hyperparathyroidism?

A Measurement of the parathyroid hormone level. Normally, in the setting of a raised calcium, parathyroid hormone levels should be low. A raised or inappropriately normal parathyroid hormone level would be diagnostic of primary hyperparathyroidism.

Q What are the causes of primary hyperparathyroidism?

A Most cases of primary hyperparathyroidism are due to a single functional parathyroid adenoma that autonomously secretes parathyroid hormone. A minority of cases are caused by hyperplasia of all four parathyroid glands for an unknown reason. Parathyroid carcinoma causing primary hyperparathyroidism has been described but is extremely rare.

Q How should this lady be treated for her primary hyperparathyroidism?

A Because she has symptomatic disease (an episode of nephrolithiasis), surgical treatment is indicated. Pre-operative localization of abnormal parathyroid tissue can be performed to highlight either a single parathyroid adenoma or four gland hyperplasia and determine the surgical treatment.

Cross-references: renal stones (p. 227), primary hyperparathyroidism (p. 321).

Case 9

A 72-year-old man presents to his GP with a history of rectal bleeding and a feeling of incomplete evacuation following defecation. The GP performs a digital rectal examination and feels a large mass in the rectum. He urgently refers the patient to a colorectal surgeon. The colorectal surgeon at the hospital performs sigmoidoscopy. He sees an ulcerated tumour in the lower rectum from which he takes multiple biopsies.

The biopsy report reads: 'These are biopsies of severely dysplastic large bowel mucosa which in places shows infiltration through the muscularis mucosae. Summary: adenocarcinoma.'

Q What is the significance of the infiltration through the muscularis mucosae?

A In colorectal neoplasia, adenocarcinoma is defined by invasion of severely dysplastic glands through the muscularis mucosae. This is because the chance of metastasis from a colorectal neoplasm confined to the mucosa is essentially zero. This contrasts with epithelial malignancies elsewhere in the body where carcinoma is defined by invasion through the *basement membrane*. If neoplastic glands are confined to the colonic mucosa, the term severely dysplastic adenoma remains appropriate.

The patient is told of the diagnosis and the surgeon organizes an MRI scan to examine the local spread of the tumour and to look for distant metastases.

Q How does rectal cancer spread? Which organ is particularly important to scrutinize on imaging for distant metastases?

A Rectal cancer spreads locally through the wall of the rectum and into mesorectal fat. An advanced tumour may infiltrate into nearby organs such as the prostate in men or the genital tract in women. Rectal cancers may also spread via lymphatic channels to local lymph nodes in the mesorectal fat. Haematogenous spread to distant organs most commonly involves the liver via the portal vein. Liver metastases should always be ruled out radiologically before considering curative surgery.

The MRI scan suggests that the tumour has infiltrated through the bowel wall into mesorectal fat but not into any adjacent organs. There are no obvious liver metastases. The surgeon lists the patient for an anterior resection with total mesorectal excision.

Q What is an anterior resection? What does total mesorectal excision mean and why is this important?

A An anterior resection is removal of the rectum and lower sigmoid colon. Total mesorectal excision refers to the surgical removal of all of the mesorectum surrounding the rectum. This is important to ensure that a wide excision of the tumour has been performed.

The surgery goes well and the anterior resection specimen is sent to histopathology for examination. The pathologist opens up the bowel away from the tumour to allow good penetration of formalin into the region of the tumour. When he opens up the bowel he notices two small dark brown mucosal polyps.

Q What type of polyp are these most likely to be? Why might you expect to find these in this patient's colon?

A These are most likely to be adenomatous polyps. The dark brown colour is typical of adenomatous polyps because the dysplastic mucosa reflects light differently from normal mucosa. Finding adenomatous polyps is not too surprising as most colorectal carcinomas arise from adenomatous polyps and these are often multiple.

Two days later, after good formalin fixation, the pathologist carefully slices the specimen and examines the tumour in the rectum macroscopically. The tumour appears to invade into the mesorectal fat but does not reach the surgical excision margin around the edge of the specimen. The areas of deepest invasion are taken for processing on to glass slides for microscopic examination. A careful lymph node search is then performed. The dark brown polyps are also sampled.

The following week, the patient is presented at the colorectal multidisciplinary meeting. The pathologist summarizes his findings from microscopic examination

of the samples: 'Moderately differentiated adenocarcinoma. Dukes C1, T3, N1. Lymphatic vessel invasion identified. No extramural vascular invasion seen. Circumferential excision margin clear of tumour.'

Q Explain the terms Dukes C1, T3, N1. Why will the surgeon be pleased to know that the circumferential margin is clear of tumour?

A Dukes C1 is related to the Dukes staging system for colorectal carcinoma. Dukes C1 means that there is lymph node involvement (regardless of the amount of local invasion by the tumour) but that the lymph node closest to the surgical margin (the 'high tie' node) is not involved by tumour. T3, N1 is related to the TNM staging system. In the rectum, T3 means that the tumour has infiltrated through the bowel wall into mesorectal fat but not into adjacent organs. N1 means that more than four lymph nodes contain metastatic adenocarcinoma. The circumferential margin refers to the true surgical margin where the surgeon has carved out the rectum from the pelvis. A clear circumferential margin means that local recurrence should not occur and the surgery has been potentially curative.

Cross-reference: colorectal neoplasia (p. 165).

Case 10

A 75-year-old woman presents to A&E following the acute loss of function of the left side of her body. The admitting medical team suspect a stroke.

Q What is a stroke and how is this different from a transient ischaemic attack?

A A stroke is a sudden neurological deficit from a vascular cause which lasts longer than 24 h. If the deficit completely resolves within 24 h, it is called a transient ischaemic attack.

Q What are the main causes of stroke?

A The most common cause of stroke is cerebral infarction due to blockage of a cerebral artery. Intracerebral haemorrhage due to rupture of a vessel within the brain substance is the second most common cause. Subarachnoid haemorrhage due to rupture of a berry aneurysm into the sub-arachnoid space accounts for a minority of cases.

An urgent head CT scan is arranged.

Q Why is a head CT required urgently?

A A CT scan can reliably distinguish between a stroke due to cerebral infarction or a stroke due to intracerebral or subarachnoid haemorrhage as the blood from the latter two causes is immediately visible. This is important as aspirin should be given for a cerebral infarct but not for a haemorrhage.

The CT scan does not reveal any haemorrhage so a cerebral infarction is presumed to be the cause.

Q What is the usual cause of a blocked cerebral artery leading to cerebral infarction?

A Most cerebral infarctions are caused by thromboembolic occlusion of a cerebral artery, from either complicated atherosclerotic plaques in the internal carotid artery or an embolus from the heart. Only a minority are due to *in situ* thrombosis over a complicated atherosclerotic plaque within a cerebral artery.

During the physical examination, you note that her pulse is irregular, and an electrocardiogram shows atrial fibrillation.

Q What is atrial fibrillation and what are the common causes?

A Atrial fibrillation is the most common sustained cardiac arrhythmia. The atria beat in an uncoordinated manner, replacing normal sinus rhythm with an irregular fast rhythm. Ischaemic heart disease, mitral valve disease, and hypertension account for most cases of atrial fibrillation.

Q Could the presence of atrial fibrillation be relevant to her stroke?

A Yes. If she is in uncontrolled atrial fibrillation and not anticoagulated, she could have developed a left atrial thrombus which embolized into the cerebral circulation, causing an embolic stroke.

An echocardiogram is performed, and this confirms the presence of a large left atrial appendage thrombus.

Q How is stroke managed?

A The management of stroke is largely supportive. Although nothing can be done to restore the brain tissue that has infarcted, much can be done with focused rehabilitation. Ideally, all patients should be cared for on dedicated stroke wards where there is suitable expertise in helping these patients regain as much function as possible.

Cross-references: stroke (p. 424), atrial fibrillation (p. 92).

Case 11

A 71-year-old retired electrician presents to you complaining of problems with breathlessness. His wife says that he has had a chesty cough for several years which she put down to his heavy smoking. He first noticed the breathlessness about 3 months ago, and it seems to be getting worse. He is now unable to take the dog for its daily walk.

Q On the basis of this information, what are the possible causes of this gentleman's breathlessness?

A Possible causes include chronic LVF, chronic obstructive pulmonary disease (COPD), lung cancer, mesothelioma, pulmonary tuberculosis, and a diffuse parenchymal lung disease. A severe anaemia can also cause breathlessness.

On examination, he is overweight and slightly breathless, having walked to your room from the waiting room. There is tar staining of the fingers of his right hand. There is no peripheral oedema. The pulse is 85 beats per min and regular. The blood pressure is 148/90 mmHg. The jugular venous pressure is not raised. Auscultation of the chest reveals occasional mild wheeze only. The electrocardiogram is normal. You arrange a chest radiograph and some routine blood tests, all of which are normal.

Q What is the implication of a normal ECG, chest radiograph, and blood tests?

A A normal ECG makes the diagnosis of chronic LVF very unlikely. A normal chest radiograph makes

pulmonary tuberculosis, lung cancer, mesothelioma, and diffuse parenchymal lung disease less
likely. The normal blood tests exclude anaemia.

You still suspect a pulmonary disease and arrange for
spirometric tests. The results are as follows:

FEV$_1$ 78 per cent of predicted
FEV$_1$/FVC ratio 67 per cent normal
No significant reversibility following inhaled bron-
chodilator

Q   What is the most likely diagnosis?

A   Chronic obstructive pulmonary disease. In the
presence of a suitable history and heavy smoking,
the presence of a reduced FEV$_1$ and FEV$_1$/FVC ratio
is strongly suggestive of COPD. Remember that in
mild COPD, the chest radiograph is often normal,
as is the peak flow.

Q   Explain the aetiology and pathogenesis of COPD.

A   COPD is almost always caused by smoking.
Smoking causes irritation of the large airways
and cough. Hyperplasia of mucus glands in the
bronchi leads to the production of plentiful
sputum. In the smaller airways, smoking causes
inflammation and eventually fibrosis. Irreversible
narrowing of the small airways is probably the
main cause of airflow obstruction in COPD. The
terminal airways also become dilated, with
destruction of the alveolar walls. This is thought to
be the result of an imbalance between proteases
and antiproteases in the distal lung spaces caused
by smoking (the protease–antiprotease hypothesis).

The following December, he becomes suddenly unwell
with a worsening of all his symptoms. His cough gets
worse, with more sputum production and he becomes
breathless at rest.

Q   This is known as an acute exacerbation of COPD.
What are the common causes of this?

A   The most common cause is infection. Other causes
to consider include a pneumothorax, LVF, a pulmonary embolus, or the development of a lung
carcinoma.

The admitting medical team take arterial blood gases.
The pO$_2$ is 7.8 kPa and the pCO$_2$ is 5.8 kPa.

Q   Explain these blood gas results.

A   This man is in respiratory failure, because his pO$_2$
is less than 8 kPa. The pCO$_2$ is within the normal
range, so this is type 1 respiratory failure.

Q   What are the implications of being in respiratory
failure?

A   Respiratory failure is defined as a pO$_2$ less than
8 kPa because this is the point at which the percentage oxygen saturation of haemoglobin leaving the lungs falls precipitously, with significant
impairment of oxygen delivery to the tissues.
Respiratory failure requires oxygen treatment to
bring the pO$_2$ back to above 8 kPa.

He is given oxygen by face mask, and a repeat blood gas
analysis 1 h later shows that he is no longer in respiratory failure. He is treated with antibiotics and makes a
good recovery.

Cross-references: chronic obstructive pulmonary disease
(p. 113), respiratory failure (p. 106).

Case 12

A 5-year-old boy is admitted urgently to hospital having
rapidly become very unwell over a period of just a few
days. He has been complaining of severe pain in his
bones and joints, and has now developed numerous
petechiae which prompted his parents to rush him into
hospital. On examination, he is extremely pale and you
think he has a palpable liver and spleen. He is not
febrile. Urgent blood tests reveal:

Haemoglobin	8 g/dl
White cell count	2 × 10^9/l
Platelets	22 × 10^9/l

The peripheral blood film shows numerous blasts. The
coagulation screen, liver function tests, and electrolytes are normal.

Q   What is going on here?

A   The full blood count reveals severe pancytopenia
with anaemia, leukopenia, and thrombocytopenia,

suggesting bone marrow failure. The presence of numerous blasts on the peripheral blood film suggest an acute leukaemia.

Q What is acute leukaemia? Why does it cause pancytopenia, bone pain, and hepatosplenomegaly?

A Acute leukaemia is a haematological malignancy in which a bone marrow haematopoietic stem cell becomes neoplastic. The neoplastic cells remain undifferentiated and proliferate in the bone marrow, rapidly overwhelming it. Production of normal blood cells by the bone marrow is quashed, causing pancytopenia. Neoplastic blasts then spill out into the blood and infiltrate organs and tissues. This explains the enlargement of the liver and spleen and the bony pain.

Q What investigations should be done next to confirm acute leukaemia?

A Definitive diagnosis requires bone marrow examination to confirm the presence of large numbers of blasts in the marrow.

A bone marrow aspirate shows large numbers of blasts. Immunophenotyping of the aspirate by flow cytometry shows them to be lymphoid blasts. A diagnosis of acute lymphoblastic leukaemia is made.

Q Explain the difference between acute lymphoblastic leukaemia and chronic lymphocytic leukaemia.

A Acute lymphoblastic leukaemia is a disorder predominantly of childhood in which the neoplastic haemopoietic stem cell remains highly undifferentiated. The primitive neoplastic cells (blasts) have a huge proliferative capacity and rapidly overwhelm the bone marrow. Acute lymphoblastic leukaemia therefore presents abruptly with bone marrow failure.

In contrast, chronic lymphocytic leukaemia is predominantly a disease of the elderly. Although the neoplastic cell is still derived from the haematopoietic stem cell, some differentiation does occur down the B lymphocyte lineage, typically halting at the stage of the circulating naïve B lymphocyte. These cells have much less proliferative capacity and so chronic lymphocytic leukaemia is a much more indolent disease which is often

picked up on the chance finding of a raised white cell count. The progression of the disease is slow, and many elderly people with chronic lymphocytic leukaemia die from other causes.

Cross-references: acute leukaemia (p. 356), chronic lymphocytic leukaemia (p. 358).

Case 13

A 44-year-old man donates blood as part of an awareness campaign launched at his office by a colleague who needed multiple blood transfusions following a road traffic accident. One week after donating a unit of blood, he receives a letter from the transfusion service telling him that one of the tests on his blood was abnormal. When he returns to the centre, a counsellor tells him that his blood sample was anti-hepatitis C virus (HCV) positive.

Q What does this result mean?

A His blood contains antibodies to HCV, meaning that at some point he has been infected with HCV.

Q How likely is it that he remains currently infected with HCV? What further test could be done to determine if he remains infected?

A Very likely. About 80 per cent of people infected with HCV fail to clear the virus and develop chronic infection. Confirming ongoing infection requires detection of HCV genetic material, such as reverse transcriptase–polymerase chain reaction (RT–PCR) for HCV RNA.

Q Does it surprise you that he does not recall an incident of acute hepatitis when he was infected?

A No. Most people with acute hepatitis C infection do not develop a clinically apparent episode of acute hepatitis (with jaundice and markedly deranged liver function tests). Most people develop a nonspecific systemic illness which they dismiss as 'flu'.

Q How is HCV transmitted, and what questions should you ask him about how he may have acquired the virus?

A HCV is transmitted via the blood. One of the most common methods of transmission is the use of contaminated needles when injecting drugs. Other sources include tattoos or ear piercings performed using infected needles. The risk of acquiring HCV from a blood transfusion is extremely low (~1 in a million transfusions) because of a window period of up to 3 months following infection with HCV before anti-HCV antibodies are measurable in the blood.

The patient admits to having injected drugs on just a few occasions when he was at university in the 1970s. He has never received a blood transfusion himself. He is referred to a hepatologist for further investigation. The following investigations are performed:

Anti-HCV (repeat)	Positive
HCV RNA	Positive
Liver function tests	All normal

Q Do the normal liver function tests imply that he has no liver disease?

A Unfortunately not. Liver 'function' tests are in reality tests of liver 'damage', as the enzymes are released into the blood following hepatocyte destruction. Patients with significant chronic liver disease with low levels of ongoing liver destruction may have completely normal biochemical liver function tests despite quite marked liver disease.

Q What investigation is required to assess the level of liver damage?

A A liver biopsy must be performed. This is the only reliable way to assess the level of inflammatory activity in the liver and to assess the degree of any liver fibrosis occurring as a result of the inflammation. The pathologist examining the liver biopsy of a patient with chronic hepatitis C will formally grade the level of inflammation and fibrosis using standardized criteria. These scoring systems are used to determine whether any treatment is indicated.

Cross-reference: hepatitis C (p. 184).

Case 14

You have just started your shift as medical SHO responsible for new admissions for the day. Your first patient is a 52-year-old lady with no significant past medical history. The GP letter says she presented in the morning with the sudden onset of severe right-sided pleuritic chest pain and breathlessness. The observations performed on arrival in hospital are: respiratory rate 30 breaths per min, pulse 105 beats per min, blood pressure normal, oxygen saturations 90 per cent on oxygen. The electrocardiogram shows a sinus tachycardia.

Q What are the characteristic features of pleuritic chest pain? What is the underlying mechanism?

A Pleuritic chest pain is typically a sharp, stabbing chest pain which is brought on by inspiration and coughing. It is due to inflammation or irritation of the richly innervated parietal pleura due to underlying lung disease.

Q What common causes of pleuritic chest pain should pass through your mind before you see this lady?

A Common causes of pleuritic chest pain in this woman would include pulmonary embolus, pneumothorax, and pneumonia.

You request a chest radiograph and take an arterial blood gas sample. The pO_2 is 9.2 kPa and the pCO_2 is 3.2 kPa.

Q Explain the results of the arterial blood gases. Is she in respiratory failure?

A The pO_2 is low, confirming that this lady is hypoxic. Although she has significant hypoxia, she is *not* in respiratory failure because the pO_2 is above 8 kPa. The pCO_2 is low because she is hyperventilating (respiratory rate 30 breaths per min) and blowing off carbon dioxide.

The chest radiograph looks normal. There is no pneumothorax and no evidence of pneumonia. You strongly suspect a pulmonary embolus.

Q What is a pulmonary embolus?

A A pulmonary embolus is a blockage of a pulmonary artery by an intravascular mass, almost always a detached thrombus from a deep vein thrombosis.

You arrange a CT pulmonary angiogram which shows a filling defect in a right-sided pulmonary artery, confirming pulmonary embolus. You start treatment with low molecular weight heparin and begin loading her with warfarin. You closely examine her legs but they both appear symmetrical and unremarkable.

The following day you present the lady's history to the consultant on the post-take ward round. He agrees with your diagnosis and management, and asks you if you have examined the breasts or performed a rectal examination.

Q Why might this be important?

A One of the risk factors for venous thrombosis is increased coagulability of the blood, which can occur in people with underlying malignancies. This should always be remembered in patients with deep vein thrombosis or pulmonary emboli, especially if they have no other clear risk factors.

Cross-references: respiratory failure (p. 106), pulmonary embolism (p. 112), deep vein thrombosis (p. 353).

Case 15

A 45-year-old woman presents to you worried about a 'mole' on her leg that seems to be growing. She is otherwise well. There is no previous personal or family history of malignant melanoma.

Q What features of this pigmented skin lesion would you be particularly interested in when you examine her?

A The ABCD guidelines have been proposed as a simple way of assessing pigmented skin lesions. Worrying features would include asymmetry, an irregular border, varying shades of colour, and a large diameter (>6 mm).

The lesion is large, measuring 7 mm in diameter, and has a notched border at one edge. However, it is uniformly pigmented and is broadly symmetrical. She has no other suspicious skin lesions elsewhere. These features worry you enough to refer her to a dermatologist for an expert opinion. The dermatologist makes a clinical diagnosis of a dysplastic nevus but does not think this is a melanoma.

Q What is a dysplastic nevus?

A A dysplastic nevus refers to a melanocytic lesion which shows some atypical features but does not fulfil criteria for a malignant melanoma. Dysplastic nevi are common lesions which may be found in up to 10 per cent of some populations.

The dermatologist offers to excise the lesion for reassurance. The patient does not like hospitals and asks you if it will develop into a melanoma if it is not removed.

Q How will you reply?

A Most dysplastic nevi are stable and do not progress into a malignant melanoma. It would probably be safe simply to monitor it, but excision is usually recommended.

The patient agrees and returns to the dermatology clinic for an excision biopsy of the lesion.

Q What is an excision biopsy? Why is it important to perform such a biopsy in this case?

A An excision biopsy means that the entire lesion is removed with a rim of normal skin using an elliptical incision. It is called an excision biopsy because the treatment is both diagnostic ('biopsy') and curative ('excision'). This contrasts with an incisional biopsy where only part of the lesion and some adjacent normal skin is removed for diagnostic purposes only. Pigmented skin lesions should *always* be removed by an excisional biopsy unless they are so large this is impossible. If only part of a pigmented lesion is removed and it turns out to be a melanoma, it then becomes impossible to assess important prognostic features.

The histopathology report comes back reading: 'Skin containing a melanocytic nevus showing a mild degree of cytological and architectural atypia. The lesion appears completely excised with a margin of 2 mm. Summary: completely excised mildly dysplastic nevus.'

Q Do you need to see this lady again?

A Probably not. Patients with a single dysplastic nevus and no personal or family history of melanoma can be safely discharged with advice about checking their skin regularly. Some dermatologists may see these patients infrequently. Only patients with multiple dysplastic nevi or a personal or family history of melanoma need close specialist follow-up.

You call in your next patient who has a very similar story. She is a 49-year-old with a pigmented skin lesion on her right leg which her GP is extremely concerned about. In the referral letter, the GP describes the lesion as 'an irregular variably pigmented 8 mm lesion with a nodular component'. When you examine the patient, you agree entirely with the GP's description. You think this is a malignant melanoma.

Q What should be done now?

A This lesion should be completely removed without delay by excisional biopsy for histopathological confirmation.

The lesion is excised that day and sent to histopathology. At the next multidisciplinary skin meeting, the pathologist presents the case. She says: 'This is an invasive superficial spreading malignant melanoma in vertical growth phase. The Breslow thickness is 2.1 mm and the melanoma reaches Clark level III.'

Q What does vertical growth phase mean and what is the implication of this?

A Invasive malignant melanomas show two stages of growth. In the radial growth phase, the growth of the tumour is parallel to the epidermis and the lesion grows radially. Clinically the melanoma appears as a flat pigmented skin lesion. After a period of time, the dominant site of growth shifts to within the dermis and the direction of growth becomes perpendicular to the epidermis; this is the vertical growth phase. Clinically a raised nodule then appears within the flat component. Once the vertical growth phase has been reached, there becomes a significant risk of distant metastasis.

Q Explain the terms Breslow thickness and Clark level.

A The Breslow thickness is the thickness of the melanoma measured from the granular layer of the epidermis down to the deepest point of the melanoma. The Clark level is a reflection of the deepest anatomical point in the skin that the melanoma has reached. Both have important prognostic information, particularly the Breslow thickness.

Cross-references: dysplastic nevus (p. 376), malignant melanoma (p. 380).

Case 16

A 58-year-old man presents to his GP following an episode of frank haematuria. He is otherwise well.

Q What causes of haematuria run through your mind?

A The top diagnosis to consider immediately with this history is a malignancy of the urinary tract. Renal cell carcinomas or transitional cell carcinomas of the urothelial tract may both present with haematuria. Other possible causes include infection, renal stones, or a renal disease such as a glomerulonephritis.

Q What tests should be done next to help narrow down a cause?

A A fresh midstream urine specimen should be sent for microscopy and culture to rule out infection. A renal ultrasound scan should be requested to rule out a renal mass. A fresh urine specimen should also be sent for cytological examination for malignant cells. This is good at picking up high grade urothelial malignancies and carcinoma in situ of the bladder. It is less good at reliably picking up low grade urothelial carcinomas, and so cystoscopy should be arranged to visualize the bladder if an alternative cause cannot be found.

The midstream urine specimen does not grow any organisms. The cytology report comes back with: 'This is a cellular specimen containing large numbers of urothelial cells, many of which are present in clusters and show mild nuclear atypia. The features are suggestive of a low grade transitional cell carcinoma.' A flexible cystoscopy shows a frond-like tumour in the bladder.

Q How would you divide up the different types of transitional cell carcinomas of the bladder?

A Bladder transitional cell carcinomas are divided into superficial, muscle invasive, and carcinoma in situ. Superficial bladder tumours are typically frond-like growths that show no, or minimal, invasion. Muscle invasive carcinomas are more solid tumours which deeply infiltrate into the muscle coat of the bladder. Carcinoma in situ is a flat lesion in which the urothelium contains frankly malignant cells but there is no invasion.

Q What other rarer types of bladder carcinomas do you know of apart from transitional cell carcinoma?

A Squamous cell carcinoma and adenocarcinoma may also develop in the bladder but these are much rarer.

The urologist resects the tumour away from the bladder wall in pieces and sends it for histopathological examination. A few days later, the report is issued: 'These are pieces of a grade 2 papillary transitional cell carcinoma. No invasion into the lamina propria is seen in this material. Summary: G2, Ta, papillary transitional cell carcinoma of the bladder.'

Q What does Ta mean? What is the prognosis for this man?

A In the bladder, Ta refers to a superficial transitional cell carcinoma that does not invade into the lamina propria. This is a confusing area, as the term 'carcinoma' usually implies invasion through the basement membrane of the epithelium into the underlying lamina propria. The reason why this term has stuck in the bladder is to reflect the well recognized fact that superficial bladder transitional cell carcinomas often show recurrence, and occasionally may recur as a muscle invasive tumour capable of wide dissemination. For this reason, the term carcinoma is used to emphasize the point that these patients should be followed-up carefully with check cystoscopies. The prognosis for most people with a grade 2 Ta superficial transitional cell carcinoma is extremely good. Although many will develop recurrences, these are easily resected, and only a small minority develop a muscle invasive tumour in the future.

Cross-reference: tumours of the urothelial tract (p. 234).

Case 17

A 20-year-old female presents to A&E after a few hours of severe right-sided upper abdominal pain. By the time you see her, the pain is easing off. On examination, she is thin, pale, and mildly jaundiced. She is mildly tender in the right upper quadrant. You suspect biliary colic. You send off routine blood tests and arrange an ultrasound scan. The ultrasound scan confirms the presence of numerous gallstones. You are going to send her home with a view to a surgical outpatient appointment to arrange cholecystectomy when you check the blood results:

Full blood count:

Hb	9.8 g/dl
MCV	102 fl
MCH	31 pg
MCHC	38 g/dl
WCC	8×10^9/l
Platelets	400×10^9/l

Biochemistry:

Na	138 mmol/l
K	4.2 mmol/l
Urea	5.6 mmol/l
Creatinine	61 µmol/l
Bilirubin	35 µmol/l
AST	25 U/l
ALT	41 U/l
ALP	90 U/l

Q What do these results suggest is going on?

A There is a macrocytic anaemia with a raised bilirubin. This suggests there may be haemolysis.

Q What further tests could be performed if one is suspecting haemolysis?

A A reticulocyte count should be performed as this should be raised in haemolysis. Lactate dehydrogenase levels are also usually raised. A blood film should also be examined to look for evidence of haemolysis and possibly the underlying cause.

The reticulocyte count is raised and the blood film shows numerous spherocytes.

Q What does this suggest?

A This picture is very typical of hereditary spherocytosis. However an immune haemolytic anaemia could give a similar picture and so a direct antiglobulin test should be performed to rule this out.

Q What is hereditary spherocytosis and why does it cause haemolysis?

A Hereditary spherocytosis is the most common inherited cause of haemolytic anaemia. Mutations in genes coding for proteins involved in maintaining the integrity of the red cell membrane lead to loss of lipid from the membrane and adoption of a spherical shape by red cells. The spherocytes are removed by macrophages in the spleen, leading to anaemia.

Q Are her gallstones related to the underlying disease?

A Yes. The increased red cell destruction leads to the production of excess quantities of unconjugated bilirubin which form pigmented gallstones. Gallstone-related disease is often what brings hereditary spherocytosis to clinical attention.

Cross-references: hereditary spherocytosis (p. 339), gallstones (p. 196).

Case 18

A 53-year-old man goes to his GP for a repeat blood pressure reading. Two previous measurements had both been raised at 148/96 and 144/94 mmHg. Today's reading is 146/97 mmHg. The GP decides to start the man on an ACE inhibitor.

Q How is hypertension defined and why is it important to take the reading on multiple occasions?

A Hypertension is defined as a blood pressure greater than 140/90 mmHg. This is the point at which the benefits of treatment outweigh the risks associated with treatment. It is important to take blood pressure readings several times to ensure a single spurious high result does not prompt lifelong drug treatment needlessly.

On the last visit, the GP had requested some routine blood tests, including renal function testing and electrolyte measurements. All of them were normal.

Q Why did the GP perform these tests?

A To rule out a secondary cause of hypertension such as chronic renal disease or Conn's syndrome. In chronic renal disease, the urea and creatinine may be raised, and in Conn's syndrome one would expect a high plasma sodium concentration and a low plasma potassium concentration.

Q What is the effect of hypertension on blood vessels?

A Hypertension causes thickening and narrowing of small arteries and arterioles, and also accelerates atherosclerosis in large and medium sized arteries.

Q What conditions may be caused by persistent untreated hypertension?

A Hypertension is a common cause of LVF (hypertensive heart disease) as the heart has to generate a higher pressure to overcome systemic blood pressure in order to produce an adequate cardiac output. Hypertension causes chronic renal failure (hypertensive nephropathy) as narrowing of renal arterioles causes ischaemic atrophy of nephrons. Hypertension is the most common cause of spontaneous intracerebral haemorrhage which causes stroke. The bleeding is usually from rupture of tiny aneurysms which form in cerebral arterioles weakened by hypertension (Charcot–Bouchard aneurysms). Hypertension is the most common cause of aortic dissection. This may be due to bleeding from vasa vasorum vessels into the wall of the aorta, causing a split to form in the wall.

Cross-reference: hypertension (p. 72).

Case 19

A 75-year-old man presents to his GP saying he has been not right for the past 5 months. He is tired all the time, has no appetite, and has lost weight. He has also had a troublesome cough which recently has become much worse. His wife booked the appointment when he coughed up some blood-tinged sputum a few days ago. Apart from noting his weight loss, you find little else on physical examination.

Q What are the possible diagnoses to consider here?

A The clinical story is suggestive of a chronic pulmonary disease. The most important diagnoses are lung cancer, pulmonary tuberculosis, and bronchiectasis.

You arrange for a chest X-ray and send off a sputum sample to the microbiology laboratory. The chest X-ray shows nodular shadowing in the left upper lobe with loss of volume, fibrosis, and evidence of cavitation. The radiology report says the features are strongly suggestive of pulmonary tuberculosis. The microbiologist then phones you to tell you that the patient has acid-fast bacilli in his sputum smear and the patient should be considered to have open pulmonary tuberculosis.

Q What is meant by open tuberculosis and what are the implications?

A Open tuberculosis means that the patient has *Mycobacterium tuberculosis* in their sputum, i.e. they are potentially infectious. Patients with open tuberculosis should be admitted to hospital and isolated in a single room for 2 weeks from the start of treatment. Adults with smear-negative or extrapulmonary disease do not need to be isolated. Active tuberculosis is a notifiable disease, and the appropriate authorities must be informed to allow contact tracing.

Q Which other organs may be affected by tuberculosis?

A Virtually any organ may be involved by tuberculosis, but the most common sites of extrapulmonary tuberculosis are the cervical lymph nodes, the genitourinary tract, and the meninges.

Q What might you expect to see histologically in an area of lung with active tuberculosis?

A The typical picture of active tuberculosis is granulomatous inflammation with caseous necrosis.

Cross-references: tuberculosis (p. 122), granulomatous inflammation (p. 15).

Case 20

You are an A&E SHO on your week of nights. At 0300, a 74-year-old man is brought in by ambulance after an episode of haematemesis. By the time he has arrived in casualty, the bleeding has stopped. His wife tells you he is otherwise well apart from an 'irregular heart rate'.

Q What are the most common causes of haematemesis?

A Haematemesis is usually caused by an acute upper gastrointestinal bleed. The most common causes are an erosive/haemorrhagic gastritis, a bleeding peptic ulcer, and bleeding oesophageal varices.

Q Why is taking a thorough drug history particularly important in this case?

A A drug history is extremely important. Non-steroidal anti-inflammatory drugs are a common cause of erosive gastritis and bleeding. He might be on medication which suggests that he has had dyspeptic symptoms before (e.g. antacids). This may indicate a chronic problem such as a peptic ulcer.

You stabilize the patient and keep him well hydrated. The following morning, the patient's care is taken over by the gastroenterologists. Endoscopy is performed once the patient is stabilized.

Q What is endoscopy and why is it useful in the management of upper gastrointestinal bleeding?

A Upper gastrointestinal endoscopy involves passing a fibreoptic scope through the mouth and into the oesophagus, stomach, and duodenum. It allows direct visualization of the mucosal surfaces. Endoscopy is performed in endoscopy suites, not on the wards. This is why it is important to ensure the patient is as stable as possible. Managing an acutely unwell patient away from the help of the wards is not easy. Endoscopy is useful to determine the cause of the bleeding, to assess prognosis by looking for stigmata suggestive of rebleeding, and to administer therapy in suitable cases.

A large peptic ulcer is seen on the posterior aspect of the first part of the duodenum with blood clot in the base.

Q Describe the features that would lead you to diagnose a peptic ulcer.

A Peptic ulcers are sharply punched out lesions of the bowel wall with clean edges.

Q What is the most likely cause of his duodenal peptic ulcer and how does this knowledge aid treatment?

A The vast majority of duodenal peptic ulcers are caused by *Helicobacter pylori*. Knowledge of the bacterial aetiology of peptic ulcers means that most can be treated with *Helicobacter* eradication regimes rather than surgery.

Cross-reference: peptic ulcer disease (p. 147).

Case 21

A 40-year-old man attends a general practice appointment for a 'well man' check up. He is found to have a positive urine dipstick test for blood with a trace of protein. His blood pressure is 152/98 mmHg.

Q What are the most likely causes of the haematuria in this gentleman?

A Haematuria may be caused by bleeding anywhere in the urinary tract. Haematuria due to a renal disorder is usually accompanied by proteinuria as well, and this is a useful clue. In young patients under 45, the most common and important causes are: glomerulonephritis (especially IgA nephropathy), urinary stones, tumours of the kidney or bladder, and autosomal dominant polycystic kidney disease.

The plasma creatinine is 185 μmol/l. Based on these results, the GP decides to refer the patient to a nephrologist at the hospital for further investigation.

Q Is this an appropriate course of action?

A Referral to a nephrologist is indeed appropriate here. The presence of hypertension, proteinuria, and haematuria are strong pointers toward renal disease. The creatinine value of 185 is a significant finding as this implies a substantial reduction in glomerular filtration rate for a man of this age.

The nephrologist suspects a glomerulonephritis and arranges a renal biopsy. A few weeks later, the patient is admitted to hospital and a renal biopsy is taken. A few days later, the histopathology report is issued, confirming a diagnosis of IgA nephropathy.

Q What features would the pathologist have seen to lead them to make a diagnosis of IgA nephropathy?

A The diagnostic feature of IgA nephropathy is the presence of deposits of IgA in the mesangium of the glomeruli. These can be demonstrated by using specific antibodies to IgA. In addition, the glomeruli show a pattern of response to the IgA deposition that can be seen on light microscopy. Usually this is in the form of focal proliferative changes in the glomeruli due to increased mesangial cellularity.

The patient comes back to the outpatient clinic and you explain the diagnosis of IgA nephropathy. He is understandably anxious and asks you 'will I need dialysis?'.

Q How would you reply?

A In about one-third of cases, IgA nephropathy causes progressive damage to the kidneys; some of these patients may need dialysis and/or transplantation in the end. IgA nephropathy tends to be very slowly progressive and so this may take 10–30 years to occur. Patients with hypertension and marked proteinuria are more likely to progress to end-stage renal failure, and so one would have a guarded approach with this chap.

Cross-reference: IgA nephropathy (p. 215).

Case 22

You are a surgical senior house officer on call. A 26-year-old female is referred to you from A&E with abdominal pain. The A&E doctor tells you that the pain came on suddenly and is localized in the right iliac fossa. She has vomited twice and feels unwell. Blood tests revealed a raised white cell count and C-reactive protein (CRP), and she is mildly pyrexial. A plain abdominal film and erect chest radiograph do not show evidence of obstruction or perforation. He thinks the diagnosis is acute appendicitis.

Q What further simple tests should the A&E doctor have performed?

A The story here is quite typical for acute appendicitis and would certainly be high on the list of differential diagnoses. However, two important and quick tests that must be performed are a pregnancy test and a urine dipstick. All women of child-bearing age with abdominal pain must have a pregnancy test. This history would fit for a complicated ectopic pregnancy, and these patients can deteriorate very rapidly if left untreated. Urinary tract infections are common in women and often give rise to lower abdominal pain which may localize to one side. A urine dipstick rules out gross infection. Isolated haematuria might suggest renal stones which could be looked for on the plain abdominal film.

When you see the patient, you confirm the history of right iliac fossa pain with nausea. Your further investigations are negative. You also suspect acute appendicitis. Your specialist registrar comes to see the patient and decides to proceed with appendicectomy. He asks you to consent her and then join him in theatre.

Q At laparotomy, what would an appendix with acute appendicitis look like?

A An inflamed appendix is dilated, congested, and covered in fibrinous exudate on the external surface. It is usually straightforward to recognize in the later stages.

You locate the appendix but it appears normal.

Q What should you do now?

A If the appendix appears normal, it is routine practice to remove it anyway. There may be microscopic inflammation. The abdomen should be then explored for any other pathology which may account for the pain.

Further exploration of the pelvis reveals a large cystic right ovary which has twisted on itself and looks very dark and congested. You remove the ovary and send it to histopathology.

A few days later the histopathology report is issued. The appendix is reported as histologically normal. The ovarian mass is reported as a mature cystic teratoma (dermoid cyst).

Q What is a mature cystic teratoma? Why is it also called a dermoid cyst?

A Mature cystic teratoma is a germ cell tumour of the ovary. It is also known as a dermoid cyst because the lining of the cyst is often composed of skin, i.e. keratinizing stratified squamous epithelium with underlying skin adnexal structures such as hair follicles and sebaceous glands. The cyst typically becomes filled with a thick greasy substance composed of keratin and sebaceous material. Hair is often present. Mature cystic teratomas are benign neoplasms.

Cross-references: acute appendicitis (p. 159), ectopic pregnancy (p. 278), mature cystic teratoma (p. 277).

Case 23

A 19-year-old university student presents with a 3 day history of severe sore throat, difficulty swallowing, and general malaise. On examination, he has a fever, his throat is inflamed, and there is a patchy white material over his tonsils. There is marked cervical lymphadenopathy. You also think you can feel some axillary lymph nodes and possibly the tip of an enlarged spleen.

Q What is the differential diagnosis?

A The picture is of a severe pharyngitis with systemic features including lymphadenopathy. The most common causes would be infection with Epstein–Barr virus, cytomegalovirus, or *Toxoplasma gondii*. The acute seroconversion illness of HIV infection may present like this and should be considered. Lymphoma is also a possibility.

Q What investigations would you perform?

A A panel of blood tests should be performed, including a full blood count and blood film, liver function tests, a Monospot test for EBV, and a throat swab.

The next day the following results return:

Haemoglobin 13.2 g/dl
White cell count 15.0 × 10⁹/l with 58 per cent lympho-
cytes and 10 per cent large unclassified cells
Blood film shows atypical lymphocytes
Other preliminary blood tests normal

Q Explain these results. What are the atypical lymphocytes?

A The blood count shows a lymphocytosis and the presence of large cells which, on examining the blood film, are shown to be atypical lymphocytes. Atypical lymphocytes are strongly suggestive of infectious mononucleosis; they represent T lymphocytes responding to the presence of EBV-infected B lymphocytes.

A few days later, some more results come back:

Monospot test: positive
Throat swab: commensal growth only

You diagnose EBV-related infectious mononucleosis.

Q What is the Monospot test?

A The Monospot test is designed to demonstrate antibodies released from EBV-infected B lympho-cytes known as 'heterophil' antibodies which agglutinate horse red blood cells.

Q If the test had been negative, what other tests could you have requested to confirm a diagnosis of EBV infectious mononucleosis?

A About 10 per cent of patients with infectious mononucleosis do not produce heterophil anti-bodies, giving a negative Monospot test. Making the diagnosis of EBV infectious mononucleosis in these people requires measurement of serum IgM antibodies to EBV or PCR testing for EBV genetic material.

Q What other conditions has EBV been associated with?

A EBV has also been linked to lymphomas in immunosuppressed people and to nasopharyn-geal carcinoma.

Cross-references: infectious mononucleosis (p. 459), nasopharyngeal carcinoma (p. 458).

Case 24

A 74-year-old man presents to his GP with a 1 month history of problems swallowing. He complains of the sensation of food getting stuck on its way down. Liquids seem to pass readily. His wife says he has lost a consid-erable amount of weight over the last few months. He has smoked about 20 cigarettes a day for most of his life.

Q What are the common causes of dysphagia?

A Dysphagia may be caused by a stricture in the lumen of the oesophagus which may be benign (e.g. peptic stricture) or malignant due to an oesophageal carcinoma. A disorder of oesophageal motility can also cause dysphagia, for example achalasia.

The GP arranges for an urgent upper gastrointestinal endoscopy. At endoscopy, an exophytic mass is seen in the middle third of the oesophagus. Biopsies are taken and sent for histopathological examination. The report comes back as showing squamous cell carcinoma.

Q What are the risk factors for squamous cell carci-noma of the oesophagus?

A Heavy smoking and alcohol intake are the strongest risk factors for oesophageal squamous cell carcinoma.

Q What is the other main carcinoma of the oesophagus and what are the risk factors for this type?

A The other main type of oesophageal carcinoma is adenocarcinoma. This tends to occur on a back-ground of Barrett's oesophagus in patients with gastro-oesophageal reflux disease.

The surgeon arranges for the patient to undergo staging to see how far the tumour has spread.

Q How does oesophageal carcinoma spread?

A Local spread is through the layers of the oesophageal wall. If it invades through the wall, it may then directly infiltrate nearby structures such as the trachea. Lymphatic spread occurs to the local lymph nodes. Haematogenous spread occurs to the liver, lungs, and adrenals most commonly.

At the upper gastrointestinal multidisciplinary meeting, the patient is discussed. The radiologist shows the staging images. The tumour has just invaded through the oesophageal wall but not into surrounding structures. There is no apparent local lymphadenopathy. No distant metastases are identified. Theoretically he would be suitable for surgical resection. The surgeon is worried that the patient's heavy smoking would place him at great anaesthetic risk.

Q What other cardiac and respiratory problems may be caused by smoking?

A Smoking is a major risk factor for atherosclerosis, so this patient could have significant ischaemic heart disease. Smoking is also a cause of chronic obstructive pulmonary disease and poor lung function. Again this poses an anaesthetic risk, especially as one lung must be deflated during surgery in order to gain access to the oesophagus.

Cross-reference: oesophageal carcinoma (p. 140).

Case 25

A 40-year-old woman with no significant past medical history is admitted to hospital with a 2 week history of arthralgia, night sweats, and a tender skin rash over the fronts of both legs. The skin rash is diagnosed as erythema nodosum.

Q What is erythema nodosum and what diseases is it associated with?

A Erythema nodosum is characterized by multiple raised erythematous nodules on the skin, typically on the lower legs, due to inflammation in the subcutaneous fat (panniculitis). Erythema nodosum may be idiopathic but has been associated with a number of underlying disorders including sarcoidosis, inflammatory bowel disease, and infections.

Blood tests reveal hypercalcaemia, and a chest radiograph shows bilateral hilar lymphadenopathy. A diagnosis of sarcoidosis is made.

Q What is sarcoidosis? Why does she have hypercalcaemia?

A Sarcoidosis is a multisystem disease of unknown aetiology in which numerous tissues become infiltrated with non-caseating granulomas. The granulomas produce the active form of vitamin D, promoting calcium absorption in the gut and causing hypercalcaemia.

Q What sort of prognosis would you expect in this case?

A One would expect a good prognosis in this lady, as she has presented with the acute form of the disease which usually spontaneously resolves without long-term complications.

Cross-references: erythema nodosum (p. 391), sarcoidosis (p. 482).

Case 26

A term male infant is noted to have blue lips and nail beds at 24 h of age. The temperature and respiratory rate are normal, but he has tachycardia. There is no significant respiratory distress. ENT examination is normal. Auscultation does not reveal a murmur, but there is a single second heart sound. His lungs are clear. The liver and spleen are normal.

Q Why is the child cyanosed?

A This infant has either a respiratory or a cardiac problem. A cardiac problem is likely as there are no respiratory signs.

Q What is the most common cyanotic congenital heart disease that can present in neonates?

A Transposition of great arteries (TGA) is the most common cyanotic congenital heart disease in the newborn infant. Tetralogy of Fallot presents later.

An echocardiogram shows the infant has transposition of the great arteries.

Q What is transposition of the great arteries?

A Transposition of the great arteries is a congenital heart disease in which the aorta is connected to the right ventricular outflow tract and the pulmonary artery is connected to the left ventricular outflow tract. Mixing of blood between the circulations occurs through a patent foramen ovale and the ductus arteriosus. As the ductus begins to close after birth, the child develops cyanosis.

Q The mother is an epileptic and was taking phenytoin during pregnancy. Is that relevant?

A Yes, it is relevant as phenytoin is a known teratogen, and a cause of cardiac malformations and neural tube defects.

Q Why is the second heart sound single?

A The single sound is caused by the coinciding aortic and pulmonary sounds.

Q How would you manage the condition?

A The first line of management is a prostaglandin infusion to maintain the patency of the ductus arteriosus and allow mixing of the systemic and pulmonary blood. Balloon atrial septostomy during cardiac catheterization also allows further mixing and maintains cardiac output over a longer period. The preferred surgical management is the arterial switch operation. The aorta and the pulmonary arteries are transected and anastomosed to the appropriate ventricles. The coronary arteries are reimplanted into the aorta, which is a critical step for the infant's survival. The arterial switch is carried out within a week or 10 days of life before the muscle mass of the left ventricle regresses to the extent of being unable to function as a systemic pump. This procedure offers the best prognosis.

Cross-reference: congenital heart disease (p. 498).

Case 27

A 76-year-old man presents to his GP with a history of worsening urinary flow. The GP performs a digital rectal examination and feels a hard craggy prostate gland. He refers him to a urologist and sends off a PSA test. The PSA level is 45 µg/l (raised). The urologist arranges for prostatic biopsies and takes four needle cores from each side of the prostate under ultrasound guidance.

One week later, the pathology report comes back: 'All of these cores are infiltrated by adenocarcinoma of Gleason sum score 8 (4+4). There is adjacent high grade PIN. Perineural infiltration is seen and there is evidence of extraprostatic spread.'

Q What is the Gleason sum score?

A The Gleason sum score is a grading system for prostate carcinoma. The architectural patterns of the tumour are examined and graded from 1 to 5 according to how well they represent normal prostate. The dominant pattern is scored, followed by the next dominant pattern, and the two patterns are added together to give the Gleason sum score. The sum score ranges from 2 to 10, with 10 being the worst.

Q What is PIN?

A PIN is prostatic intraepithelial neoplasia. It is an *in situ* form of prostate cancer which is diagnosed microscopically when neoplastic prostatic epithelial cells are seen lining the prostatic glands but there is no actual invasion. PIN is believed to be the precursor lesion of invasive prostatic adenocarcinoma.

Q How might the pathologist have known the tumour had spread outside the prostate on the basis of a tiny needle biopsy? What is the relevance of the extraprostatic spread?

A Extraprostatic spread can be presumed if the malignant glands are seen in fatty tissue at the end of the biopsy core, as there is no fat within the prostate gland. The presence of extraprostatic spread means that the tumour is no longer confined to the prostate and makes cure less likely to be achievable.

The urologist arranges for a bone scan to be performed.

Q Why is a bone scan performed?

A Prostatic carcinoma commonly spreads to bone, and a bone scan is a good way of assessing the entire skeleton for evidence of skeletal metastases.

The bone scan result shows uptake in the vertebral column and ribs suggestive of metastatic disease. The patient does not have any bony pain. He is started on injections of a gonadotrophin-releasing hormone (GnRH) agonist.

Q Why are GnRH agonists used for prostatic carcinoma?

A Proliferation of prostatic carcinoma is driven by androgens. Progression of the tumour is thus markedly depressed by blocking androgen production biochemically. GnRH agonists cause an initial surge in luteinizing hormone (LH) release from the anterior pituitary, but then a dramatic fall. The fall in LH diminishes androgen production.

Cross-reference: tumours of the prostate (p. 238).

Case 28

You are a senior house officer in obstetrics and gynaecology working in gynaecology outpatients. Your consultant asks you to see a new referral and gives you the notes. The letter from the GP tells you that this 53-year-old lady presented recently with a 2 month history of irregular vaginal bleeding. She had undergone the menopause 4 years earlier. Her last cervical smear was normal. She is married with two children and is a non-smoker. The GP found nothing on examination.

Q What are the possible causes of bleeding in this lady and which would you be most concerned about?

A Post-menopausal bleeding is a serious symptom which must be fully investigated. There are many possible causes including an endocervical polyp, cervical carcinoma, endometrial atrophy, an endometrial polyp, endometrial hyperplasia, endometrial carcinoma, or a fibroid. Clearly the most concerning diagnoses are endometrial carcinoma and cervical carcinoma. We are told her last cervical smear was negative but that does not completely rule out the possibility of cervical carcinoma.

Q What investigations would you perform in the outpatient department?

A The most important investigations are inspecting the lower genital tract with the aid of a speculum and imaging the upper genital tract with ultrasound. The vulva, vagina, and cervix should be carefully inspected. An endocervical polyp may be visible at the external os and a cervical carcinoma should be visible. A transvaginal ultrasound may be performed in the outpatient clinic, but in some hospitals this investigation may require separate referral to radiology. This technique involves passing an ultrasound probe into the vagina to visualize the uterus. The thickness of the endometrium can be measured, which may be increased in endometrial hyperplasia and endometrial carcinoma. Endometrium more than 5 mm thick, especially in a post-menopausal woman, is considered highly suspicious for carcinoma. Other lesions in the uterus that may be causing the bleeding might be seen, for instance an endometrial polyp or a fibroid. The endometrium must be sampled even if no abnormality is seen on ultrasound, and this can be achieved in the outpatient department using a pipelle sampler.

You take an endometrial sample and send it in formalin to the histopathology department. A few days later, the report is delivered to you. It reads: 'This endometrial sample shows an increase in the number of endometrial glands. There is glandular crowding and the cells show nuclear atypia. In addition, there are areas of glandular fusion and irregularity indicating invasion. No myometrial tissue is present to assess for myometrial invasion. Summary: endometrioid adenocarcinoma arising in a background of hyperplasia with cytological atypia.'

Q What is endometrial hyperplasia and how is this related to endometrial carcinoma?

A Endometrial hyperplasia refers to an increase in the ratio of endometrial glands to endometrial stroma above the normal 1:1 ratio. Microscopically, endometrial hyperplasia causes crowding of the endometrial glands together. Endometrial hyperplasia is divided into hyperplasia with or without cytological atypia depending on whether the nuclei of the glands are abnormal or not. Hyperplasia with cytological atypia has a much higher chance of progressing into an invasive endometrial carcinoma.

Following the diagnosis of endometrial adenocarcinoma, the patient is listed for total abdominal hysterectomy and bilateral oophorectomy. At laparotomy, the uterus appears externally unremarkable with no evidence of carcinoma breaching through the uterus. A 10 cm mass is present in the left ovary. The specimen is sent to histopathology for analysis. A few days later, the histopathology report is issued. The summary reads: 'Uterus: grade 2 endometrioid endometrial adenocarcinoma infiltrating inner half of myometrium. Left ovary: granulosa cell tumour.'

Q What is a granulosa cell tumour and how could this be related to the endometrial carcinoma?

A Granulosa cell tumours are a type of ovarian sex cord stromal tumour which are often oestrogen producing. Unopposed oestrogen stimulation of the endometrium leads to hyperplasia, which may progress to hyperplasia with cytological atypia and eventually endometrial adenocarcinoma.

Cross-references: endometrial hyperplasia (p. 265), endometrial carcinoma (p. 267), sex cord stromal tumours of the ovary (p. 276).

Case 29

A 1-year-old girl presents with a proven urinary tract infection. She is systemically well. The sample of urine sent to microbiology was a mid stream specimen, and it yielded a pure growth of *Escherichia coli*.

Q How will you manage the infection?

A She should be treated with a course of oral antibiotics based on the sensitivity of the *E. coli* to antibiotics.

Q Why is the collection of the urine specimen for microbiology critical?

A It is essential to diagnose urinary tract infection accurately in children. A false-positive result may

subject the child to unnecessary investigations, whilst a false-negative result may deny the child treatment which could prevent serious consequences.

Q Does she need further investigations?

A Absolutely. Any child under the age of 5 with a urinary tract infection needs thorough investigation. Urinary tract infections in children may be associated with an underlying structural anomaly of the urinary tract which should be looked for by ultrasound examination and a micturating cystourethrogram for vesicoureteric reflux. Furthermore, urinary tract infections in childhood may lead to permanent renal scarring in the kidney causing hypertension and chronic renal failure in later life without treatment. The presence of renal scars should be assessed using a radioisotope (DMSA) scan of the kidneys 6 weeks following the infection.

On micturating cystourethrography, she is found to have mild bilateral vesicoureteric reflux. No renal scars are found on DMSA scanning. She is started on prophylactic antibiotics until age 4.

Q Why is it safe to withdraw antibiotics after age 4?

A The danger with untreated reflux is the development of permanent renal scarring leading to hypertension and reflux nephropathy. The kidneys only appear to be susceptible to scarring up until age 4; beyond this age, new scars do not seem to occur in association with vesicoureteric reflux. As such, it is safe to cease antibiotic prophylaxis at this age.

Cross-references: urinary tract infection (p. 245), reflux nephropathy (p. 221).

Case 30

A 49-year-old man presents to you complaining of severe tingling and discomfort in both his hands, affecting the thumbs, second finger, and third finger. The symptoms seem to be worse at night and he has to hang his hand out of the side of the bed.

When you examine his hands, you evoke paraesthesia in the distribution of the median nerve when you tap the flexor aspect of the wrist. You make a diagnosis of carpal tunnel syndrome. Whilst examining the hands, you notice they are particularly sweaty, and the patient tells you that recently he has been troubled by excessive sweating even in the absence of exertion. As you are looking at him, you are struck by his facial appearance. His nose and ears look large and when he turns his head his lower jaw looks protuberant.

Q What diagnosis springs to mind here? What other questions might you ask the patient to confirm your suspicion and how does this tie in with his carpal tunnel syndrome?

A These features all point to a diagnosis of acromegaly, in which excessive circulating growth hormone leads to increased growth of soft tissues of the face, hands, and feet. A change in facial appearance is typical, together with increased sweating. Carpal tunnel syndrome is common due to compression of the median nerve by the soft tissue growth at the wrist. Further questions worth asking are whether he has noted his shoe size increasing or rings becoming tighter. A bitemporal hemianopia may manifest by bumping into objects when walking or, more dangerously, clipping wing mirrors when driving!

Q What other features might you expect to find on further simple examination in a general practice?

A Acromegaly is usually due to a growth hormone-secreting pituitary adenoma. Large pituitary adenomas compressing the optic chiasm typically lead to a bitemporal hemianopia. This gentleman's visual fields should therefore be tested. Acromegaly often leads to mild hypertension, and so the blood pressure should be checked. Acromegaly is also a diabetogenic state. If he has frank diabetes, there may be glycosuria on stick testing of the urine.

You refer him to an endocrinology clinic with a presumptive diagnosis of acromegaly.

The endocrinologist performs a glucose tolerance test:

| Blood glucose | 6.8 mmol/l | 2 h after glucose load | 9.5mmol/l |
| Serum GH | 22 mU/l | 2 h after glucose load | 20 mU/l |

Q What do these results show?

A The glucose tolerance test confirms the diagnosis of acromegaly. The serum growth hormone concentration is raised even before the glucose is administered, and fails to be significantly suppressed by glucose. The glucose tolerance test also shows that the patient has impaired glucose tolerance. About 25 per cent of patients with acromegaly are found to have impaired glucose tolerance and about 10 per cent have frank diabetes mellitus.

The endocrinologist also organizes a series of investigations to test for adequate levels of the other anterior pituitary hormones.

Q Why would he do this?

A Acromegaly is typically due to a growth hormone-secreting pituitary adenoma. As well as producing symptoms of hormone excess, the tumour may also cause reduction in secretion of other anterior pituitary hormones by compressing the adjacent pituitary tissue.

Cross-references: carpal tunnel syndrome (p. 444), acromegaly (p. 300), hypopituitarism (p. 301).

Case 31

A 43-year-old woman presents with a 5 month history of marked fatigue, weight loss, anorexia, and generalized pruritus. On examination, she is found to have numerous spider nevi, scratch marks, palmar erythema, and hepatomegaly. The GP suspects chronic liver disease.

Q What are the common causes of chronic liver disease? Does it surprise you that she is not jaundiced?

A Chronic liver disease may be caused by alcoholic liver disease, non-alcoholic liver disease, chronic viral hepatitis, autoimmune hepatitis, primary biliary cirrhosis, primary sclerosing cholangitis, and inherited liver diseases such as haemochromatosis, Wilson's disease, and α_1-antitrypsin deficiency. Jaundice often does not develop until very late in the history of chronic liver disease when the metabolic functions of the liver have been severely impaired.

Investigations show:

Haemoglobin	9.5 g/dl
ESR	140 mm/h
Clotting	Normal
Electrolytes	Normal
Urea and creatinine	Normal
Calcium	Normal
Albumin	41 g/l
Total protein	93 g/l
Bilirubin	18 µmol/l
ALT	152 U/l
AST	164 U/l
ALP	Normal
IgG	44 g/l
IgA	Normal
IgM	Normal

No paraprotein seen on electrophoresis
Hepatitis B surface antigen negative
Hepatitis C antibody negative

Antinuclear antibodies are strongly positive and her serum is positive for antibodies to smooth muscle. A diagnosis of autoimmune hepatitis is made.

Q What is autoimmune hepatitis?

A Autoimmune hepatitis is a liver disease caused by autoimmune attack of hepatocytes. It is associated with raised levels of IgG, antinuclear antibodies, and antibodies to smooth muscle. It typically presents with chronic liver disease but can present more acutely with markedly raised transaminases and jaundice.

She is started on prednisolone with dramatic improvement. Her serum transaminases returned to normal over the next 2 weeks. Her hepatologist then arranges for a liver biopsy to be performed.

Q Why is a liver biopsy performed?

A A liver biopsy is important in any chronic liver disease to assess the inflammatory activity in the liver and, most importantly, to determine the degree of fibrosis in the liver.

The liver biopsy shows minimal fibrosis. Her disease remains well controlled on immunosuppression. Every year she has a liver biopsy and bone densitometry.

Q Why is she sent for bone densitometry?

A Patients taking long-term glucocorticoid therapy are at risk of developing osteoporosis. Their bone density should therefore be periodically measured using bone densitometry.

Seven years later a liver biopsy comes back as showing established cirrhosis.

Q Define cirrhosis. What are the consequences of the development of cirrhosis?

A Cirrhosis is the diffuse replacement of the liver by bands of fibrosis separated by nodules of regenerating hepatocytes. It is an irreversible condition. As well as impairing the function of the liver, cirrhosis causes portal hypertension (creating portosystemic anastomoses and oesophageal varices), and is a risk factor for the development of hepatocellular carcinoma.

She is put on the list for a liver transplant and 2 years later a suitable match is found.

Cross-references: chronic liver disease (p. 185), autoimmune hepatitis (p. 188), cirrhosis (p. 192), osteoporosis (p. 401).

Case 32

A 14-year-old boy presents with a sudden onset of left-sided scrotal swelling and pain. On examination, you find erythema of the scrotum with a tender, enlarged testis on that side. Palpation of the inguinal canal reveals a thickened cord.

Q What diagnosis would you be most concerned about with this history?

A A testicular torsion.

Q What are the main differential diagnoses?

A The two main differential diagnoses are torsion of the hydatid of Morgagni and epididymo-orchitis. A hydatid of Morgagni is an embryological remnant found on the upper pole of the testis. In torsion, tenderness is localized to the upper pole of the testis. Epididymo-orchitis results in acute scrotal swelling from inflammation of the epididymis and testis.

Q How would you manage testicular torsion?

A If there is any suspicion over testicular torsion, the scrotum should be surgically explored. If the testis is torted and viable, it is unrotated and surgically fixed, as is the testis on the opposite side.

Q On scrotal exploration, the surgeon describes a 'black' testis. What does the colour indicate?

A A black testis indicates an infarcted testis. It should be excised.

Cross-reference: testicular torsion (p. 515).

Case 33

A 27-year-old female presents to her GP with a 3 week history of worsening diarrhoea. At first, she thought it was due to something she had eaten, but instead of improving the diarrhoea got worse. She has also noticed blood in the stools which worried her. She otherwise feels quite well and has no significant past medical history.

Q Name three conditions at the top of your list of differential diagnoses.

A The main three conditions to consider here are an infectious colitis, ulcerative colitis, or Crohn's disease of the colon.

Q If this was an infectious episode, which organisms would be the most likely culprits?

A The most common cause of infectious bloody diarrhoea is infection with invasive bacteria such as *Shigella*, *Salmonella*, *Campylobacter*, and *E. coli*.

The GP sends off a stool sample and refers her to a gastroenterologist at the local hospital. Three weeks later, she attends the outpatient clinic. The stool sample has not grown any pathogenic organisms. The diarrhoea has not improved. The gastroenterologist performs rigid sigmoidoscopy which shows an inflamed, bleeding, friable rectal mucosa. He suspects ulcerative colitis and takes multiple rectal biopsies.

Q What microscopic appearances would you expect in the rectal biopsy if this was indeed ulcerative colitis?

A The rectal mucosa would show architectural distortion of the crypts. Instead of normal evenly spaced straight crypts, there would be uneven spacing with branching and shortening of the crypts. In addition, there would be a diffuse inflammatory infiltrate throughout the mucosa with neutrophils collecting in crypt spaces (crypt abscesses).

A few weeks later she returns to the hospital for a colonoscopy to determine the extent of her disease. There is visible inflammation up to the splenic flexure but not beyond. The colonoscopist takes mucosal biopsies from the caecum, ascending colon, hepatic flexure, transverse colon, splenic flexure, descending colon, sigmoid colon, and rectum.

Q Why do think it is important to take biopsies from multiple points around the colon?

A This is extremely important to make absolutely sure that the diagnosis of ulcerative colitis is correct. The most important factor distinguishing ulcerative colitis from Crohn's disease affecting the colon is the *distribution of the inflammation*, being continuous in ulcerative colitis and patchy in Crohn's disease. In Crohn's colitis, one might find focal inflammation in the ascending colon, then normal mucosa in the transverse colon, then more inflammation in the descending colon. In ulcerative colitis, the inflammation is continuous, so one would not expect an intervening area of uninvolved colon. It is therefore vital that colonoscopic biopsies are correctly labelled with the site they were taken from or interpretation becomes impossible.

The biopsies corroborate a diagnosis of left-sided ulcerative colitis. She goes into remission on medical treatment and is followed-up in the inflammatory bowel disease clinic.

Q How should this patient be followed-up in the future?

A Ulcerative colitis is associated with an increased risk of colonic carcinoma, and patients should be considered for surveillance colonoscopy to look for dysplasia of the colonic mucosa. In patients with left-sided disease only, this need not start until 15–20 years after the onset of symptoms.

Ulcerative colitis is also associated with primary sclerosing cholangitis, in which large bile ducts come under immune attack. The first sign of this disease is usually a persistently raised alkaline phosphatase level, which develops long before symptoms of cholestasis occur. All patients with ulcerative colitis should therefore have regular liver function tests performed.

Cross-references: ulcerative colitis (p. 163), Crohn's disease (p. 155), primary sclerosing cholangitis (p. 189).

Case 34

A 65-year-old woman presents to her GP general practitioner complaining of extreme tiredness and breathlessness. She looks very pale. The GP requests a battery of blood tests which show:

Haemoglobin	4.2 g/dl
MCV	118 fl
Platelets	105×10^9/l
WCC	3.0×10^9/l
Na	141 mmol/l
K	4.5 mmol/l

Urea	5.0 mmol/l
Creatinine	65 µmol/l
AST	35 U/l
ALT	32 U/l
ALP	50 U/l
Bilirubin	35 µmol/l

A blood film shows hypersegmented neutrophils and oval macrocytes, suggesting a megaloblastic anaemia.

Q What is a megaloblastic anaemia? What simple tests would you request next?

A Megaloblastic anaemia strictly refers to an anaemia associated with large red cell precursors in the bone marrow (megaloblasts). In everyday life, a megaloblastic anaemia is presumed if the peripheral blood shows macrocytes and hypersegmented neutrophils, even though the bone marrow has not actually been examined to prove the presence of megaloblasts. Megaloblastic anaemias are usually due to either vitamin B12 or folate deficiency, and so measurement of these would be the next investigation.

The vitamin B12 level is low. Red cell folate is normal.

Q What are the common causes of vitamin B12 deficiency? What test would you order next?

A By far the most common cause of vitamin B12 deficiency is autoimmune gastritis caused by autoimmune attack against the parietal cells of the gastric body that produce intrinsic factor. About half of patients also develop antibodies against intrinsic factor, which should be measured. A positive anti-intrinsic factor antibody test is considered diagnostic for pernicious anaemia in this clinical setting.

A diagnosis of pernicious anaemia is made and the patient is started on vitamin B12 injections. Her symptoms improve considerably and her haemoglobin begins to normalize. Her GP intermittently measures her thyroid-stimulating hormone (TSH) level and tells her that if she develops persistent indigestion she must come back immediately.

Q Why is measurement of TSH and the advice about indigestion important?

A Patients with an organ-specific autoimmune disease such as autoimmune gastritis have an increased risk of developing other conditions such as Hashimoto's thyroiditis. Measurement of TSH allows the early diagnosis of developing hypothyroidism.

Patients with autoimmune gastritis are at increased risk of developing gastric adenocarcinoma, because the autoimmune attack causes atrophy of the gastric glands and intestinal metaplasia. One should therefore have a low threshold for performing endoscopy on patients with autoimmune gastritis with persistent upper gastrointestinal symptoms.

Cross-references: megaloblastic anaemia (p. 335), autoimmune gastritis (p. 145), gastric carcinoma (p. 147), Hashimoto's thyroiditis (p. 316).

Case 35

You are a general surgical SHO, currently on your breast and endocrine attachment. You are in the endocrine clinic with your team, and your consultant asks you to see a 34-year-old lady who presents with a lump in the neck. The lump moves on swallowing, suggesting it is a thyroid nodule.

Q What are the common causes of a solitary nodule in the thyroid?

A A dominant nodule in a multinodular goitre (the other nodules not being apparent on palpation) and a thyroid neoplasm.

You present your findings to the registrar and he proceeds to perform a fine needle aspiration of the nodule.

Q Why is fine needle aspiration cytology a useful investigation for thyroid nodules?

A Fine needle aspiration cytology is a quick, non-invasive method of sampling the nodule. Although examination of the specimen cannot always provide a precise diagnosis, it is good at triaging patients into those who can be reassured and those who should have surgical excision of the nodule.

The slide is taken to the pathology department where it is stained and examined by a pathologist. The report comes back to you in the clinic and reads: 'This is a cellular aspirate which contains little colloid. There are numerous groups of follicular epithelial cells, many in microfollicular groups. The appearances suggest a follicular neoplasm. Excision of the lesion for histological assessment is recommended.'

Q What is meant by 'follicular neoplasm' and why is surgical removal of the nodule necessary?

A Cytological examination cannot distinguish between a follicular adenoma and a follicular carcinoma as the cells look exactly the same. The cytologist can therefore only call the nodule a 'follicular neoplasm'. Surgical excision is required to distinguish the two.

A few weeks later the patient comes back into hospital to have the nodule removed. The specimen is sent to pathology in plenty of formalin. After 24 h of fixation, the pathologist examines the specimen and thoroughly samples the edge of the tumour where the surrounding capsule lies.

Q Why is it important to examine this area of the specimen thoroughly?

A It is important to look here for evidence of invasion of the capsule or for vascular invasion, as these are the defining features of a follicular carcinoma.

On microscopic examination, no capsular or vascular invasion is seen and the tumour is diagnosed as a follicular adenoma.

Cross-reference: solitary thyroid nodule (p. 318).

Case 36

A 38-year-old woman presents with a history of worsening joint pain and swelling. The symptoms are worse in the mornings and she says her hands take nearly an hour to 'get going' in the mornings. On examination, she has quite marked swelling over her metacarpophalangeal joints on both hands. The joints feel slightly warm.

Q What is a polyarthritis and what are the possible causes?

A A polyarthritis refers to inflammation within several different joints. Possible causes of a polyarthritis include rheumatoid arthritis, a seronegative arthropathy, and a multisystem disease affecting the joints such as systemic lupus erythematosus.

She is positive for antinuclear antibody (ANA), rheumatoid factor, and anti-cyclic citrullinated peptide (CCP) antibodies. A diagnosis of rheumatoid arthritis is made.

Q What are rheumatoid factor and anti-CCP antibodies?

A Rheumatoid factor is an antibody against the Fc portion of IgG which is found in about 80 per cent of patients with rheumatoid arthritis. Unfortunately it is not terribly specific, often being positive in other autoimmune conditions and in a small percentage of normal people. Antibodies to CCPs are equally as sensitive as rheumatoid factor for rheumatoid arthritis, but are much more specific for the diagnosis.

Q What is known about the aetiology and pathogenesis of rheumatoid arthritis?

A Very little is known for certain. Rheumatoid arthritis is thought to be an autoimmune condition in which inflammation within the synovium of synovial joints causes erosion of articular cartilage and irreversible joint destruction. What triggers off the inflammation in the first place is not known.

Q Why is it important to diagnose rheumatoid arthritis as early as possible?

A Early treatment of rheumatoid arthritis with disease-modifying drugs has a substantial impact on the progression to irreversible joint deformation.

Q What are some of the extra-articular features of rheumatoid arthritis?

A Rheumatoid nodules, vasculitis, pulmonary fibrosis, and amyloidosis.

Cross-reference: rheumatoid arthritis (p. 409).

Case 37

A 73-year-old man is admitted to hospital very unwell with fever, cough, and sputum. He had not seen his GP for many years. On examination, he is extremely thin, pale, and breathless at rest. His liver is palpable.

His blood results reveal:

Haemoglobin	10 g/dl
Sodium	136 mmol/l
Potassium	4.0 mmol/l
Urea	12.1 mmol/l
Creatinine	95 µmol/l
Bilirubin	25 µmol/l
ALP	875 U/l
AST	60 U/l
ALT	80 U/l
GGT	300 U/l
Calcium	2.95 mmol/l

The chest radiograph reveals an enlarged heart, pulmonary oedema, and left lower lobe consolidation.

Q Explain the blood results.

A There are a number of abnormalities in these blood results. The markedly raised alkaline phosphatase and GGT, together with the history of an enlarged liver, are highly suggestive of hepatic infiltration. The raised calcium level is also a worry, as this may be due to bony metastases which would also push up the alkaline phosphatase level (alkaline phosphatase is present in bone and liver). The raised urea is almost certainly related to his dehydration, some of which will be related to his hypercalcaemia, which causes polyuria and fluid loss through the kidneys. He does not have marked renal impairment as the creatinine is normal. The low haemoglobin is probably an anaemia of chronic disease.

You begin to suspect a disseminated malignancy in this gentleman.

Q What common malignancies would you consider?

A The most likely in a man are lung cancer, colorectal cancer, and prostate cancer.

On further questioning, he has a long history of heavy smoking. He does not have finger clubbing. The chest radiograph is difficult to interpret because of the superimposed changes of pulmonary oedema and consolidation. He gives no history of a change in bowel habit or rectal bleeding. A rectal examination reveals a smoothly enlarged prostate. No rectal mass is palpable.

You organize a CT scan of his chest, abdomen, and pelvis. A PSA test comes back normal. The CT confirms disseminated malignancy with multiple hepatic metastases, bony metastases, and a left hilar mass. Despite treatment, he deteriorates and dies 2 days later. You certify death and are asked to complete the death certificate.

Q Do you think this case needs to be referred to the Coroner? If not, how would you complete the death certificate?

A This case does not need to be referred to the Coroner. You have enough knowledge to give an accurate cause of death and there are no suspicious circumstances that would require referral to the Coroner. A reasonable 1A for the death certificate would be 'disseminated malignancy'.

That afternoon you are bleeped by the bereavement office. The relatives are keen to know what the cancer was and have asked to talk to someone from the medical team about a post-mortem examination.

Q If a post-mortem examination were to be carried out in this case, would the relatives' consent be required?

A Yes, it would. As the cause of death is known, this would be a hospital or medical interest post-mortem which requires the consent of the relatives.

The following morning, the post-mortem examination is performed by the duty pathologist. Your team is called to the mortuary to see the findings. A large tumour is present at the hilum of the left lung with nodal involvement. There is bronchiectasis and consolidation in the lung distal to the tumour. There are multiple hepatic metastases and brain metastases. The findings suggest disseminated lung carcinoma, and the pathologist tells you that he has taken a sample of the lung tumour for histological examination to type it.

Q Why is there bronchiectasis and consolidation distal to the tumour?

A The bronchiectasis and consolidation are the result of obstruction of the lung distal to the tumour predisposing to infection. Repetitive cycles of infection lead to destruction of the supporting tissue of the bronchial walls, resulting in permanent dilation of the airways (bronchiectasis).

Q Does the pathologist need specific consent to keep the piece of lung tumour for histological examination?

A Yes. The new Human Tissue Act now places strict rules on the retention of all human tissue. The relatives must have given specific consent for the retention of tissue and what they wish to be done with the tissue once it has been finished with.

The following week a supplementary report is added to the post-mortem report:

'Sections from the lung tumour confirm a small cell carcinoma, composed of small neoplastic cells with scanty cytoplasm and finely granular chromatin. Immunohistochemistry confirms this with positivity for CD56, chromogranin, synaptophysin, and TTF-1.'

Q Apart from small cell carcinoma, what are the other common types of lung carcinoma?

A Squamous cell carcinoma, adenocarcinoma, and large cell carcinoma. Microscopy is required to distinguish between them.

Q What is immunohistochemistry?

A Immunohistochemistry is an adjunctive tool in pathology which is used to help characterize the phenotype of a cell. Specific antibodies are used to see what markers a cell expresses. In this example, CD56, chromogranin, and synaptophysin are neuroendocrine markers that confirm the neuroendocrine nature of the tumour. TTF-1 is a marker that suggests the origin of the tumour is from the lung rather than a different primary site.

Cross-references: lung carcinoma (p. 130), bronchiectasis (p. 109), liver function tests (p. 179), death certification (p. 537), post-mortem examination (p. 537), immunohistochemistry (p. 536).

Glossary

Abscess A localized collection of neutrophils associated with tissue destruction.

Acanthoma A benign neoplasm derived from squamous epithelial cells.

Acute Appearing rapidly.

Adenocarcinoma A malignant neoplasm derived from glandular epithelial cells.

Adenoma A benign neoplasm derived from glandular epithelial cells.

Aetiology The underlying cause of a disease.

Allergy In Europe, synonymous with hypersensitivity reaction. In the USA, refers only to an immediate (type 1) hypersensitivity reaction.

Anaphylaxis A systemic form of immediate hypersensitivity. At its most severe, may lead to anaphylactic shock.

Aneurysm An abnormal dilation of part of a blood vessel or cardiac chamber.

Antibody A glycoprotein molecule produced by B lymphocytes which binds a specific antigen. Antibodies are the effectors of humoral immunity. Also known as immunoglobulin.

Antigen Any substance that elicits an immune response.

Antigen-presenting cell Cells of the immune system such as dendritic cells and macrophages with surface MHC class II molecules capable of presenting antigens to CD4+ helper T lymphocytes.

Apoptosis A controlled form of cell death which does not elicit any inflammation.

Atopy A predisposition to produce IgE antibodies in response to environmental antigens and develop strong immediate hypersensitivity reactions.

Atresia Failure of formation of the lumen of a hollow viscus or duct.

Atrophy Shrinkage of an organ or tissue due to a reduction in cell number and size.

Autoimmunity A hypersensitivity reaction targeted against self-antigens.

Bacteraemia The presence of bacteria in the blood.

Biopsy Removal of a piece of tissue for diagnostic purposes.

Cachexia Marked loss of body weight seen in patients with advanced diseases.

Cancer A malignant neoplasm.

Carcinoma A malignant epithelial neoplasm.

Chronic Persisting for a long period of time.

Complement A collection of circulating proteins that assist other components of the immune system in killing microorganisms.

Congenital Present at birth.

Constitutional Referring to the general state of one's health.

Cyst A cavity lined by epithelial cells.

Cytokine A secreted protein that mediates inflammatory and immune reactions.

Diffuse Widespread (compare with focal).

Dyskaryosis Nuclear abnormality of a cell.

Dysplasia Abnormal cells and architecture of an epithelium.

Erythema Abnormal redness of the skin.

Exophytic Growing outwards from a surface.

Fibrinous Rich in fibrin.

Fibrous Rich in collagen.

Focal Localized (compare with diffuse).

Granulation tissue A mixture of capillaries, fibroblasts, myofibroblasts, and inflammatory cells converted into a scar in the process of repair.

Granuloma An aggregate of epithelioid macrophages.

Granulomatous inflammation Inflammation dominated by the presence of epithelioid macrophages.

Histiocyte A tissue macrophage.

Hyperplasia Enlargement of an organ or tissue due to an increase in the number of cells within it.

Hypersensitivity reaction Disease caused by the immune system. A hypersensitivity reaction to self-antigens is also known as autoimmunity.

Hypertrophy Enlargement of an organ or tissue due to an increase in the size of cells within it.

Iatrogenic Caused by medical intervention.

Idiopathic Unknown cause.

Immunoglobulin Molecules secreted by B lymphocytes which mediate the humoral arm of the adaptive immune system.

Infarction Death of tissue due to ischaemia.

Inflammation A non-specific response to cellular injury.

Ischaemia Inadequate blood supply to a tissue.

Lesion Any visible abnormality associated with a disease.

Lewy body A solid intraneuronal inclusion composed of ubiquitin and synuclein. They are seen in the basal ganglia in Parkinson's disease and in the cerebral cortex in dementia with Lewy bodies.

Metaplasia A switch from one cell type to another.

Morbidity The extent of the reduction in the patient's health as a consequence of a particular disease.

Morphology The form and structure of a cell or tissue.

Mortality The likelihood that a patient will die from a particular disease.

Mutation Alteration in the DNA sequence of a gene resulting in the synthesis of a protein with abnormal function.

Neoplasm An abnormal mass of tissue which shows uncoordinated growth and serves no useful purpose.

Necrosis Poorly controlled form of cell death associated with an inflammatory response.

Occlusion Complete blockage of a lumen.

Oncogene A mutated form of a proto-oncogene which encodes a protein causing abnormal cell proliferation.

Organization The process by which granulation tissue removes dead tissue and replaces it with a fibrous scar.

Paroxysmal Sudden episodic attacks.

Pathogen An organism capable of causing disease.

Pathogenesis The mechanism by which an aetiological agent leads to disease.

Pathognomic A feature absolutely diagnostic of a particular disease, which is only ever seen in that condition.

Phagocyte A cell of the innate immune system which ingests and destroys foreign particles, e.g. neutrophil, macrophage.

Pleomorphic Variation in size and shape.

Polyp Any growth that projects from a body surface.

Proto-oncogene A gene encoding a protein which stimulates cell proliferation.

Reactive Reversible response to any stimulus.

Sarcoma A malignant soft tissue tumour, e.g. liposarcoma, leiomyosarcoma.

Scar Collagen-rich tissue laid down following repair of damage.

Septicaemia A clinical syndrome of bacteraemia together with evidence of a systemic response to it, such as tachycardia and hypotension.

Shock A generalized failure of tissue perfusion.

Stenosis Narrowing of a lumen.

Stroma The connective tissue framework of a tissue or organ.

Syndrome A set of symptoms and signs which, when occurring together, suggest a particular underlying cause.

Thrombosis Abnormal activation of the haemostatic system leading to the formation of a solid mass of platelets, fibrin, and entrapped blood cells (thrombus) in the circulatory system.

Ulcer A full thickness defect in an epithelial surface.

Viraemia Presence of virus in the blood.

Index

Reference intervals

Sodium	135–145 mmol/l
Potassium	3.6–5.0 mmol/l
Glucose	3.5–5.5 mmol/l
Urea	3.0–8.0 mmol/l
Creatinine	50–140 µmol/l
Bilirubin	<17 µmol/l
AST	10–40 U/l
ALT	5–35 U/l
ALP	100–300 U/l
Calcium	2.25–2.60 mmol/l
CRP	<6 mg/l
Haemoglobin	13.5–18.0 g/dl (men)
	11.5–16.0 g/dl (women)
MCV	82–98 fl
MCHC	32.0–36.0 g/dl
Platelet count	150–400 x 10^9/l
White blood cells	4.0–11.0 x 10^9/l
PT	12.0–14.0 s
APTT	26.0–33.5 s
ESR	<12 mm/hr
Arterial pH	7.35–7.45
pO_2	12.0–14.5 kPa
pCO_2	4.7–6.0 kPa